Controversies in Cancer of the Thyroid and Parathyroid Glands

Prathamesh S. Pai • Yasuhiro Ito
Ashok R Shaha • Christopher de Souza
Editors

Controversies in Cancer of the Thyroid and Parathyroid Glands

Springer

Editors
Prathamesh S. Pai
Department of Surgical Oncology
P D Hinduja Hospital & Medical
Research Centre
Khar, Mumbai, India

Ashok R Shaha
Allan H. Selig Chair in Head and Neck
Surgery, Memorial Sloan Kettering
Cancer Center
Professor of Surgery, Weill-Cornell
Medical College
New York, NY, USA

Yasuhiro Ito
Department of Surgery
Kuma Hospital
Kobe, Japan

Christopher de Souza
Lilavati Hospital
Mumbai, Maharashtra, India

ISBN 978-3-032-13129-4 ISBN 978-3-032-13130-0 (eBook)
https://doi.org/10.1007/978-3-032-13130-0

This Springer imprint is published by the registered company Springer Nature Switzerland AG
The registered company address is: Gewerbestrasse 11, 6330 Cham, Switzerland

Foreword

The steep rise in the incidence of thyroid cancer world wide in the last three decades has created a significant increase in the workload for the clinicians and a dramatic increase in the cost of care. Thyroid cancer is not one disease, but a spectrum of cancers with uniformly curable to nearly all fatal cases. Fortunately, a majority of the newly diagnosed cancers are low-risk curable cancers. The goal of modern day management of these cancers is to not "over treat" the low-risk curable cancers, or "under treat" the advanced or aggressive cancers. Coupled with advances in molecular profiling, technology in imaging, development of targeted drugs, and improved understanding of the biological behavior of these cancers, the landscape of management strategies has evolved from a "one size fits all," to more personalized, therapeutic paradigms. Development of nonsurgical ablative alternatives for indeterminate nodules or even small differentiated cancers has opened a new avenue to avoid surgery, and active surveillance of small differentiated cancers as a management option, has stood the test of time. There are arguments and debates regarding, the need for or the extent of surgery and postoperative care for low-risk cancers. The role of radioactive treatment, once a standard of care, is declining due to no benefit in low-risk patients. The indications for molecular profiling and the role of targeted therapies yet remains to be well defined.

These dynamic changes in the clinical management of thyroid cancers have generated numerous controversies, in the detection methodologies, surgical management, adjuvant therapies, and follow-up strategies for these mostly indolent cancers. Dr. Chris de Souza is to be complemented for putting together this compendium of controversial issues and advances in the management of thyroid cancer with contributions from world leaders in thyroid cancer management, sharing their experiences and opinions. Their contributions make this a "treasure trove" of the state of the art and science in the diagnosis, treatment, and surveillance of patients with thyroid cancer. Clearly, the pros and cons surrounding the controversies, and the recommendations from global leaders, make this a "must read" book for the trainees as well as practitioners in this rapidly evolving field.

Jatin P. Shah, MD, PhD (Hon), DSc. (Hon)
Attending Surgeon, Elliot W Strong Chair
in Head and Neck Oncology, Memorial Sloan
Kettering Cancer Center
New York, NY, USA

Professor of Surgery, Weill-Cornell Medical College
New York, NY, USA

Preface

While there are several well-written textbooks about thyroid and parathyroid gland disorders, we have chosen to focus exclusively on the controversies and debates surrounding their management.

The surgeon today faces a dilemma deciding the best option for his patients. This is because of the continuous change in the knowledge base and constant evolution. No other field has seen such a swing of the pendulum as in the management of thyroid cancers.

We have endeavored to present current evidence in a manner that will help the surgeon make the appropriate choice. This book includes varied subjects such as molecular biology and genetics which heretofore were on the fringe and unachievable. They are no longer a luxury and today constitute a major investigative tool that spares people from the consequences of the disease by addressing them well before they manifest themselves. This is part of precision medicine, which tailors the treatment improving the quality of not only the patient but that of their families and relatives as well.

The chapters are authored by experts in their field. They have graciously and generously shared their vast experiences in an easy-to-understand format. However, this knowledge is rapidly changing, and we want to rise to the challenge of the information age by presenting updated information in a nimble and timely manner without discarding the true and tried evidence of the past.

We, the editors and authors, owe a huge debt of gratitude to our patients who continue to teach and enrich us. It is to them that we dedicate this book. If at all we can see distant horizons well, it is because we are seated on the shoulders of giants, who have been trail blazers and have given us the tools to do the same for the generations to follow.

Mumbai, Maharashtra, India — Prathamesh S. Pai
Kobe, Hyogo, Japan — Yasuhiro Ito
New York, NY, USA — Ashok R Shaha
Mumbai, Maharashtra, India — Christopher de Souza

Contents

Contributors

Amr H. Abdelhamid Ahmed Division of Thyroid and Parathyroid Endocrine Surgery, Department of Otolaryngology-Head and Neck Surgery, Massachusetts Eye and Ear, Harvard Medical School, Boston, MA, USA

Deepak Thomas Abraham Department of Endocrine Surgery, Christian Medical College, Vellore, Tamil Nadu, India

Department of Surgery, American Mission Hospital, Manama, Bahrain

Likolani Arthurs Department of Surgery, Division of Endocrine Surgery, NYU Langone Health, New York, NY, USA

Chandrasekhar Bal Department of Nuclear Medicine, All India Institute of Medical Sciences, New Delhi, Delhi, India

Diane Bijou Holy Spirit Hospital, Mumbai, Maharashtra, India

Wanxing Chai-Ho Division of Hematology/Oncology, Department of Medicine, University of California, Los Angeles, CA, USA

Kunal Ramesh Chandekar Department of Nuclear Medicine, All India Institute of Medical Sciences, New Delhi, Delhi, India

Anish Jacob Cherian Christian Medical College, Vellore, Tamil Nadu, India

Tomohiro Chiba Department of Cytology and Department of Pathology, Cancer Institute Hospital of Japanese Foundation for Cancer Research (JFCR), Tokyo, Japan

Swapnil Deshpande Department of Cardiothoracic Surgery, Dr K.G Deshpande Memorial Hospital, Nagpur, India

Preeti Dhingra Lilavati Hospital, Mumbai, Maharashtra, India

Henning Dralle Department of General, Visceral and Transplantation Surgery, Division of Endocrine Surgery, University of Duisburg-Essen, Essen, Germany

Makoto Fujishima Department of Surgery, Kuma Hospital, Kobe, Hyogo, Japan

Neeti Kapre Gupta Department of ENT & Head & Neck Surgery, Neeti Clinics Pvt Ltd, Nagpur, Maharashtra, India

Yasuhiro Ito Department of Surgery, Kuma Hospital, Kobe, Hyogo, Japan

Sandhya Chirukandath Jayasankaran Department of Radiology, Amrita Institute of Medical Sciences and Research Centre, Amrita Vishwa Vidyapeetham, Kochi, Kerala, India

Madan Kapre Department of ENT & Head & Neck Surgery, Neeti Clinics Pvt Ltd, Nagpur, Maharashtra, India

Neeti Kapre Neeti Clinics, Nagpur, Maharashtra, India

Ken Kazahaya Division of Pediatric Otolaryngology, Children's Hospital of Philadelphia, Philadelphia, PA, USA

Department of Otorhinolaryngology-Head and Neck Surgery, University of Pennsylvania, Philadelphia, PA, USA

Sonam Khokhar Department of ENT & Head & Neck Surgery, Neeti Clinics Pvt Ltd, Nagpur, Maharashtra, India

Anuj Kumar Department of Radiation Oncology & Head & Neck Disease Management Group, Advanced Centre for Treatment, Research and Education in Cancer (ACTREC) & Homi Bhabha National Institute, Tata Memorial Centre, Mumbai, Maharashtra, India

Sarbani Ghosh Laskar Department of Radiation Oncology & Head & Neck Disease Management Group, Tata Memorial Hospital & Homi Bhabha National Institute, Tata Memorial Centre, Mumbai, Maharashtra, India

Helena Levyn Department of Otolaryngology and Head and Neck Surgery, Montefiore Medical Center, Albert Einstein College of Medicine, New York, NY, USA

Andreas Machens Medical Faculty, Department of Visceral, Vascular and Endocrine Surgery, Martin Luther University Halle-Wittenberg, Halle (Saale), Germany

Josef Madrigal Department of Surgery, Division of Head and Neck Surgery, University of California, Los Angeles, Los Angeles, CA, USA

Lakshmi Ravunniarth Menon Department of Head and Neck Surgery and Oncology, Amrita Institute of Medical Sciences and Research Centre, Amrita Vishwa Vidyapeetham, Kochi, Kerala, India

Vidula Mestry Department of Head and Neck Surgery, Apple Hospital, Kolhapur, Maharashtra, India

Akira Miyauchi Department of Surgery, Kuma Hospital, Kobe, Hyogo, Japan

Samarpita Mohanty Department of Radiation Oncology & Head & Neck Disease Management Group, Advanced Centre for Treatment, Research and Education in Cancer (ACTREC) & Homi Bhabha National Institute, Tata Memorial Centre, Mumbai, Maharashtra, India

Asif Momin PSAH Head and Neck Cancer Institute of India and Bhatia Hospital, Mumbai, India

Sir HN Reliance Foundation Hospital, HCG Hospital, Mumbai, Maharashtra, India

Prince Aly Khan Hospital, Mumbai, Maharashtra, India

Shenaz Momin Department of Radiology, Nair Hospital, Mumbai, Maharashtra, India

Sueyoshi Moritani Omi Medical Center, Center for Otolaryngology, Head and Neck Thyroid Surgery, Kusatsu, Shiga, Japan

Samantha Kass Newman Memorial Sloan Kettering Cancer Center, New York, NY, USA

Aradhya Nigam Department of Surgery, Memorial Sloan Kettering Cancer Center, New York, NY, USA

Connor H. O'Meara Division of Head & Neck Oncology and Microvascular Reconstruction, Department of Otolaryngology, Head & Neck Surgery, University of Virginia Health Services, Charlottesville, VA, USA

Prathamesh S. Pai Department of Surgical Oncology, P D Hinduja Hospital & Medical Research Centre, Khar, Mumbai, India

Mittali Shah Patani Bhatia Hospital Tardeo, Mumbai, Maharashtra, India

Kepal N. Patel Department of Surgery, Division of Endocrine Surgery, NYU Langone Health, New York, NY, USA

Snehal Patel Department of Surgery, Memorial Sloan Kettering Cancer Center, New York, NY, USA

Aishan Patil Spr, Vascular Surgery, Scotland, UK

Anish Patil GP Trainee, Manchester, UK

Armando Patrizio Memorial Sloan Kettering Cancer Center, New York, NY, USA

Lina Pedraza-Sanchez Memorial Sloan Kettering Cancer Center, New York, NY, USA

Muhammad S. Quraishi Doncaster Royal Infirmary, Doncaster, UK

Natasha Quraishi Bradford Royal Infirmary, Bradford, UK

Gregory W. Randolph Division of Thyroid and Parathyroid Endocrine Surgery, Department of Otolaryngology-Head and Neck Surgery, Massachusetts Eye and Ear, Harvard Medical School, Boston, MA, USA

Karthik N. Rao Department of Head and Neck Oncology, Sri Shankara Cancer Hospital and Research Center, Bangalore, India

Shubha Gadde Ravindra Department of Nuclear Medicine, All India Institute of Medical Sciences, New Delhi, Delhi, India

Marika D. Russell Division of Thyroid and Parathyroid Endocrine Surgery, Department of Otolaryngology-Head and Neck Surgery, Massachusetts Eye and Ear, Harvard Medical School, Boston, MA, USA

Shawn Thomas Sam Department of Endocrine Surgery, Christian Medical College, Vellore, Tamil Nadu, India

Swayamjeet Satapathy Department of Nuclear Medicine, All India Institute of Medical Sciences, New Delhi, Delhi, India

Supriya Sen Christian Medical College, Vellore, Tamil Nadu, India

Ashok R Shaha Allan H. Selig Chair in Head and Neck Surgery, Memorial Sloan Kettering Cancer Center, Professor of Surgery, Weill-Cornell Medical College, New York, NY, USA

David C. Shonka Jr. Division of Head & Neck Oncology and Microvascular Reconstruction, Department of Otolaryngology, Head & Neck Surgery, University of Virginia Health Services, Charlottesville, VA, USA

Sanjog Singh Department of ENT & Head & Neck Surgery, Neeti Clinics Pvt Ltd, Nagpur, Maharashtra, India

Shwetabh Sinha Department of Radiation Oncology & Head & Neck Disease Management Group, Advanced Centre for Treatment, Research and Education in Cancer (ACTREC) & Homi Bhabha National Institute, Tata Memorial Centre, Mumbai, Maharashtra, India

Christopher de Souza Lilavati Hospital, Holy Family Hospital, Holy Spirit Hospital, Mumbai, Maharashtra, India

Rosemarie de Souza Department of Internal Medicine, and Medical Intensive Care, TN Medical College and Nair Hospital, Mumbai, Maharashtra, India

Preethi Srikanthan UCLA Research Center at Alhambra, Alhambra, CA, USA

Department of Medicine, Division of Endocrinology, University of California, Los Angeles, Los Angeles, CA, USA

Maie St. John Department of Head and Neck Surgery, UCLA David Geffen School of Medicine, Los Angeles, CA, USA

Brendan C. Stack Department of Otolaryngology-Head and Neck Surgery, Southern Illinois University School of Medicine, Springfield, IL, USA

Chad K. Sudoko Division of Pediatric Otolaryngology, Children's Hospital of Philadelphia, Philadelphia, PA, USA

Department of Otorhinolaryngology-Head and Neck Surgery, University of Pennsylvania, Philadelphia, PA, USA

Kyung Tae Department of Otolaryngology-Head and Neck Surgery, College of Medicine, Hanyang University, Seoul, Republic of Korea

Krishnakumar Thankappan Department of Head and Neck Surgery and Oncology, Amrita Institute of Medical Sciences and Research Centre, Amrita Vishwa Vidyapeetham, Kochi, Kerala, India

Vishal N. Tyagi ENT Department V N Desai Hospital (Santacruz), Fortis Hospital (Mulund), Holy Family Hospital (Bandra, West), Holy Spirit Hospital (Andheri East), P D Hinduja Hospital (Khar), Mumbai, Maharashtra, India

Abhishek Vaidya National Cancer Institute, Nagpur, Maharashtra, India

Deborah J. Wong Division of Hematology/Oncology, Department of Medicine, University of California, Los Angeles, CA, USA

Alice Yu David Geffen School of Medicine at UCLA, Los Angeles, CA, USA

Kevin J. Zhang Division of Endocrinology, Department of Medicine, University of California, Los Angeles, CA, USA

Embryology, Anatomy, and Applied Anatomy of the Thyroid and Parathyroid Glands

1

Abhishek Vaidya and Neeti Kapre

Editorial

Thorough and accurate knowledge of the surgical anatomy of the thyroid, parathyroid gland, and surrounding structures, with their key surgical landmarks (e.g., triangles and planes), are important guideposts that help surgeons in performing a safe and effective thyroid surgery. The thyroid lies in the visceral compartment of the neck deep to the infrahyoid "strap" muscles. The thyroid gland is enclosed by a thin fibro-elastic "true capsule" and is invested in the pretracheal layer of deep cervical fascia ("false capsule"). Thus, the gland may be considered to be covered by two capsules:

- Inner true capsule: This is a thin fibro-elastic layer formed by the condensation of connective tissue of the gland itself. This layer sends septa (partitions) deep into the parenchyma, dividing the gland into lobules. These septa also carry blood vessels, nerves, and lymphatic vessels into the gland.
- Outer false capsule: This is external to the true capsule and is formed by pretracheal fascia, which is a broader layer of deep cervical fascia. The false capsule is not part of the thyroid gland itself, but rather a layer of surrounding tissue. The thyroid has a rich arterial supply from paired superior and inferior thyroid arteries. The *superior thyroid arteries (STAs)* are the first branches of the external carotid arteries. The *inferior thyroid arteries (ITAs)* arise from the thyrocervical trunks (branches of the subclavian arteries) and ascend behind the carotid sheath toward the lower poles of the thyroid. *Recurrent laryngeal nerves (RLNs)* course intimately along the thyroid lobes and must be preserved to maintain vocal cord function. The superior laryngeal nerve, a branch of the vagus high in the neck,

A. Vaidya (✉)
National Cancer Institute, Nagpur, India

N. Kapre
Neeti Clinics, Nagpur, India

P. S. Pai et al. (eds.), *Controversies in Cancer of the Thyroid and Parathyroid Glands*, https://doi.org/10.1007/978-3-032-13130-0_1

divides into internal and external branches. The internal branch pierces the thyrohyoid membrane and is sensory to the larynx. The external branch of the superior laryngeal nerve (EBSLN) provides motor innervation to the cricothyroid muscle, which tenses the vocal cords.

Several anatomical–surgical triangles in the neck have been described to facilitate safe thyroidectomy. These triangles are tissue planes bounded by important structures, serving as roadmaps to find key nerves and vessels:

- Joll's triangle (sternothyro-laryngeal triangle) (Fig. 1.11): This triangle is used to locate the external branch of the superior laryngeal nerve (EBSLN) near the superior pole of the thyroid. It is formed by the following borders:
  - Superiorly: the attachment of the strap muscles to the thyroid cartilage (at the oblique line).
  - Medially: the midline of the neck.
  - Laterally: the upper pole of the thyroid gland along with the superior thyroid vessels.

The floor of Joll's triangle is the cricothyroid muscle, into which the EBSLN inserts. Identifying this triangle intraoperatively is done by retracting the superior pole of the thyroid downward and laterally, which exposes the space between the sternothyroid muscle and larynx. The EBSLN can often be seen or stimulated here, running in the fascia on the surface of the cricothyroid muscle (in the triangle's floor).

Opening the avascular *Reeves' space* (*cricothyroid space of Reeves*, just deep to the sternothyroid muscle at the upper pole, medial to STA) corresponds to entering Joll's triangle and is a technique to protect the EBSLN.

- Beahr's triangle: An important landmark for the recurrent laryngeal nerve (RLN), this triangle lies in the lateral aspect of the tracheoesophageal groove after the thyroid lobe is retracted medially. Its borders are base—the common carotid artery; superiorly—the inferior thyroid artery; and medial side—the RLN itself. Within Beahr's triangle, the inferior thyroid artery typically crosses the RLN. Recognizing this triangle helps the surgeon anticipate where the RLN will appear as it ascends. In practice, once the inferior pole is mobilized and the thyroid lobe is pulled medially, Beahr's triangle is visualized and the surgeon will often find the RLN coursing obliquely upward through it.
- Lore's triangle: Another triangle used to find the RLN, described by John Lore. The boundaries are medially—the trachea and esophagus; laterally—carotid; and superiorly—the inferior pole of the thyroid gland. Lore's triangle lies essentially at the level of the lower thyroid pole, deep in the neck. The RLN is commonly found within this triangle as it travels in the tracheoesophageal groove, making this a useful window for nerve identification.

Simon's triangle (triangle of safety): This classic triangle is also referenced for locating the RLN low in the neck. Its borders are the common carotid artery laterally, the trachea/esophagus medially, and the inferior thyroid artery superiorly. It overlaps with the lower part of Beahr's triangle. Essentially, Simon's triangle describes the space in which the RLN can be found as it loops upward, before reaching the ligament of Berry.

Triangle of concern: The triangle of concern is a crucial anatomical region in thyroidectomy, as it is the most common site for postoperative bleeding and recurrent laryngeal nerve (RLN) injury.
Medial border: trachea
Lateral border: recurrent laryngeal nerve (RLN)
Base: thyrothymic ligament and loose fat above the sternum
Apex: Berry's ligament

The parathyroid glands are small, oval endocrine glands usually found on the posterior aspect of the thyroid. Typically, there are four parathyroids—two *superior* and two *inferior*—each measuring about 3–8 mm and weighing 30–40 mg [15]. They are soft, tan-brown glands with a delicate capsule and are often imbedded in fat. The superior parathyroid glands derive embryologically from the fourth pharyngeal pouch, whereas the inferior glands originate from the third pharyngeal pouch (descending with the thymus). This developmental origin explains their final locations: the superior glands tend to remain higher and more posterior, while the inferior glands migrate further and can end up in more anterior–inferior positions.

Christopher de Souza

Introduction

The thyroid and parathyroid glands are integral components of the endocrine system, critically involved in metabolic regulation, calcium homeostasis, and overall physiological equilibrium. Thyroid and parathyroid glands have an intricated developmental origin and anatomical relationships that underpin safe surgical practice. Historically, thyroid surgery has evolved substantially from the era before the early nineteenth century, when it was fraught with complications and mortality as much as 40% [1]. Advances in embryological and anatomical understanding, surgical techniques, anesthesia, and postoperative care have dramatically improved patient outcomes. The pioneering works of Theodor Kocher and William Halsted laid the foundational principles of meticulous surgical technique, accurate anatomical dissection, and careful hemostasis, transforming thyroid surgery into a procedure with very low morbidity and mortality rates [1, 2]. The modern thyroid surgeon must have a thorough understanding of the developmental origin, detailed anatomy, and applied anatomy of the thyroid and parathyroid glands to execute safe and standard surgery, while avoiding complications such as nerve injury or hypoparathyroidism during neck surgery. This chapter reviews the embryology of the thyroid and parathyroid glands, details their surgical anatomy (including important classifications of laryngeal nerves and embryologic remnants), and highlights key surgical landmarks (e.g., triangles and planes) that guide surgeons in performing safe and effective thyroid surgery.

Embryology

Thyroid Gland Embryology (Fig. 1.1)

The thyroid gland is the first endocrine organ to develop, beginning around the third to fourth week of gestation. It originates in the form of median anlage and two lateral anlagen as follows [3–6]:

Median anlage begins as a median endodermal thickening in the floor of the primordial pharynx at the site of the future *foramen cecum* of the tongue. The foramen cecum is located at the junction of the anterior two-thirds and posterior one-third of the tongue. By the fourth week, a bilobed thyroid diverticulum forms and descends in front of the pharyngeal gut as the embryo's head and tongue develop.

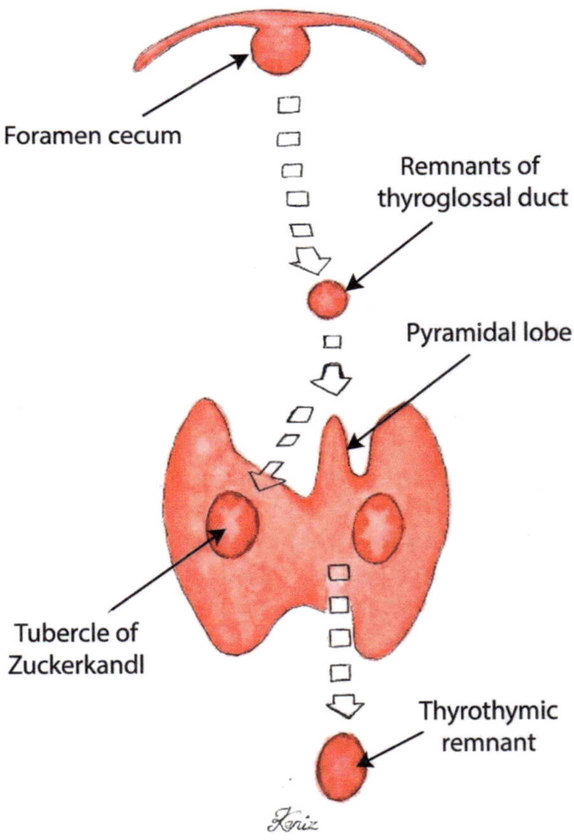

Fig. 1.1 Embryology of thyroid

This descent carries the thyroid anlage from the tongue base to the anterior neck. As it migrates caudally along the midline, the thyroid remains connected to the foramen cecum by the *thyroglossal duct*, a transient embryonic structure. During its descent, the thyroid anlage passes anteriorly to the developing hyoid bone and laryngeal cartilages, ultimately reaching its definitive anatomical position in the anterior cervical region, anterior and lateral to the trachea, by approximately the seventh week of gestation.

The thyroglossal duct typically involutes completely by the eighth to tenth week of gestation. Failure of this duct to regress fully can result in clinically significant anomalies such as thyroglossal duct cysts or fistulas (see below). A pyramidal lobe (present in ~50% of individuals) represents a remnant of the distal thyroglossal duct and typically arises from the isthmus or adjacent lobe, pointing upward toward the foramen cecum.

Lateral Thyroid Anlagen In addition to the median thyroid primordium, the thyroid gland has contributions from the neural crest that form the lateral anlagen. The neural crest cells from the fourth pharyngeal pouch form the *ultimobranchial bodies*. These fuse with the developing thyroid lobes and give rise to the parafollicular C-cells (calcitonin-producing cells). An embryological remnant of this fusion is the tubercle of Zuckerkandl, a consistent posterior projection of the thyroid lobe. Zuckerkandl's tubercle (if prominent) is an important surgical landmark—it is attached to the thyroid capsule near the ligament of Berry, and the superior parathyroid gland often lies just superior to it.

The descent and morphological maturation of the thyroid gland are governed by an interplay of molecular signals and transcription factors. Notable among these is thyroid transcription factor-1 (TTF-1 or Nkx2–1), paired box gene 8 (Pax8), forkhead box protein E1 (Foxe1), and hexose kinase domain-containing protein-2 (Hhex) [7–9]. Each of these factors plays a distinct role:

- *Nkx2–1 (TTF-1):* essential for thyroid specification and differentiation; its expression marks the initial stages of thyroid organogenesis and continues throughout gland maturation.
- *Pax8:* vital for thyroid follicular cell differentiation and survival; mutations can lead to thyroid dysgenesis, often associated with congenital hypothyroidism.
- *Foxe1:* involved in thyroid gland morphogenesis, particularly in the formation and degeneration of the thyroglossal duct.
- *Hhex:* important for early gland specification and overall growth of the thyroid anlage.

Molecular signaling pathways, such as fibroblast growth factor (FGF) and bone morphogenetic protein (BMP) signaling, significantly influence thyroid migration and differentiation. Aberrations in these pathways can lead to ectopic thyroid tissue or complete agenesis.

Developmental Anomalies of Thyroid and Thyroglossal Duct Tract

Developmental anomalies involving the thyroid gland and thyroglossal duct tract are significant due to their clinical implications and surgical management complexities.

1. Thyroglossal Duct Cysts and Fistulae [10, 11]

As stated previously, the thyroglossal duct normally degenerates by the tenth week of embryonic life. However, incomplete involution of this duct can result in the formation of a thyroglossal duct cyst, typically manifesting as a painless, midline cervical mass. These cysts are predominantly located at or below the hyoid bone, frequently moving superiorly with tongue protrusion or swallowing. Infection or inflammation may complicate cysts, prompting the development of thyroglossal duct fistulae—tracts communicating with the skin surface. Surgical management typically involves the Sistrunk procedure, entailing complete excision of the cyst, the central portion of the hyoid bone, and a tract of tongue musculature to minimize recurrence.

2. Lingual Thyroid and Ectopic Thyroid Tissue [12, 13] (Fig. 1.2)

Lingual thyroid represents ectopic thyroid tissue remaining at the base of the tongue due to arrested descent of the gland during embryogenesis. Clinically, this anomaly can manifest symptoms ranging from asymptomatic masses to dysphagia, dysphonia, or airway obstruction. It becomes particularly evident during periods of hormonal stimulation such as puberty, pregnancy, or stress. Diagnostic evaluation typically involves imaging modalities such as ultrasound, computed tomography (CT), or scintigraphy with technetium-99 m or iodine-123, essential for confirming thyroid tissue presence and functionality. Management may include hormonal suppression, radioiodine ablation, or surgical excision, with the critical caveat that lingual thyroid tissue often constitutes the patient's only functional thyroid tissue.

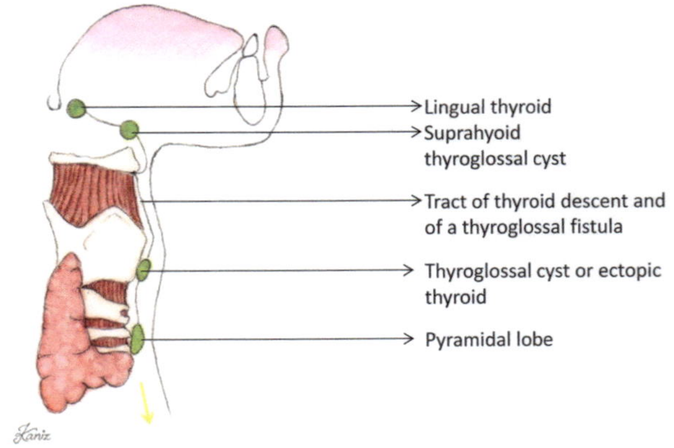

Fig. 1.2 Thyroglossal tract developmental anomalies

Other less common ectopic locations of thyroid tissue include intratracheal, intrathymic, and mediastinal regions. Surgical recognition and preservation are vital, especially in cases of total thyroidectomy for benign or malignant conditions, to prevent inadvertent hypothyroidism.

3. Thyroid Agenesis and Hemiagenesis [8, 14]

Complete agenesis or hemiagenesis of the thyroid gland represents rare congenital conditions characterized by the absence or significant hypoplasia of thyroid tissue. Complete thyroid agenesis manifests clinically as congenital hypothyroidism, typically identified through neonatal screening programs. Such patients necessitate lifelong thyroid hormone replacement therapy.

Hemiagenesis involves the unilateral absence of a thyroid lobe, predominantly affecting the left lobe. Often asymptomatic, it may be detected incidentally during imaging studies or thyroid surgery. However, patients with thyroid hemiagenesis have an increased propensity for developing pathology in the contralateral lobe, such as benign nodules or malignancies, necessitating vigilant long-term follow-up [14].

As noted above, genetic mutations implicated in thyroid dysgenesis involve transcription factors such as PAX8, TTF1, FOXE1, and NKX2-1 [7, 9]. Genetic syndromes such as Pendred syndrome, characterized by congenital hearing loss and thyroid dysfunction, highlight the intricate genetic-environmental interplay underpinning thyroid anomalies.

Parathyroid Glands Embryology (Fig. 1.3)

Parathyroid development is closely related to the formation and migration of the branchial apparatus and commences around the fifth week of gestation. The glands are derived from endodermal cells of the third and fourth pharyngeal pouches.

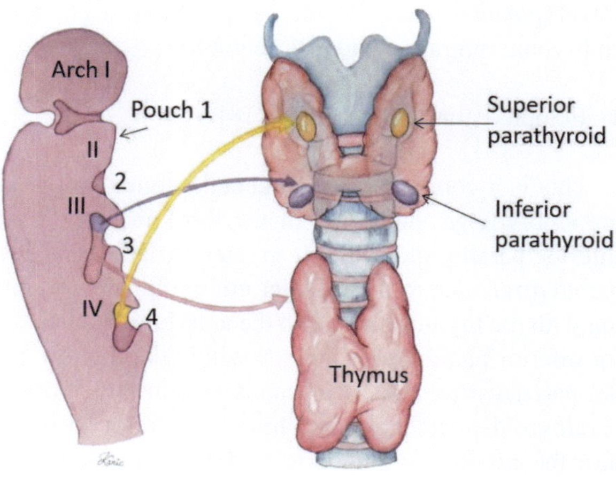

Fig. 1.3 Parathyroid embryology

Specifically, the superior parathyroid glands originate from the dorsal wing of the fourth pharyngeal pouch, whereas the inferior parathyroid glands arise from the dorsal wing of the third pharyngeal pouch. This distinction in embryological origin is clinically significant, accounting for differences in the anatomical localization and susceptibility to ectopic positions of these glands [5, 6, 15].

As development progresses, the third pharyngeal pouch elongates and differentiates into two distinct structures: the inferior parathyroid gland (from its dorsal portion) and the thymus (from its ventral portion) [5, 6, 15]. This dual differentiation contributes significantly to the inferior parathyroid glands' variable positions, as they migrate caudally alongside the developing thymus gland into the thoracic cavity, occasionally descending into the mediastinum.

In contrast, the superior parathyroid glands exhibit relatively limited migration and remain closely associated with the posterior aspect of the developing thyroid gland, near the cricoid cartilage [5, 6, 15]. As such, their final anatomical location is more consistent compared to the inferior glands.

The migration and differentiation processes of parathyroid glands are regulated by complex molecular signaling pathways, including those mediated by transcription factors and molecular signals such as Gcm2 (Glial cells missing homolog 2), Hoxa3, Pax1, and Pax9 [16, 17]. These factors are crucial in the differentiation and survival of parathyroid progenitor cells. For instance, Gcm2 is essential for parathyroid gland development, and its absence leads to agenesis or severe hypoplasia of these glands. Similarly, mutations in Hoxa3 and Pax genes have been associated with malformations involving the parathyroid glands and thymus, notably observed in clinical syndromes such as *DiGeorge syndrome*. In DiGeorge syndrome, failure of the third and fourth pouches to differentiate leads to the absence of thymus and parathyroids, underscoring the common developmental origins of these structures.

Developmental Anomalies of Parathyroids

Developmental anomalies of the parathyroid glands arise from variations during embryonic migration and differentiation.

1. Ectopic Parathyroid Glands [18]

This is a common developmental anomaly, originating from deviations during the embryologic migration of the third and fourth pharyngeal pouch derivatives. Inferior parathyroids exhibit greater variability in location compared to superior parathyroids due to their longer embryological migratory pathway, often descending with the thymus gland into the anterior mediastinum. Frequent ectopic locations for inferior parathyroids include within the thymus, mediastinal tissue, intrathyroidal parenchyma, and occasionally within the carotid sheath. Conversely, superior parathyroids, with their more limited migratory distance, typically occupy positions near the cricothyroid junction, with fewer instances of ectopia.

Clinically, ectopic glands are significant in patients with hyperparathyroidism, particularly primary hyperparathyroidism, complicating preoperative localization and surgical intervention. Preoperative imaging modalities such as ultrasound, Sestamibi scintigraphy, and computed tomography (CT) play critical roles in accurately identifying ectopic parathyroids, thus guiding successful surgical management.

2. Supernumerary Parathyroid Glands [19]

Supernumerary parathyroid glands result from additional embryonic branching or fragmentation of the migrating parathyroid tissue. These glands occur in approximately 5–13% of the general population and are clinically significant primarily in hyperparathyroidism, where undetected supernumerary glands may lead to persistent or recurrent disease following surgical intervention.

3. Parathyroid Agenesis and Hypoplasia

Complete agenesis or hypoplasia of the parathyroid glands represents a rare but clinically significant anomaly. These conditions are primarily associated with genetic syndromes such as DiGeorge syndrome (22q11 deletion syndrome), characterized by thymic hypoplasia, congenital heart defects, and parathyroid gland anomalies [20]. DiGeorge syndrome results from a microdeletion on chromosome 22q11, disrupting normal development of the third and fourth pharyngeal pouch derivatives. Patients typically present with hypocalcemia shortly after birth, necessitating lifelong calcium and vitamin D supplementation.

4. Intrathyroidal Parathyroid Glands [21]

Intrathyroidal parathyroid glands occur due to close anatomical associations during embryological development. These glands may embed within the thyroid parenchyma, complicating both diagnosis and surgical management, especially in thyroidectomy procedures.

Embryological Remnants Relevant to Surgery The thyroid's embryologic journey leaves behind three main potential remnants that surgeons must recognize:

- *Pyramidal lobe* [22]: The pyramidal lobe is a cone of thyroid tissue extending upward from the isthmus (often left of midline). It is seen in about 12–80% [23, 24] of individuals, with a pooled average of incidence of 42% [24], and is considered to be a residual of the thyroglossal tract. In thyroidectomy, a prominent pyramidal lobe should be removed to avoid leaving functional thyroid tissue. The pyramidal lobe may be attached to the hyoid by a fibrous or muscular band (levator glandulae thyroideae), which is another vestige of the developmental descent. Persistence of the thyroglossal duct itself can cause thyroglossal cysts or sinus tracts along this path, requiring surgical excision as described earlier.

- *Tubercle of Zuckerkandl* [25, 26]: This posterior projection of the thyroid lobe is found in up to 40–90% of people [27]. It is essentially a fusion nodule where the lateral anlage (from the ultimobranchial contribution) joined the median thyroid anlage. The tubercle can vary in its shape and size. Surgically, it is an important landmark because the recurrent laryngeal nerve (RLN) typically runs just medial or behind this tubercle. During thyroid lobectomy, identifying the tubercle of Zuckerkandl helps trace the RLN and superior parathyroid, and ensures completeness of surgery.
- *Thyrothymic thyroid "rests":* The thyrothymic ligament is a ligamentous band (sometimes containing thyroid tissue) that may extend inferiorly from the lower pole of the thyroid to the thymus. Small nodules of thyroid tissue can be present here, known as thyrothymic thyroid rests. Such thyrothymic thyroid rests or extensions may be seen in as much as 33–46% of thyroid lobes [28, 29]; however, these rests were completely separate from the gland in only about 6–9% [28, 30]. Sackett et al. [28] classified these remnants into four grades based on their relationship to the thyroid's inferior pole (Fig. 1.4):

Grade I: a small protuberance of thyroid tissue at the lower pole, within the thyrothymic ligament, easily distinguishable from the normal thyroid margin.

Grade II: a larger projection of thyroid tissue extending along the thyrothymic tract and attached to the thyroid pole by a narrow pedicle of thyroid tissue.

Grade III: a thyroid rest similar to grade II but connected to the thyroid pole only by a thin fibrovascular stalk (minimal thyroid tissue in the connection).

Grade IV: a completely separate focus of thyroid tissue in the thyrothymic tract, with no thyroid tissue connection to the main gland (only a fibrous attachment).

Surgically, these grades predict how firmly attached the rest is. Grades III and IV represent essentially autonomous thyroid tissue that can be missed during total thyroidectomy. If viable thyroid rests are left behind, they can hypertrophy and recur, defeating the purpose of total thyroidectomy. Therefore, careful inspection of the inferior pole region and along the thyrothymic ligament is needed.

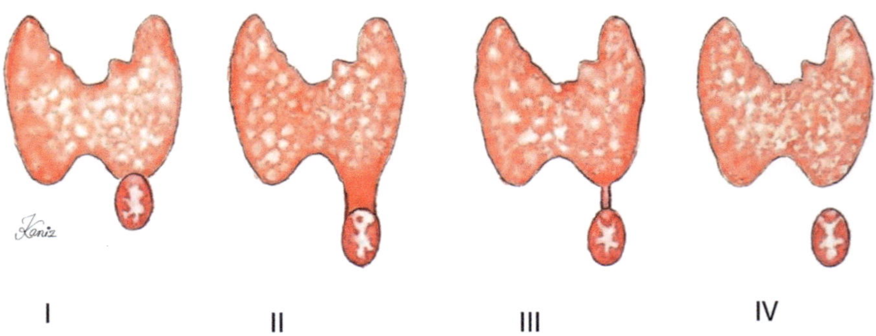

Fig. 1.4 Types of thyrothymic thyroid rests [28]

Thyroid Gland: Surgical Anatomy

Gross Anatomy

The thyroid gland is a brownish-red vascular gland situated in the lower anterior neck, between the level of the fifth cervical vertebra down to the first thoracic vertebra [31]. It consists of two lateral lobes joined by a midline isthmus. Each lobe is roughly conical, about 4–6 cm in length and extends from the level of the oblique line of thyroid cartilage lamina to the fourth to fifth tracheal rings. The isthmus typically lies anterior to the upper trachea at the level of the second to third tracheal rings. It usually weighs about 20–30 g in adults, but these dimensions may be significantly altered in thyroid pathologies. In about 12–80% [23, 24] of individuals, a pyramidal lobe (a remnant of the thyroglossal duct; described above) projects upward from the isthmus or adjacent lobe, more commonly from the left side. Posterolaterally the thyroid lobes usually show a protuberance known as the tuberculum of Zuckerkandl (described below).

Relations The thyroid lies in the visceral compartment of the neck deep to the infrahyoid "strap" muscles.

- The gland's anterior surface is covered by the sternothyroid ("inner strap muscle"), and the sternohyoid ("outer strap muscle") is more superficially, extending from the hyoid to the sternum.
- Laterally, each thyroid lobe is related to the carotid sheath and may partially overlap the common carotid artery. Further antero-lateral is sternocleidomastoid muscle.
- Medially, the lobes abut the larynx and trachea, wrapping around the anterolateral surfaces of these structures. More postero-medial to the lobes are the pharynx and esophagus, which is closer on the left side.
- Posteriorly the lobes lie on the prevertebral fascia.

The superior poles of the lobes reach the level of the cricothyroid muscle and inferior constrictor muscle. Here, the external branch of superior laryngeal nerve (EBSLN) lies medial to the superior pole as it passes to the cricothyroid muscle.

Fascial Anatomy

The thyroid gland is enclosed by a thin fibro-elastic "true capsule" and is invested in the pretracheal layer of deep cervical fascia ("false capsule"). Thus, the gland may be considered as covered by two capsules:

- Inner true capsule: This is a thin fibro-elastic layer formed by the condensation of connective tissue of the gland itself. This layer sends septa (partitions) deep

into the parenchyma, dividing the gland into lobules. These septa also carry blood vessels, nerves, and lymphatic vessels into the gland.
- Outer false capsule: This is external to the true capsule and is formed by pretracheal fascia, which is a broader layer of deep cervical fascia. The false capsule is not part of the thyroid gland itself, but rather a layer of surrounding tissue.

This is important during surgery: Surgeons perform *capsular dissection* (Fig. 1.5) between the true and false capsules to remove the gland. In this technique, an avascular plane is developed between the true thyroid capsule and the overlying pretracheal fascia (false capsule), staying immediately on the gland surface. This allows tertiary branches of the thyroid arteries to be ligated on the capsule itself. The true capsule is typically removed with the gland as it contains a dense capillary plexus.

Posteriorly, the prevertebral fascia condenses into the *ligament of Berry* (lateral suspensory ligament) (Fig. 1.6), which firmly anchors each thyroid lobe to the cricoid cartilage and upper tracheal rings. It serves as a suspensory ligament, holding the thyroid gland in place. The ligament's firm attachment to the trachea causes the thyroid's upward movement during deglutition.

The clinical significance of the ligament of Berry is that the recurrent laryngeal nerve passes lateral or through the fibers of Berry's ligament [32], making this site a critical zone during thyroidectomy. Excessive medial traction on the thyroid can kink or stretch the RLN at this fixed point. Further, small perforating arteries (laryngeal or tracheal branches of inferior thyroid artery) run alongside Berry's ligament—if not ligated close to the gland, they can cause troublesome bleeding; and blind clamping of them risks RLN injury [33].

Arterial Supply

The thyroid has a rich arterial supply from paired superior and inferior thyroid arteries. The *superior thyroid arteries (STAs)* are the first branches of the external carotid arteries. Each STA descends along the external surface of inferior constrictor

Fig. 1.5 Capsular dissection plane

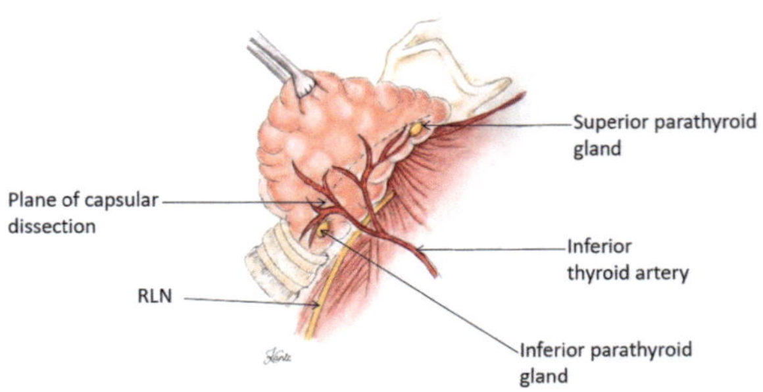

Fig. 1.6 Ligament of berry

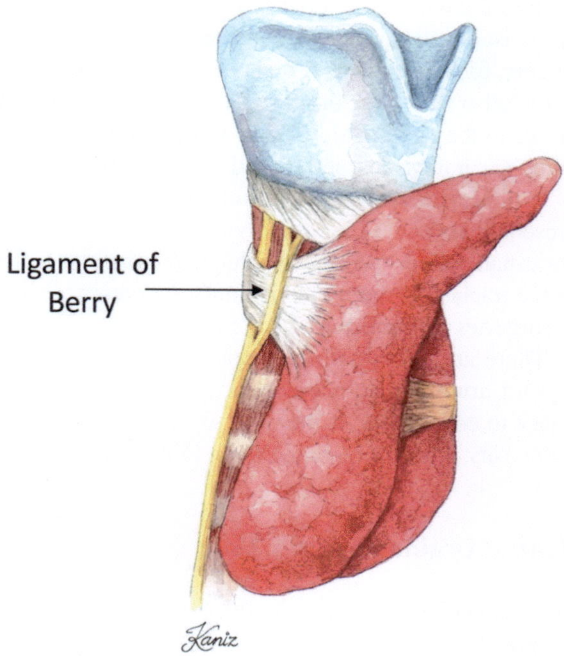

muscle toward the superior pole of a thyroid lobe, accompanied by the superior thyroid vein [5]. It gives off the superior laryngeal artery, which pierces the thyrohyoid membrane alongside the internal laryngeal nerve; other important branches being infrahyoid, sternocleidomastoid, and cricothyroid branches. At the superior pole, STA lies superficial to the EBSLN. Here, the STA divides into anterior and posterior glandular branches. The anterior (or ventral medial) branch is larger and communicates with its counterpart from the other side across or superior to the isthmus [5]. The posterior (or dorsal lateral) branch descends and communicates with branches of the inferior thyroid artery. Occasionally, the STA may arise from the common carotid artery just proximal to the carotid bifurcation [32].

At surgery, the STA and its branches are ligated close to the thyroid capsule to prevent injury to the EBSLN.

The *inferior thyroid arteries* (ITAs) arise from the thyrocervical trunks (branches of the subclavian arteries) and ascend behind the carotid sheath toward the lower poles of the thyroid. Each ITA typically reaches the thyroid at the level of the junction of the middle and inferior thirds of the lobe's lateral border. The ITA then divides into several ascending and descending branches supplying the posterior–inferior aspect of the gland and sending tiny twigs to the parathyroids. A notable relationship is that the RLN intersects the terminal part of the ITA near the thyroid gland. The relation of RLN with ITA is quite variable and does not follow a constant. However, some authors have reported that *right* RLN more often passes *anterior* to the ITA branches, whereas the left RLN usually runs *posterior* to the artery [34, 35]. In a minority, the nerve courses *between* the arterial branches. This anatomic variation means the surgeon must visually identify the RLN rather than assume its position relative to the artery. At surgery, for safety, the ITA branches are ligated on the thyroid capsule (capsular ligation), rather than tying off the main ITA trunk, to preserve blood flow through anastomoses to the parathyroid glands. Indeed, the ITA is the primary vascular source for both the parathyroids, and truncal ligation can jeopardize their perfusion.

An occasional additional artery, the *thyroid ima artery (Neubauer's artery)*, is present in about 3.3 [36] of individuals. When present, it may have a variable origin, but usually arises from the brachiocephalic trunk or aortic arch and ascends in front of the trachea to supply the isthmus. Its presence should be anticipated, especially in surgeries for retrosternal goiter.

There are also small collateral anastomoses between the superior and inferior thyroid arteries within the gland. This rich anastomotic network can allow one artery to compensate if the other is ligated, but it also contributes to the thyroid's propensity for brisk bleeding if cut improperly.

Venous Drainage (Fig. 1.7)

Thyroid venous outflow is via three paired veins forming a plexus on the surface of the gland.

- The *superior thyroid veins* are constant veins draining the upper poles. They accompany the STA upward and usually empty into the internal jugular vein bilaterally [37].
- The *middle thyroid veins* are present in about 29–62% of individuals [37, 38]. They emerge from the lateral surfaces of the lobes, are often short stubby, and

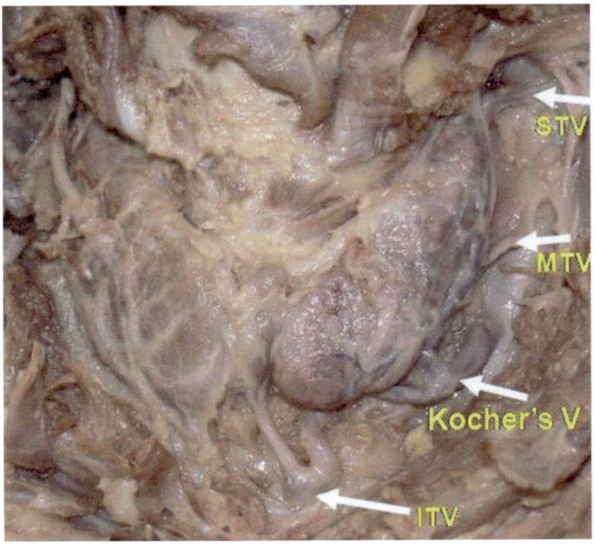

Fig. 1.7 Cadaveric dissection demonstration of venous anatomy of thyroid

drain into the internal jugular vein. These superior and middle veins are often thin-walled and tortuous; they must be carefully ligated to prevent avulsion during surgery.

- The *inferior thyroid veins* draining the lower poles and isthmus may be variable or multiple and form a pretracheal venous plexus or plexus thyroidea impar anterior to the trachea. They descend anterior to the trachea and typically empty into the brachiocephalic veins behind the manubrium. Often, the right and left inferior veins converge into a common trunk (especially into the left brachiocephalic vein) [37]. These veins are a common source of bleeding in low tracheostomy or thyroidectomy if not secured. Notably, the inferior thyroid veins also provide venous drainage for the parathyroid glands.
- Occasionally, a fourth vein of Kocher may be present between the middle and inferior thyroid vein [37]. When present, it usually drains directly into the IJV.

Lymphatic Drainage

The thyroid's lymphatic network is rich and drains to both central and lateral nodal basins. The lymphatic drainage usually follows the venous drainage.

The central nodal basin consists of the left and right paratracheal nodes, pretracheal nodes, and prelaryngeal nodes. The lateral nodal basin comprises nodes along the IJV (levels II–IV). Overall, the superior portion of the gland tends to drain to the *upper jugular nodes*, whereas the inferior thyroid regions drain to the *lower jugular and paratracheal nodes***.** The superior aspect of the gland drains into the superior pretracheal nodes, prelaryngeal nodes, and jugular nodes along the internal jugular vein (levels II–IV). The lateral lobes of the thyroid drain both into paratracheal nodes and laterally to the jugular lymph nodes. Lymphatic drainage from the thyroid isthmus and lower poles drains primarily to the *central compartment nodes*, which include the prelaryngeal, pretracheal, and paratracheal lymph nodes (level VI). A notable node in front of the laryngeal prominence is the *Delphian node* (prelaryngeal).

Nerve Supply and Relations

The thyroid gland is primarily innervated by autonomic fibers that regulate its blood flow. Sympathetic nerves from the superior, middle, and inferior cervical ganglia reach the thyroid along the arterial supply as periarterial plexuses. Parasympathetic input comes from branches of the vagus nerve (primarily the laryngeal branches). These autonomic fibers *do not control hormone secretion*, but rather modulate vasomotor tone and perhaps glandular blood volume.

Nerves in Relation to the Thyroid

Of critical importance to thyroid surgeons are the nearby *laryngeal nerves.*

Recurrent laryngeal nerves (RLNs) course intimately along the thyroid lobes and must be preserved to maintain vocal cord function. The right and left RLNs arise from the vagus nerves but take asymmetric paths [5, 32]. The right RLN loops around the subclavian artery at approximately the T1–T2 level, then ascends superiorly in the neck. The left RLN branches off the vagus in the upper chest, looping under the aortic arch (just behind the ligamentum arteriosum at T4–T5) before turning upward. Both RLNs travel in the tracheoesophageal groove as they ascend to the larynx, with the left RLN usually staying more consistently in the groove. In the neck, the RLN lies just deep to the thyroid's posterior suspensory fascia and often immediately posterior to the thyroid lobe. Within about 2–3 cm of the larynx, the RLN typically runs immediately behind the tubercle of Zuckerkandl and Berry's ligament. It then enters the larynx just inferior to the inferior constrictor muscle at the level of the cricothyroid joint. The RLN supplies all the intrinsic muscles of the larynx except the cricothyroid and provides sensory innervation to the mucosa below the vocal folds. Injury to one RLN causes ipsilateral vocal cord paralysis (hoarseness and risk of aspiration), whereas bilateral injury can cause airway obstruction.

Right vs. Left RLN The two RLNs have distinct anatomical differences, summarized in Table 1.1. These differences impact surgical strategy and risk profile during thyroid and parathyroid operations.

Nonrecurrent Laryngeal Nerve (NRLN) In rare cases (0.3–0.8% of thyroid operations on the right), the right RLN does not loop at all and instead travels directly from the vagus to the larynx in a horizontal course [39]. This *nonrecurrent RLN* occurs when an embryologic vascular anomaly (e.g., an aberrant right subclavian artery arising from the descending aorta) eliminates the subclavian loop. A nonrecurrent nerve is at high risk of accidental transection if an index of suspicion is not maintained. On the left side, a nonrecurrent laryngeal nerve is exceedingly rare (about 0.004%, reported only in situations of situs inversus and an aberrant right aortic arch) [39]. Surgeons need to be alert to the possibility of NRLN, especially if preoperative imaging shows an aberrant subclavian artery. In such a case, the RLN should be sought in an unusual lateral location at the level of the cricoid instead of the tracheoesophageal groove. If intraoperative nerve monitoring is used at surgery, right V1 signal will have short latency because the nonrecurrent nerve enters the larynx earlier and directly [40]. The classification of such a nonrecurrent RLN is as follows:

Table 1.1 Differences between the right and left RLN

Feature	Right RLN	Left RLN
Origin and loop	Loops around the right subclavian artery (T1–T2 level).	Loops around aortic arch, behind ligamentum arteriosum (T4–T5 level). Longer intrathoracic course.
Typical course in neck	Ascends more obliquely, often entering the tracheoesophageal groove higher up.	Ascends vertically in the tracheoesophageal groove for a longer distance.
Relation to inferior thyroid artery (ITA)	*More likely to be anterior* to the ITA or its branches; in ~30% runs posterior to it. A nonrecurrent variant (direct vagal branch in neck) occurs ~1% (usually with aberrant subclavian artery).	*More likely to be posterior* to the ITA; ~32% anterior to it. Nonrecurrent laryngeal nerve is extremely rare on the left (seen only in situs inversus with aberrant vessels).
Branching pattern	Often gives 2–5 extralaryngeal branches (to the larynx, trachea, esophagus) before entering cricothyroid area. May bifurcate near larynx into anterior (motor) and posterior (sensory) divisions.	Tends to have 2–3 extralaryngeal branches. Also often bifurcates into terminal branches near laryngeal entry.
Vulnerability	Injury usually occurs in the lower neck (e.g., at berry's ligament or ITA crossing). A nonrecurrent RLN, if present, is at risk of misidentification.	Longer course makes it susceptible to mediastinal pathology (e.g., lung tumors or aortic aneurysms). In surgery, its predictable groove location aids identification, but it is equally at risk near Berry's ligament.

- Type 1: the NRILN arises from the cervical vagus directly and descends into the larynx at the level of the superior thyroid pole along with vessels of the superior thyroid pedicle.
- Type 2A: the NRILN assesses from the cervical vagus directly and follows a transverse path parallel to and over the trunk of the ITA, at the level of the isthmus.
- Type2B: the NRILN follows a transverse path parallel to and under the trunk of ITA, marking a downward curve.

External Branch of the Superior Laryngeal Nerve (EBSLN)

The superior laryngeal nerve, a branch of the vagus high in the neck, divides into internal and external branches. The internal branch pierces the thyrohyoid membrane and is sensory to the larynx. The external branch of the superior laryngeal nerve (EBSLN) provides motor innervation to the cricothyroid muscle, which tenses the vocal cords. Injury to the EBSLN causes loss of high-pitch phonation and voice fatigue, which are subtle but significant deficits for voice professionals. EBSLN is usually a small nerve that runs a short course in the neck. It descends close to the superior thyroid vessels toward the upper pole of the thyroid gland. Usually, it travels along or within the inferior pharyngeal constrictor muscle and approaches the cricothyroid muscle from a lateral–superior position. Since it often courses with the superior thyroid artery (STA) and its branches, surgeons must be cautious when ligating the superior thyroid vascular pedicle. The nerve may be anywhere from well above the superior pole (in which case it is safe from harm) to running posterior to the superior pole and along the artery into the gland's capsule (in which case it is at high risk if not identified).

Cernea's Classification of EBSLN To predict the EBSLN's position relative to the superior pole, Cernea et al. (1992) [41] proposed a widely used classification: (Fig. 1.8)

- Type 1: The EBSLN crosses the STA more than 1 cm above the upper border of the superior thyroid pole. In this case, the nerve runs high and is usually not in the surgical field when the thyroid pole is being ligated; risk of injury is low.
- Type 2a: The EBSLN crosses the STA less than 1 cm above the upper pole. Being close to the gland, here the nerve is in proximity to where the surgeon is working and is at risk during vessel ligature.
- Type 2b: The EBSLN crosses below the upper border of the thyroid. In type 2b, the nerve is effectively at the greatest risk—it is low-lying and often intimately associated with the superior thyroid vessels or the capsule of the gland at the apex. Without careful dissection, a Cernea type 2b nerve is easily injured when the superior pole is clamped or tied.

Cernea's original data indicated type 2 nerves (near or below the pole) were much more common in larger goiters, presumably because an enlarged gland extends upward closer to the nerve. Subsequent studies have found variable prevalence; however, the largest clinical study has shown a distribution of type 1: 17.1%; type IIa: 57.2%; and type IIb: 18.8% [42].

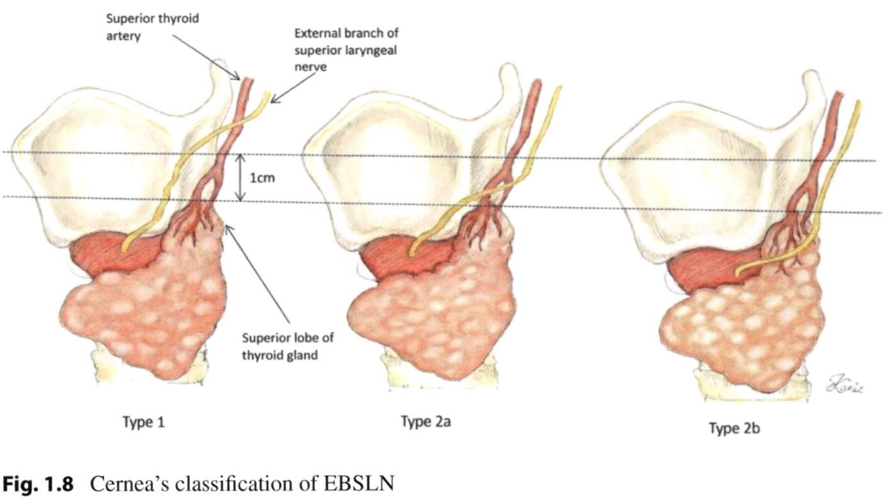

Fig. 1.8 Cernea's classification of EBSLN

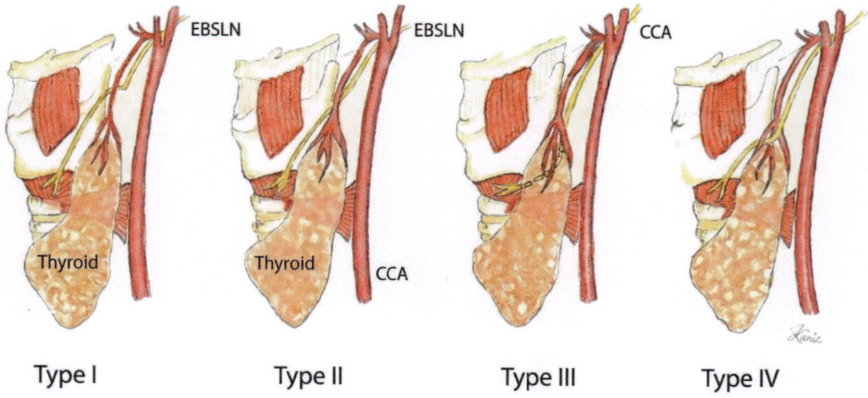

Fig. 1.9 Kierner's classification of EBSLN

Kierner's Classification of EBSLN [43] Kierner et al. in 1998 expanded on Cernea by adding a fourth category. In Kierner's system, types 1, 2, and 3 correspond essentially to Cernea's 1, 2a, and 2b (Fig. 1.9).

– Type 4 (Kierner): The EBSLN runs dorsally to the superior thyroid artery and its branches. In this variant, instead of coursing superficially and crossing the artery, the nerve goes behind the artery and approaches the cricothyroid muscle from a deeper plane. A type 4 EBSLN is considered high risk because it might not be seen superficially at all—it could be mistaken for a small branch of the STA or hidden until the vessel is ligated.

For practical purposes, surgeons usually reference Cernea types. However, being aware of Kierner's type 4 is important—it reminds the surgeon that occasionally the EBSLN is not found in the cricothyroid space since it may be deep along the vessels.

Triangles in Thyroid Surgery (Fig. 1.10)

Several anatomical–surgical triangles in the neck have been described to facilitate safe thyroidectomy. These triangles are tissue planes bounded by important structures, serving as roadmaps to find key nerves and vessels:

- Joll's triangle (sternothyro-laryngeal triangle) (Fig. 1.11): This triangle is used to locate the external branch of the superior laryngeal nerve (EBSLN) near the superior pole of the thyroid. It is formed by the following borders:
  - Superiorly: the attachment of the strap muscles to the thyroid cartilage (at the oblique line).
  - Medially: the midline of the neck.
  - Laterally: the upper pole of the thyroid gland along with the superior thyroid vessels.

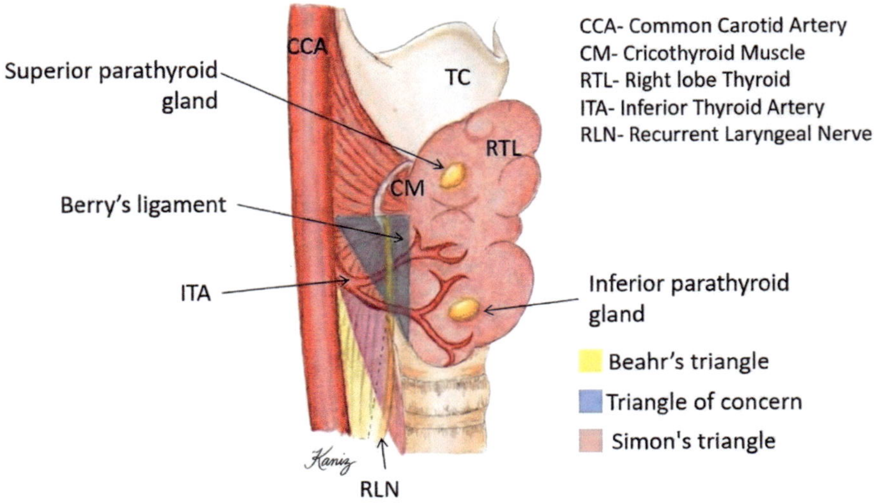

Fig. 1.10 Triangles in thyroid Surgery

Fig. 1.11 Joll's triangle

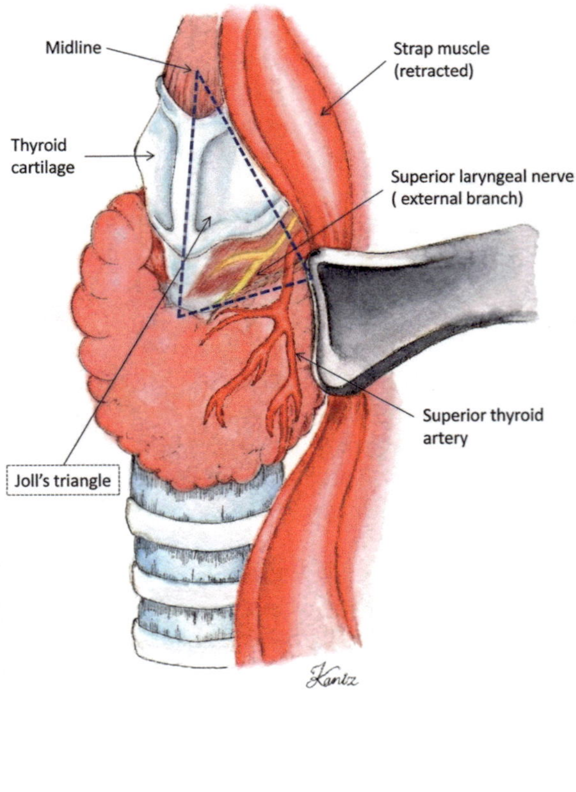

The floor of Joll's triangle is the cricothyroid muscle, into which the EBSLN inserts. Identifying this triangle intraoperatively is done by retracting the superior pole of the thyroid downward and laterally, which exposes the space between the sternothyroid muscle and larynx. The EBSLN can often be seen or stimulated here, running in the fascia on the surface of the cricothyroid muscle (in the triangle's floor).

Opening the avascular *Reeves' space (cricothyroid space of Reeves*, just deep to the sternothyroid muscle at the upper pole, medial to STA) corresponds to entering Joll's triangle and is a technique to protect the EBSLN.

- Beahr's triangle: An important landmark for the recurrent laryngeal nerve (RLN), this triangle lies in the lateral aspect of the tracheoesophageal groove after the thyroid lobe is retracted medially. Its borders are base—the common carotid artery; superiorly—the inferior thyroid artery; and medial side—the RLN itself. Within Beahr's triangle, the inferior thyroid artery typically crosses the RLN. Recognizing this triangle helps the surgeon anticipate where the RLN will appear as it ascends. In practice, once the inferior pole is mobilized and the thyroid lobe is pulled medially, Beahr's triangle is visualized and the surgeon will often find the RLN coursing obliquely upward through it.
- Lore's triangle: Another triangle used to find the RLN, described by John Lore. The boundaries are medially—the trachea and esophagus; laterally—carotid; and superiorly—the inferior pole of the thyroid gland. Lore's triangle lies essentially at the level of the lower thyroid pole, deep in the neck. The RLN is commonly found within this triangle as it travels in the tracheoesophageal groove, making this a useful window for nerve identification.
- Simon's triangle (triangle of safety): This classic triangle is also referenced for locating the RLN low in the neck. Its borders are the common carotid artery laterally, the trachea/esophagus medially, and the inferior thyroid artery superiorly. It overlaps with the lower part of Beahr's triangle. Essentially, Simon's triangle describes the space in which the RLN can be found as it loops upward, before reaching the ligament of Berry.
- Triangle of concern: The triangle of concern is a crucial anatomical region in thyroidectomy as it is the most common site for postoperative bleeding and recurrent laryngeal nerve (RLN) injury.

  Medial border: trachea
  Lateral border: recurrent laryngeal nerve (RLN)
  Base: thyrothymic ligament and loose fat above the sternum
  Apex: Berry's ligament

This region contains small branches of the inferior thyroid artery, which require careful ligation or cauterization to prevent postoperative hematoma.

These triangles are mainly heuristic aids; in practice they overlap.

Anatomic Landmarks for RLN Identification In addition to the triangles already described (Beahr's, Lore's, etc.), surgeons use several consistent landmarks to find and verify the RLN:

- Inferior thyroid artery crossing: As noted, the ITA's intersection with the RLN is a key location. Often, the RLN can be found just inferior to where the ITA branches cross toward the thyroid. Ligation of the ITA trunk is usually done after identifying the RLN either just above or below this crossing to avoid inadvertent injury. The artery can be double-looped or branching; the nerve may run between the arterial branches (this is common especially on the right). Meticulous dissection here will reveal the nerve, which typically has a distinctive white, striated appearance and sometimes a slight neural sheen compared to blood vessels or fibrous tissue.
- Ligament of Berry and laryngeal entry point: One very reliable landmark is where the RLN enters the larynx. Both RLNs pass under the inferior constrictor muscle to reach the larynx, typically at the level of the cricothyroid joint, just behind the cricothyroid muscle. This point is just deep to Berry's suspensory ligament. Often, the RLN runs immediately behind the cricothyroid joint and then angles medially into the larynx. Some surgeons, however, locate the RLN first at its insertion (e.g., just below the cricoid cartilage where it enters the larynx) by finding the cricothyroid junction and Berry's ligament area—here, the nerve is usually within a few millimeters, often slightly lateral to the ligament.
- Tubercle of Zuckerkandl: (detailed above in embryology context) A prominent tubercle can be followed medially to find the RLN. In thyroidectomy, once the superior pole is dissected and the lobe is rolled back, the surgeon often encounters the tubercle at the posterolateral aspect. The RLN almost invariably runs in the groove just medial to this structure. The tubercle of Zuckerkandl also points to the superior parathyroid. Recognizing the tubercle and skeletonizing, it can provide a visual cue for finding the nerve. The tubercle may be variable in size. Pelizzo et al [25] gave a classification system for the size of the tubercle as follows:

  0: unrecognizable
  1: only a thickening of the lateral edge of the thyroid lobe
  2: smaller than 1 cm
  3: larger than 1 cm

Given these landmarks, the common teaching is to expose the RLN either in the lower neck (near the root of neck—inferior approach to the nerve) or near Berry's ligament (laryngeal entry—superior approach to the nerve) or from lateral to medial (lateral approach to the nerve). Identifying the nerve early in the dissection is highly recommended. The use of nerve monitoring (discussed later) has complemented these visual cues by providing functional confirmation.

Pyrtek's plane (relation of parathyroids to RLN): In 1964, Pyrtek and Painter [44] described a helpful conceptual "cleavage plane" using the RLN as a dividing line to distinguish the typical locations of the superior vs. inferior parathyroid glands. If one considers a coronal plane through the RLN in the neck, the superior parathyroid gland is almost always located dorsal (posterior) to the plane of the nerve, whereas the inferior parathyroid gland is usually found ventral (anterior) to that plane.

Parathyroid Glands: Anatomy

The parathyroid glands are small, oval endocrine glands usually found on the posterior aspect of the thyroid. Typically, there are four parathyroids—two *superior* and two *inferior*—each measuring about 3–8 mm and weighing 30–40 mg [15]. They are soft, tan-brown glands with a delicate capsule and are often imbedded in fat. The superior parathyroid glands derive embryologically from the fourth pharyngeal pouch, whereas the inferior glands originate from the third pharyngeal pouch (descending with the thymus). This developmental origin explains their final locations: the superior glands tend to remain higher and more posterior, while the inferior glands migrate further and can end up in more anterior–inferior positions.

Typical Location In most individuals, the superior parathyroid glands lie in the *tracheoesophageal groove* at the level of the cricoid cartilage or just below, roughly 1 cm above the crossing of the RLN and inferior thyroid artery [5, 15]. They are usually attached to the posterior aspect of the upper thyroid lobe, just outside the thyroid capsule (often near the tubercle of Zuckerkandl). In contrast, the inferior parathyroid glands are more variable in location. Commonly, an inferior gland is found near the inferior pole of the thyroid or in the thyrothymic ligament (a fibrofatty band between the thyroid and thymus). They may reside anterior to the tracheoesophageal groove, often in closer proximity to the inferior thyroid vein plexus or thymus.

A useful concept is *Pyrtek's plane* [44], which considers the RLN as a vertical divider: The inferior parathyroid is almost always located *anterior/ventral* to the RLN (toward the surface of the neck), whereas the superior parathyroid lies *posterior/dorsal* to the RLN (deeper in the neck). In practical terms, surgeons expect to find the superior glands at the back of the thyroid (near or behind the nerve), and the inferior glands on the front or lateral aspect of the thyrothymic ligament area (often in front of the nerve). Another way to describe this: The superior parathyroid is usually *posterior to the inferior thyroid artery*, while the inferior parathyroid is *anterior to the artery*, reflecting the same anatomical plane separation.

Surface and Deep Relations Parathyroid glands are intimately associated with the thyroid but are separated by a thin fascial plane. They are usually encased in fat and are *extracapsular* (outside the thyroid's true capsule). Occasionally, a gland may be *intrathyroidal* [21] (embedded within thyroid tissue)—this occurs in a small percentage of individuals (most often an inferior gland that failed to separate during development). The *deep (medial)* relations of the parathyroids include the pharynx/esophagus and recurrent laryngeal nerve in the tracheoesophageal groove. The *surface (lateral)* relations include the thyroid lobe itself (for a superior gland) or the inner aspect of the carotid/jugular complex (for an inferior gland that may be more anterior). Both gland pairs lie in the visceral compartment deep to the sternothyroid muscle. A well-known landmark for superior glands is the intersection of the *inferior thyroid artery and RLN*—the superior parathyroid is usually found just above and dorsal to that intersection. Inferior glands have no single reliable landmark, but about 50–60% are within 1 cm of the lower thyroid pole, and others track along the thymus into the upper mediastinum [15].

Blood Supply The arterial supply of the parathyroids is predominantly from the inferior thyroid artery [31, 45, 46]. Small arterioles branch from the ITA to each gland—in fact, the inferior thyroid artery may be considered the "parathyroid artery" in most cases. If the ITA is absent (occurring in about 5–10% of people, more often on the left), a branch of the superior thyroid artery may supply the inferior parathyroid gland in its place [45, 46]. The superior parathyoids receive blood supply from the ITA in 77% of cases, from the STA in 15%, and from anastomoses between the two arteries, running posteriorly to the thyroid in 8%. The inferior PGs were supplied by the ITA in 90.3% of cases and by the STA in 5% [46]. An inferior parathyroid that has descended into the chest may be supplied by thymic branch of the internal thoracic artery or by a branch from the arch of aorta [47]. Venous drainage from the parathyroids is via the thyroid venous plexus (primarily into the inferior and middle thyroid veins).

Lymphatic Drainage Lymphatic drainage of the parathyroids follows paths similar to the thyroid—predominantly to the central compartment (pretracheal/paratracheal) nodes and to adjacent deep cervical nodes [31]. The parathyroid glands have fewer lymphatics compared to thyroid.

Nerve Supply Parathyroid gland innervation is primarily autonomic, receiving sympathetic input from the cervical sympathetic ganglia, specifically the superior cervical ganglion, via periarterial plexuses accompanying the thyroid arteries [31]. Parasympathetic fibers, originating from branches of the vagus nerve, contribute minimally to the glandular innervation. Autonomic innervation primarily regulates parathyroid gland blood flow rather than hormone secretion.

Surgical Identification Differentiating parathyroid glands from surrounding fat or lymph nodes is a crucial skill in endocrine surgery. Experienced surgeons use several visual and tactile cues. *Color* is a key factor: normal parathyroids are usually beige, tan, or light brown, whereas fat is yellow and lymph nodes are white-gray to pink. Parathyroid usually have a *vascular pedicle*, while nodes and fat do not. Since parathyroids have well-defined encapsulated appearance, manipulation of the fat surrounding the parathyroids, causes a distinct gliding or rowboat like motion of the parathyroid: this is known as "glide sign." Table 1.2 depicts the differences between parathyroid and other structures encountered in neck.

Table 1.2 Differentiating features between parathyroid and other structures in neck

Structure	Color	Shape	Immersion in saline	Gliding movement	Vascular hilum
Parathyroid	Tan brown	Kidney shaped or elliptical	Sinks	Yes	Yes
Node	White-gray, pink	Ovoid or spherical	Sinks	Usually not	No
Fat	Bright yellow	Irregular	Floats	No	No
Thymus	Yellowish, brownish	Irregular	Sinks	No	No

Acknowledgments The authors thank Mrs. Fatema Akolawala (Kaniz) for providing hand-painted diagrams to accompany the text of this chapter.

References

1. Hanbury EM Jr, Boyd DP. History of thyroid surgery. Surgery. 1963;54:550–6. https://www.ncbi.nlm.nih.gov/pubmed/14057426
2. Hegner CF. A history of thyroid surgery. Ann Surg. 1932;95(4):481–92. https://doi.org/10.1097/00000658-193204000-00001.
3. Fagman H, Nilsson M. Morphogenesis of the thyroid gland. Mol Cell Endocrinol. 2010;323(1):35–54. https://doi.org/10.1016/j.mce.2009.12.008.
4. Gray SW, Skandalakis JE, Akin JT Jr. Embryological considerations of thyroid surgery: developmental anatomy of the thyroid, parathyroids and the recurrent laryngeal nerve. Am Surg. 1976;42(9):621–8. https://www.ncbi.nlm.nih.gov/pubmed/949130
5. Mansberger AR Jr, Wei JP. Surgical embryology and anatomy of the thyroid and parathyroid glands. Surg Clin North Am. 1993;73(4):727–46. https://doi.org/10.1016/s0039-6109(16)46082-2.
6. Sadler TW. Langman's medical embryology. 12th ed. Philadelphia: Wolters Kluwer/Lippincott Williams & Wilkins; 2012.
7. Fernandez LP, Lopez-Marquez A, Santisteban P. Thyroid transcription factors in development, differentiation and disease. Nat Rev Endocrinol. 2015;11(1):29–42. https://doi.org/10.1038/nrendo.2014.186.
8. Nilsson M, Fagman H. Mechanisms of thyroid development and dysgenesis: an analysis based on developmental stages and concurrent embryonic anatomy. Curr Top Dev Biol. 2013;106:123–70. https://doi.org/10.1016/B978-0-12-416021-7.00004-3.
9. Trueba SS, Auge J, Mattei G, et al. PAX8, TITF1, and FOXE1 gene expression patterns during human development: new insights into human thyroid development and thyroid dysgenesis-associated malformations. J Clin Endocrinol Metab. 2005;90(1):455–62. https://doi.org/10.1210/jc.2004-1358.
10. Allard RH. The thyroglossal cyst. Head Neck Surg. 1982;5(2):134–46. https://doi.org/10.1002/hed.2890050209.
11. Chou J, Walters A, Hage R, et al. Thyroglossal duct cysts: anatomy, embryology and treatment. Surg Radiol Anat. 2013;35(10):875–81. https://doi.org/10.1007/s00276-013-1115-3.
12. Huang NS, Wei WJ, Qu N, Wang YL, Wang Y, Ji QH. Lingual ectopic papillary thyroid carcinoma: two case reports and review of the literature. Oral Oncol. 2019;88:186–9. https://doi.org/10.1016/j.oraloncology.2018.11.019.
13. Noussios G, Anagnostis P, Goulis DG, Lappas D, Natsis K. Ectopic thyroid tissue: anatomical, clinical, and surgical implications of a rare entity. Eur J Endocrinol. 2011;165(3):375–82. https://doi.org/10.1530/EJE-11-0461.

14. Lesi OK, Thapar A, Appaiah NNB, et al. Thyroid hemiagenesis: narrative review and clinical implications. Cureus. 2022;14(2):e22401. https://doi.org/10.7759/cureus.22401.
15. Fancy T, Gallagher D 3rd, Hornig JD. Surgical anatomy of the thyroid and parathyroid glands. Otolaryngol Clin N Am. 2010;43(2):221–7. https://doi.org/10.1016/j.otc.2010.01.001.
16. Liu Z, Yu S, Manley NR. Gcm2 is required for the differentiation and survival of parathyroid precursor cells in the parathyroid/thymus primordia. Dev Biol. 2007;305(1):333–46. https://doi.org/10.1016/j.ydbio.2007.02.014.
17. Zajac JD, Danks JA. The development of the parathyroid gland: from fish to human. Curr Opin Nephrol Hypertens. 2008;17(4):353–6. https://doi.org/10.1097/MNH.0b013e328304651c.
18. Noussios G, Anagnostis P, Natsis K. Ectopic parathyroid glands and their anatomical, clinical and surgical implications. Exp Clin Endocrinol Diabetes. 2012;120(10):604–10. https://doi.org/10.1055/s-0032-1327628.
19. Pattou FN, Pellissier LC, Noel C, Wambergue F, Huglo DG, Proye CA. Supernumerary parathyroid glands: frequency and surgical significance in treatment of renal hyperparathyroidism. World J Surg. 2000;24(11):1330–4. https://doi.org/10.1007/s002680010220.
20. McDonald-McGinn DM, Sullivan KE. Chromosome 22q11.2 deletion syndrome (DiGeorge syndrome/velocardiofacial syndrome). Medicine (Baltimore). 2011;90(1):1–18. https://doi.org/10.1097/MD.0b013e3182060469.
21. Mazeh H, Kouniavsky G, Schneider DF, et al. Intrathyroidal parathyroid glands: small, but mighty (a Napoleon phenomenon). Surgery. 2012;152(6):1193–200. https://doi.org/10.1016/j.surg.2012.08.026.
22. Geraci G, Pisello F, Li Volsi F, Modica G, Sciume C. The importance of pyramidal lobe in thyroid surgery. G Chir. 2008;29(11–12):479–82. https://www.ncbi.nlm.nih.gov/pubmed/19068184
23. Irawati N, Vaish R, Chaukar D, Deshmukh A, D'Cruz A. Surgical anatomy of the pyramidal lobe in cancer patients: a prospective cohort in a tertiary Centre. Int J Surg. 2016;30:166–8. https://doi.org/10.1016/j.ijsu.2016.04.051.
24. Ostrowski P, Bonczar M, Iwanaga J, et al. The prevalence and anatomy of the pyramidal lobe of the thyroid gland: a meta-analysis with implications for thyroid surgery. Clin Anat. 2023;36(6):937–45. https://doi.org/10.1002/ca.24062.
25. Pelizzo MR, Toniato A, Gemo G. Zuckerkandl's tuberculum: an arrow pointing to the recurrent laryngeal nerve (constant anatomical landmark). J Am Coll Surg. 1998;187(3):333–6. https://doi.org/10.1016/s1072-7515(98)00160-4.
26. Pezillo AA, Greco F, Gurrado A, et al. The tubercle of Zuckerkandl: anatomical landmark in thyroid surgery. Clinical study based on 200 cases and literature review. Langenbecks Arch Surg. 2003;388(5):306–9.
27. Henry BM, Sanna B, Vikse J, et al. Zuckerkandl's tubercle and its relationship to the recurrent laryngeal nerve: a cadaveric dissection and meta-analysis. Auris Nasus Larynx. 2017;44(6):639–47. https://doi.org/10.1016/j.anl.2017.03.013.
28. Sackett WR, Reeve TS, Barraclough B, Delbridge L. Thyrothymic thyroid rests: incidence and relationship to the thyroid gland. J Am Coll Surg. 2002;195(5):635–40. https://doi.org/10.1016/s1072-7515(02)01319-4.
29. Sheahan P, O'Duffy F. Thyroid thyrothymic extension: an anatomic study in a surgical series. Head Neck. 2016;38(5):732–5. https://doi.org/10.1002/hed.23954.
30. Gurleyik E, Gurleyik G. Separate thyrothymic thyroid remnant; clinically crucial anatomic variation. Ann Surg Treat Res. 2020;98(3):111–5. https://doi.org/10.4174/astr.2020.98.3.111.
31. Standring S. Gray's anatomy: the anatomical basis of clinical practice. 42nd ed. New York: Elsevier; 2021.
32. Mohebati A, Shaha AR. Anatomy of thyroid and parathyroid glands and neurovascular relations. Clin Anat. 2012;25(1):19–31. https://doi.org/10.1002/ca.21220.
33. Bhargav PR. Salient anatomical landmarks of thyroid and their practical significance in thyroid surgery: a pictorial review of thyroid surgical anatomy (revisited). Indian J Surg. 2014;76(3):207–11. https://doi.org/10.1007/s12262-013-0856-x.

34. Thomas AM, Fahim DK, Gemechu JM. Anatomical variations of the recurrent laryngeal nerve and implications for injury prevention during surgical procedures of the neck. Diagnostics (Basel). 2020;10(9) https://doi.org/10.3390/diagnostics10090670.
35. Yalcin B. Anatomic configurations of the recurrent laryngeal nerve and inferior thyroid artery. Surgery. 2006;139(2):181–7. https://doi.org/10.1016/j.surg.2005.06.035.
36. Yurasakpong L, Nantasenamat C, Janta S, et al. The decreasing prevalence of the thyroid ima artery: a systematic review and machine learning assisted meta-analysis. Ann Anat. 2022;239:151803. https://doi.org/10.1016/j.aanat.2021.151803.
37. Singh R. Variations of venous drainage of the thyroid gland and their surgical implications: a narrative review. J Vasc Bras. 2023;22:e20220163. https://doi.org/10.1590/1677-5449.202201632.
38. Dionigi G, Congiu T, Rovera F, Boni L. The middle thyroid vein: anatomical and surgical aspects. World J Surg. 2010;34(3):514–20. https://doi.org/10.1007/s00268-009-0350-6.
39. Mahmodlou R, Aghasi MR, Sepehrvand N. Identifying the non-recurrent laryngeal nerve: preventing a major risk of morbidity during thyroidectomy. Int J Prev Med. 2013;4(2):237–40. https://www.ncbi.nlm.nih.gov/pubmed/23543847
40. Donatini G, Carnaille B, Dionigi G. Increased detection of non-recurrent inferior laryngeal nerve (NRLN) during thyroid surgery using systematic intraoperative neuromonitoring (IONM). World J Surg. 2013;37(1):91–3. https://doi.org/10.1007/s00268-012-1782-y.
41. Cernea CR, Ferraz AR, Nishio S, Dutra A, Cruz O. Surgical anatomy of the external branch of the superior laryngeal nerve. Head Neck. 1992;14(5):380–3.
42. Ravikumar K, Sadacharan D, Muthukumar S, Mohanpriya G, Hussain Z, Suresh RV. EBSLN and factors influencing its identification and its safety in patients undergoing Total thyroidectomy: a study of 456 cases. World J Surg. 2016;40(3):545–50. https://doi.org/10.1007/s00268-015-3383-z.
43. Kierner AC, Aigner M, Burian M. Surgical anatomy of the external branch of the superior laryngeal nerve. Arch Otolaryngol Head Neck Surg. 1998;124(3):301–3.
44. Pyrtek L, Painter RL. An anatomic study of the relationship of the parathyroid glands to the recurrent laryngeal nerve. Surg Gynecol Obstet. 1964;119:509–12. https://www.ncbi.nlm.nih.gov/pubmed/14210149
45. Delattre JF, Flament JB, Palot JP, Pluot M. Variations in the parathyroid glands. Number, situation and arterial vascularization. Anatomical study and surgical application. J Chir Paris. 1982;119(11):633–41. https://www.ncbi.nlm.nih.gov/pubmed/7153263
46. Sadowski SM, Vidal Fortuny J, Triponez F. A reappraisal of vascular anatomy of the parathyroid gland based on fluorescence techniques. Gland Surg. 2017;6(Suppl 1):S30–7. https://doi.org/10.21037/gs.2017.07.10.
47. Wang C. The anatomic basis of parathyroid surgery. Ann Surg. 1976;183(3):271–5. https://doi.org/10.1097/00000658-197603000-00010.

Contemporary Workup of Thyroid Nodules

2

Helena Levyn and Snehal Patel

Editorial
Patel and Levyn have extensively discussed the workup of thyroid nodules. Clearly, much of the emphasis is focused on history and physical examination. The ultrasound of the thyroid has become a mainstay in the evaluation of the thyroid nodules. Various organizations have developed risk factors in the evaluation of thyroid nodules; these are commonly called TIRADS. The most important findings in the ultrasound include punctate calcification, irregular margins, extrathyroidal extension, taller than wider thyroid nodules, and suspicious lymph nodes in the central compartment or lateral neck. Fine-needle aspiration is very critical in the evaluation of thyroid nodules. Approximately one-third of the needle biopsies may be Bethesda III or IV, which typically warrant additional diagnostic workup in the United States—often involving molecular analysis. This is obviously an expensive study; however, it is quite helpful when available. Still, the clinical evaluation and sonographic features direct our decision-making. CT scan is quite helpful to evaluate the extent of the disease and three-dimensional review of the entire thyroid. It also helps to evaluate paratracheal and lateral neck nodes. The workup also depends upon individual institutional practices and the available expertise.

The authors have done a fantastic job in this chapter related to radiomics and artificial intelligence (AI). The future of evaluation of thyroid nodules is going to be the application of AI. I have a feeling the majority of the patients with thyroid nodules will increasingly rely on tools like ChatGPT and other forms of artificial

H. Levyn
Department of Otolaryngology and Head and Neck Surgery, Montefiore Medical Center, Albert Einstein College of Medicine, New York, NY, USA
e-mail: hlevyn@montefiore.org

S. Patel (✉)
Department of Surgery, Memorial Sloan Kettering Cancer Center, New York, NY, USA
e-mail: patels@mskcc.org

P. S. Pai et al. (eds.), *Controversies in Cancer of the Thyroid and Parathyroid Glands*, https://doi.org/10.1007/978-3-032-13130-0_2

intelligence for their evaluation. Many patients are already reviewing their own ultrasound results in the portal and making their own decisions regarding follow-up care. Despite these technological shifts, thorough clinical examination, good history-taking, and fine-needle aspiration remain the cornerstone of evaluation for thyroid nodules.

Ashok R Shaha

This chapter aims to provide a systematic approach to thyroid nodule evaluation while addressing thought-provoking dilemmas encountered during workup of thyroid nodules. Additionally, it highlights recent publications that enhance clinicians' understanding and decision-making in this dynamic field.

As defined in the American Thyroid Association (ATA) guidelines, a thyroid nodule is a distinct lesion within the thyroid gland that appears radiologically different from the surrounding thyroid tissue. Some palpable lesions may not show corresponding radiologic abnormalities and therefore do not meet the formal definition of thyroid nodules. Nonpalpable nodules identified through ultrasound or other imaging techniques are referred to as incidentally discovered nodules, or "incidentalomas" [1]. Nonpalpable nodules carry the same malignancy risk as palpable nodules of similar size when confirmed via ultrasound [2].

Initial Patient Encounter

Despite technological advancements such as comprehensive molecular testing and radiomics becoming gradually more accessible in many parts of the world, the management of thyroid nodules remains fundamentally grounded in the clinical encounter. There is no substitute for traditional assessment skills, including thorough history-taking, physical examination, and, when feasible, performing an office ultrasound (US).

Table 2.1 entails the recommended baseline history-taking in the first encounter for workup for a thyroid nodule. Asking simple yet focused questions can significantly enhance the accuracy of a patient's workup. For instance, identifying symptoms such as diarrhea may prompt the clinician to include calcitonin and Carcinoembryonic Antigen (CEA) in the diagnostic algorithm, while a prior history of radiation exposure warrants heightened vigilance and meticulous evaluation of the nodule for potential malignancy.

In the age of electronic medical records, it is essential to review key test results and clinical notes, as outlined in Table 2.2. A quick review of the patient's laboratory data not only provides insight into their thyroid function status but can also reveal the need for further evaluation, such as assessing for a concurrent parathyroid adenoma in cases of elevated calcium levels.

Table 2.1 Recommended history-taking in first encounter for workup of a thyroid nodule

1. Patient demographics and medical background:
Patient's age, gender, comorbidities, and medications
Prior thyroid surgery or biopsy history
2. Nodule history:
Mode of nodule discovery (incidental finding on imaging, self-palpation, or clinical exam)
Duration of nodule presence
3. Symptom evaluation:
Symptoms related to voice change/swallowing/breathing
Symptoms aggravated in specific positions (e.g., breathiness or pressure when lying supine)
Local symptoms: Pain, tenderness, or rapid growth (suggesting possible recent hemorrhage or malignancy)
4. Thyroid function/hormone-related symptoms:
Hyperthyroidism: Heat intolerance, palpitations, unexplained weight loss, increased appetite, tremor, or irritability
Hypothyroidism: Cold intolerance, fatigue, dry skin, hair thinning, constipation, unexplained weight gain, or menstrual irregularities
Presence of diarrhea, palpitations, or flushing (specific for conditions like calcitonin-secreting medullary thyroid carcinoma or thyrotoxicosis)
5. Family and social history:
Family history of thyroid cancer, other endocrine neoplasias, or autoimmune thyroid disease
History of childhood, environmental, or therapeutic radiation exposure
Residence/recent immigration from iodine-deficient areas

Table 2.2 Recommended review of patient record upon initial encounter

1. Latest thyroid function tests:
Include TSH, free T4, free T3, and thyroglobulin (if relevant)
2. Imaging records:
All neck and chest imaging (ultrasound, CT, MRI, PET scans)
Review findings such as nodule size, intrathyroidal location, characteristics (solid, cystic, calcifications), and lymphadenopathy
3. Pathology:
Any prior biopsy results [e.g., fine-needle aspiration (FNA)] or cytology reports
4. Endocrine-related tests:
Calcium, PTH levels (if ever done), and calcitonin (if medullary thyroid cancer is suspected)
5. Growth timeline:
Previous nodule measurements to assess growth or changes over time
6. Clinical notes:
Previous clinician assessments and treatment plans related to the thyroid

The physical exam should be a comprehensive head and neck exam, including

1. *Voice evaluation:*
   - A simple subjective voice assessment
2. *Thyroid examination:*
   - Assess size, consistency (soft, firm, hard), mobility, tenderness, and any nodularity of the thyroid
   - Look for thrills or bruits over the gland, which may indicate hyperthyroidism
3. *Neck evaluation:*
   - *Lymph node assessment:* Palpate all cervical lymph node groups systematically (submental, submandibular, jugular, supraclavicular).
   - Dilated superficial veins may indicate venous congestion from thoracic inlet obstruction. Pemberton's sign is a clinical finding seen in patients with large goiters or mediastinal masses causing thoracic inlet obstruction. It is elicited by having the patient raise their arms until they touch the sides of their head for 30 s. A positive sign is marked by facial congestion, jugular vein distention, respiratory distress, or cyanosis, resulting from compression of the thoracic inlet structures.
   - *Substernal assessment:* If extension into the thorax is suspected, try to palpate the inferior border of the thyroid upon neck extension, and check for tracheal deviation.
4. *General habitus, eyes, and skin:*
   - Inspect for exophthalmos, lid retraction, or periorbital edema (hyperthyroidism signs).
   - Look for dry or coarse skin, or a hyperpigmented pretibial rash (Graves' dermopathy).
5. *Vital signs:*
   - Check for tachycardia and bradycardia, which can signal thyroid dysfunction.

In-Office Thyroid Ultrasound Examination

Recent studies emphasize the value of ultrasound in assessing thyroid nodules by nonradiologists, highlighting the unique advantages of dynamic evaluations performed by treating physicians [3, 4]. With their understanding of head and neck anatomy and the patient's differential diagnosis, clinicians can integrate imaging into the physical exam. Slough et al. underscored that routine office-based ultrasonography is a critical extension of history and physical examination, improving diagnostic efficiency and enabling prompt decision-making [3].

In their publication, the authors suggested a focused yet systematic approach that would include US of the central and lateral compartments, focusing on thyroid, concomitant parathyroid pathology, and central and lateral neck node assessment. A hypoechoic thyroid nodule has a greater likelihood of malignancy compared to iso- or hyperechoic nodules. Solid nodules often indicate malignancy, whereas predominantly cystic nodules are usually benign, with entirely cystic nodules considered benign. Irregular or blurred margins suggest malignancy. While the "taller-than-wide" shape is debated, spherical nodules might also carry increased malignancy risk. Intranodular blood flow correlates with malignancy risk, and microcalcifications significantly raise suspicion, often warranting fine-needle aspiration for further evaluation [1].

The use of in-office ultrasound enables clinicians to perform ultrasound-guided FNA when indicated, offering patients the convenience of a single visit that includes the clinical assessment, imaging, and cytologic sampling. When performed by a surgeon, the US also gives the provider a good sense of what to expect in case of potential surgery—nodule location, relation to the trachea, esophagus, and major vessels, suspicion of invasion of nearby structures, particularly the trachea or esophagus—all allow for proper presurgical planning.

Clinicians intending to perform office-based head and neck ultrasonography are advised to pursue formal training through certification or accreditation programs. Various certification options are available, including courses offered by the American College of Surgeons, the American Association of Clinical Endocrinologists (AACE), and the Endocrine Society. In the United States, the primary accreditation pathways include the American Institute of Ultrasound in Medicine (AIUM) in collaboration with the AAO-HNS and the Endocrine Certification in Neck Ultrasound (ECNU). Accreditation may also be required by some insurers for reimbursement of ultrasound services [3].

The primary drawbacks of in-office clinician-performed ultrasonography include its time-consuming nature, subsequently requiring appropriate prescheduling, and the high cost of equipment. Additionally, clinicians must undergo specialized training to develop the required skills. In the United States, providers cannot bill for these services unless they have obtained formal accreditation.

When to Investigate: The Threshold for Thyroid Nodule Assessment

Nodules larger than 1 cm are typically evaluated due to their greater likelihood of clinical significance. Smaller nodules, under 1 cm, may warrant further investigation if associated with symptoms or lymphadenopathy. Rarely, nodules under 1 cm without warning signs can still lead to morbidity or mortality, though such cases are exceedingly uncommon. Diagnosing all small thyroid cancers may do more harm than good, given the unfavorable cost–benefit ratio [5]. The clinical approach should acknowledge the low risk of most thyroid nodules and the minimal threat posed by many thyroid cancers, which are most often fully curable [1].

Structural Assessment

Recommendation 6 of the ATA guidelines strongly recommends that a diagnostic thyroid or neck ultrasound should be performed for all patients with a suspected thyroid nodule, nodular goiter, or when a thyroid nodule is incidentally identified on imaging studies such as CT, MRI, or FDG-PET scans indicating thyroidal uptake [1]. The sonographic features of a nodule, in combination with its size, determine its risk of malignancy and inform the decision to proceed with FNA.

The features with the highest specificities (median >90%) for thyroid cancer include microcalcifications, irregular margins, and a taller than wider shape on transverse view; however, the sensitivities of these individual features are considerably lower [6, 7, 8]. It is important to clarify that poorly defined margins—where the sonographic interface between the nodule and the surrounding thyroid parenchyma is challenging to distinguish—are not the same as irregular margins. Irregular margins mean the demarcation between the nodule and the surrounding thyroid is clearly seen, yet the pattern of this margin is either lobulated, spiculated, or infiltrative [1].

It is noteworthy that follicular thyroid carcinoma (FTC) exhibits distinct ultrasound characteristics compared to papillary thyroid carcinoma (PTC), often appearing more rounded, iso- or hyperechoic, with smooth, regular margins [9]. Similarly, the follicular variant of papillary thyroid carcinoma (FVPTC) is more likely than conventional PTC to share these features with FTC. Distant metastases are rarely seen in follicular cancers smaller than 2 cm in diameter, supporting the rationale for a higher size threshold when evaluating hyperechoic nodules [10].

There are three main validated ultrasonographic classification systems used to stratify malignancy risk and guide the need for fine-needle aspiration (FNA) [1, 11, 12]. The revised American Thyroid Association (ATA) guidelines classify risk into five categories: benign, very low, low, intermediate, and high suspicion. The AACE/ACE/AME system groups nodules into three categories: low, intermediate, and high risk. The most recent system, the American College of Radiology (ACR) TI-RADS, assigns points based on sonographic features, categorizing nodules from benign to highly suspicious and determining biopsy thresholds based on total scores and size. Figure 2.1 depicts the assessment parameters used in the TI-RADS system, their correlating points, and subsequent TI-RADS classification of suspicion of malignancy.

In a study by Pantano et al., the TI-RADS system demonstrated the highest concordance with high-risk cytology findings while also successfully classifying all nodules. In contrast, the other two systems left up to 5% of nodules unclassified [13]. A recent meta-analysis comparing ultrasound classifications with surgical pathology concluded that TI-RADS is a reliable tool, particularly for detecting papillary thyroid carcinoma, which accounts for approximately 95% of thyroid cancers. However, its utility is more limited in diagnosing follicular and medullary thyroid carcinomas [14].

Indications for Cross-Sectional Imaging (CT or MRI) During Thyroid Nodule Workup

- Retrosternal or substernal extension of the thyroid.
- Clinical or sonographic suspicion of regional spread to lymph nodes or adjacent structures.
- Signs or symptoms of airway or esophageal compression, such as dyspnea, stridor, dysphagia, or tracheal deviation.

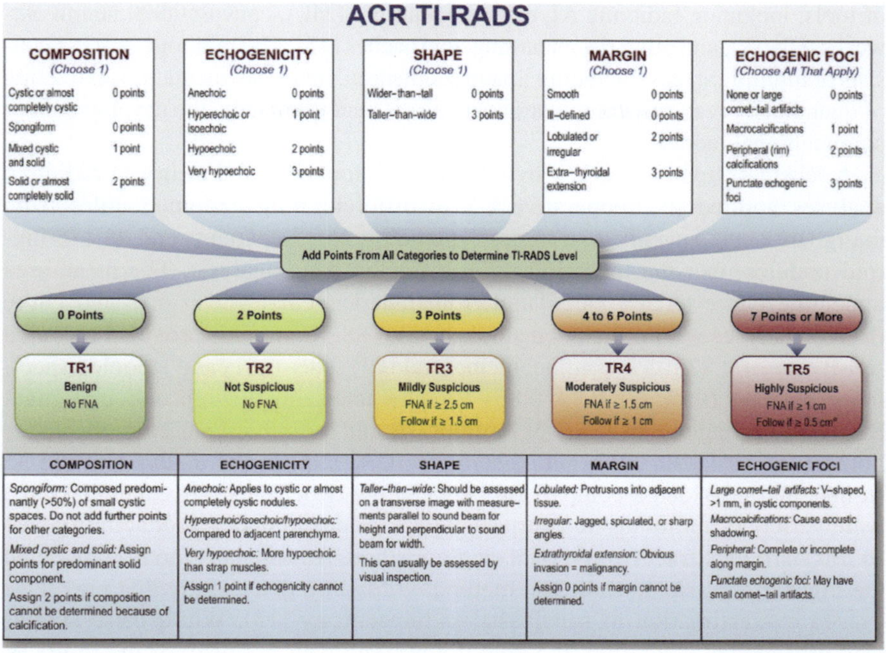

Fig. 2.1 ACR TI-RADS classification. (From Tessler et al. [12])

- Large, bulky, or posteriorly located nodules where ultrasound visualization is limited.
- Suspected invasive disease, including extrathyroidal extension into strap muscles, trachea, esophagus, or suspected RLN involvement.
- Preoperative planning in patients with distorted or complex anatomy, such as prior neck surgery or radiation.
- Lymph node assessment in areas poorly visualized by ultrasound, including retropharyngeal, retrosternal or mediastinal.
- Suspected aggressive thyroid histology, such as anaplastic thyroid carcinoma, particularly with rapidly enlarging masses.

The Role of Radiomics in the Workup of Thyroid Nodules

Radiomics, also known as radiogenomics, is an emerging and rapidly advancing field that leverages artificial intelligence (AI) to extract large volumes of data from medical imaging. This approach provides a quantitative perspective on medical imaging by mathematically analyzing the spatial distribution of signal intensities and the relationships between pixels, thereby quantifying textural information using AI-driven analysis techniques. Current radiomic methodologies encompass a range of tools, including radiomic AI, machine learning (ML), convolutional neural networks (CNNs), and other deep learning approaches [15]. The radiomic process consists of multiple stages, including image acquisition, image segmentation, extraction of quantitative features, computational analysis, and ultimately, the development of computational models.

A recent systematic review by Cleere et al. looked at the utility of radiomic analyses applied to preoperative US in differentiating benign nodules from malignant ones. Seventy-five studies, including 26,373 patients and 46,175 thyroid nodules, met the inclusion criteria for the meta-analysis. The mean area under the curve (AUC) calculated from independent receiver-operated curve (ROC) analyses within included studies was 0.88. Radiomics provided a pooled sensitivity of 0.87 [95% confidence interval (CI) 0.86–0.87] and a pooled specificity of 0.84 (95% CI 0.84–0.85) for characterizing benign and malignant lesions. The diagnostic ability of radiologists and radiomics was comparable for both sensitivity (OR 0.98) and specificity (OR 0.95) in the analysis of the 35 studies that provided a comparison between the two. The study encompassed a wide variety of radiomics techniques, with variance in data reproducibility, and so it is hard to extract from it on a single method. Additionally, authors selected the highest performing radiomic method within any given study that may have caused overestimation of sensitivity and specificity [15]. While these studies lack prospective validation, the field holds significant promise for the future of structural assessment in thyroid nodules.

Functional Assessment

Serum thyrotropin (TSH) should be evaluated during the initial workup of a thyroid nodule. Subnormal TSH is an indication for a radionuclide thyroid scan (^{123}I), as "hot," hyperfunctional nodules are unlikely to be malignant and do not need to undergo FNA [1]. Conversely, elevated serum TSH levels, even within the higher end of the reference range, are linked to an increased risk of malignancy in thyroid nodules and are associated with more advanced stages of thyroid cancer [16]. One study reported significantly increased adjusted odds ratios (AORs) for the diagnosis of malignancy in subjects with serum TSH 1.0–1.7 mU/liter compared with TSH less than 0.4 mU/liter [AOR 2.72, 95% confidence interval (CI) 1.02–7.27, $P = 0.046$], with further increases evident in those with TSH 1.8–5.5 mU/liter (AOR 3.88, 95% CI 1.48–10.19, $P = 0.006$, compared with TSH < 0.4 mU/liter) and greater than 5.5 mU/liter (AOR 11.18, 95% CI 3.23–8.63, $P < 0.001$, compared with TSH < 0.4 mU/liter) [16]. Another study showed that a higher TSH also correlates with a more advanced disease stage in differentiated thyroid cancer (DTC), with the mean TSH found to be 4.9+/−1.5 mIU/liter in patients with stage III/IV disease vs. 2.1+/−0.2 mIU/liter in patients with stage I/II disease ($P = 0.002$) [17]. Figure 2.2 illustrates the ATA algorithm for the workup and management of suspected thyroid nodules with a normal or elevated TSH.

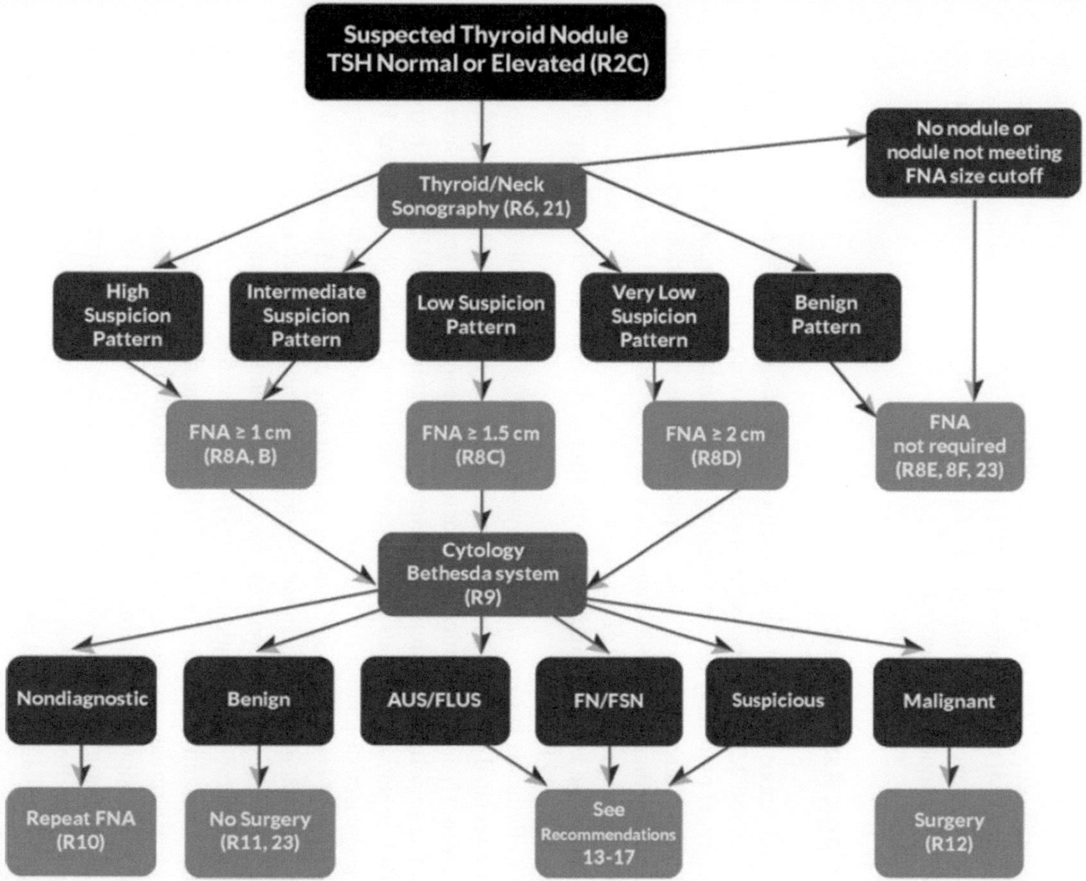

Fig. 2.2 Algorithm for the evaluation and management of patients with thyroid nodules based on US pattern and FNA cytology. *R*, recommendation in ATA guidelines [1]

While serum thyroglobulin levels are not routinely recommended for the workup of thyroid nodules since it is an insensitive and nonspecific test for thyroid cancer, the ATA guidelines do not recommend for or against routine measurement of calcitonin [1]. We believe this is reasonable in cases of a patient presenting with a thyroid nodule and diarrhea or a family history of thyroid cancer of unknown/nonrecorded histology. Serum calcitonin can also be considered for a subset of patients with suspicious cytology inconsistent with papillary thyroid carcinoma (PTC) or patients with indeterminate cytology whose molecular diagnostic (MD) test identified a RET mutation. When unstimulated serum calcitonin levels exceed 50–100 pg/mL, a diagnosis of medullary thyroid carcinoma (MTC) is frequently observed [1].

Cytologic Assessment

The indications for cytologic assessment per sonographic features are shown in Figs. 2.1 and 2.2 and are based on suspicious sonographic features and nodule size. FNA should preferably be performed under US guidance, especially for lesions that are partly cystic or nonpalpable. Palpable lesions with a correlating solid nodule observed on diagnostic sonography may be biopsied without US guidance [1].

The cytologic findings of thyroid nodule FNA should be classified according to the diagnostic categories defined by the Bethesda System for Reporting Thyroid Cytopathology [18, 19].

The Bethesda system classifies thyroid cytology into six diagnostic categories, each associated with an estimated cancer risk based on literature reviews and expert consensus: (i) nondiagnostic/unsatisfactory; (ii) benign; (iii) atypia of undetermined significance/follicular lesion of undetermined significance (AUS/FLUS); (iv) follicular neoplasm/suspicious for follicular neoplasm (FN/SFN), including Hürthle cell neoplasm/suspicious for Hürthle cell neoplasm; (v) suspicious for malignancy (SUSP); and (vi) malignant. Studies utilizing the criteria and terminology of the Bethesda system in large patient cohorts have demonstrated relatively high concordance in FNA cytology reporting. Between 89% and 95% of samples were deemed satisfactory for interpretation, with 55–74% classified as definitively benign and 2–5% as definitively malignant [20, 21]. The remaining samples fell into cytologically indeterminate categories, including atypia of undetermined significance (AUS) /follicular lesion of undetermined significance (FLUS) in 2–18% of nodules, follicular neoplasm (FN) in 2–25%, and SUSP in 1–6%. It is worth mentioning that although the Bethesda system includes estimated malignancy rates for each category, the actual risk varies based on population and institution. The ATA guidelines further recommend that the risk of malignancy should be independently defined at each cytologic canter or institution to guide clinicians [1].

For a nodule with an initial nondiagnostic cytology result, FNA should be repeated under ultrasound guidance, ideally with on-site cytologic evaluation for adequacy if available. The established criteria for cytologic adequacy include the presence of at least six groups of well-visualized follicular cells, with each group comprising a minimum of 10 well-preserved epithelial cells, ideally on a single slide [18, 22]. If repeat FNA is also nondiagnostic, consideration of the nodule's sonographic features weighs more in the decision-making process. Other practices are performing a core biopsy of the nodule and MD testing [23, 24, 25], although the latter is only relevant if sufficient quantity of cytologic material is present.

For an initially benign nodule, repeat FNA is advised when there is significant nodule growth, defined as a volume increase exceeding 50%, a size increase of more than 20%, or an increase of over 2 mm in at least two dimensions for solid nodules or the solid component of mixed cystic-solid nodules [1, 11].

Workup for Indeterminate Cytology: AUS/FLUS FN

Approximately 20–30% of thyroid FNA procedures yield a diagnosis of indeterminate thyroid nodules (ITNs), which fall into the categories of AUS/FLUS (Bethesda III) or FN (Bethesda IV). To accurately assess the current risk of malignancy associated with Bethesda III or IV nodules, it is essential to introduce the concept of noninvasive follicular thyroid neoplasm with papillary-like nuclear features (NIFTP). In 2016, a multidisciplinary team of pathologists, endocrinologists, and other specialists examined the clinical behavior of the encapsulated follicular variant of papillary thyroid carcinoma (EFVPTC) [26]. This group established diagnostic criteria for EFVPTC and demonstrated that, in a cohort of 109 patients with noninvasive EFVPTC, there were no recurrences or disease-related deaths. Based on these favorable outcomes, the term "noninvasive follicular thyroid neoplasm with papillary-like nuclear features" (NIFTP) was introduced, suggestings that this entity should not be classified as cancer due to its indolent nature.

Excluding NIFTP from the pool of thyroid cancers significantly lowers the estimated malignancy risk for ITNs, with rates adjusted to 6–18% for Bethesda III and 10–40% for Bethesda IV, as opposed to traditional estimates [27]. Table 2.3 illustrates the risk of malignancy for each Bethesda category, comparing scenarios where NIFTP is considered benign versus when it is classified as malignant. Understanding that 60–94% of ITNs are benign nodules highlights the importance of continuing a thoughtful and evidence-based evaluation of these cases.

As is the case for any ancillary tests, MD testing for ITN should also be considered in the context of the overall clinical picture and not be done reflexively, especially considering their high cost and weak evidence on improving patient outcomes

Table 2.3 2017 Bethesda system for reporting thyroid cycopathology

Diagnostic category	Risk of malignancy if NIFTP ≠ CA (%)	Risk of malignancy if NIFTP = CA (%)
Nondiagnostic or unsatisfactory	5–10	5–10
Benign	0–3	0–3
Atypia of undetermined significance Or follicular lesion Of undetermined significance	6–18	~10–30
Follicular neoplasm or suspicious For a follicular neoplasm	10–40	25–40
Suspicious for malignancy	45–60	50–75
Malignant	94–96	97–99

Adapted with permission for Ali and Cibas [7], CA= carcinoma

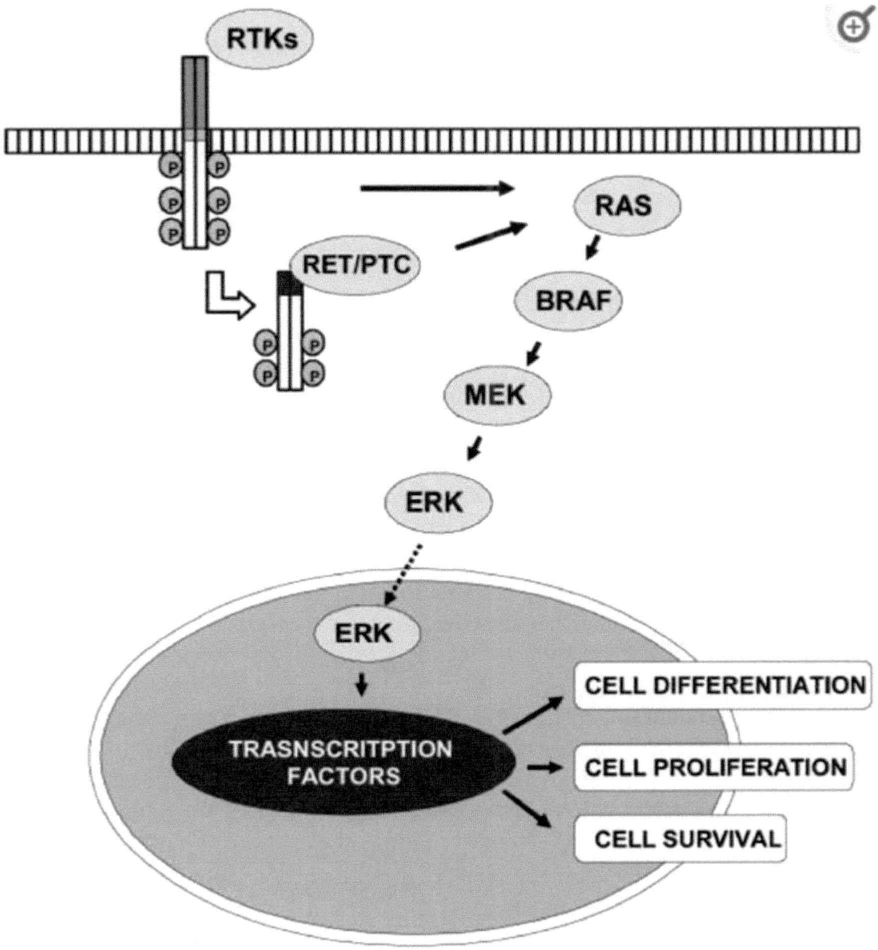

Fig. 2.3 Mitogen-activated protein kinase (MAPK) pathway. (Reproduced from Nikoforov [29])

or reducing the number or extent of thyroidectomies [28]. For instance, MD may offer limited value for a patient with a large nodule causing compressive symptoms and ITN cytology, as surgery would be indicated regardless. Similarly, it would be unnecessary for a patient unwilling to observe a nodule, even if the reported risk of malignancy is minimal.

The basic principle of MD testing is identifying/ruling out mutations associated with thyroid cancer. Gaining a basic understanding of the mitogen-activated protein kinase (MAPK) pathway provides valuable insight into the rationale behind testing for these specific mutations (Fig. 2.3). The MAPK pathway is a gene regulation pathway that controls cell differentiation, multiplication, and death [29]. Activation of this pathway can result from genetic alterations in various genes, some of which are associated with the development of thyroid cancer. Certain genetic markers, such as the BRAF V600E point mutation (valine to glutamate), are highly diagnostic for malignancy and can be particularly valuable in cases where cytopathology results are inconclusive.

Approximately 75% of papillary carcinomas harbor mutations in one of three primary genes involved in the MAPK pathway [29]. The most common mutation occurs in the BRAF oncogene (v-raf murine sarcoma viral oncogene homolog B1), which is implicated in nearly half of all papillary thyroid cancers, yet not seen in follicular thyroid carcinoma. BRAF is perhaps the most useful of the molecular markers assayed and is also associated with a poorer prognosis. The next most common gene mutation seen in papillary thyroid cancer is in the RET/PTC gene. A rearrangement of this gene results in uncontrolled activation of the extracellular signal-regulated kinase (ERK) signaling cascade and is present in approximately 20% of all papillary thyroid cancers. This gene mutation is typically observed in younger patients, is associated with a higher incidence of lymph node metastases, yet carries a more favorable prognosis [29]. The RAS gene is less frequently detected in papillary thyroid carcinomas, comprising only about 10% of cases. In contrast, it is the most commonly identified genetic mutation in follicular thyroid cancer, occurring in approximately 45% of cases [29]. Another notable genetic alteration is the PAX8-PPARγ rearrangement, which is implicated in approximately one-third of follicular carcinomas. This mutation is commonly associated with smaller tumors that exhibit more frequent vascular invasion and typically present in younger patients [29]. The presence of the TERT promoter gene, now included in multigene panels, is associated with aggressive tumor behavior and appears to synergize with BRAF, significantly worsening the prognosis. The combination of BRAF and TERT is often found in more aggressive carcinomas, such as the tall cell variant of papillary carcinoma [30, 31].

The basic technical requirement of MD testing for thyroid nodules is to acquire and preserve enough material during the performance of FNA biopsy, which, in the case of ITN cytology, can be used for the assessment of several genes that aid in defining the risk of an underlying neoplasm. The goal of these tests is to avoid thyroid lobectomy for diagnostic purposes [27]. MD thyroid tests can generally be divided into two primary categories: those aimed at "ruling out" malignancy to enable safe observation of ITN (Affirma), and those intended to "rule in" malignancy by identifying nodules with a high likelihood of harboring cancer, warranting surgical treatment (ThyroSeq v3). Two of the most widely recognized commercial tests are the Afirma Genomic Sequencing Classifier (Afirma GSC) and ThyroSeq v3, which utilizes next-generation sequencing of 112 genes. Each genetic expression report is usually accompanied by an assessment, often presented as a percentage, indicating the likelihood of malignancy. Clinicians should recognize the considerable disparity between company-sponsored reports of these tests' negative predictive value (NPV) and positive predictive value (PPV) and independent clinical research. This discrepancy is largely attributable to the distinction between efficacy (performance under ideal circumstances) and effectiveness (performance in real-world conditions) [32]. In a

Table 2.4 Predictive values of molecular assays for indeterminate thyroid nodules [32]

Assay result	Probability stated on clinical report	Probability observed in real-world data
Molecular assay negative	95% NPV	85–90% NPV
Molecular assay positive	40–90% PPV	20–40% PPV

Abbreviations: *NPV* negative predictive value, *PPV* positive predictive value

recent review of the predictive values of MD assays for ITN, the PPV observed in real-world data was 20–50% lower than the companies' clinical report (Table 2.4) [28]. There are many plausible explanations to these discrepancies in predictive values, including the different pre-test probability among distinct populations, that is, the rates of PTC in a given community [28].

Table 2.4 Comparison of probabilities stated on clinical reports vs observations in real-world data for the Afirma Gene Expression Classifier and ThyroSeq v2 assays.

Although originally designed as a tool to reduce diagnostic lobectomies for ITNs, the reflexive implementation of MD tests failed to show a reduction in the amount or even the extent of thyroidectomies performed. Furthermore, studies have shown the reflexive use of these tests was associated with more *total* thyroidectomies, as surgeons had the intuitive urge to act more aggressively on mutations associated with poorer prognosis, although the evidence for these practices is lacking [33, 34].

As with any diagnostic tool, clinicians are encouraged to thoroughly understand the test's strengths and limitations, applying careful judgment in its use.

The Role of PET CT in the Workup of Indeterminate Cytology

Commercial diagnostic MD panels are not widely available outside the United States, prompting the investigation of [18F]FDG-PET/CT as a tool for distinguishing ITN. [18F]FDG-PET/CT avidity or lack thereof can effectively rule out malignancy in ITN with a 94% sensitivity, and some studies reported its cost-effectiveness in preventing 40% of unnecessary diagnostic surgeries for benign nodules [35, 36]. However, its specificity is only 40%, as many noncancerous ITNs also exhibit increased [18F]FDG uptake [35].

In a European multidisciplinary study by de Koster et al., the study group compared the diagnostic performance of MD tests and [18F]FDG-PET/CT in ITN and assessed the efficacy of their combined use. Of the 132 patients included, MD provided a diagnostic result in 115 cases (87%). The sensitivity, specificity, NPV, PPV, and benign call rate (BCR) for MD were 80%, 69%, 91%, 48%, and 57%, respectively. For [18F]FDG-PET/CT, these metrics were 93%, 41%, 95%, 36%, and 32%, respectively. When combined, a double-negative test (negative MD and negative [18F]FDG-PET/CT) yielded a sensitivity of 95% and specificity of 44%, while a double-positive test had a sensitivity of 68% and specificity of 86%. Concordance between MD and [18F]FDG-PET/CT was observed in 63% of cases (82/130). While both tests appear suitable as rule-out tools, their combined use did not demonstrate significant added benefit. Instead, each test should be selected based on the overall clinical necessity, local diagnostic availability, clinical expertise, and cost-effectiveness considerations.

References

1. Haugen BR, Alexander EK, Bible KC, et al. 2015 American Thyroid Association Management Guidelines for adult patients with thyroid nodules and differentiated thyroid cancer: the American Thyroid Association Guidelines Task Force on Thyroid Nodules and Differentiated Thyroid Cancer. Thyroid. 2016;26(1):1–133. https://doi.org/10.1089/thy.2015.0020.
2. Hagag P, Strauss S, Weiss M. Role of ultrasound-guided fine-needle aspiration biopsy in evaluation of nonpalpable thyroid nodules. Thyroid. 1998;8(11):989–95. https://doi.org/10.1089/thy.1998.8.989.
3. Slough CM, Kamani D, Randolph GW. In-office ultrasonographic evaluation of neck masses/thyroid nodules. Otolaryngol Clin N Am. 2019;52(3):559–75. https://doi.org/10.1016/j.otc.2019.02.012.
4. Hamill C, Ellis P, Johnston PC. Ultrasound for the assessment of thyroid nodules: an overview for non-radiologists. Br J Hosp Med (Lond). 2022;83(7):1–7. https://doi.org/10.12968/hmed.2022.0071.
5. Force USPST, Bibbins-Domingo K, Grossman DC, et al. Screening for thyroid cancer: US Preventive Services Task Force Recommendation Statement. JAMA. 2017;317(18):1882–7. https://doi.org/10.1001/jama.2017.4011.
6. Kwak JY, Han KH, Yoon JH, et al. Thyroid imaging reporting and data system for US features of nodules: a step in establishing better stratification of cancer risk. Radiology. 2011;260(3):892–9. https://doi.org/10.1148/radiol.11110206.
7. Moon WJ, Jung SL, Lee JH, et al. Benign and malignant thyroid nodules: US differentiation—multicenter retrospective study. Radiology. 2008;247(3):762–70. https://doi.org/10.1148/radiol.2473070944.
8. Salmaslioglu A, Erbil Y, Dural C, Issever H, Kapran Y, Ozarmagan S, Tezelman S. Predictive value of sonographic features in preoperative evaluation of malignant thyroid nodules in a multinodular goiter. World J Surg. 2008;32(9):1948–54. https://doi.org/10.1007/s00268-008-9600-2.
9. Jeh SK, Jung SL, Kim BS, Lee YS. Evaluating the degree of conformity of papillary carcinoma and follicular carcinoma to the reported ultrasonographic findings of malignant thyroid tumor. Korean J Radiol. 2007;8(3):192–7. https://doi.org/10.3348/kjr.2007.8.3.192.
10. Machens A, Holzhausen HJ, Dralle H. The prognostic value of primary tumor size in papillary and follicular thyroid carcinoma. Cancer. 2005;103(11):2269–73. https://doi.org/10.1002/cncr.21055.
11. Gharib H, Papini E, Garber JR, et al. American Association of Clinical Endocrinologists, American College of Endocrinology, and Associazione Medici Endocrinologi Medical Guidelines for Clinical Practice for the Diagnosis and Management of Thyroid Nodules—2016 Update. Endocr Pract. 2016;22(5):622–39. https://doi.org/10.4158/EP161208.GL.
12. Tessler FN, Middleton WD, Grant EG, et al. ACR Thyroid Imaging, Reporting and Data System (TI-RADS): White Paper of the ACR TI-RADS Committee. J Am Coll Radiol. 2017;14(5):587–95. https://doi.org/10.1016/j.jacr.2017.01.046.
13. Lauria Pantano A, Maddaloni E, Briganti SI, et al. Differences between ATA, AACE/ACE/AME and ACR TI-RADS ultrasound classifications performance in identifying cytological high-risk thyroid nodules. Eur J Endocrinol. 2018;178(6):595–603. https://doi.org/10.1530/EJE-18-0083.

14. Trimboli P, Castellana M, Piccardo A, Romanelli F, Grani G, Giovanella L, Durante C. The ultrasound risk stratification systems for thyroid nodule have been evaluated against papillary carcinoma. A meta-analysis. Rev Endocr Metab Disord. 2021;22(2):453–60. https://doi.org/10.1007/s11154-020-09592-3.
15. Cleere EF, Davey MG, O'Neill S, et al. Radiomic detection of malignancy within thyroid nodules using ultrasonography-a systematic review and meta-analysis. Diagnostics (Basel). 2022;12(4) https://doi.org/10.3390/diagnostics12040794.
16. Boelaert K, Horacek J, Holder RL, Watkinson JC, Sheppard MC, Franklyn JA. Serum thyrotropin concentration as a novel predictor of malignancy in thyroid nodules investigated by fine-needle aspiration. J Clin Endocrinol Metab. 2006;91(11):4295–301. https://doi.org/10.1210/jc.2006-0527.
17. Haymart MR, Repplinger DJ, Leverson GE, Elson DF, Sippel RS, Jaume JC, Chen H. Higher serum thyroid stimulating hormone level in thyroid nodule patients is associated with greater risks of differentiated thyroid cancer and advanced tumor stage. J Clin Endocrinol Metab. 2008;93(3):809–14. https://doi.org/10.1210/jc.2007-2215.
18. Baloch ZW, LiVolsi VA, Asa SL, et al. Diagnostic terminology and morphologic criteria for cytologic diagnosis of thyroid lesions: a synopsis of the National Cancer Institute Thyroid Fine-Needle Aspiration State of the Science Conference. Diagn Cytopathol. 2008;36(6):425–37. https://doi.org/10.1002/dc.20830.
19. Crippa S, Mazzucchelli L, Cibas ES, Ali SZ. The Bethesda system for reporting thyroid fine-needle aspiration specimens. Am J Clin Pathol. 2010;134(2):343–4; author reply 345. https://doi.org/10.1309/AJCPXM9WIRQ8JZBJ.
20. Theoharis CG, Schofield KM, Hammers L, Udelsman R, Chhieng DC. The Bethesda thyroid fine-needle aspiration classification system: year 1 at an academic institution. Thyroid. 2009;19(11):1215–23. https://doi.org/10.1089/thy.2009.0155.
21. Sughayer MA, Abdullah N. The Bethesda system for reporting thyroid cytopathology: a meta-analysis. Acta Cytol. 2017;61(2):172. https://doi.org/10.1159/000455116.
22. Ali SZ, Baloch ZW, Cochand-Priollet B, Schmitt FC, Vielh P, VanderLaan PA. The 2023 Bethesda system for reporting thyroid cytopathology. Thyroid. 2023;33(9):1039–44. https://doi.org/10.1089/thy.2023.0141.
23. Na DG, Kim JH, Sung JY, Baek JH, Jung KC, Lee H, Yoo H. Core-needle biopsy is more useful than repeat fine-needle aspiration in thyroid nodules read as nondiagnostic or atypia of undetermined significance by the Bethesda system for reporting thyroid cytopathology. Thyroid. 2012;22(5):468–75. https://doi.org/10.1089/thy.2011.0185.
24. Nam SY, Han BK, Ko EY, et al. BRAF V600E mutation analysis of thyroid nodules needle aspirates in relation to their ultrasongraphic classification: a potential guide for selection of samples for molecular analysis. Thyroid. 2010;20(3):273–9. https://doi.org/10.1089/thy.2009.0226.
25. Yip L, Nikiforova MN, Carty SE, et al. Optimizing surgical treatment of papillary thyroid carcinoma associated with BRAF mutation. Surgery. 2009;146(6):1215–23. https://doi.org/10.1016/j.surg.2009.09.011.
26. Nikiforov YE, Seethala RR, Tallini G, et al. Nomenclature revision for encapsulated follicular variant of papillary thyroid carcinoma: a paradigm shift to reduce overtreatment of indolent tumors. JAMA Oncol. 2016;2(8):1023–9. https://doi.org/10.1001/jamaoncol.2016.0386.
27. Richmond BK, Gallimore J. Genetic considerations in the tumorigenesis, diagnosis, and treatment of differentiated thyroid cancer: current state of the science. Am Surg. 2023;89(11):4853–9. https://doi.org/10.1177/00031348231180952.
28. Morris LGT. Molecular profiling of thyroid nodules-are these findings meaningful, or merely measurable?: a review. JAMA Otolaryngol Head Neck Surg. 2020;146(9):845–50. https://doi.org/10.1001/jamaoto.2020.1851.
29. Nikiforov YE. Thyroid carcinoma: molecular pathways and therapeutic targets. Mod Pathol. 2008;21 Suppl 2(Suppl 2):S37–43. https://doi.org/10.1038/modpathol.2008.10.
30. Yip L. Molecular markers for thyroid cancer diagnosis, prognosis, and targeted therapy. J Surg Oncol 2015;111(1):43–50. doi:https://doi.org/10.1002/jso.23768.

31. Yip L, Sosa JA. Molecular-directed treatment of differentiated thyroid cancer: advances in diagnosis and treatment. JAMA Surg. 2016;151(7):663–70. https://doi.org/10.1001/jamasurg.2016.0825.
32. Lee M, Valero C, Morris LGT, Marti JL. Association of Study Methods and Industry Sponsorship with Inconsistent Performance of molecular assays for indeterminate thyroid nodules. JAMA Otolaryngol Head Neck Surg. 2020;147(1):101–3. https://doi.org/10.1001/jamaoto.2020.3252.
33. Valderrabano P, Khazai L, Thompson ZJ, et al. Impact of oncogene panel results on surgical management of cytologically indeterminate thyroid nodules. Head Neck. 2018;40(8):1812–23. https://doi.org/10.1002/hed.25165.
34. Fazeli SR, Zehr B, Amraei R, et al. ThyroSeq v2 testing: impact on Cytologic diagnosis, management, and cost of care in patients with thyroid nodule. Thyroid. 2020;30(10):1528–34. https://doi.org/10.1089/thy.2019.0191.
35. de Koster EJ, de Geus-Oei LF, Brouwers AH, et al. [(18)F]FDG-PET/CT to prevent futile surgery in indeterminate thyroid nodules: a blinded, randomised controlled multicentre trial. Eur J Nucl Med Mol Imaging. 2022;49(6):1970–84. https://doi.org/10.1007/s00259-021-05627-2.
36. de Koster EJ, Vriens D, van Aken MO, et al. FDG-PET/CT in indeterminate thyroid nodules: cost-utility analysis alongside a randomised controlled trial. Eur J Nucl Med Mol Imaging. 2022;49(10):3452–69. https://doi.org/10.1007/s00259-022-05794-w.

Imaging in Thyroid Diseases and Cancer

3

Asif Momin, Shenaz Momin, and Mittali Shah Patani

Editorial

Dr. Momin and his colleagues, Dr. Shenaz and Dr. Mittali Shah have discussed the Imaging of thyroid disease and cancer extensively. They have appropriately discussed the American Thyroid Association (ATA) guidelines. The authors have emphasized the workup, including the ultrasound of the thyroid as a cornerstone modality for diagnosis. They have also emphasized the Thyroid Imaging Reporting and Data System system, as well as the implications of cross-sectional imaging. They have also included elastography, even though it is not very popular in the United States. They have emphasized molecular testing and summarized a patient-centered, evidence-based approach. They have also guided the personalized treatment planning. The chapter also emphasizes on active surveillance. Different types of thyroid cancers are well described in this chapter. The final section of the chapter includes evaluation and management of recurrent thyroid cancer. This is an excellent introduction to thyroid cancer, evaluation, and management.

The new ATA guidelines published in 2025 represent the fourth version of thyroid nodule evaluation and management. This is an excellent document, which

A. Momin (✉)
PSAH Head and Neck Cancer Institute of India and Bhatia Hospital, Mumbai, India

Sir HN Reliance Foundation Hospital, HCG Hospital, Mumbai, India

Prince Aly Khan Hospital, Mumbai, India

S. Momin
Department of Radiology, Nair Hospital, Mumbai, India

M. Shah Patani
Bhatia Hospital Tardeo, Mumbai, India

P. S. Pai et al. (eds.), *Controversies in Cancer of the Thyroid and Parathyroid Glands*, https://doi.org/10.1007/978-3-032-13130-0_3

describes the major paradigm shift in the management of thyroid cancer. The principle behind the treatment of thyroid cancer today is "less is better" or let the punishment fit the crime. We need to adhere to the principle "primum non nocere"—First, do no harm!

Ashok R Shaha

Introduction

Thyroid disorders are common and include many entities. The incidence of thyroid cancer has dramatically increased in the past five decades, with it ranking as the 13th most common cancer worldwide and the sixth most common in women.

The major contributing factor to the rise in incidence is the early diagnosis of small, localized tumors owing to incidentally picked-up lesions. The majority being solid and hypoechoic tend to stand out against the echogenic background of normal thyroid on ultrasound, which is the most common imaging tool. Other advanced and sensitive diagnostic tools like computed tomography (CT) and positron emission tomography (PET) also contribute to numbers.

Primary thyroid carcinomas include papillary, follicular, medullary, and anaplastic carcinomas. Lymphoma and metastasis of other primary malignancies to the thyroid gland represent a minority of thyroid carcinomas.

However, the most common papillary (PTC) tends to behave like a good cancer compared to other more sinister, but fortunately uncommon thyroid cancer makes up the majority. One of the major controversies in thyroid cancers lies in the fact that most early thyroid cancers have an indolent course, with an impressive overall survival rate. Most patients with low-risk differentiated thyroid cancer will do exceptionally well, having disease-specific survival rates of over 97% and recurrence rates of less than 5–10%.

The American Thyroid Association (ATA) guidelines recommend active surveillance (AS) for PMCs (micropapillary cancers); however, there are challenges in convincing the patient to adopt a "wait-and-watch policy" and ensuring follow-up scans at regular intervals by a similar set of experienced radiologists.

Imaging is fundamental in managing thyroid malignancies, including preoperative staging, operative planning, post-treatment surveillance, and evaluation of suspected recurrences. Ultrasound (US) is the primary imaging modality in evaluating palpable thyroid nodules or known thyroid malignancies. Additionally, thyroid abnormalities are often first detected incidentally on computed tomography (CT) or magnetic resonance imaging (MRI), which may be employed to assess unknown neck masses or further characterize thyroid lesions (Table 3.1).

Table 3.1 Thyroid imaging modalities

Modality	Role	Limitations
Duplex US [2]	Most suitable modality for diagnosis with elastography and built in AI application Guided fine needle aspiration cytology (FNAC)/biopsy and ablations	Difficult assessment of exact extent and deep invasion
Radionuclide scan [2]	IF thyroid stimulating hormone (TSH) is low/lower limit of normal in the presence of thyroid nodules Iodine deficiency To search for ectopic thyroid tissue / residual thyroid tissue after surgery To decide upon suitability if radioiodine treatment	Contraindicated in pregnancy Poor resolution Cannot be performed if contrast enhanced computed tomography (CECT) done <3 weeks ago
CECT [3] CEMR	Better staging of extrathyroidal disease (anaplastic carcinoma) Distant metastasis Multiple endocrine neoplasia (MEN) syndrome screening	Morphology of thyroid nodules and smallest lymph node mets cannot be assessed
PET CT [4]	Treatment response assessment Recurrent disease not seen on other imaging MEN syndrome screening	Expensive Not for initial workup

However, there are various challenges and discrepancies in thyroid imaging. This chapter will focus on the difficulties and mimics encountered in the imaging of thyroid malignancies in clinical practice, emphasizing the importance of a thorough and nuanced approach to thyroid imaging.

Referral for Imaging (Indications)

Indications for thyroid imaging according to the American Association of Clinical Endocrinologists (AACE) and Association of Medical Endocrinology (AME) recommendations are

Confirm and characterize a thyroid nodule
Differentiate between benign and malignant
Differentiate from other cervical masses
Evaluate diffuse changes
Detect postoperative residual or recurrent tumor
Screen high-risk patients for thyroid malignancy
Diagnostic (FNA cytology/biopsy) and therapeutic interventional procedures

Available Guidelines for Risk Stratification (RSS) and Their Role in Management

Qualtitiative assesment	Quantitative assesment
SRU	Kwak *et al.* TIRADS
TIRADS	Choi *et al.* Web-based malignancy risk stratification system
F-TIRADS	ACR-TIRADS
BTA guidelines	TMC-RSS
ATA guidelines	
K-TIRADS	

SRU: Society of radiologists in ultrasound, TIRADS: Thyroid imaging reporting and data system, F-TIRADS: French TIRADS, BTA: British Thyroid Association, ATA: American Thyroid Association, K-TIRADS: Korean TIRADS, ACR: American College of Radiology, TMC-RSS: Thyroid Multimodal-imaging Comprehensive Risk Stratification Scoring

* Used with kind permission from' The Journey of Ultrasound-based Thyroid Nodule Risk Stratification Scoring Systems: Do All Roads Lead to Thyroid Imaging, Reporting and Data System (TIRADS)? Journal of Head & Neck Physicians and Surgeons; Mahajan, Abhishek; Vaidya, Tanvi; Vaish, Richa1; Sable, Nilesh. 5(2): p 57–65, Jul–Dec 2017. | DOI: 10.4103/jhnps.jhnps_40_17 [1] (1) K-TIRADS, ACR-TIRADS, and EU-TIRADS all performed well in differentiating thyroid nodules, among which K-TIRADS and ACR-TIRADS showed a better diagnostic efficiency in differentiating nodules >10 mm, but they cannot simultaneously achieve high sensitivity and specificity. (2) Multiple RSS aims at reducing the number of unnecessary interventions and providing high NPV diagnosis of clinically significant thyroid carcinoma; however, establishing a universally applicable risk stratification system will benefit the clinicians and patients.

TIRADS vs. ATA

- Among the multiple Thyroid Imaging Reporting and Data System (TIRADS) and ATA guidelines available, the 2017 TIRADS has the highest diagnostic performance, followed by the 2018 ATA guidelines.
- The American College of Radiology (ACR TIRADS) has a higher biopsy yield of malignancy due to a small number of biopsies of benign nodules. However, the confusion of multiple RSS and the cost–benefit ratio is a variable factor across the globe. ATA is pattern-based recognition, so it is easier but may not be able to classify all the nodules, while TIRADS is more comprehensive. TIRADS, however, encourages follow-up scans.

ATA guidelines, when followed, have the following goals:

1. For decision-making
2. Minimize harm from overtreatment (in low-risk patients)
3. Treat and monitor patients at higher risk

However, the purpose of these guidelines is to supplement clinical decision-making, not to replace it.

Preoperative Staging and Diagnostic Imaging and Laboratory Tests [5]

Recommendation number	ATA guidance
32 A	Preoperative neck ultrasound for cervical(central and lateral) lymph nodes is recommended for all patients undergoing thyroidectomy for malignancy cytologic or molecular findings(strong evidence, moderate quality evidence)
32B	Ultrasound guided fine needle aspiration or sonographically suspicious nodes ≥8-10mm in the smallest diameter should be performed to confirm malignancy if this would change management(strong recommendation, moderate quality evidence)
32C	The addition of fine needle aspiration thyroglobulin in washout in the evaluation of suspicious cervical lymph nodes is appropriate in selected patients , but interpretation maybe difficult in patients with an intact thyroid gland(weak recommendation, low quality evidence)
33A	Preoperative use of cross sectional imaging studies (CT,MRI) with intravenous contrast is recommended as adjunct to ultrasound for patients with clinical suspicion for advanced disease, including invasive primary tumor , or clinically apparent multiple or bulky lymph node involvement(strong recommendation, low quality evidence)
33B	Routine preoperative 18 FDG-PET scanning is not recommended(strong recommendation, moderate quality evidence)

Ultrasound of Thyroid Nodule

The objectives are

- Differentiate benign from malignant
- Identify the most abnormal nodule
- Obtain tissue diagnosis with guided procedures
- Staging

The following points are given due consideration during thyroid ultrasound:

- Nodule evaluation using ACR TIRADS or ATA guidelines
- Background thyroid parenchymal changes
- Choosing two most suspicious nodules for FNAC if more than three nodules qualify
- If serum TSH is low and iodine scan is available, FNAC should be done from the hypo functioning nodule if suspicious on ultrasound

US features of benign and malignant nodules applicable in all RSS are as shown in Table 3.2.

Table 3.2 US features of benign and malignant nodules

Benign thyroid nodule	Malignant thyroid nodule
Comet tail artifact in cystic thyroid nodule	Marked hypoechogenicity
Cystic, total, or near total	Solid/complex
Calcifications—Rim or large coarse	Irregular margins
Complete halo s/o complete well-defined wall	Taller than wider
Echogenic or isoechoic to normal tissue	Microcalcifications
Avascular or hypovascular with a surrounding ring of vessels	Abnormal vascularity

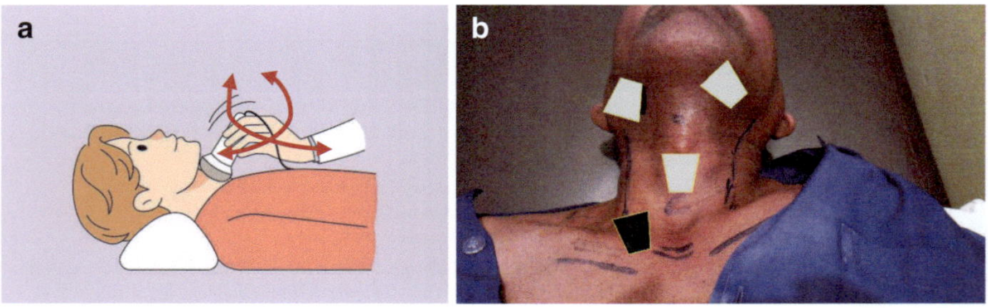

Fig. 3.1 (**a**) Optimal patient position for thyroid ultrasound (with extended neck). Arrows indicating direction of sweep of the probe (**b**) Detailed nodal evaluation and probe positions for central and lateral compartments

Technique of ultrasonography (USG)

US of the neck is generally done in a supine hyperextended position with a linear high-frequency transducer using thyroid preset (Fig. 3.1a, b). Sometimes, additionally a small footprint probe is used for checking retrosternal extension. Wideview imaging can assist in capturing the entire thyroid image in the axial plane (Fig. 3.2a, b), and it also aids in the early identification of needle entry during FNACs performed using the "in-plane" technique. The other "out-of-plane technique" can be used for FNAC and aspiration of larger cystic nodules. Longitudinal and multiple recurrent views are essential to complete coverage.

Panoramic views when used can help to capture the entire thyroid gland. If available, various tools such as microvascular flow and elastography (Fig. 3.3a–d), *along* with an AI-based TIRADS calculator, aid in the systematic US evaluation of thyroid nodules and produce a structured report

US is noninvasive, has good patient tolerance, and has superior near-field resolution compared with MRI or CT. On the other hand, US can have difficulty in depicting deeper structures, and the images may be difficult to comprehend compared to cross-sectional imaging to a referring clinician.

Evaluation of neck nodes should be done for the central compartment, from the submental region to the sternal notch, with additional inferiorly angled views to evaluate the upper mediastinal nodes (Fig. 3.4a, b).

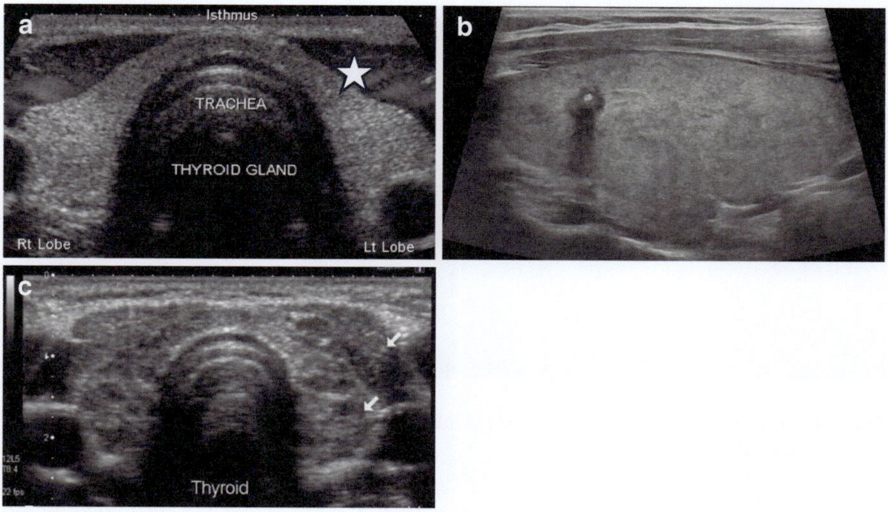

Fig. 3.2 (**a**) Ultrasound representation of axial section of normal thyroid with visceral relations. Note: echogenicity of normal thyroid parenchyma is brighter compared to the strap muscles (*), (**b**) Longitudinal section, wideview of thyroid lobe with smooth convex outlines. Note: most abnormal lesions tend to stand out being darker compared to adjacent normal thyroid, (**c**) Diffuse thyroiditis. Note: reduced thyroid echogenicity, like strap muscles (⟹:thyroid, *: strap muscles)

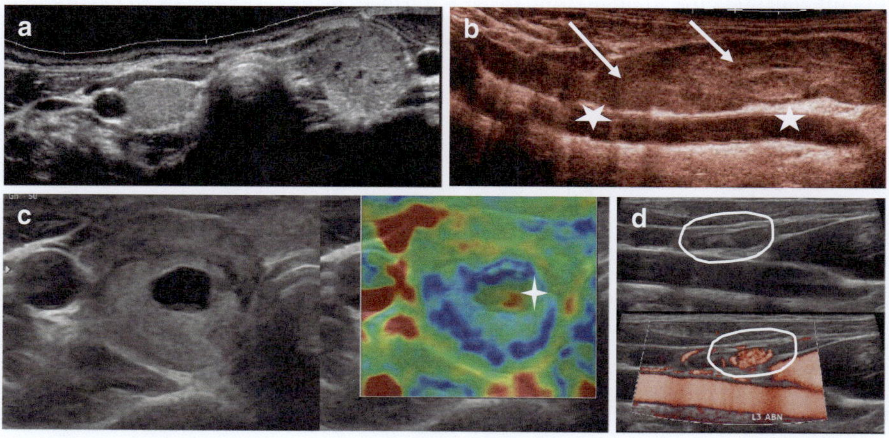

Fig. 3.3 (**a**) Panoramic view in axial plane, to demonstrate entire thyroid with spongiform nodule in the left lobe and both carotid sheaths. (**b**) Extended view in longitudinal plane, along the carotid sheath depicting tumor thrombus in internal jugular vein (IJV) (arrow) and normal carotid artery (*). (**c**) Strain elastography of right thyroid nodule, showing hard (blue) peripheral area, and cystic (red) central zone (*). (**d**) Comparative image of proven PTC nodal metastasis in left level III node (encircled) depicting abnormal microvascular flow (bottom image) in an otherwise flatter lymph node seen with difficulty on B mode (top image)

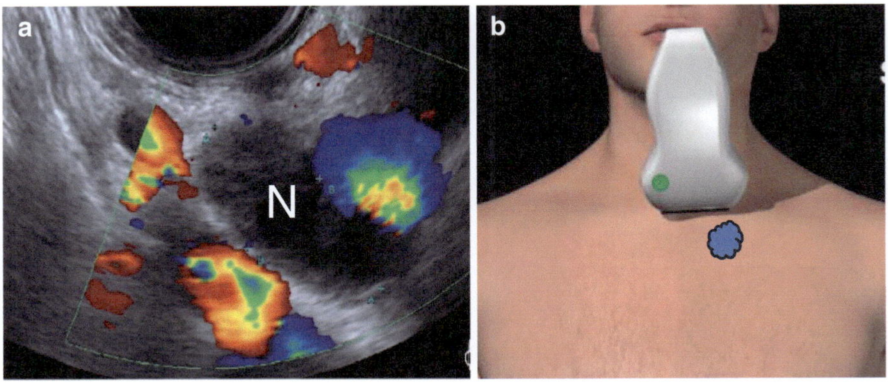

Fig. 3.4 (**a**, **b**) Ultrasound image of abnormal infraclavicular lymph node (N), level VII, by using angled/small footprint probe

The lateral compartment is separately evaluated from levels 2–4, followed by the entire posterior triangle. Additional views behind the proximal carotid sheaths are rewarding for picking up small, deep-seated metastatic nodes (Fig. 3.2d).

Special attention should be given to checking retrothyroidal areas if a lesion extends close to the trachea or near the expected position of the recurrent laryngeal nerve.

Routine scanning of the midline area around the hyoid is done to look for incidental thyroglossal duct cyst (TGDC) or prominent pyramidal lobe (Fig. 3.5b–e). Finally, evaluate the jugular veins for any intrinsic lesion. Tubercle of Zuckerkandl can mimic as a thyroid nodule (Fig. 3.5a).

TIRADS Challenges

These are related to some of the assumptions in ACR-TIRADS categories.

Composition

If the rim calcification obscures the nodule completely, composition is to be assigned as solid, and echogenicity is to be assumed isoechoic (Fig. 3.6a).

1. Overlooking a peripheral hypoechoic solid-looking abnormal area within the large isoechoic nodule, as FNAC from this specific area can change the diagnosis (Fig. 3.7).
2. Similarly, solid abnormal components can get obscured in a predominantly cystic nodule.
3. In the absence of prior aspiration or ablative treatment of a cystic nodule, it can make it look suspicious at the time of follow-up (mummified nodule) (Fig. 3.8a, b).

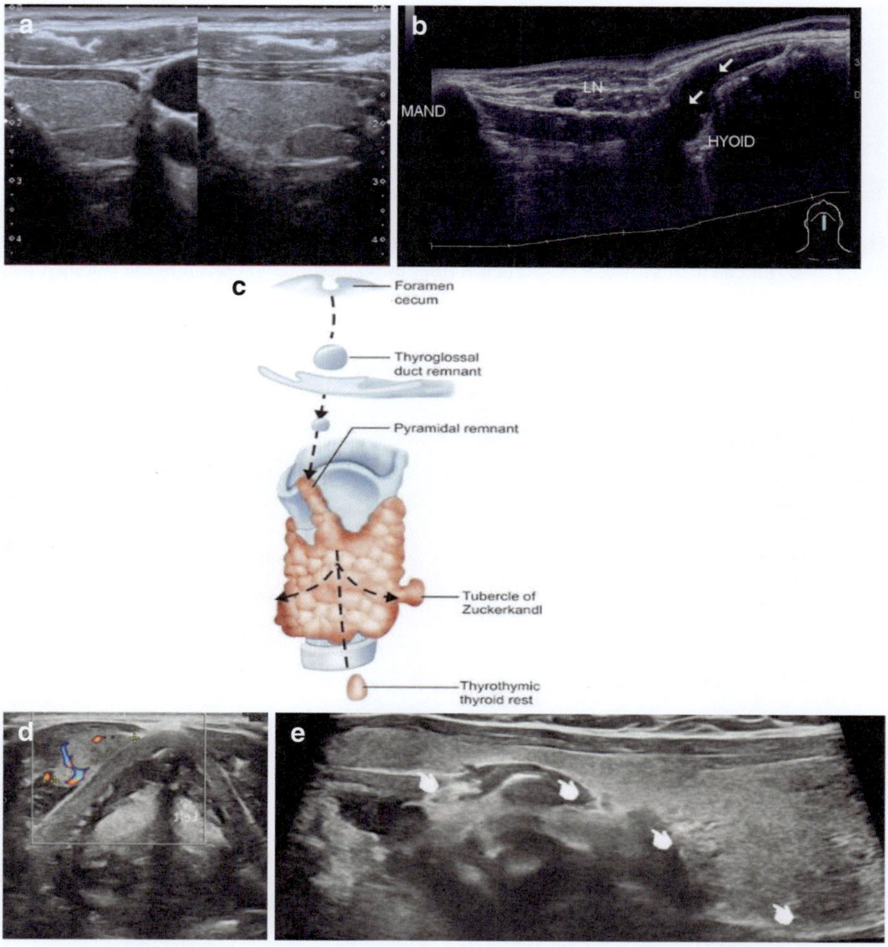

Fig. 3.5 (**a**) Transverse and longitudinal scan of the left lobe of normal thyroid, showing tubercle of Zuckerkandl, which can mimic a thyroid nodule (*), (**b**) Incidental thyroglossal duct cyst seen at the level of hyoid in midline extended field of view, (**c**) Anatomical depiction of thyroid and its embryology, (**d, e**) Transverse (d) and longitudinal views (e) at the level of thyroid cartilage demonstrating pyramidal lobe extending upward from the thyroid, anterior to the right thyroid cartilage with internal vascularity (finger pointers)

Shape

Using both longitudinal and transverse sections helps in characterizing the shape of the nodule more precisely rather than judging it only in a single-axial section. An AI-based TIRADS calculator based on single-section analysis can misinterpret this information (Fig. 3.9a, b).

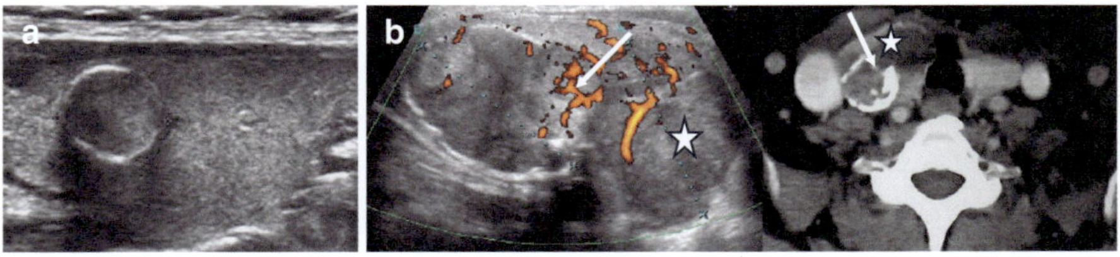

Fig. 3.6 (**a**) Rim calcified thyroid nodule obscuring the internal details, (**b**) Ultrasound and CT image of a rim calcified proven PTC needed further evaluation due to breach in the calcified rim (arrow) and solid component (asterix)

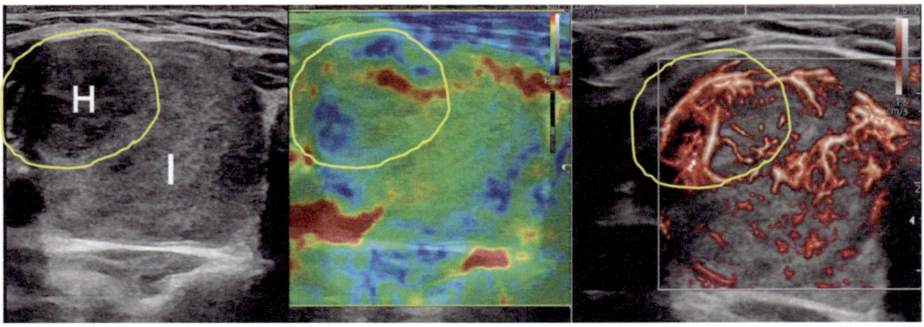

Fig. 3.7 B-mode, elastography, and microvascular flow imaging, FNAC from peripheral area (I) was negative, while from hypoechoic solid area (H) was positive for PTC

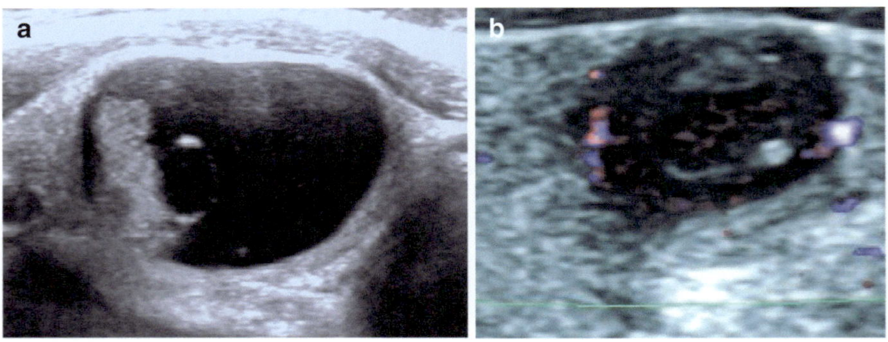

Fig. 3.8 (**a**) Pre-aspiration, cystic nodule (TIRADS 1), (**b**) Post-aspiration-mummified, solid nodule (TIRADS 4)

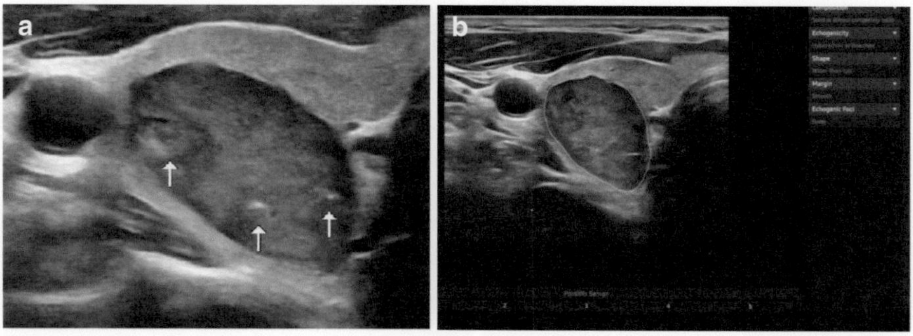

Fig. 3.9 (**a**) Oblique view showing abnormal punctate calcification—suspicious finding, (**b**) Axial view of the same nodule not showing calcification when subjected to AI calculator downgrading to TIRADS 3

Punctate Calcification

Identifying true punctate echogenic foci (PEF) is an important diagnostic clue. Comet tail artifacts (Fig. 3.10d) are considered as a benign finding; however, they can coexist with punctate echogenic foci.

True punctate echogenic foci (<1 mm, without comet tail artifact) are psammoma bodies with high specificity and sensitivity of 85–95% in PTC; hence, it is an important diagnostic marker (Fig. 3.10a, b).

On the other hand, true comet-shaped artifacts in solid suspicious lesions may not be a sign of benign nature (Fig. 3.10e).

Diffuse spread of echogenic foci in the entire thyroid gland (Fig. 3.11a) without a typical solid hypoechoic lesion can be occasionally seen in PTC (Fig. 3.11a), even with extensive nodal metastasis showing similar punctate echogenic foci (Fig. 3.11b).

Other TIRAD problem areas and possible solutions are given in Table 3.3 [6] (Fig. 3.12).

Does the Size Matter

With the increasing use of ATA guidelines and ACR TIRADS calculators, active surveillance has gained significant evidence-based support, which has justification because PTC less than 1 cm are seen in up to 10% of surgical specimens and up to 30% of autopsies; however, malignant lesions of less than 1 cm can show the evidence of extensive nodal metastasis and invasion. The bottom line is all cancers at one time in their life where small nodules; hence, clinical decision-making will depend on institutional and patient-related factors.

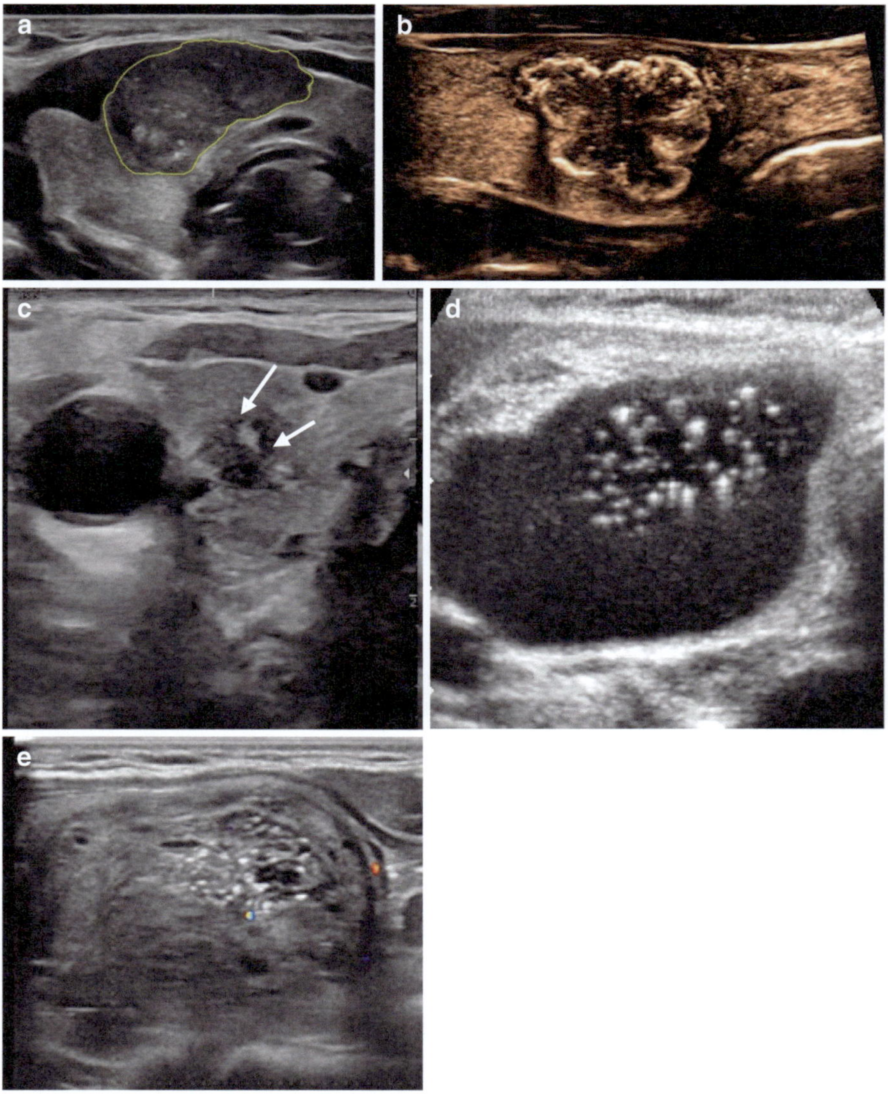

Fig. 3.10 (**a**, **b**) Punctate echogenic foci in proven PTC, subtle (**a**), and extensive (**b**), (**c**) Pseudo-echogenic foci (arrows) in a benign nodule with colloidal degeneration, (**d**) True comet tail artifact in a benign cystic nodule (bright echogenic speck with a tapering tail of echoes), (**e**) Proven follicular variant of PTC, with comet tail artifact in a solid nodule

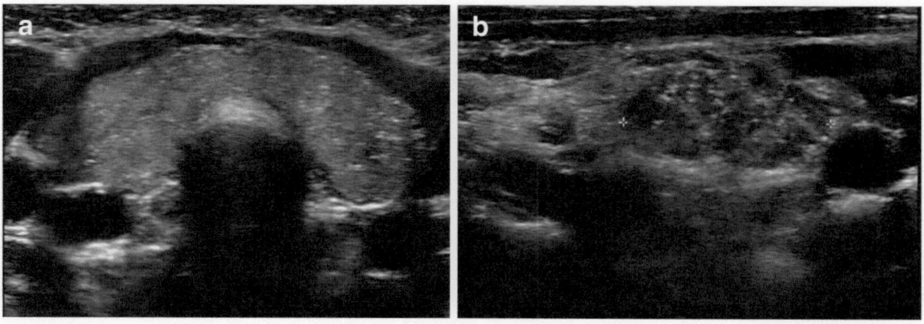

Fig. 3.11 (**a**) Normal-looking thyroid gland, (**b**) Abnormal right supraclavicular node with extensive echogenic foci in the same patient

Table 3.3 TIRAD problems and solutions

Problem	Solution
Consistently characterize spongiform nodules	Nodule with at least >50%cystic spaces declared as true spongiform nodule (TIRADS-1)
lack of uniform global model for radiologists and clinicians alike	Merging multiple guidelines with more diagnostic parameters
Identifying the index nodule amongst multiple nodules of similar morphology	Largest nodule is index nodule
Punctate foci vs calcification in wall vs comet tail artifact	Solid nodules with comet tail artefact should be scrutinized on other parameters.

Papillary microcarcinoma (PMC) is defined as a type of PTC less than 1 cm in greatest dimension. Recent guidelines have updated the approach as follows:

- Fine-needle aspiration biopsy (FNAB) is no longer recommended for nodules smaller than 5 mm.
- FNAB is not advised for nodules between 5 and 10 mm unless they are:
  - Classified as TIRADS 4b or 5
  - In subcapsular or superolateral locations (Fig. 3.13b)
  - With elevated calcitonin levels
  - Found in patients under 40 years of age with evidence of multifocality or associated lymphadenopathy (Fig. 3.13a)
  - Show pathological FDG uptake and show abnormal grades on elastography

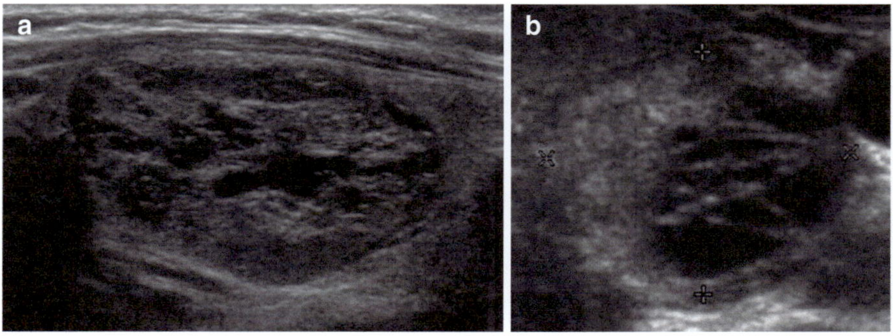

Fig. 3.12 (**a**) Typical spongiform nodule., (**b**) Spongiform component less than 50%

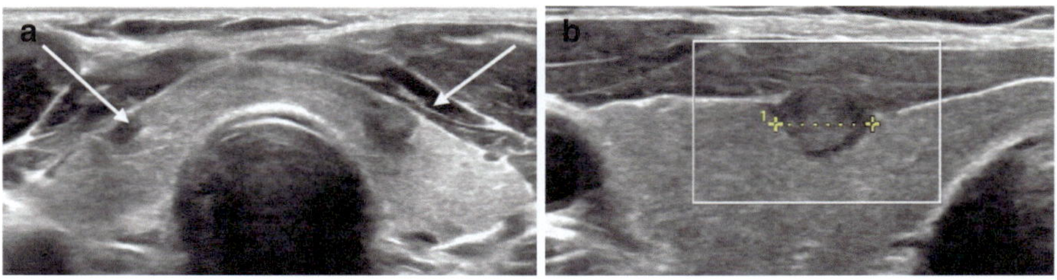

Fig. 3.13 (**a**) Proven bilateral FV-PTC, 3 mm sized on the right and 7 mm on the left (arrows), (**b**) Subcapsular nodule with focal breach in the thyroid capsule

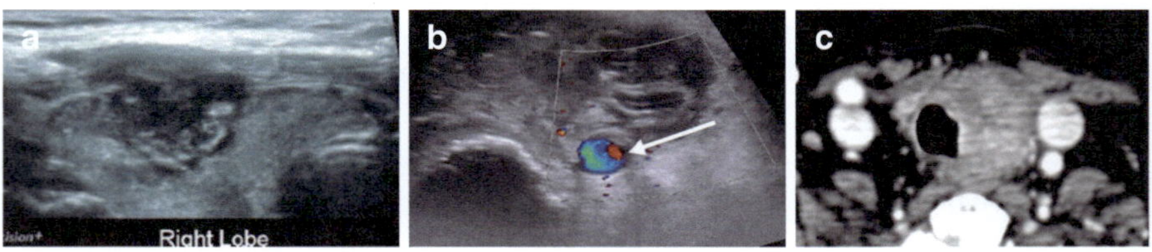

Fig. 3.14 (**a**) Capsular breach with adherence to strap muscles anteriorly, (**b**) Extrathyroidal extension with encasement of left carotid artery (⟹), (**c**) Transverse CT section showing extrathyroidal extension with tracheal invasion extending posteriorly increasing possibility for RLN involvement

Extrathyroidal Extension (ETE)

Assessment of ETE is important for the accurate staging of thyroid cancer and preoperative decision-making. US is beneficial for diagnosing ETE in relation to the strap muscle/ trachea and the location of RLN for posteriorly located lesions (Fig. 3.14a–c). Some of the hypothesized predictors of ETE are tumor diameter, lesion site, LN metastasis extent, and thyroglobulin concentration.

Both poorly differentiated thyroid carcinoma and anaplastic thyroid carcinomas are aggressive lesions that are commonly present with ETE, which necessitates cross-sectional imaging. In general, on US, poorly differentiated thyroid carcinoma can show a significantly higher incidence of a circumscribed margin and an oval-to-round shape than anaplastic thyroid carcinoma with gross ETE.

Venous Spread and Tumor Thrombus

Thyroid malignancies, especially follicular lesions and rarely PTC/MTC, are known to cause tumor thrombus through draining thyroid vein to the IJV (Fig. 3.15a). This hematogenous spread could lead to distant bony, pulmonary, and rarely metastatic spread to other organs. Diagnosis of thyroid cancer and jugular thrombus sometimes is detected during the workup of a bony lytic expansile lesion (Fig. 3.15b).

Tumor spread through any of these draining thyroidal veins can mimic enlarged metastatic nodes. However, intravenous spread is not considered extrathyroidal extension, but it should be documented for appropriate management like venous extirpation (Fig. 3.15c).

Occult Primary, Primary Thyroid Malignancy in TGDC, or Pyramidal Lobe

Significant PTC LN metastasis without an identifiable primary tumor even after extensive histological thyroid sampling is a rare but known phenomenon (burntout primary). However, 2/3 rd of these metastases were BRAF positive, as seen in one series. However, this should alert the radiologist to look for primary DTC in remote areas like the pyramidal lobe or thyroglossal duct cyst harboring an internal abnormal solid portion with typical punctate calcification (Fig. 3.16).

Thyroglossal duct (TGD)-associated malignancy is rare (about 1%), with most cases being papillary thyroid carcinoma. Metastasis to the regional lymph nodes has been reported in 7.7–12.9% of TGD-associated PTCs, much less frequently than primary papillary carcinomas of the thyroid gland (Fig. 3.17a, b). According to the literature, 88% of TGD-associated malignancies are PTC, 6% are squamous cell carcinoma, and the rest include Hürthle cell, follicular, and anaplastic carcinomas [4, 8–10]. Medullary thyroid carcinoma has not been reported in TGDCs.

Lymph Node Mapping

Lymph node mapping with ultrasound before surgical planning is an evidence-based, effective tool for staging to plan the exact method of elective lymph node dissection both during initial and postoperative treatment of recurrent cancers. Ultrasound is the recommended imaging modality in preoperative screening, as ATA management guidelines (2015) do not advocate neck dissection without evidence of metastasis (Fig. 3.18). Routine computed tomography is not recommended. The majority of the most common DTCs have lymph node metastasis with an

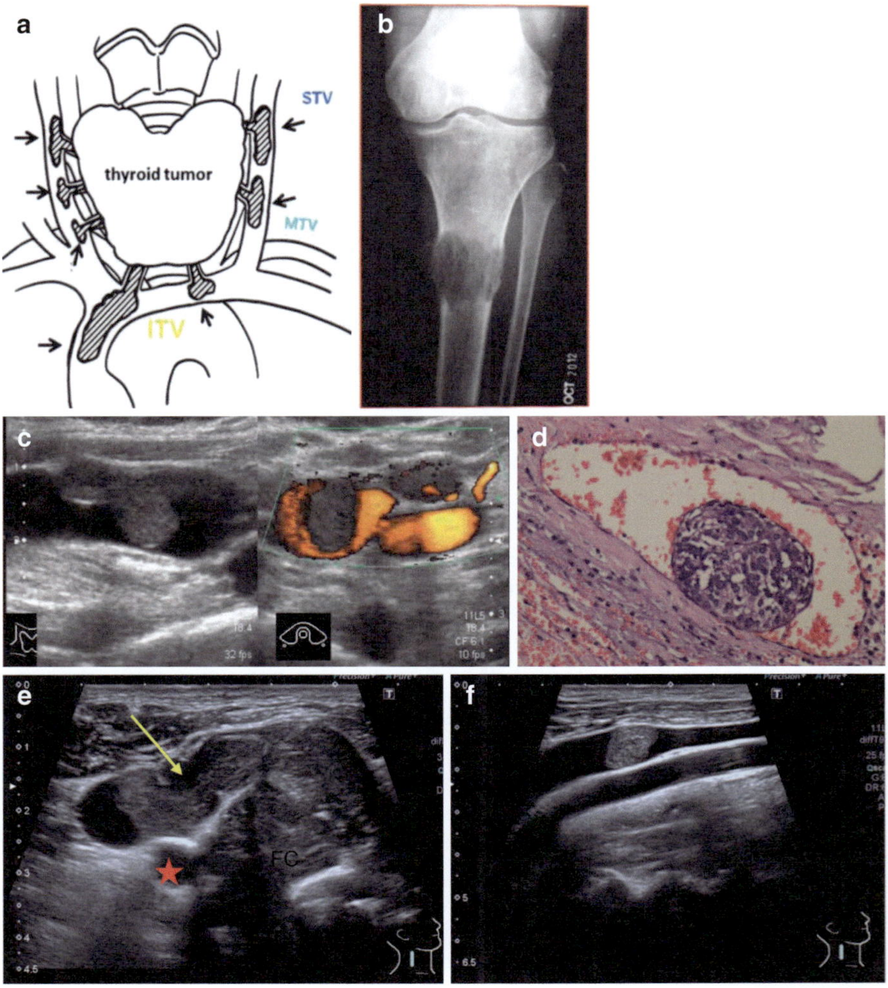

Fig. 3.15 (**a**) Schematic picture depicting thyroid cancer causing tumor thrombosis extending to the jugular vein and superior vena cava through thyroidal veins, (**b**) Lytic lesion in left proximal tibia proven to be metastatic lesion due to primary thyroid cancer, (**c**) Tumor thrombosis in right middle thyroidal vein and IJV, (**d**) Histopathological section of right IJV showing tumor thrombus of follicular cancer, (**e**) FC-follicular cancer. *Common carotid artery, ⟹ thrombus in the IJV, (**f**) Well-defined echogenic filling defect suggesting thrombus in the internal jugular vein. (*Image courtesy—Prof Dr. Roshan Chinoy, MD, Head of Pathology, Prince Aly Khan hospital, Mumbai)

increased risk of recurrence, leading to up to 20% cases requiring additional treatment. Up to 40% of small PTCs and 75% of large PTCs are known to have nodal metastasis, though as discussed earlier both the burntout tumors and the smallest of the PTCs can present extensive metastasis. Medullary cancer (MTC) LN metastasis can look like PTC but tend to be larger, solid, with absent hilum and fewer PEF; however, high serum calcitonin levels will be the deciding factor [7].

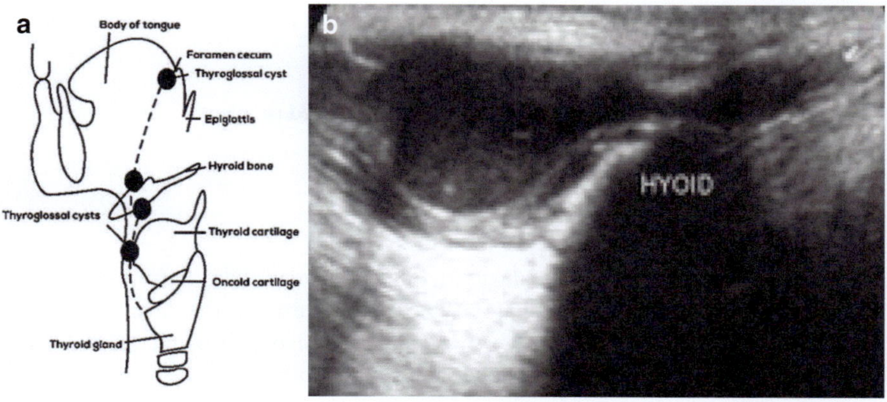

Fig. 3.16 (**a**) Anatomical line diagram showing various locations for thyroglossal duct cyst, (**b**) Incidental benign thyroglossal duct cyst without any solid component

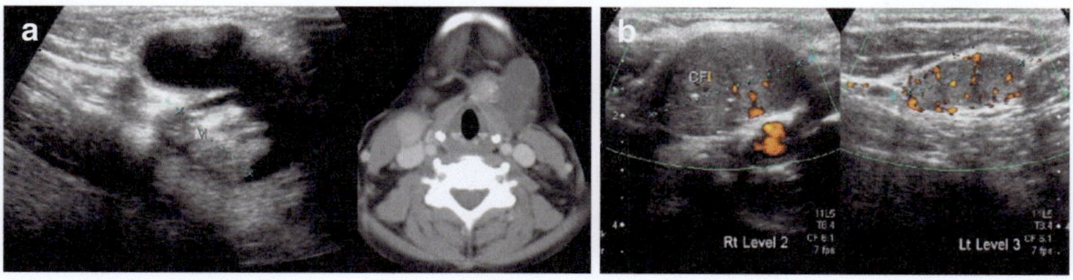

Fig. 3.17 (**a**, **b**) Ultrasound and CECT of thyroglossal duct cyst harboring solid calcified nodule, proven PTC with bilateral level II and III nodal metastasis

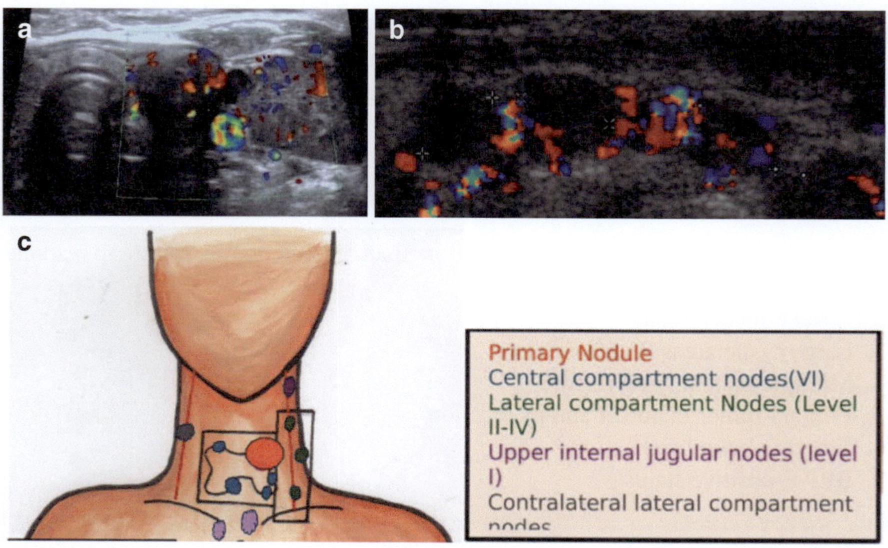

Fig. 3.18 (**a**) Axial view of post-total thyroidectomy thyroid bed showing abnormal level VI nodes, (**b**) Proven PTC metastatic lymph nodes, (**c**) Schematic diagram showing routes of spread of thyroid cancer in ipsilateral and contralateral cervical and mediastinal lymph nodes

Table 3.4 Ultrasound features of nodes

Ultrasound feature of nodes	Incidence
Microcalcifications	5–69%
Cystic change	10–34%
Abnormal or increased/peripheral vascularity	40–86%
Hyperechogenicity	30–87%
Round shape	37%

Thyroid cancer follows a typical pattern of nodal spread, starting from the central compartment (level 6) to the ipsilateral lateral compartment (by levels 2–5), followed by the contralateral side; level 1A and 1B involvement is uncommon. Skip metastasis to the lateral compartment without central compartment disease is known in up to 20% of cases, especially when the tumor is in the upper poles or TGDC. Lateral compartment nodes are easier to identify than central ones, probably due to less ultrasound-friendly structures crowded in the midline region. CECT with early arterial phase tends to be superior (Table 3.4).

Levels of Lymph Nodes (Fig. 3.19)

7th Edition AJCC TNM Staging nodal status is simply N0, N1A (ipsilateral) N1B (bilateral, midline or contralateral nodes).

Varying Features of PTC and MTC Lymph Nodal Metastasis (Figs. 3.20a, 3.20b, 3.20c, 3.20d, 3.20e, and 3.20f)

Extranodal extension (ENE) is a less commonly discussed parameter in thyroid cancers compared to SCC. Although ENE is not recognized in American Joint Committee on Cancer (AGCC) UICC TNM staging system (UICC) staging, it has direct correlation with recurrence in thyroid bed. Extracapsular extension is invasion of tumor cells beyond the nodal capsule in the surrounding tissue.

Factors associated with ENE are:

1. Nodal burden—number and extent (more than 5 could predict failure to respond to complete treatment)
2. Level 6 involvement
3. Large cystic areas (Fig. 3.20b)
4. Multiple matted lymph nodes
5. Primary tumor diameter and its location
6. Thyroglobulin levels
7. BRAF-positive status

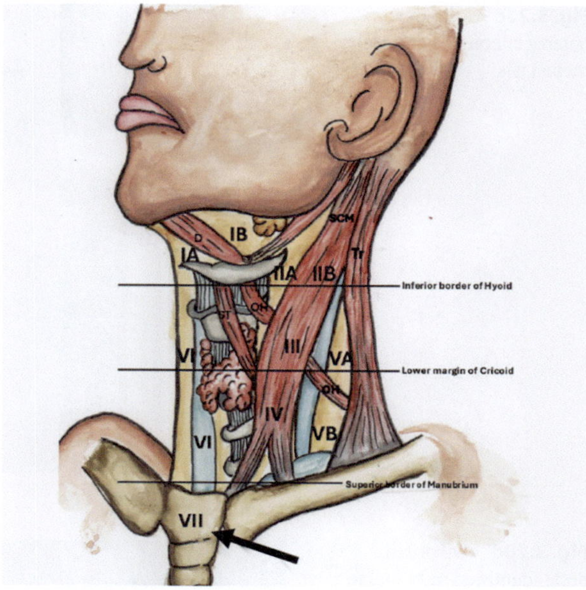

Fig. 3.19 Diagrammatic representation of normal cervical lymph nodal groups

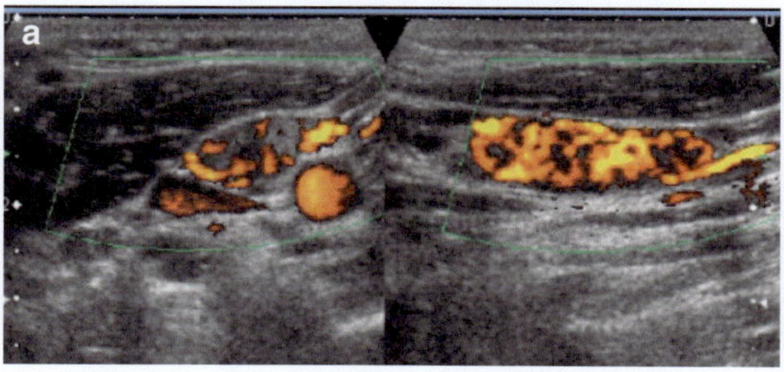

Fig. 3.20a Longitudinal and transverse views of oval elongated proven PTC lymph node metastasis with disorganized abnormal vascularity on power doppler

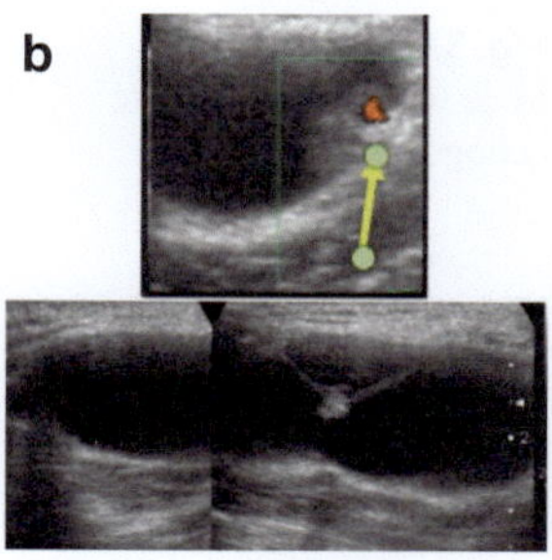

Fig. 3.20b Composite image of cystic right-V a node, earlier mistaken as lymphangioma. However, repeat FNAC from peripheral nodule with vascularity (⟹) proved PTC lymph node metastasis

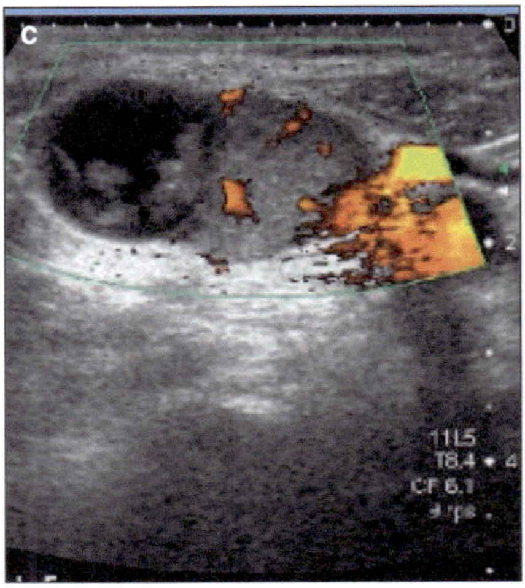

Fig. 3.20c Solid cystic heterogeneous PTC nodal metastasis

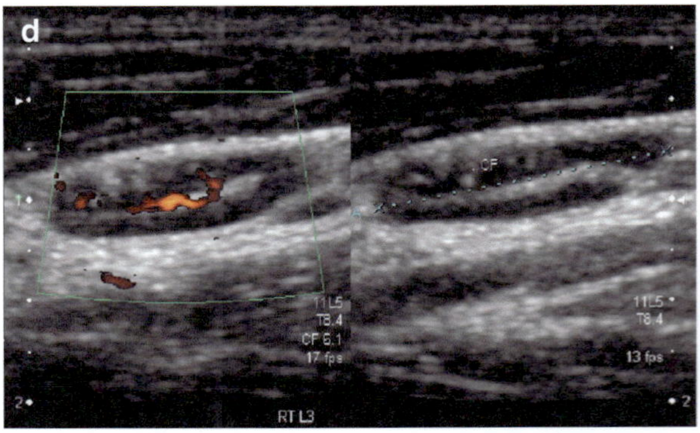

Fig. 3.20d Abnormal node identified only due to the presence of punctate echogenic foci

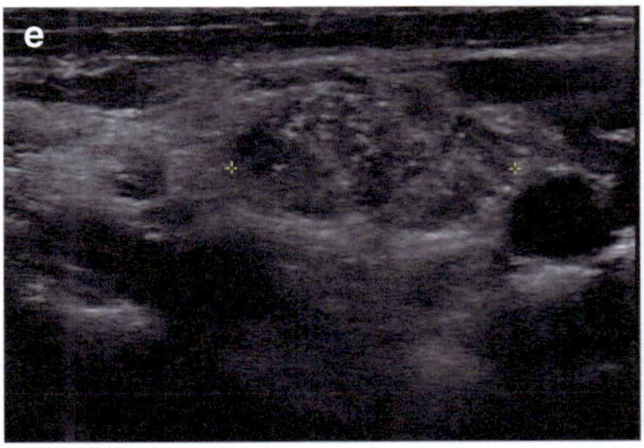

Fig. 3.20e Abnormal node with gross punctate echogenic foci

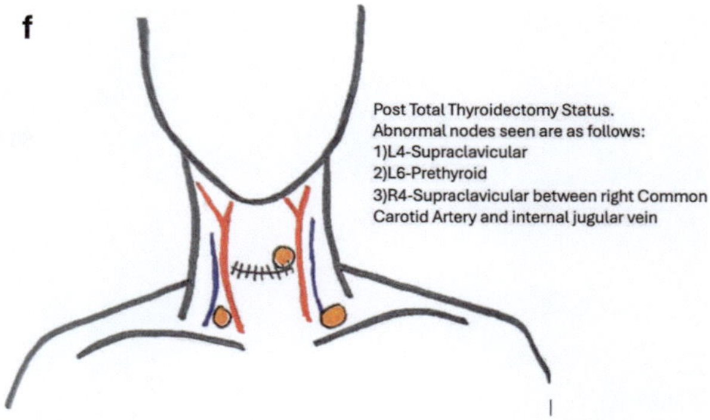

Fig. 3.20f Example of hand drawn sketch is often used to convey exact location of abnormal neck nodes/residual disease in a post total thyroidectomy follow up patient. Diagrammatic documentation of nodes helps for better surgical planning and location of the abnormal nodes/masses

Table 3.5 Lymph nodes with pitfalls and solutions

Pitfall	Solution
1. Tuberculous lymph nodes with coarse calcifications can look like metastatic PTC nodes (Fig. 3.21a)	Calcification in tuberculous nodes is coarser and clump-like, generally found after antituberculous treatment and can show echogenic cystic necrosis due to caseation
2. Incidental cervical nodal metastasis from PTC in known squamous cell carcinoma	Nodal metastasis patterns are different even if SCC and PTC coexist, allowing simultaneous management of both cancers (Fig. 3.21b)
3. Hashimoto's thyroiditis may have abnormal lymph nodes present, which may lead to false positive ultrasound (Fig. 3.21c)	Lack of abnormal calcification/vascularity or cystic changes favors lymph nodes associated with thyroiditis
4. DTC nodes metastasis at unusual sites like retropharyngeal, intraparotid, axillary, and dermal spread (superficial to strap muscles) are rarely known	Cross-sectional imaging will help when extensive nodal burden is suspected

Pitfalls in lymph node mapping with possible solutions (Table 3.5).

Structures that can look like abnormal lymph node:

1. Muscle belly/tortuous vessel
2. Ligated vessels with slow flow
3. Thrombosed vein (Fig. 3.22c)
4. Cartilage
5. F B granuloma/Warthin's tumor (Fig. 3.22a, b)
6. Other neoplasms like schwannoma (Fig. 3.31f)
7. Epidermal inclusion cyst/second branchial cleft cyst

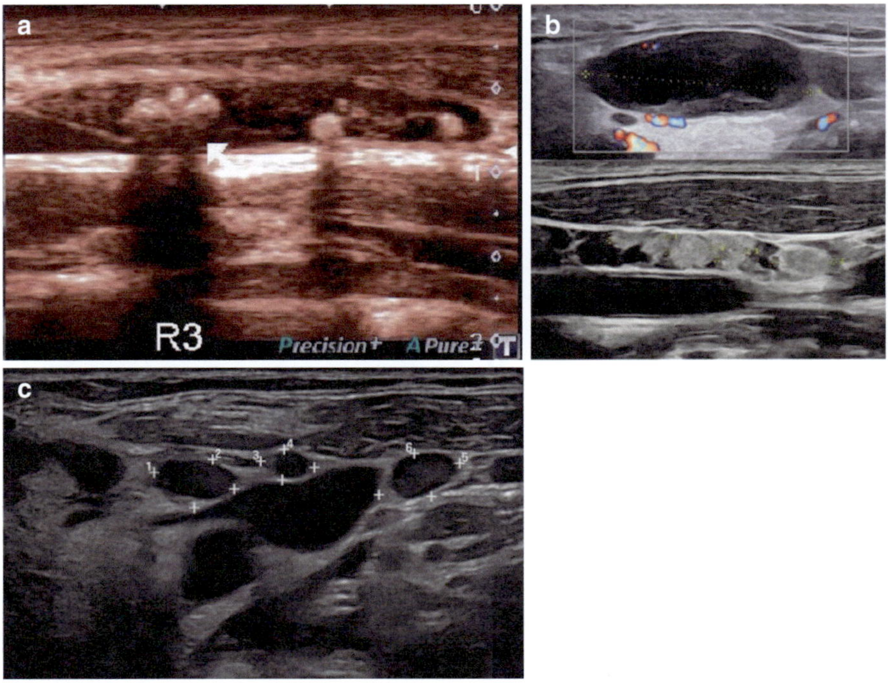

Fig. 3.21 (**a**) Proven nodal Koch's with coarse calcification, (**b**) Known Ca tongue squamous cell carcinoma with necrotic level 2 nodal mets and incidental level 3 lymph node PTC mets with second look ultrasound having small left lobe PTC (P/S it is possible to differentiate between the two if they coexist), (**c**) Multiple normal level 6 node are often seen in thyroiditis

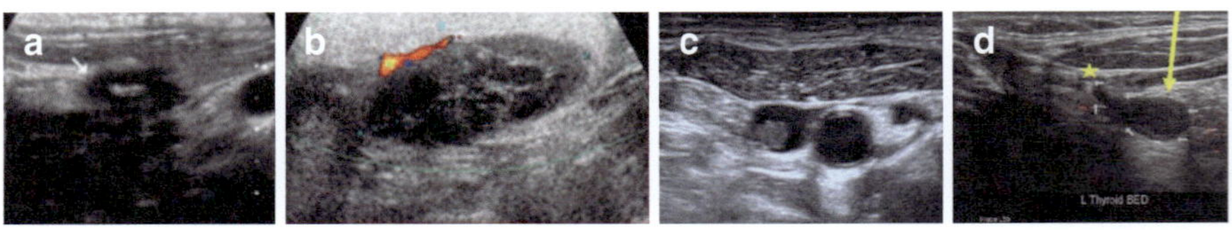

Fig. 3.22 (**a**) Suture granuloma with central echogenic speck, (**b**) Palpable Warthin's tumor can mimic abnormal lymph node, (**c**) Partial jugular thrombus mimics abnormal lymph node, (**d**) Ligated thrombosed supraclavicular vein can mimic suspicious lymph nodes

Demographics of Various Thyroid Cancers (Table 3.6)

Imaging Features of Various Types of Thyroid Cancers (Table 3.7)

Table 3.6 Thyroid cancers

Type of cancer [8]	Frequency	Key pointers	Gene / Tumor markers	Routes of spread	Prognosis
Papillary (PTC) Follicular Insular Tall cell Diffuse sclerosing	70% [1]	Younger age, M: F = 1:2.5 Can be associated with prior Hashimoto's	NTRK RET BRAF Thyroglobulin	Lymphatic Local>pulmonary and skeletal	Overall good
Follicular (FTC) Hürthle cell (now renamed as oncocytic carcinoma)[a]	10–20%	Older age (40 years) Three times more common in females	RAS oncogene Thyroglobulin	Hematogenous Pulmonary and skeletal and brain Neck nodes	Good if early detection, poorer than papillary
Medullary carcinoma (MTC) MEN IIA MEN IIB FMTC	1–5%	25% familial Asso with MEN II Resistant to CT/RT	RET gene Calcitonin, CEA Calcitonin>200 being a poor prognostic factor	Distant spread is known Local, liver lung skeletal	Depends on stage and age at onset
Anaplastic	<3%	Peak age 65 yrs. Highly aggressive		Hematogenous and lymphatic	Poor, median survival 3–8 months
Lymphoma	2%	Associated with prior Hashimoto's thyroiditis (after more than 20 yrs) [9] MC subtype is diffuse large B-call lymphoma (DLBCL) Highly chemo/radio sensitive	TPO and antithyroid antibodies LDH	Can be either primary or associated with Hashimoto's thyroiditis (after 20–30 yrs) [9]	Varied

Ref [a]WHO classification of endocrine tumors 2022

Table 3.7 Imaging features of thyroid cancer

	Ultrasound						
	Appearance	Margins	Vascularity	Calcifications	Characteristic features	CT	MRI
PTC	Hypoechoic Cystic changes in 50%	Well defined / spiculated/ Irregular	Hypervascular	Microcalcification (punctate) Coarse calcifications rarely	Microcalcifications (PEF)	Hypo to isodense solid (NCCT) Microcalcifications (<2 mm) in nodules and lymph nodes Clear, cystic necrosis commo Post-contrast enhancement clear sign (nodule enhances more than native thyroid hence seen better) [10]	Iso- to hypointense on T2WI. Well defined to irregular spiculated margins Low ADC values but higher than ATC
FTC	Hypoechoic Homogeneous	Well defined	Variable	Uncommon	Pseudo-testes sign Tubercle in nodule appearance Trabecular /spoke wheel-like scar within nodule	Rounded/oval Well demarcated No/rare lymph nodal extension Skeletal/distant mets can be a presenting feature	Well defined (round/oval) Iso-/hypointense on T2 Mild enhancement Local spread Skeletal mets
Medullary	More homogeneous and solid than PTC Larger at the time of presentation than PTC	Regular margins	Highly vascular, More than PTC	Coarse calcifications	Coarse calcifications Metastatic nodes hypoechoic *(+calcified) compared to PTC*	Hypodense solid ±coarse/ psammomatous calcification Necrosis rare Cervical nodal mets (50% cases)	Coarse calcifications (T2 hypointense) Well defined Lower ratio compared to PTC Smooth margins

Anaplastic	Heterogeneous hypoechoic, Infiltrative Large masses	Irregular with soft tissue invasion	Intralesional and peripheral vascularity	Variable	Invasion of multiple fascial planes Invasion in adjacent structures Aggressive extrathyroidal extension	Bulky heterogeneous Ill-defined Necrosis Nodular calcification Direct extrathyroidal extension ± nodal metastasis [11]. Extrathyroidal extension, tracheal invasion, esophageal invasion, vascular invasion Venous thrombosis	Hyperintense on T2WI Ring-shaped hypointensity on T2 (Ca++) Very low ADC values due to hypercellularity
Lymphoma	Markedly hypoechoic homogeneous Necrosis= > post CT/RT	Lobulated	Hypovascular	Absent	Increased through transmission	Homogeneous Isodense to strap muscles Necrosis/ca++ rare Adjacent lymph nodal involvement Hypoenhancing compared to normal gland [12]	Markedly hypointense on T1 and T2WI imaging Intense restricted diffusion and corresponding drop on ADC Hyperenhancing on CEMRI

Follicular Carcinoma vs Adenoma Imaging

Follicular neoplasms amount to 10–20% of thyroid cases, although it varies by age, sex, race, and iodine levels in the region. Ultrasound (US) is commonly used to characterize thyroid nodules, although challenges remain in using it to evaluate follicular neoplasms.

Although follicular carcinoma can be confirmed after surgery through histological examination for capsular or vascular invasion, distinguishing it from benign follicular lesions preoperatively has long been a diagnostic challenge in thyroid cytology due to overlapping cytomorphological features. Some researchers attempted using US-guided core biopsy through the capsular wall for better sampling; however, the results are erratic.

US characteristics such as ill-defined margins, solid composition, no halo, non-parallel shape, mild to moderate hypoechogenicity compared to normal thyroid parenchyma and calcification have been associated with malignant thyroid nodules, but none have been shown to be specific to follicular neoplasms (Fig. 3.23c).

The "tubercle-in-nodule" feature, which describes multiple nodule-like solid masses within a thyroid nodule, and the "trabecular formation" feature, which refers to spoke-wheel-like central scars or network-like extensions within the nodules. These features are more commonly observed in follicular thyroid carcinomas than in benign adenomas [13].

Anaplastic Carcinoma

Accounts for 1–2% of all cancers and is a highly aggressive lesion frequently presenting with airway compression and vascular encasement in almost 30% of patients. On ultrasound, a large hypoechoic heterogeneous lesion with few necrotic and calcific areas is a common feature. This tumor has a propensity for extracapsular spread along with nodal and distant metastasis in almost two-thirds of patients. Part of the lesion tends to extend in the retrocricoid/tracheoesophageal groove.

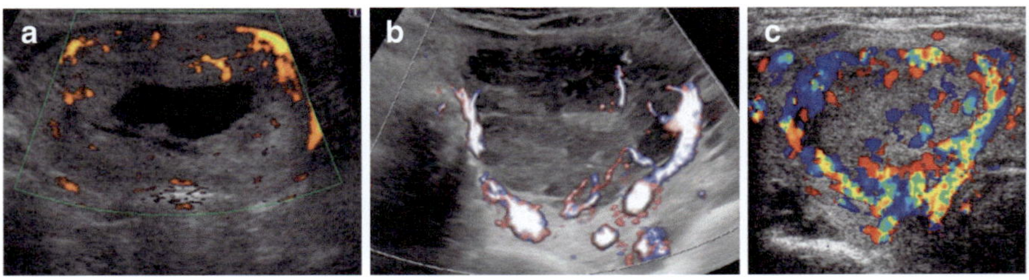

Fig. 3.23 (**a**) Benign follicular adenoma with central cystic change. An adenomatoid lesion can have similar appearance. It tends to be more echogenic compared to heterogeneous follicular carcinoma, (**b**) Patient presented as a lung mass, biopsy was s/o oncocytic carcinoma of thyroid. Thyroid left lobe space-occupying lesion, Histopathology was oncocytic carcinoma with diffuse infiltration of left lobe with vascular emboli, (**c**) Femoral metastatic SOL proven as follicular cancer with histopathology s/o widely invasive follicular cancer with no extrathyroidal extension or vascular invasion

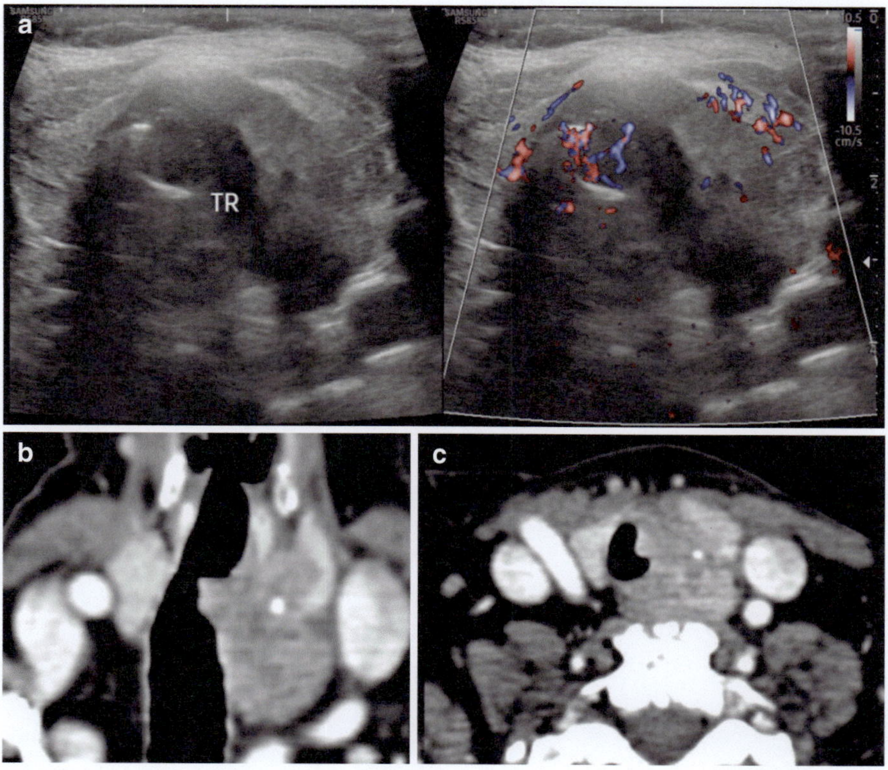

Fig. 3.24 (**a**) Axial scan of thyroid shows a large heterogeneous infiltrative lesion with tracheal invasion identified with focal intraluminal vascularity suggesting its invasive nature, (**b**, **c**) Coronal and axial CT shows clear intra- and retrotracheal invasion. CT depicts the extent more precisely, though high-resolution ultrasound can be useful to suspect it. This was a proven case of anaplastic carcinoma

Tracheal invasion can also be identified on ultrasound (Fig. 3.24a); however, for overall extrathyroidal staging cross-sectional imaging is the modality of choice (Fig3.24b, c, 3.25, and 3.26).

Lymphoma

It is a rare form of thyroid malignancy (less than 5%). Nodular, diffuse, or mixed varieties are known, with the presence of irregular infiltrative lesions involving the entire thyroid gland being the most common feature. There is association with prior Hashimoto's thyroiditis. Serum antimicrosomal and antithyroglobulin antibodies are elevated in up to 90% of patients, and serum LDH levels are also raised in one-third of patients with high-grade lymphoma. Extrathyroidal spread and vascular invasion is known in 50% and 25% cases, respectively; associated abnormal hypoechoic solid lymphomatous node with reticular pattern is an additional clue. Fine-needle aspiration biopsy is generally recommended on which DLBCL and

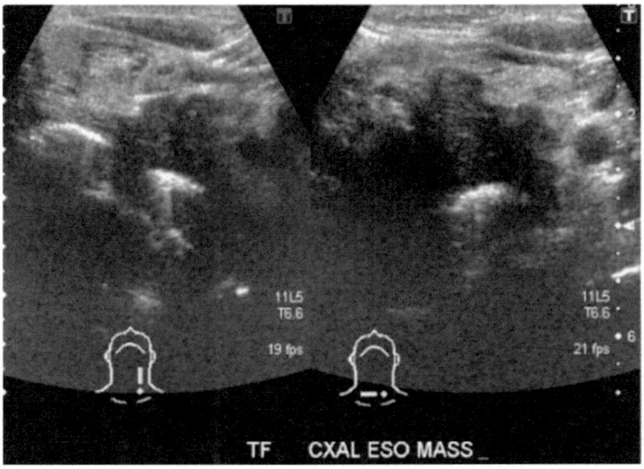

Fig. 3.25 Proven case of retrocricoid esophageal malignancy. Ultrasound of the lower neck at the level of thyroid showing hypoechoic lesion invading the thyroid

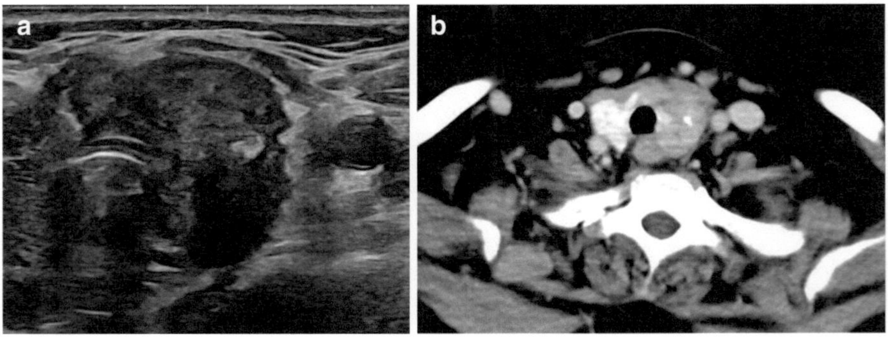

Fig. 3.26 (**a**, **b**) Similar appearance is seen; however, this was nonanaplastic hyalinizing trabecular tumor (HTT). Tracheal adherence was suspected; however, no invasion was seen on surgery

mucosa associated lymphoid tissue (MALT) are the most common subtypes on histopathology. Nodular form may mimic anaplastic thyroid carcinoma; however, calcification, necrosis, and cystic changes are uncommon. Thyroid lymphoma can less commonly cause tracheal and esophageal compression; rarely SVC syndrome is known with mediastinal extension (Fig. 3.27).

CT or MRI would be useful to stage the disease due to its invasive nature. Most cases are treated with chemotherapy; surgical approach is limited to cases with tracheal invasion. FDG PET is useful for staging and assessing treatment responses (Fig. 3.28a–c).

PET scan can be helpful with using the Deauville score for prognostication.

Differentiating it from Hashimoto's thyroiditis and Riedel's thyroiditis remains a challenge on imaging; hence, biopsy is considered definitive.

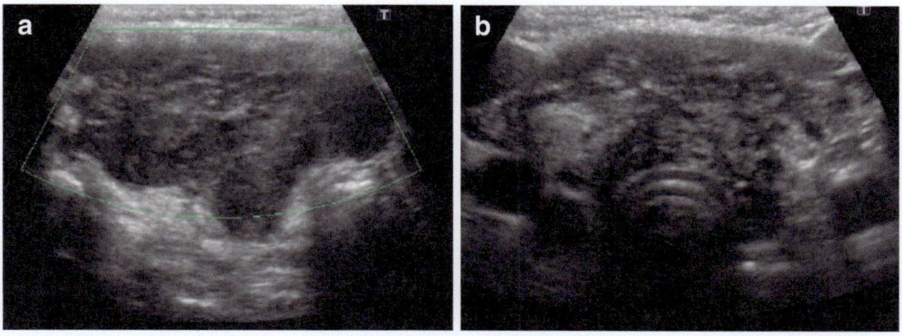

Fig. 3.27 (**a**) Axial ultrasound image of thyroid shows diffuse thyroid enlargement with heterogeneous nodular involvement with marked hypoechoic echogenicity, (**b**) Similar pattern but diffuse involvement is noted

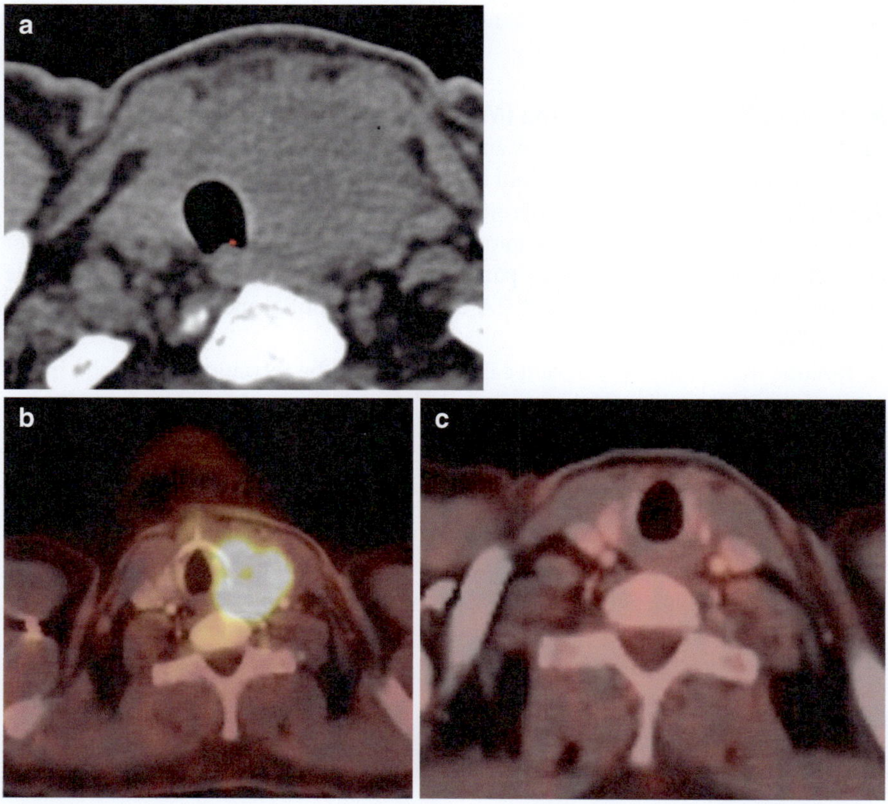

Fig. 3.28 (**a**, **b**) NCCT and PET of the thyroid showing avid uptake with a Deauville score of 5 in the left lobe of thyroid corresponding to left lobe focal hypodense expansile area on CT, (**c**) Post-chemotherapy follow-up PET CT showing complete remission of disease

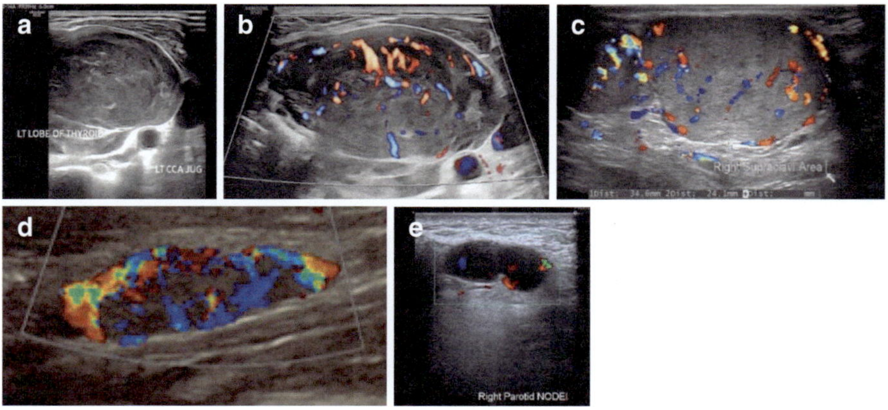

Fig. 3.29 (**a**, **b**) Lobulated well-defined hypoechoic solid lesion with intense vascularity in a proven MTC. Even the metastatic node (**c**, **d**) tends to be solid with increased vascularity but without any cystic change, (**e**) Another patient showing intraparotid metastatic node in a known case of MTC (feature not seen in PTC)

Medullary Thyroid Carcinoma (MTC)

Medullary thyroid cancer (MTC) is an endocrine tumor arising from thyroid C cells and accounts for about 5% of thyroid malignancy. It has a more aggressive behavior than PTC, with up to 13.4% of thyroid cancer-related deaths due to MTC [14].

Differentiation from more common PTC is based on features described earlier and can occur sporadically or as part of hereditary syndromes, such as multiple endocrine neoplasia (MEN) types 2A and 2B or familial medullary thyroid cancer (FMTC).

Routine measurement of serum calcitonin should be recommended in the initial evaluation of thyroid nodules to avoid delayed diagnosis and achieve better prognosis.

Due to its tendency for metastatic spread, clinical lymphadenopathy and distant metastatic disease are more common in MTC.

Disease recurrence was negatively associated with biochemical cure (Sr calcitonin and CEA) and positively associated with extrathyroidal extension, central node metastasis, N staging, and preoperative serum calcitonin level.

MTC may also be associated with symptoms related to elevated calcitonin levels (e.g., diarrhea or flushing), ectopic Cushing syndrome, or positive familial screening (Fig. 3.29).

Mimics (Figs. 3.30, 3.31a, 3.31b, 3.31c, 3.31d, 3.31e, 3.31f, 3.31g, 3.31h)

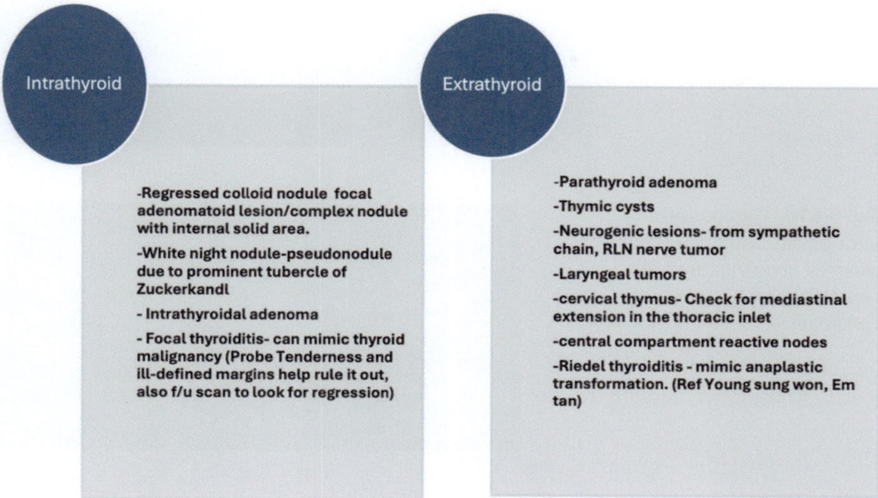

Fig. 3.30 Mimica

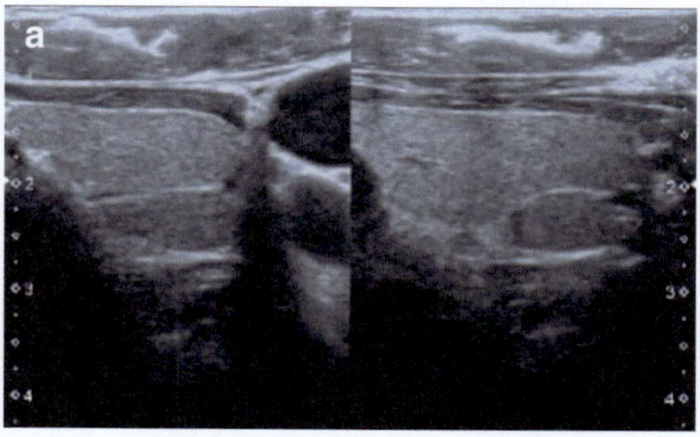

Fig. 3.31a Tubercle of Zuckerkandl can mimic a nodule in the inferior pole of thyroid

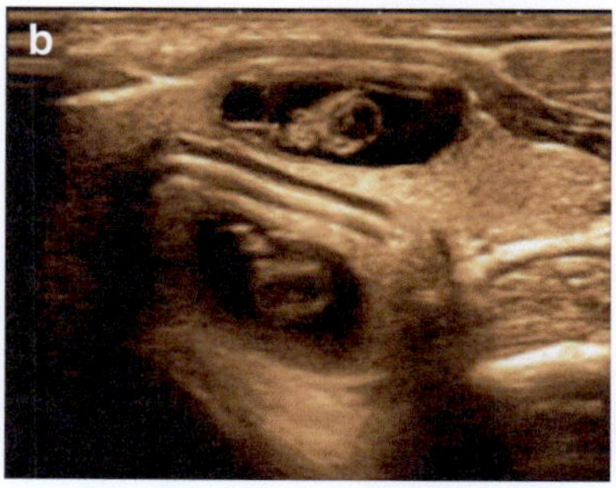

Fig. 3.31b Mirror image of isthmic nodule due to tracheal interface gives appearance of false nodule in trachea

Fig. 3.31c White knight pseudonodule in a case of Hashimoto's thyroiditis

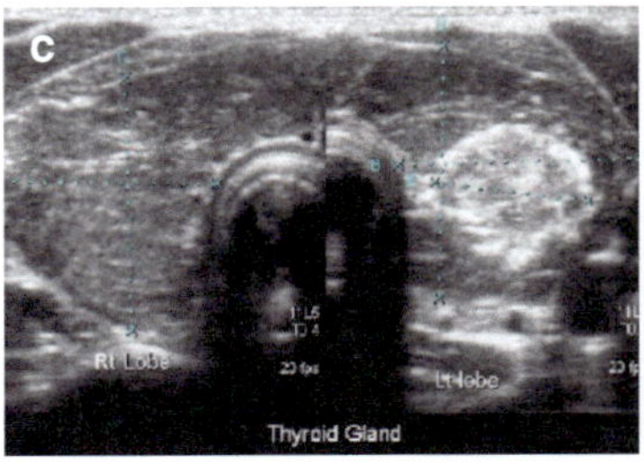

Fig. 3.31d Carotid sheath schwannoma mimicking an enlarged nodule in thyroid bed. (VN: vagus nerve, *nodule)

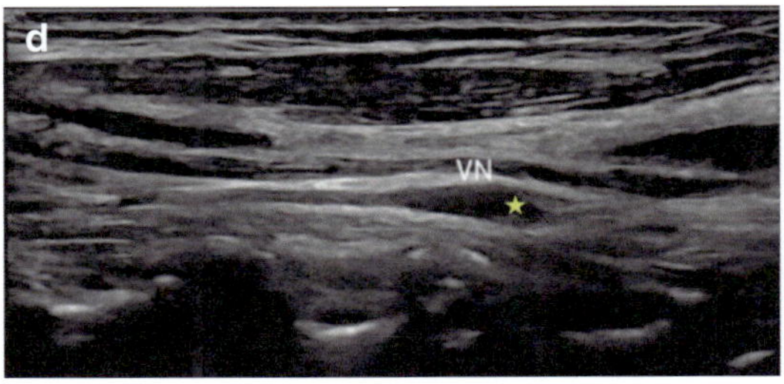

Fig. 3.31e Left- focal thyroiditis can mimic a neoplasm; Right- follow-up scan after 6 weeks shows complete resolution of this nodule

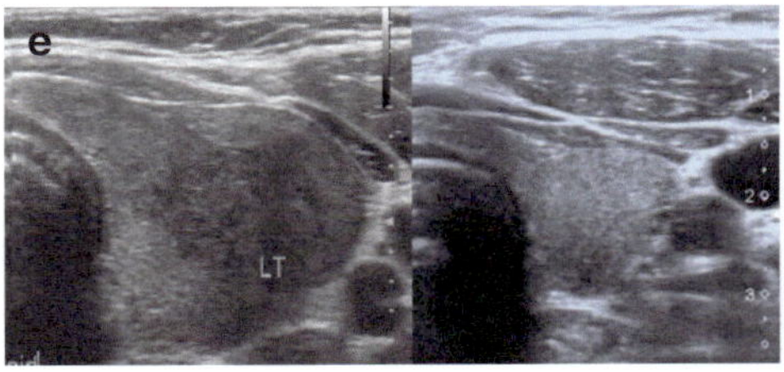

Fig. 3.31f Sympathetic ganglion in thyroid bed can mimic a recurrent nodule

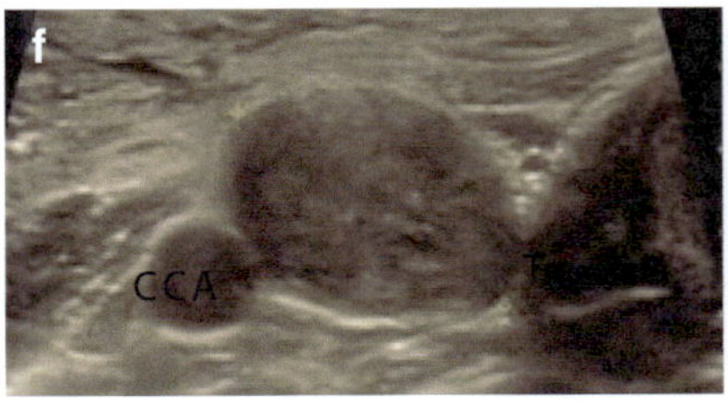

Fig. 3.31g Parathyroid adenoma can mimic a thyroid nodule

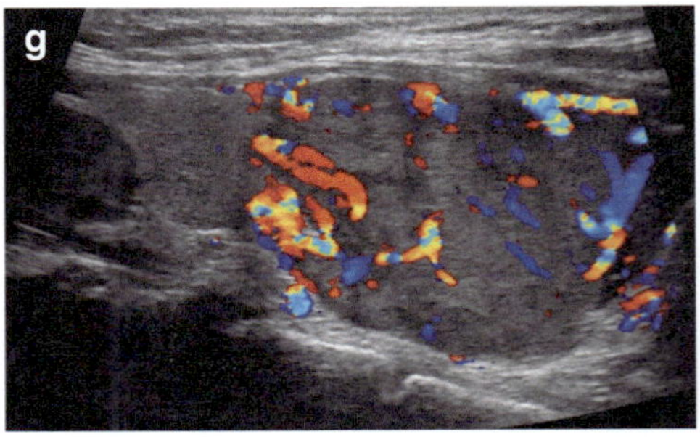

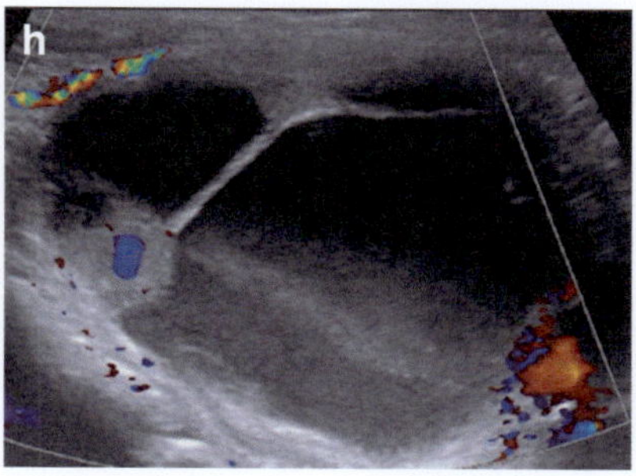

Fig. 3.31h Proven cystic parathyroid adenoma was mistaken as a cystic thyroid nodule

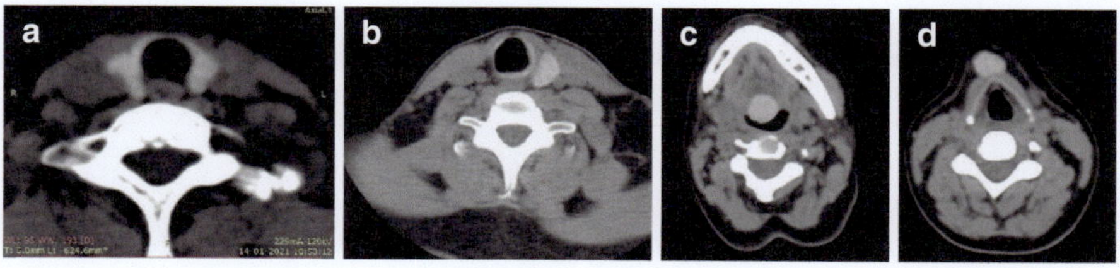

Fig. 3.32 (**a**) Normal thyroid is well seen (hyperdense) due to iodine content, (**b**) Right hemi agenesis, only left lobe is visualized, (**c**, **d**) Typical location of lingual thyroid at the base of tongue(c) and midline ectopic thyroid(d)in the same patient at the lower level

CT/MRI Role in Thyroid Imaging

Despite its operator dependency, ultrasound is a highly sensitive modality for thyroid imaging. The primary limitation of ultrasound is when there is a deeper extent of the tumor, especially invasion posterior to the trachea and nodal invasion.

If there is extrathyroidal extension of the tumor or nodal disease, then CT/MRI has a crucial role to define the disease extent, especially for preoperative planning (Fig. 3.32).

Plain CT Axial Sections of the Neck

Primary indications of CT/MRI in thyroid imaging:

- Extrathyroid extent
- Enhancement pattern and cystic changes in the tumor
- Lymph nodal disease with staging of tumor
- Mediastinal extension of mass
- Evaluation of recurrent disease (Fig. 3.33)

CT/MRI, although not the initial imaging modality of choice for imaging of thyroid neoplasms, has an advantage over ultrasound in the following scenarios:

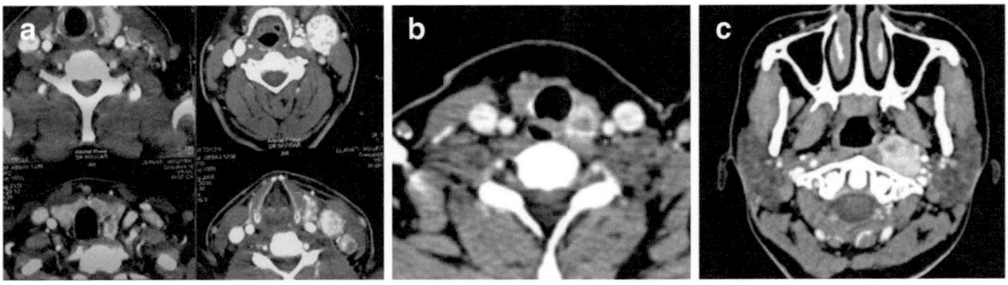

Fig. 3.33 (**a**) Multilevel axial contrast sections of the neck in early arterial contrast phase useful to detect PTC nodal met depict clockwise (top right) to top left. Large intensely enhancing left level II lymph node, partially necrotic left 5B node. Thyroid left lobe hyperdense primary lesion and small central compartment preisthmic/pretracheal lymph node, (**b**, **c**) Post-total thyroidectomy follow-up evaluation in a case of MTC shows a partially necrotic lesion in the left lobe, suggesting residual disease with another necrotic lesion in the left retropharyngeal region (beyond the scope of neck ultrasound)

1. Extrathyroidal extension:

   Cross-sectional imaging can reliably stage the extrathyroidal extension of the tumor with local and distant metastasis. Evaluation of the involvement of retro-cricoid/retrotracheal extension, vascular invasion prediction of the recurrent laryngeal nerve by documenting effacement of tracheoesophageal groove fat on CT /MRI holds an edge over ultrasound evaluation.
2. Recurrence of tumors if.

   – High thyroglobulin, negative neck ultrasound, and inconclusive radionuclide imaging-CECT in combination with FDG PET can reliably detect recurrent and metastatic deposits.
   – Ultrasound is unable to document the extent.
   – Presence of pulmonary micrometastases-HRCT chest with FDG PET in investigation of choice to pick up active nodule [15].

For extrathyroidal invasion, there are limitations of every modality; hence, a cumulative approach to imaging diagnosis should be considered for accurate staging and treatment planning.

- CT has the lowest sensitivity and specificity to predict tracheal and esophageal wall and luminal invasion [16]
- Compared to CT and MR, endoscopic ultrasound is a more reliable investigation for the depth of tracheal and esophageal wall invasion [17]
- MR is better than CT to predict RLN involvement due to beam hardening artifacts (Fig. 3.34)

Value of cross-sectional imaging in identifying tracheal invasion (Fig. 3.35).

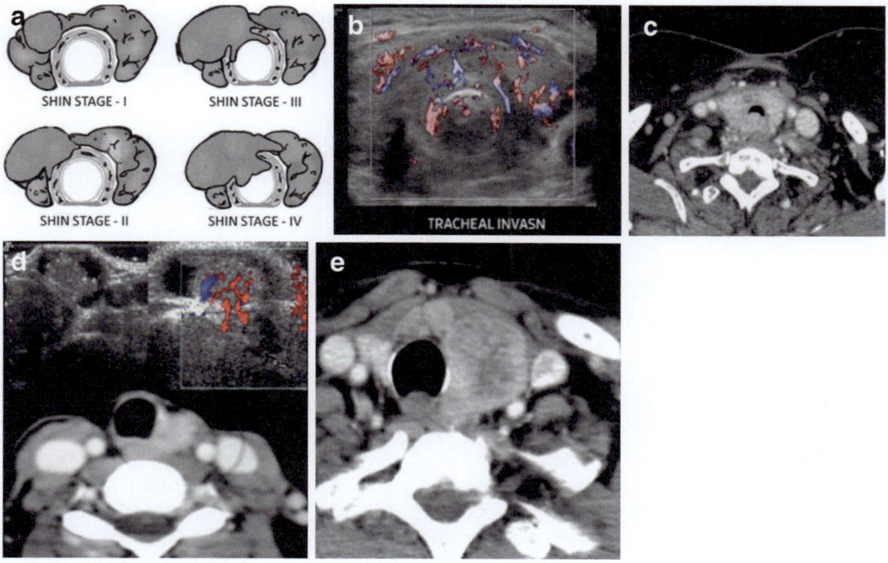

Fig. 3.34 (**a**) Shin classification staging, (**b**, **c**) Ultrasound can pick up anterior tracheal invasion. However, CECT axial scan (**c**) accurately demonstrated posterior tracheal involvement in the same patient. Shin stage IV, (**d**) Post-total thyroidectomy thyroid bed CECT evaluation shows tracheal Shin stage I. Ultrasound can also help to identify typical punctate echogenic foci and cystic change as well as abnormal vascularity extending to the tracheal wall, (**e**) CECT axial scan showing mild tracheal invasion, seen along the left anterior aspect (Shin stage II)

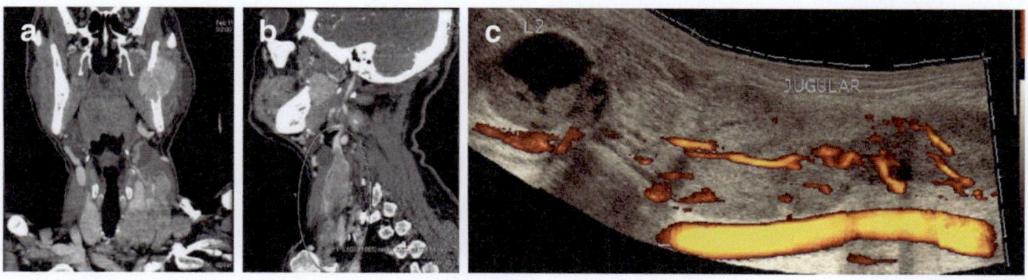

Fig. 3.35 (**a**) CECT neck coronal view showing mandibular destruction due to metastatic lesion and primary left lobe thyroid PTC, (**b**, **c**) Extensive jugular tumor thrombus well seen on neck CECT, ultrasound also helps to pick up abnormal vascularity within the jugular tumor thrombus

CT Imaging Protocol [18] (Table 3.8, Fig. 3.36)

Table 3.8 CT imaging

CT phase	Timing	Scan area	Slice thickness	What to detect
Precontrast	0 sec	Base of skull to tracheal bifurcation[b]	5 mm	Ectopic thyroid tissue Calcified nodes
Arterial (parathyroid protocol-4D-CT)[a]	25–30 s post injection at rate of 3–3.5 ml/sec	Base of skull to aortic arch	3 mm	Increased detection of primary PTC and LN mets [19] due to increased tumor perfusion owing to neo-angiogenesis and capsular vessels involving lymph nodes
Venous phase	60–70 s delay	Base of skull to tracheal bifurcation (scan extended to upper abdomen, if suspicious of MEN syndrome/MTC/ extensive mediastinal extension of tumor / nodes	3 mm	Cystic change in lesions Lymph nodal involvement Extrathyroidal extension Staging of tumor Retroesophageal/ retrotracheal invasion Mediastinal extension with vascular invasion

[a]CT protocol for PTC is slightly different than conventional imaging for thyroid malignancies and involves the parathyroid protocol with acquisition of an early arterial phase at 25 s to enhance the contrast of hyperenhancing primary PTC nodules and lymph nodal mets
[b]Maneuvers to avoid beam hardening artifacts in the lower neck can help not miss lymph nodes in the lower neck and thoracic inlet

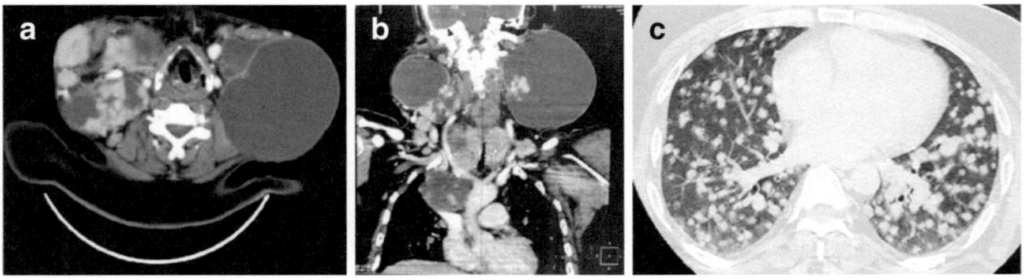

Fig. 3.36 Axial (**a**) and coronal (**b**) CECT and CT thorax in pulmonary window (**c**); demonstrates extensive papillary cancer disease involving multiple ballooned cystic SOL in both central and lateral compartment, except level I with extensive pulmonary hematogenous parenchymal metastasis

MRI Imaging Protocol [18] (Table 3.9)

Predictors of Local Invasion on CT/MRI [16] (Table 3.10, Figs. 3.37, 3.38, and 3.39)

Table 3.9 MRI imaging

Sequence	What to detect
Axial and coronal T1	Hyperintense normal thyroid tissue Local invasion into adjacent soft tissue
Axial T2	Normal thyroid: Iso- to hypointense
Diffusion WI with ADC mapping	Benign tumors have higher ADC values than malignant lesions Metastatic lymph nodes show diffusion restriction
Postcontrast study	Normal thyroids show uniform Gd contrast enhancement
Spectroscopy	Thyroid tumors show a choline peak (absent in normal thyroid tissue Choline/creatinine ratio ranging from 1.6 to 9.4 from DTC to de-differentiated thyroid tumors

Table 3.10 Predictor of local invasion

Organ	Criteria of invasion
Trachea	At least one of - =180° contact Deformity of lumen at level of mass Focal irregularity, thickening, or bulge in the mucosa adjacent to the mass
Esophagus	One of the following on CT: - =180° contact Loss of normal esophageal wall and lumen On MRI, the most suspicious finding for esophageal invasion is a focal T2 signal in the outer layer of the esophageal wall
Artery/vein	=180° contact
Recurrent laryngeal nerve	Two of the following: Completely effaced fat in the tracheoesophageal groove > 25% abutment at the posterior portions of the thyroid (posterior extracapsular invasion) Ipsilateral vocal cord palsy on CT seen as paramedian cord, anteromedial deviation of the arytenoid cartilage, enlarged pyriform sinus Enlarged laryngeal ventricle

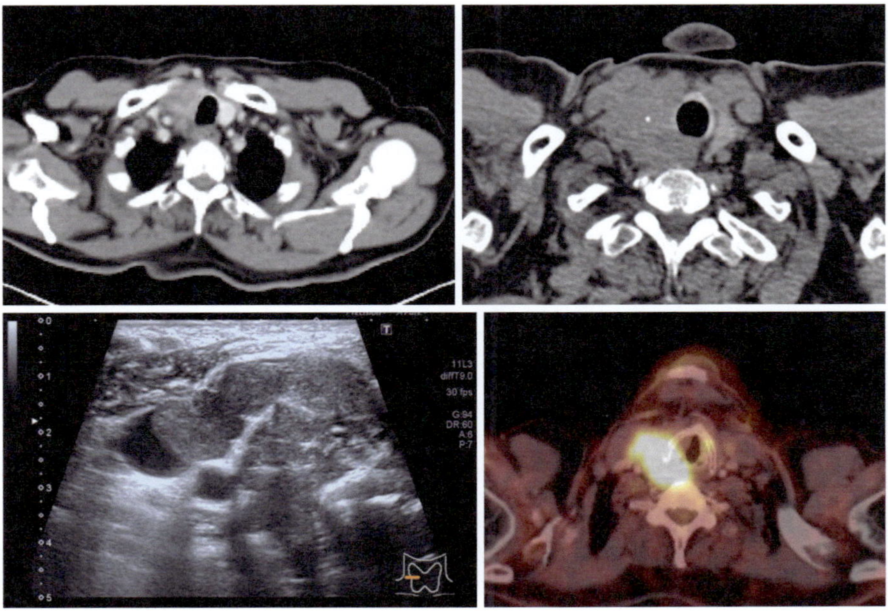

Fig. 3.37 (Clockwise) Axial contrast and plain CT neck shows mass lesion in the right lobe of thyroid with tracheal and retrotracheal extrathyroidal extension. Ultrasound demonstrating tumor thrombus extension in the right internal jugular vein. PET CT shows avid uptake in the corresponding mass lesion. This was a proven case of high-grade follicular non-anaplastic carcinoma

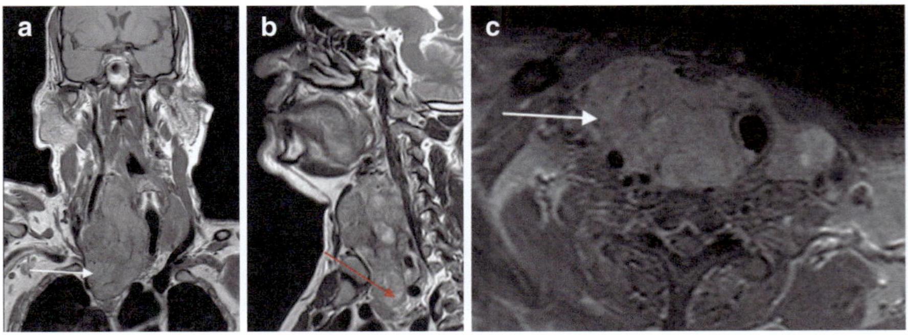

Fig. 3.38 Coronal (**a**) Sagittal (**b**) T1WI demonstrating a heterogenous mass lesion in the right lobe. White and red arrow shows mediastinal extension. T1 fat sat post contrast axial MRI image (**c**) white arrow shows enhancing lesion with similar enhancement of the left lobe

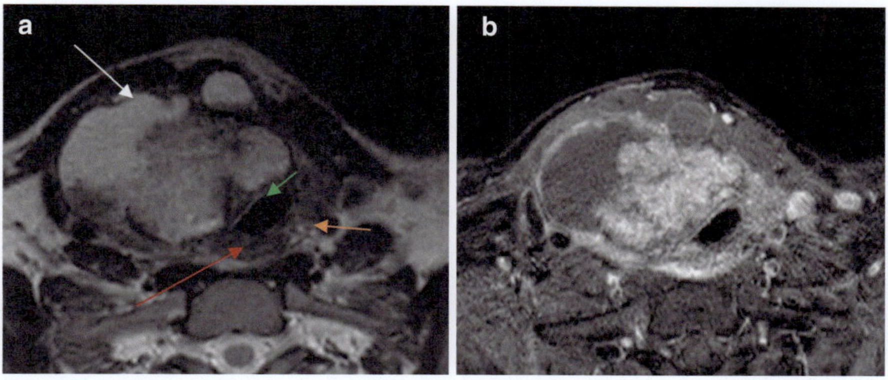

Fig. 3.39 (**a**) Axial T2WI image of MRI of thyroid shows a complex hyper- to isointense solid cystic mass involving the right lobe of thyroid with extrathyroidal extension to involve the trachea and tracheoesophageal groove without invasion of the esophagus. Red arrow: TE groove; orange arrow: esophagus; green arrow: Trachea; white arrow: thyroid mass, (**b**) Postcontrast T1WI showing moderate heterogeneous enhancement of the solid components of the mass. (*Image courtesy: Dr. Nitin Panchal, Dr. Suman Kumar Ankathi-Asso. Professor dept. of Radiology, Tata Memorial hospital, Mumbai)

Role of PET

PET/CT has a limited role in the initial diagnosis but plays a crucial role in the postsurgery management of patients with thyroid cancer.

The intensity of FDG uptake is correlated with progressive dedifferentiation and a more aggressive tumor suggesting that well-differentiated iodine-avid lesions may not absorb 18F-FDG, and a reciprocal relationship between iodine and FDG uptake, called the "flip-flop relationship" [4].

Elevated Tg levels suggest recurrence or metastasis, and I-131 whole-body scans (WBS) can help localize the tumor. When I-131 WBS results are negative, other imaging modalities, especially neck ultrasound (US), CT, and MRI, help to pinpoint recurrent disease. Therefore, combining functional and anatomical imaging methods enhances the ability to detect recurrence and metastatic disease [3].

PET/CT has 81–82% sensitivity and 64–89% specificity for the detection of recurrent tumors in the setting of increased serum thyroglobulin level and negative whole-body iodine scan.

A pitfall of PET is that most thyroid nodal metastases are typically small and may be missed by the resolution of PET/CT.

PET/CT can detect regional as well as unrecognized distant metastases in the lungs and bones (Fig. 3.40).

Serum calcitonin and carcinoembryonic antigen (CEA) are markers used for the detection of even subclinical MTC recurrence. FDG uptake is variable for MTC, and even large metastases can be FDG negative (Fig. 3.41).

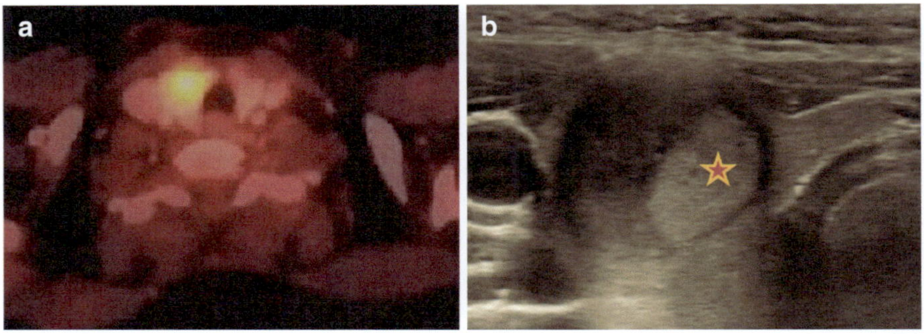

Fig. 3.40 Incidental PET-positive nodule in a k/c/o breast CA (**a**); corresponding ultrasound image (**b**) shows predominantly echogenic nodule (asterix) within peripheral hypoechoic area from which FNAC was done. This was proven to be PTC

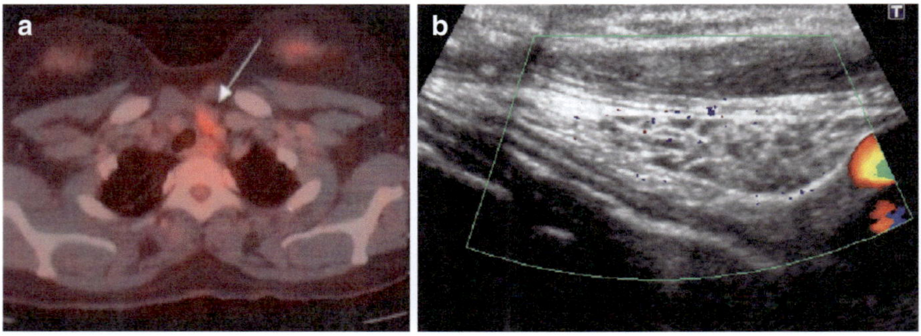

Fig. 3.41 Post-total thyroidectomy in a k/c/o PTC showed focal uptake in the left supraclavicular region (**a**). On ultrasound evaluation (**b**), this corresponded to focal cervical thymic tissue. There was no abnormal metastatic lesion

Recurrent or Residual Disease After Thyroidectomy

Recurrent or residual disease after thyroidectomy occurs most frequently in the cervical and mediastinal lymph nodes (74%), thyroid bed (20%), and trachea or adjacent muscles (6%). The thyroid bed evaluation can be challenging. Small nodules seen in up to one-third of patients, mostly (>90%) are not malignant, and do not progress over time. The 2013 European Thyroid Association guidelines for postoperative US management suggest waiting 3 months postoperactively before imaging the surgical bed to allow for resolution of postoperative changes. US evaluation of recurrent disease is done with increasing level of thyroglobulin, lesion on whole-body "I" scan or PET with CT/MRI (Figs. 3.42 and 3.43).

As most of these lesions are nonpalpable, often subcentimeter size, duplex ultrasound is highly reliable and the easiest modality in postoperative surveillance and

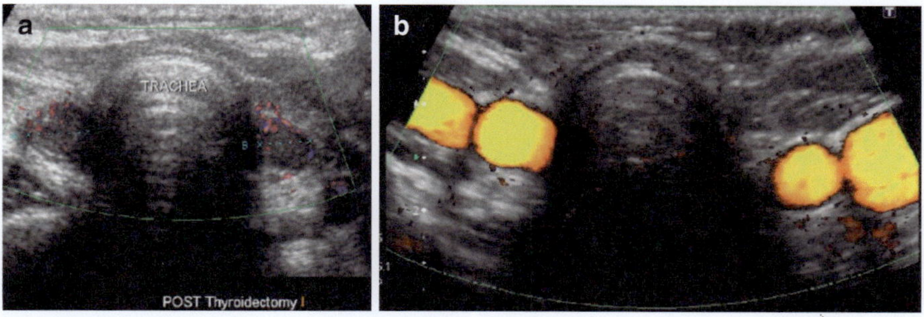

Fig. 3.42 (**a**) Bilateral normal residual thyroid tissue seen in region of ligament of Bary, (**b**) Typical ultrasound appearance of post-total thyroidectomy

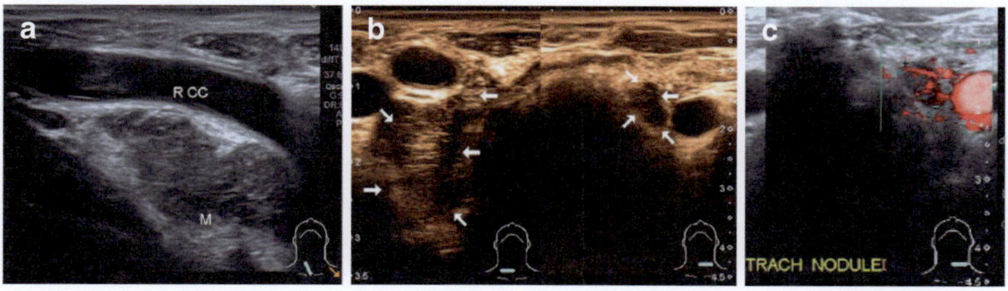

Fig. 3.43 (**a**, **c**) Abnormal nodular lesion (M) seen posterior to the right common carotid (R CC) and left paratracheal region with vascularity (c) is a suspicious finding for residual/recurrent disease, (**b**) Post-total thyroidectomy thyroid bed evaluation showing bilateral nodular lesions (⇨)

detection. One needs to distinguish between true recurrent/metastatic lesions or pseudolesions that need to be ignored. Without thyroiditis or radioiodine therapy, residual unresected thyroid tissue will have a US appearance like that of normal thyroid tissue preoperatively. Residual thyroid tissue in a patient who has been treated with radioiodine therapy will appear hypoechoic and heterogeneous, which can be a potential pitfall and mimic a suspicious nodule. US features that favor malignancy in thyroid bed nodules are like those seen in malignant thyroid nodules: Irregular margins, increased vascularity, microcalcifications, and cystic components. Serum thyroglobulin levels can be a useful correlate with the imaging findings when assessing the patient for disease recurrence. The ATA recommends serum thyroglobulin level measurements every 6–12 months after treatment for thyroid cancer, with more frequent measurements for high-risk patients. In patients receiving thyroid hormone replacement therapy, a thyroglobulin level of 0.2–0.3 ng/mL has the best accuracy for detecting persistent disease. However, after a hemithyroidectomy, neck US is the mainstay for surveillance as the serum thyroglobulin level will be of limited value. Even when TG level is undetectable, LN metastasis can exist, and loss of fatty hilum is a less sensitive US marker compared to other

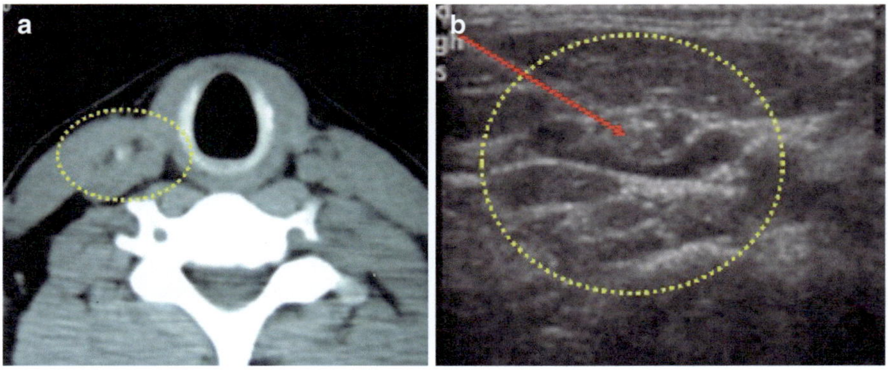

Fig. 3.44 Post-total thyroidectomy status plain axial CT shows focal calcification in right mid neck. Corresponding ultrasound image shows this to be abnormal FNAC-proven PTC metastasis

pointers like abnormal intranodal intense vascularity, tiny calcific specks or cystic change. FNAC can be diagnostic in such situations.

Postop suture or clip granulomas ligated thrombosed venous channels, small normal lymph nodes, thymic tissue, or parathyroid gland can mimic unusual nodes or recurrent nodules. Thyroid bed nodules on surveillance ultrasound may warrant fine-needle aspiration cytology if they increase in size and number, are persistent, and are associated with suspicious features on ultrasound with elevated Tg levels, depending on the patient and primary tumor factors. These patients may undergo a biopsy with repeat surgery and/or active surveillance. Suspicious nodules located posteromedially near the expected position of the recurrent laryngeal nerve should be highlighted because their presence may influence patient counseling and surgical strategy. If recurrent disease is detected, it should be denoted to either the central neck (either thyroid bed or central compartment lymph node) or the lateral neck to guide management (Fig. 3.44).

Role of Imaging in Ablations

Thermal and chemical ablation is an accepted method in symptomatic benign nodules and autonomously functioning nodules when surgery is refused or when the patient would not tolerate surgery. PMC and recurrent lesions also are being ablated (Fig. 3.45). Ultrasound-guided ablation allows precise visualization of the tip of electrode, safeguarding critical vessels and nerves (RLN, brachial plexus, vagus and other neck nerves, and the sympathetic chain).

In our experience, the real-time ultrasound has an unparalleled role:

1. "Moving shot technique and continuous hydrodissection" are two most important steps to achieve satisfactory ablation without thermal injuries to the important nerves in the thyroid bed and in the vicinity (Fig. 3.45).

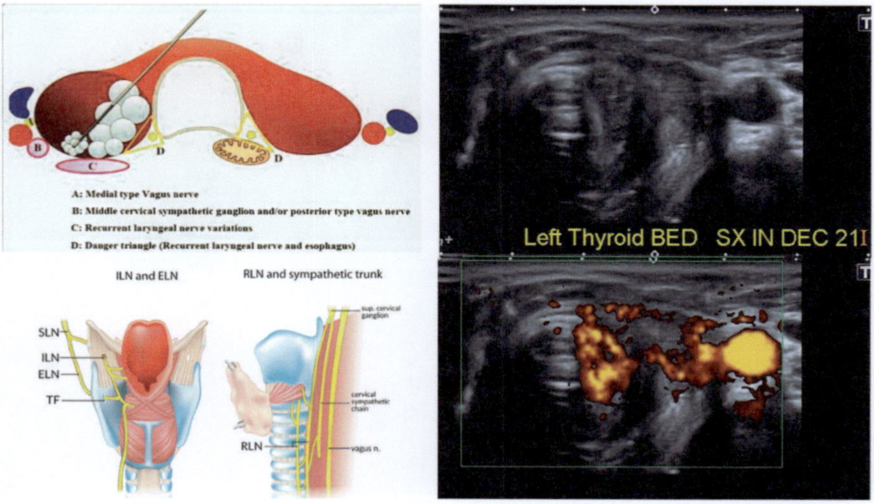

Fig. 3.45 Post-total thyroidectomy status with incomplete resection due to left tracheal wall invasion. The patient was offered thermal ablation as a treatment option

2. Vocal cord movements can also be monitored using real-time ultrasound if patients were to be under anesthesia.
3. To document near-total eradication of tumoral vascularity as an end point.
4. Preprocedural identification of danger triangles and using elastography can help in judicious case selection.
5. Monitoring post-ablation volume reduction rate.

From Present Status to Future Directions

Imaging is pivotal in managing DTC and guiding the diagnostic, staging, and treatment planning processes. While US remains the first-line imaging modality for most cases, CT and MRI are indispensable tools in evaluating advanced disease, local invasion, and recurrence. The selection of the appropriate imaging modality should be tailored to the specific clinical scenario to optimize patient outcomes (Fig. 3.46).

Importance of Multimodality Imaging

Use of radiomics and real-time AI-based tools on datasets will lead to robust algorithms. Molecular testing of the tissue sample with the help of gene sequencing classifier (GSC) differentiating benign from malignant lesions, contrast-enhanced ultrasound, and elastography will further help in better multidisciplinary team management of thyroid malignancies.

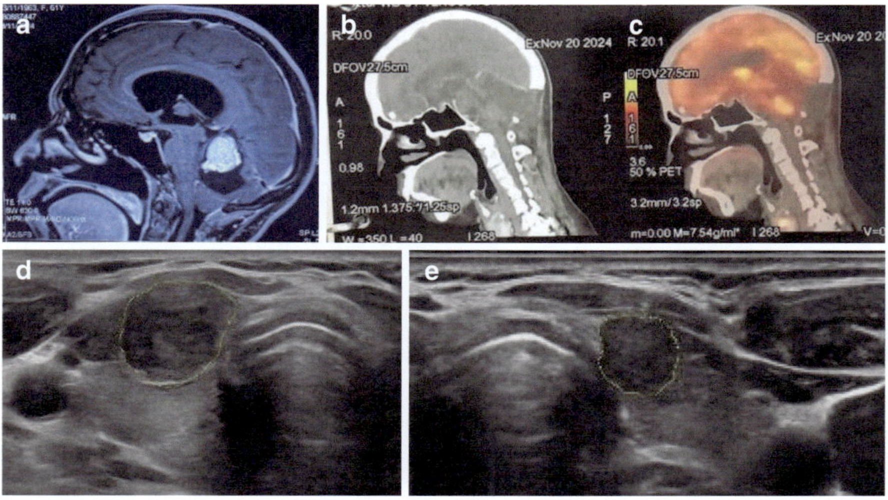

Fig. 3.46 (**a**) MRI sagittal image showing large intraventricular SOL causing obstructive hydrocephalus, (**b**, **c**) Postoperative sagittal PET CT images showing a craniotomy defect and an abnormal uptake in the thyroid region (arrow), (**d**, **e**) Axial thyroid ultrasound shows bilateral thyroid nodules-proven follicular cancer, leading to solitary intraventricular metastasis

Acknowledgments We thank Dr. Sultan Pradhan, MS, FRCS, FACS, FCPS, Surgical Oncologist and Chairman of Head and Neck Cancer Institute of India (HNCII), Mumbai. Staff and Department of Imaging and Department of Pathology, Prince Aly Khan Hospital and HNCII Mumbai for images and clinical data contribution.

References

1. Mahajan A, Vaidya T, Vaish R, Sable N. The journey of ultrasound-based thyroid nodule risk stratification scoring systems: do all roads lead to thyroid imaging, reporting and data system (TIRADS)? J Head Neck Phys Surg. 2017;5(2):57.
2. Lee JY, Baek JH, Ha EJ, Sung JY, Shin JH, Kim J Hoon, et al. 2020 imaging Guidelines for Thyroid Nodules and Differentiated Thyroid Cancer: Korean Society of Thyroid Radiology. Korean J Radiol 2021;22(5):840–860.
3. Zampella E, Klain M, Pace L, Cuocolo A. PET/CT in the management of differentiated thyroid cancer. Diagn Interv Imaging. 2021;102(9):515–23.
4. Larg MI, Barbus E, Gabora K, Pestean C, Cheptea M, Piciu D. 18F-FDG PET/CT in differentiated thyroid carcinoma. Acta Endocrinol (Buchar). 2019;15(2):203–8.
5. ATA Guidelines & Statements [Internet]. American Thyroid Association. [cited 2025 Jun 26]. Available from: https://www.thyroid.org/professionals/ata-professional-guidelines/
6. Tappouni RR, Itri JN, McQueen TS, Lalwani N, Ou JJ. ACR TI-RADS: pitfalls, solutions, and future directions. Radiographics. 2019;39(7):2040–52.
7. Ultrasonographic features of cervical lymph node metastases from medullary thyroid cancer: a retrospective study | BMC Medical Imaging | Full Text [Internet]. [cited 2025 Jun 26]. Available from: https://bmcmedimaging.biomedcentral.com/articles/10.1186/s12880-022-00882-7

8. RV L, RY O, G K, J R. WHO Classification of Tumors of Endocrine Organs [Internet]. [cited 2025 Jun 26]. Available from: https://publications.iarc.fr/Book-And-Report-Series/Who-Classification-Of-Tumours/WHO-Classification-Of-Tumours-Of-Endocrine-Organs-2017
9. Walsh S, Lowery AJ, Evoy D, McDermott EW, Prichard RS. Thyroid lymphoma: recent advances in diagnosis and optimal management strategies. Oncologist. 2013;18(9):994–1003.
10. Value of CT Features in the Diagnosis of Papillary Thyroid Tumors in Incidental Thyroid Nodules—Zhang—2020—International Journal of Endocrinology—Wiley Online Library [Internet]. [cited 2024 Dec 26]. Available from: https://onlinelibrary.wiley.com/doi/10.1155/2020/9342317
11. Lee JW, Yoon DY, Choi CS, Chang SK, Yun EJ, Seo YL, et al. Anaplastic thyroid carcinoma: computed tomographic differentiation from other thyroid masses. Acta Radiol. 2008;49(3):321–7.
12. Kim HC, Han MH, Kim KH, Jae HJ, Lee SH, Kim SS, et al. Primary thyroid lymphoma: CT findings. Eur J Radiol. 2003;46(3):233–9.
13. Kuo TC, Wu MH, Chen KY, Hsieh MS, Chen A, Chen CN. Ultrasonographic features for differentiating follicular thyroid carcinoma and follicular adenoma. Asian J Surg. 2020;43(1):339–46.
14. Valderrabano P, Klippenstein DL, Tourtelot JB, Ma Z, Thompson ZJ, Lilienfeld HS, et al. New American Thyroid Association sonographic patterns for thyroid nodules perform well in medullary thyroid carcinoma: institutional experience, systematic review, and meta-analysis. Thyroid. 2016;26(8):1093–100.
15. Johnson NA, Tublin ME. Postoperative surveillance of differentiated thyroid carcinoma: rationale, techniques, and controversies. Radiology. 2008;249(2):429–44.
16. Seo YL, Yoon DY, Lim KJ, Cha JH, Yun EJ, Choi CS, et al. Locally advanced thyroid cancer: can CT help in prediction of extrathyroidal invasion to adjacent structures? Am J Roentgenol. 2010;195(3):W240–4.
17. Tracheal Invasion by Thyroid Carcinoma [Internet]. [cited 2024 Dec 25]. Available from: https://www.ajronline.org/doi/epdf/10.2214/ajr.177.4.1770929
18. Mahajan A, Agarwal U, Padashetty S, Shukla S, Smriti V, Rastogi S, et al. A narrative review of the role of cross-sectional imaging in the management of thyroid carcinoma: imaging guidelines and T-CIRADS. Cancer Res Stat Treat. 2022;5(3):490.
19. Park JE, Lee JH, Ryu KH, Park HS, Chung MS, Kim HW, et al. Improved diagnostic accuracy using arterial phase CT for lateral cervical lymph node metastasis from papillary thyroid cancer. AJNR Am J Neuroradiol. 2017;38(4):782–8.

Molecular Testing in FNA in Thyroid Cancer

4

Alice Yu, Preethi Srikanthan, and Maie St. John

Editorial

Thyroid cancers have grown significantly, with almost a threefold rise. Incidentally detected nodules are increasingly being investigated with ultrasound and fine-needle aspiration cytology (FNAC). The sensitivity and specificity of ultrasound sonography (USG) are around 80% while FNAC reports it as Bethesda 3 and 4 in up to 30% of patients, ensuing in more debates over need for surgery. The risk of malignancy is around 15% in Bethesda 3 and up to 30% in Bethesda 4, which may result in unnecessary surgery in almost 75% of cases. Further clarity is required to make treatment decisions. Molecular testing on the FNAC samples has emerged as a troubleshooting tool. However, it is not discussed by the authors in this chapter. The various molecular tests in use are laid out, with the newer iterations showing better specificity and negative predictive value. The sensitivity is still not high enough and can result in unnecessary or inappropriate treatment plans. These tests being expensive are not universally followed and in some regions of the world a diagnostic lobectomy might

A. Yu
David Geffen School of Medicine at UCLA, Los Angeles, CA, USA
e-mail: AlYu@mednet.ucla.edu

P. Srikanthan
UCLA Research Center at Alhambra, Alhambra, CA, USA
e-mail: PSrikanthan@mednet.ucla.edu

M. St. John (✉)
Department of Head and Neck Surgery, UCLA David Geffen School of Medicine, Los Angeles, CA, USA
e-mail: MStJohn@mednet.ucla.edu

P. S. Pai et al. (eds.), *Controversies in Cancer of the Thyroid and Parathyroid Glands*, https://doi.org/10.1007/978-3-032-13130-0_4

be more cost-effective. It is highly debatable at this stage to make the molecular testing mandatory as it involves a higher degree of follow-up and a bigger burden on the resources. Besides these controversies, molecular testing may help in decision-making, diagnosis, prognosis, and therapy in the years to come.

Prathamesh S. Pai

Introduction

Thyroid cancer is the seventh most prevalent cancer worldwide as of 2022 [1]. In recent decades, there has been an increase in the incidence of thyroid cancer, though mortality has remained unchanged [2]. The rise in diagnosis without a corresponding rise in mortality is due in large part to improved diagnostic and surveillance strategies capable of detecting early-stage disease, the increasing availability of thyroid ultrasound, and earlier therapeutic interventions [2]. Though the wealth of information provided by pretreatment clinical tests such as ultrasounds or fine-needle aspirations (FNA) can greatly aid clinical decision-making, there are patients for whom the ideal course of treatment may not be well defined [3]. In these cases, clinicians may turn to the use of molecular testing in FNA.

Background

With more than 800,000 new cases and 47,000 deaths in 2022, thyroid cancer is the seventh highest cancer in incidence globally, but only the 24th highest in mortality. As these statistics demonstrate, many patients who have thyroid cancer will not die due to complications of their thyroid cancer [1, 2]. As such, this cancer is one where, for most patients with treatable disease, clinical conversations regarding treatment revolve around preserving function and quality of life [2].

The diagnosis of thyroid cancer encompasses four primary histological subtypes: papillary, follicular, medullary, and anaplastic thyroid cancers [4]. Particularly in the case of thyroid nodules harboring papillary and follicular neoplasms, a key clinical decision is whether surgery would confer survival risk without unnecessary morbidity. However, while surgery is the most definitive method of both diagnosis and treatment for many thyroid cancers, many patients have concerns regarding undergoing anesthesia, potential risks of surgery, and need for thyroid hormone replacement [2, 4].

This prioritization of quality of life in the context of improved survival outcomes is reflected in both American Thyroid Association (ATA) and National Comprehensive Cancer Network (NCCN) guidelines, wherein eligibility criteria for hemithyroidectomy were expanded to include low-risk thyroid cancers under 4 centimeters [5]. Increasingly, patients with additional comorbidities or advanced age may choose to observe FNA-positive thyroid cancers under 1.5 centimeters in a clinical strategy known as active surveillance [6]. As such, it is important to understand the interplay between current guidelines regarding thyroid cancer diagnosis and workup, surgical indications, and the role molecular testing plays in guiding treatment [3, 5].

Ultrasound

The workup of thyroid cancers generally includes both ultrasound and, when indicated, FNA. Ultrasound usually serves as the initial screening commonly ordered by primary care providers. This inexpensive and rapid test can provide a wealth of information regarding the characteristics and malignant potential of thyroid nodules.

To provide a standardized method of grading these images, the American College of Radiology published the "White Paper" in 2017 detailing the TI–RADS/ACR TI-RADS (TR scoring system), which examines five categories of characteristics of thyroid nodules: composition, echogenicity, shape, margin, and echogenic foci to stratify thyroid nodules into five categories based on risk of malignancy [7]. Under this system, TR1 strongly suggests the lesion described possesses benign characteristics, TR2 suggests not suspicious, TR3 lesions are mildly suspicious, TR4 lesions are moderately suspicious, and TR5 suggests highly suspicious features [7].

Similarly, comprehensive guidelines regarding the risk stratification of thyroid nodules based on ultrasound markers were released by the American Thyroid Association in 2015 [6]. This guideline also subdivides categories of risk into five tiers. However, in practice, ACR TI-RADS criteria are more frequently used by radiologists and are commonly encountered in a clinical setting (Fig. 4.1) [8].

For either of these grading systems, studies have suggested sensitivities ranging from 49% to 85%, along with specificities of 79–85%. As such, when concerning findings are noted on these imaging modalities, they are supplemented by tissue biopsy, which is obtained using fine-needle aspiration (FNA) [9]. The ACR TI-RADS system suggests different size thresholds depending on risk classification. While FNA is not recommended for lesions that are TR1 or TR2, follow-up or FNA is recommended of TR3–5 lesions that meet size criteria. Size thresholds for both follow-up and FNA diminish as the TI-RADS grading increases (Image 1) [9]. Similar thresholds for FNA/follow-up exist for the ATA nodule classification system.

Fine-Needle Aspiration

The preferred method of tissue biopsy for thyroid nodules is fine-needle aspiration (FNA). In this procedure, a thin needle, usually of 22- to 27-gauge caliber, is passed several times under ultrasound guidance into lesions of interest. This technique results in a collection of cells that are examined cytologically; however, FNA also loses aspects of tissue architecture and dimension analysis that may be

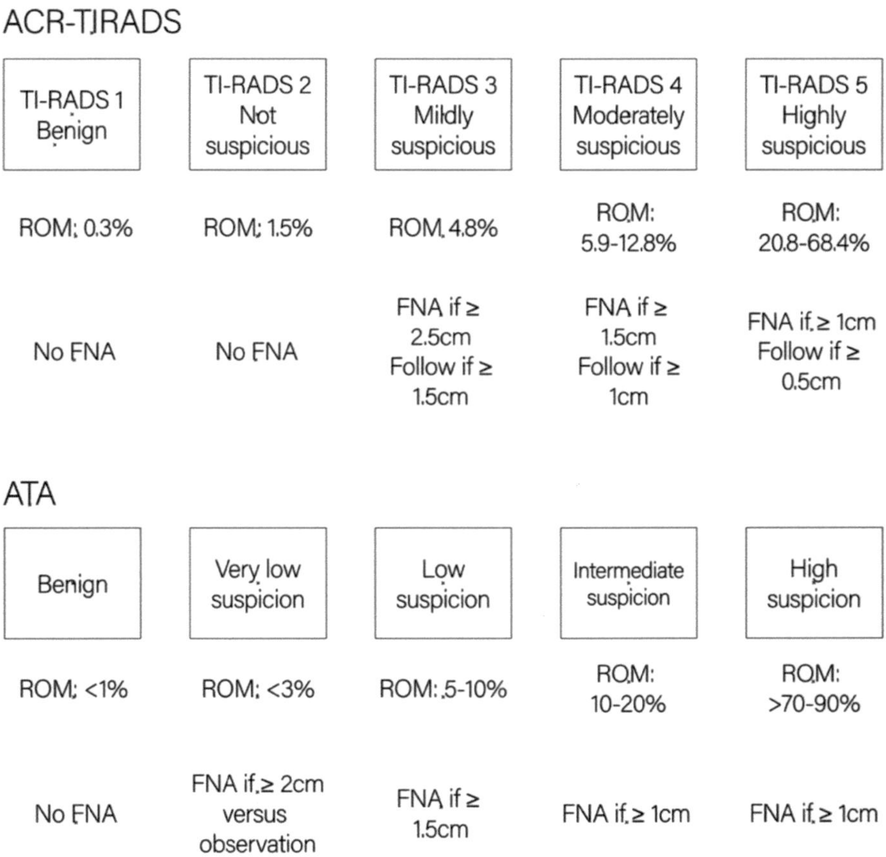

Fig. 4.1 Diagram of FNA recommendations of ACR TIRADS reporting system versus ATA system

gleaned from a traditional biopsy [10, 11]. Notably, FNA molecular testing is predominantly useful in clinical decision-making connected with papillary and follicular cancers and has a far more limited clinical role in medullary and anaplastic thyroid cancers [6].

The method by which these samples are evaluated is the Bethesda System for Reporting Thyroid Cytopathology, most recently updated in 2023. Under this system, results of thyroid FNA are classified under six categories: (I) nondiagnostic, (II) benign, (III) atypia of undetermined significance, (IV) follicular neoplasm, (V) suspicious for malignancy, and (VI) malignant. Treatment recommendations for surgery versus observation vary depending on category [10–12].

Benign lesions (Bethesda class II) are the most straightforward in management, as they may be observed without the need for additional FNA if the lesion does not evolve in appearance over time [6, 11]. For nondiagnostic FNA (Bethesda class I), repeat FNA is generally recommended, as either sample quantity or quality was not sufficient to formulate a diagnosis. While some have stated in the past that clinicians should wait at least 3 months prior to performing repeat FNA in order to avoid additional nondiagnostic tests, guidelines now state that there is no need to wait before repeating. Moreover, FNA success is operator dependent; a multicenter study performed by Houdek et al. showed that high-volume providers and institutions with capabilities for bedside evaluation had significantly reduced rates of nondiagnostic results [6, 11, 13]. For patients with lesions of both suspicious for malignancy as well as malignant classifications, surgery is generally recommended. In both cases, the diagnosis is given when there is sufficient evidence to be reasonably certain of the presence of thyroid cancer or other malignancy [11].

The two categories with greatest uncertainty are atypia of unknown significance (AUS; Bethesda class III) and follicular neoplasm (FN; Bethesda class IV). Patients with FNA showing AUS have an average risk of malignancy of 22%, while those with the diagnosis of follicular neoplasm have an average risk of 50% [11]. For patients with AUS, certain features may suggest a higher risk of malignancy; for example, nuclear atypia is associated with a significantly higher risk of malignancy (ROM). Nevertheless, those who receive the diagnosis of AUS are also advised to repeat FNA. Most nodules identified as AUS or follicular neoplasm on FNA will be rediagnosed as benign on repeat FNA, 10–30% of cases will be reclassified in an indeterminate category. If the diagnosis of AUS is obtained twice, a discussion is warranted between clinician and patient (and if available presented at multidisciplinary conference) after which molecular testing may be offered for more diagnostic information or the patient may choose to either continue to observe or undergo surgery [6, 11].

The category of follicular neoplasm is reserved for FNA samples that are composed of follicular cells with some architectural atypia. Thirty percent of tumors diagnosed as "follicular neoplasm" on FNA are noted to be benign nodular disease. It also acts as the category for suspected noninvasive follicular thyroid neoplasm with papillary-like nuclear features (NIFTP), which is a low-risk thyroid tumor usually treated conservatively with limited surgery such as hemithyroidectomy [4, 10]. Roughly 8% of Bethesda class IV FNA results are NIFTP [14]. As such, some patients may elect to pursue molecular testing to avoid surgery unless the risk of malignancy is greater (Fig. 4.2) [6, 11].

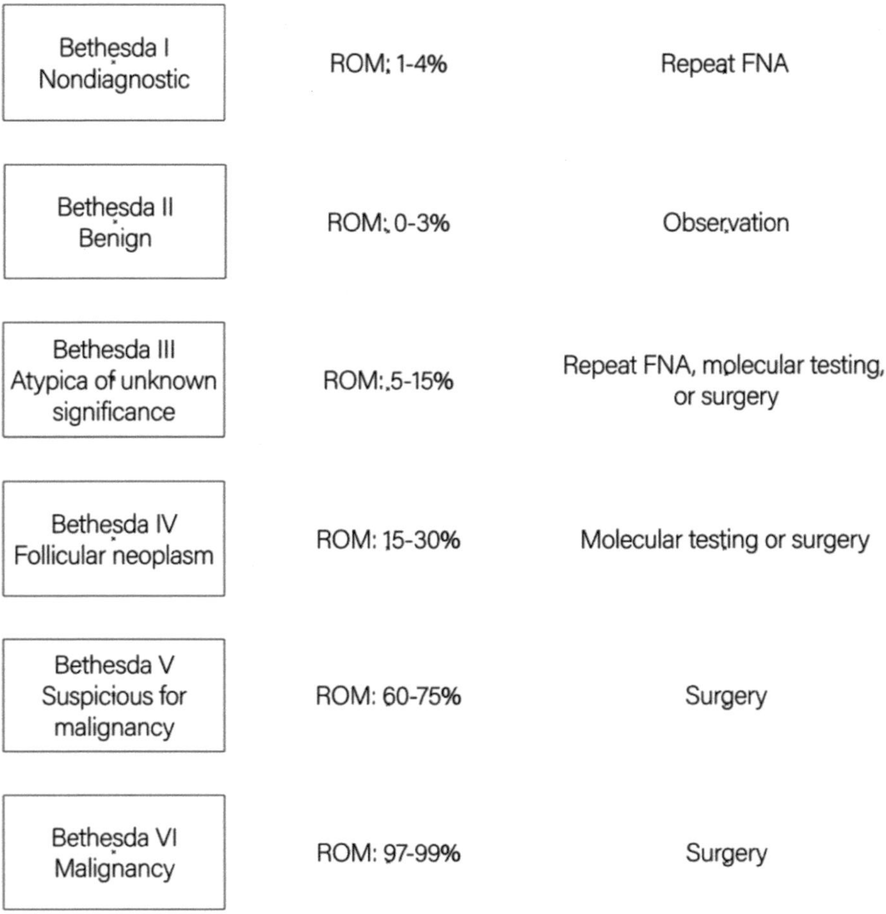

Fig. 4.2 Risk stratification and management based on Bethesda classification [11]

The diagnostic uncertainty in the AUS/FN Bethesda classification categories often requires additional information for clinicians to make appropriate clinical decisions. As such, molecular testing is utilized to fill the gap of knowledge in these Bethesda categories.

Molecular Testing

As noted above, 15–30% of all FNAs will have indeterminate diagnoses that require further workup with molecular testing [3]. Molecular testing can provide necessary information to tilt clinical decision-making in favor of or away from surgical management. Moreover, certain mutations that are associated with more aggressive cancers, bilateral disease spread, or metastasis may suggest patients may benefit from more extensive surgery. Molecular panels, including thyroid cancer genetic markers, were first introduced in the American Thyroid Association management guidelines in 2015.

Common Mutations

Prevalent mutations differ across the four types of thyroid cancers. While well-differentiated thyroid cancer (papillary and follicular) accounts for 90% of all cancers, medullary and anaplastic thyroid cancer can also be tested for through molecular testing [4]. The most commonly assessed genetic mutations are mentioned next.

Well-Differentiated Thyroid Cancer

One of the earliest genetic markers identified in thyroid cancer was the *BRAFV600E* mutation in papillary thyroid cancer. BRAF is a member of the RAF kinase family that regulates the RAS/MAPK signaling pathway, which regulate cell division and differentiation. This marker is highly specific, yet poorly sensitive, as it is found in <10% of indeterminate thyroid FNAs. Interestingly, this gene mutation was found to be associated with bilateral malignancy in patients with papillary thyroid cancer [3, 15].

Other known genetic causes of thyroid cancer include point mutations in *RAS, TERT* promoter, *RET, PIK3CA,* and *TP53* genes. Fusion genes *RET/PTC, PAX8/PPARγ,* and *NTRK* are also associated with the development of thyroid cancer. In particular, follicular adenomas and follicular variants of papillary thyroid cancer show overrepresentation of *PAX8/PPARγ* mutations [3, 15].

Importantly, certain gene combinations are more associated with thyroid cancer recurrence or lower life expectancy. A study published in 2014 noted that the presence of a BRAF or TERT mutation was associated with more than three times higher risk of recurrence. Patients with either mutation were found to have a lower life expectancy, with the lowest life expectancy found in patients with both mutations [16]. The co-occurrence of both mutations was associated with larger tumors as well as extrathyroidal or extranodal extension. An estimated 69% of patients had recurrent cancer [16]. Patients with these mutations may choose to have more extensive surgery.

Other important avenues of molecular diagnosis include the identification of microRNA (miRNAs), which function as gene regulators in controlling processes of cell growth, differentiation, and apoptosis. Specifically, miR-221 and 222 have been noted to be elevated in papillary thyroid cancer compared to benign tissue. miRNA-146 has also been noted to be overexpressed in most studies, while miRNA-138, 345, and 130b were downregulated in several studies [17].

Medullary

Medullary thyroid cancer (MTC) is a neuroendocrine tumor that accounts for 3–5% of all thyroid cancers. The majority of MTCs are sporadic (75–80%), while the rest are familial cases caused by multiple endocrine neoplasia syndromes, usually MEN2a and MEN2b. Most cases of familial medullary thyroid cancer are caused by mutations of the *RET* oncogene, which is a tyrosine receptor kinase important in regulating cell proliferation and differentiation [18].

Diagnosis of MTC can often be challenging, as more than 50% of cases can be missed on FNA. One study noted that only 44% of MTCs were identified via cytology, while 26% had cytological diagnoses of AUS or follicular neoplasm [19]. As patients with MTC have poorer outcomes compared to those with well-differentiated thyroid cancer, appropriate preoperative identification is critical to ensure patients do not receive inappropriate de-escalation of surgery (i.e., observation or hemithyroidectomy). RNA-sequencing and molecular testing can appropriately augment preoperative assessment of MTCs [20].

Of *RET* mutations, the M918T mutation is the most typical of MEN2b syndrome and is associated with the development of aggressive disease at a young age with the worst prognosis; patients develop metastases within the first year of life [18, 21]. The most common mutation is C634R, which is also associated with an aggressive form of disease, where patients develop MTC before 10 and present with lymph node metastases after 14 years of age. Other mutations generally present with milder disease, with extended time until the presentation of medullary thyroid cancer [18, 21].

In sporadic cases of MTC, *RET* mutations are the most common drivers of malignancy and are similarly associated with increased risk of locoregional and distant metastasis. However, *RAS* mutations are also seen and are generally associated with improved clinical performance. *RAS* mutations are quoted as being present in 10–60% of *RET*-negative MTC. [18, 21] Importantly, many de novo germline RET mutations can be detected in sporadic MEN 2b and 2a patients, which illustrates the importance of genetic testing in all MTC patients [22].

Anaplastic

Anaplastic thyroid cancer (ATC) is the rarest form of thyroid cancer, accounting for 1–2% of cases. However, it is also associated with the poorest outcomes, with disease-specific mortality approaching 100%. The putative theory of the development of anaplastic cancer is the accumulation of additional mutations in well-differentiated thyroid cancer, causing increased disease aggressiveness [12].

As such, the most common mutation in ATC is *BRAF V600E*, the same as in well-differentiated thyroid cancer. *RAS* mutations are also commonly seen. In ATC, the presence of *P53* mutations has also been reported, as have gain-of-function mutations in *PIK3CA* and loss-of-function mutations in *PTEN* [23].

Commercially Available Assays

Testing for the most common genetic mutations has been commercialized by a few companies. Three are most commonly used in practice: ThyroSeq TSv3, Afirma Genome Sequencing Classifier (GSC), and ThyGeNEXT/ThyraMIR (MPTX) [24].

ThyroSeq

One commonly used molecular testing assay is ThyroSeq, most recently released in its third iteration. The ThyroSeq v3 is a DNA- and RNA-based next-generation sequencing assay that analyzes 112 genes. As described by Nikiforova et al., the new version diagnostic test was validated on a training set of 238 tissue samples and 175 FNA samples with final surgical pathology [25]. Mutations testing includes BRAF, RAS, TERT, and DICER1 mutations. Final diagnostic sensitivity was quoted to be 98% sensitivity, 81.8% specificity, and 90.9% accuracy for FNA samples [25]. A key point of differentiation between ThyroSeq version 3 and version 2 was improved testing performance in oncocytic thyroid nodules. The initial study by Nikiforova reported a sensitivity of 92.9% and specificity of 69.3% in oncocytic nodules [25].

Additional validation studies at other institutions in Bethesda III/IV nodules noted a positive predictive value of 66–78.2% and negative predictive value of 75.9–97% [26, 27]. Sensitivity was quoted to be 94%, whereas specificity was noted to be 82% [26, 27]. These independent validation studies also noted 100% risk of malignancy from nodules reported to have BRAFV600E mutations [26, 27]. RAS-like mutations were associated with a 77.5% risk of malignancy [27]. Interestingly, additional studies have noted that over 68% of patients with Bethesda class III and IV nodules were classified as negative by ThyroSeq, indicating a significant proportion of patients were spared from unnecessary surgery by using molecular testing [28].

Studies investigating accuracy of ThyroSeq testing in Bethesda V nodules noted that ThyroSeq showed a sensitivity of 89.6% and a specificity of 77.3%. Assuming a cancer prevalence of 50–75%, the negative predictive value was lower in the suspicious for malignancy category at 71.2–88.1%. The positive predictive value increased in a category with increased risk of malignancy, with a reported range of 79.8–92.2% [29].

Afirma Genomic Sequencing Classifier

The Afirma Genomic Sequencing Classifier (GSC) is an update of the Afirma Gene Expression Classifier (GEC), intended to improve sensitivity and positive predictive value. This test relies upon machine learning algorithms to interpret nuclear and mitochondrial RNA expression, RNA sequencing, and copy number analysis data to stratify FNA samples into high- and low-risk categories [24].

In the initial publication introducing the results of Afirma GSC, 183 patients with Bethesda class III and IV nodules were tested with both the previous GEC and the GSC. The GSC was reported to have sensitivity of 91%, specificity of 68%, negative predictive value (NPV) of 96%, and positive predictive value (PPV) of 47%. The GSC was noted to have significantly higher specificity than the GEC. [30]

In subsequent single-institution papers published from academic centers, the reported sensitivity was 100%, specificity was 92.6%, positive predictive value was 57.1–60%, and negative predictive value was 100%. The benign call rate was noted to be 81% in Bethesda class III nodules, while it was 78.9% in follicular neoplasm nodules [31, 32]. Benign call rate was noted to be 61–68.2% in the GSC [32–34]. Notably, these studies found that the benign call rate was significantly higher in the GSC compared to the GEC in the AUS FNA category [32–34].

Meta-analyses of the performance of Afirma GSC published from different institutions noted that the benign call rate of Hurthle cell nodules was elevated compared to the prior Afirma GEC, with 73.7% BCR reported. Two meta-analyses noted greater than 90% of both sensitivity and negative predictive values of Afirma GSC [35, 36].

MPTX

The MPTX is a combination of ThyGeNEXT—a next-generation targeted DNA and RNA sequencing panel—and ThyraMIR, a microRNA risk classifier test. The genes examined in ThyGeNEXT include *BRAF, KRAS, NRAS, PIK3CA, PTEN, RET,* and *TERT*. The RNA panel assesses for mutations in *ALK, BRAF, PPARg, RET, THADA*, and presence of *PAX8*. ThyraMIR risk classification test detects expression changes of multiple promoter and suppressor miRNAs, including miR-29,155, 31, and 375 [24, 37].

Independent analysis of the MPTX has reported 95% sensitivity, 90% specificity, and 97% negative predictive value when the MPTX reported benign findings, and 75% positive predictive value when the results were findings concerning for malignancy [37]. Notably, in this study, NIFTP was combined with thyroid cancer as a diagnostic group. As such, the MPTX was effective at ruling out the possibility of cancer but was less effective as a "rule-in" test [37].

Notably, only 40% of tumors were proven to be cancer in patients with intermediate MPTX results. This is due in part to the presence of RAS mutations, which can also appear in benign adenomas that do not require surgery. Presence of RAS mutations can present a clinical challenge as the intermediate risk presented by these mutations (and subsequently reported in molecular testing) does not lend diagnostic clarity to patients [37, 38].

As reported by Lupo et al., the percentage of patients reported with positive, negative, and moderate MPTX results varies with the expected percentage malignancy—as it does with any of the genetic assays available [37]. In general, for the rate of 14% reported from Bethesda class III or IV nodules (AUS or FN), approximately 20% of MPTX results are expected to be positive, 20% intermediate, and 60% negative, suggesting that a significant proportion of patients may receive more definitive guidance from molecular testing [37].

Additional assessment of the accuracy of MPTX used in indeterminate thyroid nodules also noted that negative MPTX results predicted durable cancer-free status, where 94% of patients, regardless of whether they underwent surgery or not, remained disease-free [38]. While the MPTX was less accurate at predicting presence of cancer (high-risk results showed a 70% probability of malignancy), it offered more information than FNA and thyroid ultrasound alone [38]. [39]

Comparison of Molecular Testing Assays

A meta-analysis done by Lee et al. noted that, in Bethesda category III and IV patients, Afirma GSC and ThyroSeq v3 were noted to have particularly high sensitivity and NPV, but that no statistically significant difference existed between Afirma and ThyroSeq [39]. Individual studies vary in reporting of benign call rate, as well as reports of diagnostic statistics, including sensitivity, specificity, and predictive value [40–42].

Kandil et al. noted that Afirma GSC, with the addition of Xpression Atlas, an additional panel reporting on 761 genomic variants and 130 fusion pairs, outperformed both the ThyroSeq and MPTX cohorts in terms of PPV and NPV. This study also noted that this combination testing was able to decrease the rate of surgery by 75%. However, less data exists in the literature regarding the addition of Atlas to improve results, likely due to its infrequent clinical use [43].

An additional study by Şilaghi et al. stated that, after a meta-analysis of thyroid molecular testing studies, ThyroSeq v3 and Afirma GSC were superior to their earlier versions—namely, ThyroSeq v2 and Afirma GEC [44]. Additionally, this paper remarked that ThyroSeq v3 had superior "rule-in" abilities, or a lower positive likelihood ratio, compared to Afirma GSC. However, in these compiled studies, ThyroSeq v2 had the lowest negative likelihood ratio compared to both updated studies [44].

However, not all aspects of thyroid molecular testing have been optimized. Specifically, specificity in molecular testing has been reported to be around 40–60%, indicating that, even when positive, final diagnostic surgery may not show cancer [45]. Notably, one systematic review reported a specificity of 41% for ThyroSeq v3 and a specificity of 38% for Afirma GSC. Nevertheless, the high reported sensitivity of these tests of 92% for ThyroSeq and 94% for Afirma GSC reaffirms their clinical use, which is predominantly as a method of eliminating surgery as a necessity for patients [45].

Cost of Molecular Testing

Important in the consideration of the use of molecular testing is the additional cost burden associated with genetic send-out tests. In a study investigating the cost burden on reflexively ordering molecular testing for indiscriminate thyroid nodules, the authors estimated that each avoided surgery saved an estimated cost of $20,600 [46]. Given an average benign call rate of over 50%, this results in significant healthcare savings by reducing unnecessary surgery. As such, the relative amount saved with the ThyroSeq—or any molecular—testing is determined by the pricing of the assay [46]. Notably, molecular testing of FNA samples is not commonly used outside of the United States due to issues with insurance reimbursement [47, 48].

Another study investigating the cost-effectiveness of Afirma, utilizing the cost estimates based on medical reimbursements, noted that Afirma was less cost-effective than diagnostic thyroid lobectomy [49]. Though the upfront cost of surgery provided a higher cost to surgery at first, the repeated surveillance required for molecular testing posed a higher cumulative cost [49].

Conclusion

Uncertainty inherent in the workup of thyroid nodules can often lead to unnecessary or inappropriate treatment plans. This can occur both because masses that appear suspicious on FNA are benign or because high-risk tumor mutations are undertreated with thyroid lobectomy alone. Molecular testing with FNA can provide useful clinical information to bolster decision-making and guide intervention. The most commonly utilized commercially available assays—ThyroSeq v3, Afirma GSC, and MPTX—demonstrate a strong sensitivity and negative predictive value. These tests demonstrate benign call rates of greater than 50%, suggesting that many patients may avoid unnecessary diagnostic thyroidectomy. However, cost remains an important factor in considering whether routine use of molecular testing is necessary, as both the upfront cost of genetic testing assays and continued disease monitoring after a negative diagnosis on genetic testing may ultimately prove less cost-effective than surgery.

References

1. Bray BF, Laversanne M, Hyuna S, et al. Global cancer statistics 2022: GLOBOCAN estimates of incidence and mortality worldwide for 36 cancers in 185 countries. CA Cancer J Clin. 2024;74(3):229–63. https://doi.org/10.3322/CAAC.21834.
2. Lubitz CC, Sosa JA. The changing landscape of papillary thyroid cancer: epidemiology, management, and the implications for patients. Cancer. 2016;122(24):3754–9. https://doi.org/10.1002/CNCR.30201.
3. Ferrari SM, Fallahi P, Ruffilli I, et al. Molecular testing in the diagnosis of differentiated thyroid carcinomas. Gland Surg. 2018;7(Suppl 1):S19. https://doi.org/10.21037/GS.2017.11.07.
4. Chen DW, Lang BHH, McLeod DSA, Newbold K, Haymart MR. Thyroid cancer. Lancet. 2023;401(10387):1531–44. https://doi.org/10.1016/S0140-6736(23)00020-X.
5. Addasi N, Fingeret A, Goldner W. Hemithyroidectomy for thyroid cancer: a review. Medicina (B Aires). 2020;56(11):1–12. https://doi.org/10.3390/MEDICINA56110586.

6. Haugen BR, Alexander EK, Bible KC, et al. 2015 American Thyroid Association management guidelines for adult patients with thyroid nodules and differentiated thyroid cancer: the American Thyroid Association guidelines task force on thyroid nodules and differentiated thyroid cancer. Thyroid. 2016;26(1):1. https://doi.org/10.1089/THY.2015.0020.
7. Tessler FN, Middleton WD, Grant EG, et al. ACR thyroid imaging, reporting and data system (TI-RADS): white paper of the ACR TI-RADS Committee. J Am Coll Radiol. 2017;14(5):587–95. https://doi.org/10.1016/j.jacr.2017.01.046/asset/dbde62ac-462f-4718-b795-f58d5267276f/main.assets/figs3.jpg.
8. Dunya G, Dance L, Grimmer JF. Comparing ATA guidelines vs TI-RADS for evaluation of pediatric thyroid lesions. Int J Pediatr Otorhinolaryngol. 2023;164:111411. https://doi.org/10.1016/J.IJPORL.2022.111411.
9. Torshizian A, Hashemi F, Khoshhal N, et al. Diagnostic performance of ACR TI-RADS and ATA guidelines in the prediction of thyroid malignancy: a prospective single tertiary center study and literature review. Diagnostics. 2023;13(18) https://doi.org/10.3390/DIAGNOSTICS13182972.
10. Cibas ES, Ali SZ. The 2017 Bethesda system for reporting thyroid cytopathology. Thyroid. 2017;27(11):1341–6. https://doi.org/10.1089/THY.2017.0500.
11. Ali SZ, Baloch ZW, Cochand-Priollet B, Schmitt FC, Vielh P, Vanderlaan PA. The 2023 Bethesda system for reporting thyroid cytopathology. Thyroid. 2023;33(9):1039–44. https://doi.org/10.1089/THY.2023.0141.
12. Bible KC, Kebebew E, Brierley J, et al. American Thyroid Association Guidelines for Management of Patients with Anaplastic Thyroid Cancer: American Thyroid Association Anaplastic Thyroid Cancer Guidelines Task Force. Thyroid. 2021;31(3):337. https://doi.org/10.1089/THY.2020.0944.
13. Houdek D, Cooke-Hubley S, Puttagunta L, Morrish D. Factors affecting thyroid nodule fine needle aspiration non-diagnostic rates: a retrospective association study of 1975 thyroid biopsies. Thyroid Res. 2021;14(1) https://doi.org/10.1186/S13044-021-00093-2.
14. Strickland KC, Howitt BE, Marqusee E, et al. The impact of noninvasive follicular variant of papillary thyroid carcinoma on rates of malignancy for fine-needle aspiration diagnostic categories. Thyroid. 2015;25(9):987–92. https://doi.org/10.1089/THY.2014.0612.
15. Macerola E, Poma AM, Vignali P, et al. Molecular genetics of follicular-derived thyroid cancer. Cancers (Basel). 2021;13(5):1–12. https://doi.org/10.3390/CANCERS13051139.
16. Xing M, Liu R, Liu X, et al. BRAF V600E and TERT promoter mutations cooperatively identify the most aggressive papillary thyroid cancer with highest recurrence. J Clin Oncol. 2014;32(25):2718–26. https://doi.org/10.1200/JCO.2014.55.5094.
17. Celano M, Rosignolo F, Maggisano V, et al. MicroRNAs as biomarkers in thyroid carcinoma. Int J Genomics. 2017;2017 https://doi.org/10.1155/2017/6496570.
18. Pavlidis E, Sapalidis K, Chatzinikolaou F, Kesisoglou I. Medullary thyroid cancer: molecular factors, management and treatment. Romanian J Morphol Embryol. 2020;61(3):681. https://doi.org/10.47162/RJME.61.3.06.
19. Thomas CM, Asa SL, Ezzat S, Sawka AM, Goldstein D. Diagnosis and pathologic characteristics of medullary thyroid carcinoma—review of current guidelines. Curr Oncol. 2019;26(5):338. https://doi.org/10.3747/CO.26.5539.
20. Randolph GW, Maniar D. Medullary carcinoma of the thyroid. Cancer Control. 2000;7(3):253–61. https://doi.org/10.1177/107327480000700305.
21. Taccaliti A, Silvetti F, Palmonella G, Boscaro M. Genetic alterations in medullary thyroid cancer: diagnostic and prognostic markers. Curr Genomics. 2011;12(8):618–25. https://doi.org/10.2174/138920211798120835.
22. Younis E. Oncogenesis of Thyroid Cancer. Asian Pac J Cancer Prev. 2017;18(5):1191–9. https://doi.org/10.22034/APJCP.2017.18.5.1191.
23. Rashid M, Agarwal A, Pradhan R, et al. Genetic alterations in anaplastic thyroid carcinoma. Indian J Endocrinol Metab. 2019;23(4):480. https://doi.org/10.4103/IJEM.IJEM_321_19.

24. Patel J, Klopper J, Cottrill EE. Molecular diagnostics in the evaluation of thyroid nodules: current use and prospective opportunities. Front Endocrinol (Lausanne). 2023;14 https://doi.org/10.3389/FENDO.2023.1101410.
25. Nikiforova MN, Mercurio S, Wald AI, et al. Analytical performance of the ThyroSeq v3 genomic classifier for cancer diagnosis in thyroid nodules. Cancer. 2018;124(8):1682–90. https://doi.org/10.1002/CNCR.31245.
26. Nikiforov YE, Baloch ZW. Clinical validation of the ThyroSeq v3 genomic classifier in thyroid nodules with indeterminate FNA cytology. Cancer Cytopathol. 2019;127(4):225–30. https://doi.org/10.1002/CNCY.22112.
27. Sirotnikov S, Griffith CC, Lubin D, et al. ThyroSeq overview on indeterminate thyroid nodules: an institutional experience. Diagn Cytopathol. 2024;52(7):353–61. https://doi.org/10.1002/DC.25311.
28. Chiosea S, Hodak SP, Yip L, et al. Molecular profiling of 50 734 Bethesda III-VI thyroid nodules by ThyroSeq v3: implications for personalized management. J Clin Endocrinol Metab. 2023;108(11):2999–3008. https://doi.org/10.1210/CLINEM/DGAD220.
29. Skaugen JM, Taneja C, Liu JB, et al. Performance of a multigene genomic classifier in thyroid nodules with suspicious for malignancy cytology. Thyroid. 2022;32(12):1500–8. https://doi.org/10.1089/THY.2022.0282.
30. Patel KN, Angell TE, Babiarz J, et al. Performance of a genomic sequencing classifier for the preoperative diagnosis of Cytologically indeterminate thyroid nodules. JAMA Surg. 2018;153(9):817–24. https://doi.org/10.1001/JAMASURG.2018.1153.
31. Endo M, Nabhan F, Porter K, et al. Afirma gene sequencing classifier compared with gene expression classifier in indeterminate thyroid nodules. Thyroid. 2019;29(8):1115–24. https://doi.org/10.1089/THY.2018.0733/ASSET/IMAGES/LARGE/FIGURE3.JPEG.
32. Wei S, Veloski C, Sharda P, Ehya H. Performance of the Afirma genomic sequencing classifier versus gene expression classifier: an institutional experience. Cancer Cytopathol. 2019;127(11):720–4. https://doi.org/10.1002/CNCY.22188.
33. Geng Y, Aguilar-Jakthong JS, Moatamed NA. Comparison of Afirma gene expression classifier with gene sequencing classifier in indeterminate thyroid nodules: a single-institutional experience. Cytopathology. 2021;32(2):187–91. https://doi.org/10.1111/CYT.12920.
34. Angell TE, Heller HT, Cibas ES, et al. Independent comparison of the Afirma genomic sequencing classifier and gene expression classifier for Cytologically indeterminate thyroid nodules. Thyroid. 2019;29(5):650–6. https://doi.org/10.1089/THY.2018.0726.
35. Nasr CE, Andrioli M, Endo M, et al. Real-world performance of the Afirma genomic sequencing classifier (GSC)—a meta-analysis. J Clin Endocrinol Metab. 2023;108(6):1526–32. https://doi.org/10.1210/CLINEM/DGAC688.
36. Vuong HG, Nguyen TPX, Hassell LA, Jung CK. Diagnostic performances of the Afirma gene sequencing classifier in comparison with the gene expression classifier: a meta-analysis. Cancer Cytopathol. 2021;129(3):182–9. https://doi.org/10.1002/CNCY.22332.
37. Lupo MA, Walts AE, Sistrunk JW, et al. Multiplatform molecular test performance in indeterminate thyroid nodules. Diagn Cytopathol. 2020;48(12):1254–64. https://doi.org/10.1002/DC.24564.
38. Sistrunk JW, Shifrin A, Frager M, et al. Clinical performance of multiplatform mutation panel and microRNA risk classifier in indeterminate thyroid nodules. J Am Soc Cytopathol. 2020;9(4):232–41. https://doi.org/10.1016/J.JASC.2020.02.002.
39. Lee E, Terhaar S, McDaniel L, et al. Diagnostic performance of the second-generation molecular tests in the assessment of indeterminate thyroid nodules: a systematic review and meta-analysis. Am J Otolaryngol. 2022;43(3) https://doi.org/10.1016/J.AMJOTO.2022.103394.
40. Gortakowski M, Feghali K, Osakwe I. Single institution experience with Afirma and Thyroseq testing in indeterminate thyroid nodules. Thyroid. 2021;31(9):1376–82. https://doi.org/10.1089/THY.2020.0801.
41. Kim NE, Raghunathan RS, Hughes EG, et al. Bethesda III and IV thyroid nodules managed nonoperatively after molecular testing with Afirma GSC or Thyroseq v3. J Clin Endocrinol Metab. 2023;108(9):E698–703. https://doi.org/10.1210/CLINEM/DGAD181.

42. Jug RC, Datto MB, Sara JX. Molecular testing for indeterminate thyroid nodules: performance of the Afirma gene expression classifier and ThyroSeq panel. Cancer Cytopathol. 2018;126(7):471–80. https://doi.org/10.1002/CNCY.21993.
43. Kandil E, Metz TA, Issa PP, et al. Diagnostic performance of Afirma and Interpace diagnostics genetic testing in indeterminate thyroid nodules: a single center study. Cancers (Basel). 2023;15(7) https://doi.org/10.3390/CANCERS15072098.
44. Silaghi CA, Lozovanu V, Georgescu CE, et al. Thyroseq v3, Afirma GSC, and microRNA panels versus previous molecular tests in the preoperative diagnosis of indeterminate thyroid nodules: a systematic review and meta-analysis. Front Endocrinol (Lausanne). 2021;12 https://doi.org/10.3389/FENDO.2021.649522.
45. Digennaro C, Vahdatzad V, Jalali MS, et al. Assessing bias and limitations of clinical validation studies of molecular diagnostic tests for indeterminate thyroid nodules: systematic review and meta-analysis. Thyroid. 2022;32(10):1144–57. https://doi.org/10.1089/THY.2022.0269.
46. Dharampal N, Smith K, Harvey A, Paschke R, Rudmik L, Chandarana S. Cost-effectiveness analysis of molecular testing for cytologically indeterminate thyroid nodules. J Otolaryngol Head Neck Surg. 2022;51(1) https://doi.org/10.1186/S40463-022-00604-7.
47. Durante C, Hegedüs L, Czarniecka A, et al. 2023 European thyroid association clinical practice guidelines for thyroid nodule management. Eur Thyroid J. 2023;12(5) https://doi.org/10.1530/ETJ-23-0067.
48. Nishino M. Less is more meets do more with less: exploring differences in thyroid FNA molecular testing between Asian and Western practices. Cancer Cytopathol. 2023;131(7):421–3. https://doi.org/10.1002/CNCY.22700.
49. Balentine CJ, Vanness DJ, Schneider DF. Cost-effectiveness of lobectomy versus genetic testing (Afirma) for indeterminate thyroid nodules: considering the costs of surveillance. Surgery. 2018;163(1):88. https://doi.org/10.1016/J.SURG.2017.10.004.

Nonsurgical Approaches to the Thyroid Nodule

5

Likolani Arthurs and Kepal N. Patel

Editorial

Most thyroid nodules are benign and asymptomatic and are incidentally found on physical exam or imaging for an unrelated workup. Several studies have shown the efficacy of chemical and thermal ablation, with high success rates and a low complication profile.

Various sclerosing agents have been used to treat thyroid cysts with agents such as sodium tetradecyl sulfate, hydroxypolyethoxydodecan, tetracycline, or ethanol. The most recent guidelines from the American Thyroid Association recommend aspiration with or without ethanol ablation (EA) for large or symptomatic purely cystic thyroid nodules.

Ethanol acts by causing cellular dehydration and protein denaturation, which leads to necrosis, fibrosis, and small vessel thrombosis. Ethanol ablation (EA) can reduce the volume of completely cystic thyroid nodules by 72–95%, but is less successful with large cystic nodules, or those with a solid component.

EA has also been studied as a treatment for hyperfunctioning nodules. The size and functioning of these nodules have been shown to decrease after EA; however, increasing size hinders therapeutic effect.

Another minimally invasive treatment option is thermal ablation, which utilizes high temperatures to ablate the thyroid tissue. There are multiple forms of thermal ablation that deliver heat to thyroid nodules through different techniques, all leading to irreversible cellular damage, resulting in shrinkage of the nodule. Of the various forms of thermal ablation, laser ablation, microwave and radiofrequency ablation (RFA) are the most studied and most available.

L. Arthurs · K. N. Patel (✉)
Department of Surgery, Division of Endocrine Surgery, NYU Langone Health, New York, NY, USA
e-mail: Likolani.arthurs@nyulangone.org; Kepal.Patel@nyulangone.org

P. S. Pai et al. (eds.), *Controversies in Cancer of the Thyroid and Parathyroid Glands*, https://doi.org/10.1007/978-3-032-13130-0_5

A single radiofrequency ablation (RFA) session has been shown to adequately achieve the desired volume reduction in benign thyroid disease of less than 20 mL. For larger nodules (greater than 20 mL), multiple RFA sessions may be needed to achieve peak volume reduction. Regardless of the number of RFA sessions, there can be significant volume reduction (50–80%) within the first 6–12 months of treatment in nonfunctioning thyroid nodules. Long-lasting nodule volume reduction (67–93.4%), along with improvement in compressive symptoms, has been seen when followed at 2-, 4-, and 5-year post treatment. The reported low recurrence rate of 4.1–5.6% appears to be due to regrowth from undertreated peripheral margins. Currently, there are little data on the role of RFA for the curative treatment of primary malignant disease greater than 1 cm.

Christopher de Souza

Introduction

Over the last two decades, the incidence of thyroid cancer in the United States has increased from 7.7 to 13.6/100,000 from 2000 to 2021, while over the same time period, the age-adjusted mortality rate has remained unchanged at 0.5/100,000 [1]. A partial explanation for this increased incidence is the increased use of imaging, resulting in increased discovery of incidental thyroid nodules [2]. Up to 90% of these incidentally found nodules are benign, and the majority are asymptomatic [3]. The management of these incidental thyroid nodules is controversial [4]. Although surgery remains the gold standard for treating symptomatic benign and malignant thyroid nodules, chemical and thermal percutaneous ablation techniques have emerged as promising outpatient minimally invasive procedures for treating select patients with thyroid nodules [5]. Percutaneous treatment options are appealing for those unable or unwilling to undergo surgery. These interventional procedures are low risk and often performed with only local anesthesia or sedation [6].

Chemical Ablation

Various sclerosing agents have been trialed to treat thyroid cysts, such as sodium tetradecyl sulfate, hydroxypolyethoxydodecan, tetracycline, or ethanol [7]. The most recent guidelines from the American Thyroid Association recommend aspiration with or without ethanol ablation (EA) for large or symptomatic purely cystic thyroid nodules [8]. First performed in 1985, injection of ethanol as a sclerosing agent into thyroid cysts causes volume reduction and prevents recurrence [9, 10]. Ethanol acts by causing cellular dehydration and protein denaturation, leading to necrosis, fibrosis, and small vessel thrombosis [11]. EA can reduce the volume of completely cystic thyroid nodules by 72–95% [12], but is less successful with large cystic nodules, or those with a solid component [12, 13]. EA has also been studied as a treatment for hyperfunctioning nodules [9]. Both size and function of these nodules have been shown to decrease after EA [11]; however, increasing size hinders therapeutic effect [14, 15]. Evidence is lacking for the use of EA to treat primary thyroid cancer [9]. It has been proposed as a treatment strategy for recurrent thyroid carcinoma. Though surgery is the primary treatment strategy for locally recurrent thyroid cancer, if surgical resection is not possible for various reasons, ablation can be an alternative. EA may be recommended for select patients with recurrent disease or for palliative management in patients who have distant metastasis [9].

Thermal Ablation

Another minimally invasive treatment option is thermal ablation that utilizes high temperatures to ablate the thyroid tissue. There are multiple forms of thermal ablation that deliver heat to thyroid nodules through different techniques, all leading to irreversible cellular damage, resulting in the shrinkage of the nodule. Of the various forms of thermal ablation, laser ablation, microwave, and radiofrequency ablation (RFA) are the most studied and most available [15].

First described as an alternative treatment for nonfunctional, benign thyroid nodules, RFA has also been studied as a potential treatment for autonomously functioning thyroid nodules (AFTNs) [16–18], primary differentiated thyroid microcarcinomas [19–21], and recurrent well-differentiated thyroid carcinoma (WDTC) [22–26].

RFA for Benign Nonfunctional Nodules

A single RFA session has been shown to adequately achieve the desired volume reduction in benign thyroid disease of less than 20 mL. For larger nodules (greater than 20 mL), multiple RFA sessions may be needed to achieve peak volume reduction [27]. Regardless of the number of RFA sessions, there can be significant volume reduction (50–80%) within the first 6–12 months of treatment in nonfunctioning thyroid nodules [17, 25, 28–30]. Long-lasting nodule volume reduction (67–93.4%), along with improvement in compressive symptoms, has been seen when followed at 2-, 4-, and 5-year post treatment. The reported low recurrence rate of 4.1–5.6% appears to be due to regrowth from undertreated peripheral margins [17, 29, 31, 32].

When compared to thyroidectomy, RFA results in similar symptom improvement, but lower incidences of hoarseness, hypothyroidism, pain, and hospitalization time [33]. Those treated with RFA also have higher thyroid-specific QoL, total social well-being, and total psychological well-being scores and are more likely to recommend thermal ablation than those who underwent thyroidectomy [34].

RFA for AFTN

For those patients unable to undergo surgery or who have contraindications to radioactive iodine [11] therapy, RFA may be a treatment option for AFTN. RFA had similar nodule volume reduction rates, similar rates of euthyroid restoration, and decreased rates of clinical hypothyroidism (0% vs. 20%, $P < 0.05$) compared to a fixed dose of RAI (15 mCi of ^{131}I) [35]. RFA can also result in significant AFTN volume reduction (50–86%) [16–18, 36]. However, a wide range of hormonal normalization rates have been seen after RFA treatment for AFTN and is hypothesized to be due to incomplete ablation of possibly functional nodule margins. It remains unclear whether preoperative nodule volume size is associated with successful achievement of euthyroid state after RFA [32, 36, 37]. Due to the variable response rates in treating AFTN, current guidelines cautiously recommend RFA as a therapeutic alternative when first-line therapies (RAI or surgery) are contraindicated. While there are no definitive size cutoffs, all recommendations specifically acknowledge that RFA may be less effective in large AFTNs.

RFA for Malignant Nodules

Currently, there are little data on the role of RFA for the curative treatment of primary malignant disease greater than 1 cm. However, if the treatment intent is palliative, patients with larger tumors may be candidates for RFA to relieve compressive symptoms [6]. For patients with papillary thyroid microcarcinomas (PTMCs), defined as papillary thyroid carcinoma less than 1 cm, without clinical evidence of unfavorable features (proximity to trachea/recurrent laryngeal nerve, clinical nodal disease or high-grade "suspicious" features on biopsy), "active surveillance," where patients are serially monitored with US for progression of disease, is a viable option [38, 39]. RFA has been studied as an alternative option, showing promising results. Complete resolution of PTMC has been shown in 79–100% of patients treated with RFA with only rare complications [20, 21]. Currently, both the Task Force Committee of the Korean Society of Thyroid Radiology RFA guidelines [40] and an international multidisciplinary consensus statement [6] cautiously recommend RFA as a treatment strategy in well-selected patients with low-risk PTMC who refuse or are otherwise unfit to undergo surgery and do not want to undergo active surveillance. Additionally, the international consensus statement [6] specifies that primary PTMC candidates must be (i) unifocal and confined to the thyroid gland, (ii) cytologically confirmed to be malignant without aggressive subtype, and (III) without evidence of metastatic lymphadenopathy.

Similar to primary PTMC, studies have suggested that RFA may have a role as an interventional treatment option in patients with local regional recurrences of WDTC. When a locally recurrent disease is identified, resection with RAI remains the standard of care. However, studies have shown that RFA can lead to ultrasonographic and/or repeat FNA disappearance or significant volume reduction of recurrent tumor burden [22–24].

When retrospectively compared to surgery, RFA has shown comparable 3-year recurrence-free rates (92.2% vs 92.6%, respectively) in patients with recurrent WDTC less than 2 cm [24]. RFA may have a role in recurrent disease even if radiological complete ablation is not possible as symptom relief can be achieved with volume reduction [41]. Current recommendations agree that RFA may be considered in well-selected patients with recurrent WDTC who are not amenable to or unable to tolerate surgery [6, 40, 42]. However, when considering RFA for recurrent disease, the treatment intent needs to be discussed with the patient in order to set clear expectations [6]. For those hoping for curative outcome, patients with small lesions (less than 2 cm) confined to the neck are ideal candidates, while a palliative strategy may be more amenable for patients with larger lesions.

Summary

Both chemical and thermal ablation techniques provide a good alternative treatment for thyroid nodules when surgery is not an option. EA is a safe and effective treatment strategy for cystic nodules of the thyroid, while RFA has been shown to result in consistent volume reduction and improvement in symptoms for those with benign thyroid nodules. With growing evidence to support the use of these minimally invasive techniques, societal and international guidelines and consensus statements agree that both chemical and thermal ablation can be viable options for select patients. Although surgery remains the standard treatment for those with index and/or recurrent malignant disease, ablation may have a therapeutic and palliative role in patients who decline or are not surgical candidates.

References

1. SEER*Explorer: an interactive website for SEER cancer statistics [internet]. Surveillance Research Program, National Cancer Institute; 2024.
2. Jin J, McHenry CR. Thyroid incidentaloma. Best Pract Res Clin Endocrinol Metab. 2012;
3. Durante C, et al. The diagnosis and management of thyroid nodules: a review. JAMA. 2018;319(9):914–24.
4. Dean DS, Gharib H. Epidemiology of thyroid nodules. Best Pract Res Clin Endocrinol Metab. 2008;22(6):901–11.
5. Lui MS, Patel KN. Current guidelines for the application of radiofrequency ablation for thyroid nodules: a narrative review. Gland Surg. 2023;13(1):59–69.
6. Orloff LA, et al. Radiofrequency ablation and related ultrasound-guided ablation technologies for treatment of benign and malignant thyroid disease: an international multidisciplinary consensus statement of the American Head and Neck Society Endocrine Surgery Section with the Asia Pacific Society of Thyroid Surgery, Associazione Medici Endocrinologi, British Association of Endocrine and Thyroid Surgeons, European Thyroid Association, Italian Society of Endocrine Surgery Units, Korean Society of Thyroid Radiology, Latin American Thyroid Society, and Thyroid Nodules Therapies Association. Head Neck. 2022;44(3):633–60.
7. Kanotra SP, Lateef M, Kirmani O. Non-surgical management of benign thyroid cysts: use of ultrasound-guided ethanol ablation. Postgrad Med J. 2008;84(998):639–43.

8. Haugen BR, et al. 2015 American Thyroid Association Management Guidelines for Adult Patients with Thyroid Nodules and Differentiated Thyroid Cancer: The American Thyroid Association Guidelines Task Force on Thyroid Nodules and Differentiated Thyroid Cancer. Thyroid. 2016;26(1):1–133.
9. Hahn SY, et al. Ethanol ablation of the thyroid nodules: 2018 consensus statement by the Korean Society of Thyroid Radiology. Korean J Radiol. 2019;20(4):609–20.
10. Rozman B, B.Z., Tomicbrzac H, Skreb F, Pavlinovic Z, Simonovic I. Sclerosation of thyroid cysts by ethanol. 1990;91:453.
11. Livraghi T, et al. Treatment of autonomous thyroid nodules with percutaneous ethanol injection: preliminary results. Work in progress. Radiology. 1990;175(3):827–9.
12. Bennedbaek FN, Hegedus L. Treatment of recurrent thyroid cysts with ethanol: a randomized double-blind controlled trial. J Clin Endocrinol Metab. 2003;88(12):5773–7.
13. Jang SW, Baek JH, Kim JK, et al. How to manage the patients with unsatisfactory results after ethanol ablation for thyroid nodules: role of radiofrequency ablation. Eur J Radiol. 2012;81(5):905–10.
14. Di Lelio A, et al. Treatment of autonomous thyroid nodules: value of percutaneous ethanol injection. AJR Am J Roentgenol. 1995;164(1):207–13.
15. Papini E, et al. 2020 European thyroid association clinical practice guideline for the use of image-guided ablation in benign thyroid nodules. Eur Thyroid J. 2020;9(4):172–85.
16. Baek JH, et al. Radiofrequency ablation for the treatment of autonomously functioning thyroid nodules. World J Surg. 2009;33(9):1971–7.
17. Deandrea M, et al. US-guided percutaneous radiofrequency thermal ablation for the treatment of solid benign hyperfunctioning or compressive thyroid nodules. Ultrasound Med Biol. 2008;34(5):784–91.
18. Cesareo R, et al. Efficacy of radiofrequency ablation in autonomous functioning thyroid nodules. A systematic review and meta-analysis. Rev Endocr Metab Disord. 2019;20(1):37–44.
19. Kim JH, et al. Radiofrequency ablation of low-risk small papillary thyroidcarcinoma: preliminary results for patients ineligible for surgery. Int J Hyperth. 2017;33(2):212–9.
20. Lim HK, et al. US-guided radiofrequency ablation for low-risk papillary thyroid microcarcinoma: efficacy and safety in a large population. Korean J Radiol. 2019;20(12):1653–61.
21. Cho SJ, et al. Long-term follow-up results of ultrasound-guided radiofrequency ablation for low-risk papillary thyroid microcarcinoma: more than 5-year follow-up for 84 tumors. Thyroid. 2020;30(12):1745–51.
22. Dupuy DE, et al. Radiofrequency ablation of regional recurrence from well-differentiated thyroid malignancy. Surgery. 2001;130(6):971–7.
23. Baek JH, et al. Locoregional control of metastatic well-differentiated thyroid cancer by ultrasound-guided radiofrequency ablation. AJR Am J Roentgenol. 2011;197(2):W331–6.
24. Kim JH, Yoo WS, Park YJ, et al. Efficacy and safety of radiofrequency ablation for treatment of locally recurrent thyroid cancers smaller than 2 cm. Radiology. 2015;276:909–18.
25. Kim YS, et al. Radiofrequency ablation of benign cold thyroid nodules: initial clinical experience. Thyroid. 2006;16(4):361–7.
26. Ha EJ, et al. Radiofrequency ablation of benign thyroid nodules: recommendations from the Asian Conference on Tumor Ablation Task Force. Ultrasonography. 2021;40(1):75–82.
27. Huh JY, et al. Symptomatic benign thyroid nodules: efficacy of additional radiofrequency ablation treatment session--prospective randomized study. Radiology. 2012;263(3):909–16.
28. Jeong WK, et al. Radiofrequency ablation of benign thyroid nodules: safety and imaging follow-up in 236 patients. Eur Radiol. 2008;18(6):1244–50.
29. Spiezia S, et al. Thyroid nodules and related symptoms are stably controlled two years after radiofrequency thermal ablation. Thyroid. 2009;19(3):219–25.
30. Jung SL, et al. Efficacy and safety of radiofrequency ablation for benign thyroid nodules: a prospective multicenter study. Korean J Radiol. 2018;19(1):167–74.
31. Lim HK, et al. Radiofrequency ablation of benign non-functioning thyroid nodules: 4-year follow-up results for 111 patients. Eur Radiol. 2013;23(4):1044–9.

32. Bernardi S, et al. 12-month efficacy of a single radiofrequency ablation on autonomously functioning thyroid nodules. Endocrine. 2017;57(3):402–8.
33. Guan SH, Wang H, Teng DK. Comparison of ultrasound-guided thermal ablation and conventional thyroidectomy for benign thyroid nodules: a systematic review and meta-analysis. Int J Hyperth. 2020;37(1):442–9.
34. Jin H, et al. Conventional thyroidectomy vs thyroid thermal ablation on postoperative quality of life and satisfaction for patients with benign thyroid nodules. Eur J Endocrinol. 2021;184(1):131–41.
35. Cervelli R, Mazzeo S, Boni G, et al. Comparison between radioiodine therapy and single-session radiofrequency ablation of autonomously functioning thyroid nodules: a retrospective study. Clin Endocrinol. 2019;90:608–16.
36. Cesareo R, Naciu A, Iozzino M, et al. Nodule size as predictive factor of efficacy of radiofrequency ablation in treating autonomously functioning thyroid nodules. Int J Hyperth. 2018;34:617–23.
37. Kim HJ, et al. Efficacy and safety of thermal ablation for autonomously functioning thyroid nodules: a systematic review and meta-analysis. Eur Radiol. 2021;31(2):605–15.
38. Ito Y, Uruno T, Nakano K, et al. An observation trial without surgical treatment in patients with papillary microcarcinoma of the thyroid. Thyroid. 2003;13:381–7.
39. Ito Y, et al. An observational trial for papillary thyroid microcarcinoma in Japanese patients. World J Surg. 2010;34(1):28–35.
40. Kim JH, B.J., Lim HK, et al. 2017 Thyroid radiofrequency ablation guideline: Korean Society of Thyroid Radiology. Korean J Radiol. 2018;19:632–55.
41. Park KW, et al. Inoperable symptomatic recurrent thyroid cancers: preliminary result of radiofrequency ablation. Ann Surg Oncol. 2011;18(9):2564–8.
42. Dietrich CF, Müller T, Bojunga J, et al. Statement and recommendations on interventional ultrasound as a thyroid diagnostic and treatment procedure. Ultrasound Med Biol. 2018;44:14–36.

Active Surveillance for Low-Risk Papillary Thyroid Microcarcinoma

6

Yasuhiro Ito, Akira Miyauchi, and Makoto Fujishima

Editorial

Ito, Miyauchi, and Fujishima have done a fantastic job on their approach to active surveillance for papillary microcarcinoma. Akira Miyauchi was the earliest to consider active surveillance for microcarcinoma in Kobe, Japan. The incentive for this was the commonality of papillary microcarcinoma in the general population and slow growth of these tumors. Their experience now extends to over 2000 patients. Similar studies have been undertaken in Korea and the United States. Even though the authors have used 1 cm as the arbitrary cutoff, Tuttle et al. have used 1.5 cm, and researchers at UCLA are using 2 cm. The results of active surveillance are quite promising, and as described by the authors, the increase in the size of the tumor under active surveillance is 5–10%, while the risk of developing nodal metastasis is 2–3%. It is important for the patient and the family to understand the reasoning behind active surveillance and the risk and complications of surgical intervention. It does require an excellent team of physicians to undertake active surveillance, which generally involves ultrasound at the interval of 6 months and detailed discussion with the patient and the family.

The location of the tumor is very critical, especially tumors against the trachea or posterior capsule. The tumor volume may be a better parameter than the size alone. The understanding of the patient's minimalist or maximalist approach is very critical in the decision-making process, and it requires a team-based approach with a surgeon, endocrinologist, and devoted radiologist. Patients can be divided into ideal, appropriate, and inappropriate for active surveillance. The patients need to be aware of the rising incidence of microcarcinoma with no impact on long-term survival. In certain

Y. Ito (✉) · A. Miyauchi · M. Fujishima
Department of Surgery, Kuma Hospital, Kobe, Hyogo, Japan
e-mail: ito01@kuma-h.or.jp; miyauchi@kuma-h.or.jp; fujishima@kuma-h.or.jp

P. S. Pai et al. (eds.), *Controversies in Cancer of the Thyroid and Parathyroid Glands*, https://doi.org/10.1007/978-3-032-13130-0_6

select patients, especially in older individuals or in patients with high-risk comorbidities, we have used active surveillance even in patients presenting with limited nodal metastasis. I am sure many other institutions will adopt this approach and consider active surveillance in the management schema of micropapillary carcinoma.

Ashok R Shaha

History of Active Surveillance for Papillary Thyroid Microcarcinoma

Low-risk papillary thyroid microcarcinoma (PTMC) is cT1aN0M0 papillary thyroid carcinoma (PTC) with a ≤10-mm maximum diameter, no invasion to the adjacent organs, and no clinical node metastasis or distant metastasis on imaging studies. PTMC was originally identified in autopsy studies as a latent carcinoma or was occasionally detected by a pathological examination for thyroid specimens dissected for thyroid disease other than thyroid carcinoma as an incidental carcinoma. However, the development of ultrasound technology and ultrasound-guided fine-needle aspiration cytology (FNAC) enabled clinicians to detect PTMC much more easily.

Many autopsy studies of individuals who died of nonthyroid diseases have indicated that the incidence of latent PTMCs ≥3 mm was as high as 5.2%, which was >1000 times the prevalence of clinical thyroid carcinoma in Japanese women at that time [1]. Takebe et al. reported that as much as 3.5% of otherwise healthy women had thyroid carcinoma (cytologically diagnosed), and ~75% of the tumors were ≤15 mm in size [2]. These findings suggested that (i) a majority of PTMC cases remain asymptomatic and stable, and (ii) a very small percentage of cases progress and become a clinical problem. Performing surgery for all patients with PTMC would thus result in more harm than good.

With these considerations, in 1993, Dr. Akira Miyauchi proposed active surveillance (AS) management for PTMC at a medical meeting at Kuma Hospital (Kobe, Japan) [1]. He thought that since only a small percentage of patients experience progression of the disease, surgery for only those patients would be sufficiently effective. A prospective clinical trial of AS for patients with PTMC was thus initiated at Kuma Hospital for the first time worldwide. Dr. Miyauchi suspected that progressive cases could be identified during AS by ultrasound and that conversion surgery (CS) at the time of slight disease progression would be a safe and appropriate management for PTMC [1]. At that time and even today, no markers suggestive of the growth of PTMC have been identified. In 1995, the Cancer Institute Hospital (CIH; Tokyo) also started AS for patients with PTMC based on a concept that is similar to that applied by Kuma Hospital.

Active surveillance was adopted as a management option in the guidelines issued by the Japan Association of Endocrine Surgeons/Japanese Association of Thyroid Surgery (presently the Japan Association of Endocrine Surgery) in 2010, 2018, and 2024 [3–5], and the recommended grade of AS has become stronger with time. The 2015 American Thyroid Association (ATA) management guidelines for adult patients with thyroid nodules and differentiated thyroid cancer stated that AS may be considered [6]. Thereafter, prospective and retrospective studies from Japan and other countries have been published, and consensus statements and a position paper issued by the Japan Association of Endocrine Surgeons and the Japan Thyroid Association, respectively, have described the safe implementation of AS [7, 8].

Wide Disparities in Thyroid Cancer Incidence and Mortality

A rapid increase in the incidence of thyroid carcinoma over time with a stable thyroid cancer mortality rate has been reported around the world. Two reports from the United States stated that the incidence of thyroid carcinoma increased by 2.4-fold between 1973 and 2002 and by 2.9-fold between 1975 and 2009, while the thyroid cancer mortality rate over those years has remained stable [9, 10]. This increased incidence of thyroid carcinoma was due mainly to the increase in the incidence of small PTC, that is, those ≤20 mm (including PTMC). A study from South Korea demonstrated that the incidence of thyroid carcinoma in that country and increased 15-fold between 1993 and 2011 with a stable mortality rate, based on thyroid screening using ultrasound as a national policy [11]. That study also noted that the incidences of patients who acquired hypoparathyroidism and vocal cord paralysis were increased, confirming the possibility that surgery for these cancers resulted in more harm than good, as alluded to by Dr. Miyauchi. Similar findings have been obtained in Italy, France, England, Scotland, Australia, Spain, and Nordic countries [9, 12]. These increases in the identification of thyroid carcinoma occurred because of the eventual widespread availability of ultrasound and ultrasound-guided FNAC, revealing the unnecessary surgical treatment for harmless small carcinomas.

The Clinical Practice of Active Surveillance for PTMC

Case Selection

We must note that not all PTMCs are suitable for AS. Of course, tumors that have high-risk features such as clinical node metastasis (or, although rare, distant metastasis) or aggressive cytology (also very rare) are strong candidates for immediate surgery (IS). Patients who have recurrent laryngeal nerve paralysis due to tumor invasion and patients whose tumors invade the trachea should undergo IS. No evidence is available regarding the effectiveness of active surveillance for PTMCs among patients <20 years old.

In addition to the abovementioned factors, the tumor's location is important in decisions regarding the management strategy. A solitary tumor with no possibility of invasion to extrathyroidal organs is ideal for AS (Fig. 6.1a). At our institution, we do not exclude multiple tumors (Fig. 6.1b) or tumors suspected of invasion to the ventral thyroid capsule (Fig. 6.1c) as candidates for AS. Multiple PTMCs are not necessarily associated with disease progression (as described below), and if immediate surgery is

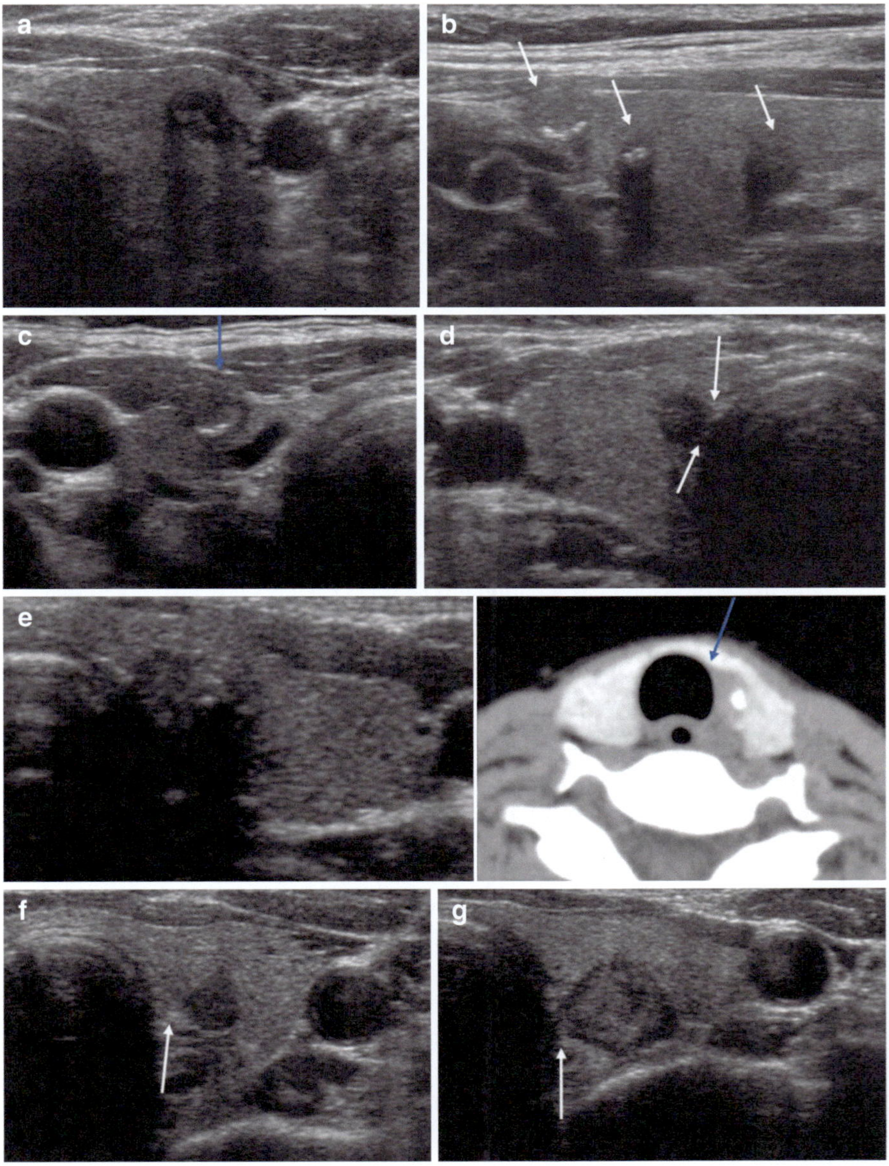

Fig. 6.1 (**a**) A solitary papillary thyroid microcarcinoma (PTMC) buried in the thyroid (ideal). (**b**) Multiple PTMCs in thyroid tissue (see *arrows*) (appropriate). (**c**) PTMC suspected of anterior invasion (appropriate). (**d**) PTMC attached to the trachea with an acute angle (*arrows*) (appropriate). (**e**) PTMC attached to the trachea with an obtuse angle (*arrow*) (inappropriate). For this case, a CT examination was better for the evaluation than ultrasound. (**f**) PTMC located at the dorsal side but with normal thyroid tissue (*arrow*) along the course of the recurrent laryngeal nerve (appropriate). (**g**) PTMC located at the dorsal side, without normal thyroid tissue along the course of the recurrent laryngeal nerve (inappropriate). (Cited from Ref. [13] with permission)

being considered for patients with multiple PTMCs, a total thyroidectomy would be necessary, resulting in a higher incidence of surgical complications.

For tumors attached to the trachea, the angle between the tumor and the trachea is a deciding factor regarding whether the tumor is suitable for AS or IS [13]. As shown in Fig. 6.1e, a tumor forming an obtuse angle between its surface and tracheal cartilage is an IS candidate as it has been reported that 24% of such tumors ≥7 mm had tracheal invasion requiring the dissection of tracheal cartilage or the whole thickness of the trachea for curative surgery [14]. None of the tumors showing acute angles or right angles showed tracheal invasion on intraoperative findings (Fig. 6.1d). Ito et al. also proposed a simple technique for deciding the application of AS for PTMCs located at the dorsal side of the trachea. The presence of normal thyroid tissue between the tumor and the course of the recurrent laryngeal nerve indicates that no risk of the tumor invading the recurrent laryngeal nerve is present (Fig. 6.1f). However, the tumor in Fig. 6.1g was at risk of invading the recurrent laryngeal nerve because the presence of normal thyroid tissue between the tumor and the course of the recurrent laryngeal nerve was not detected; according to Ito's data, 9.2% of such tumors ≥7 mm exhibited recurrent laryngeal nerve invasion requiring a partial layer resection or nerve resection with nerve reconstruction [14].

Cytological Examination

The ATA guidelines do not recommend a cytological examination for tumors ≤10 mm unless the patient has malignant findings such as clinical node metastasis or distant metastasis [15]. However, this policy might be based on our AS data. When we initiated the world's first AS trial, there were no guidelines about performing FNAC for thyroid nodules. If we did not perform FNAC for small suspicious nodules, those patients might have visited other hospitals, undergone a cytological examination, and been told, "You have thyroid cancer. Kuma Hospital failed to diagnose the cancer. You should undergo surgery immediately." This would be an unpleasant situation for both the patient and our hospital. Since 2015, we have performed a cytological examination for suspicious nodules ≥5 mm in accordance with the guidelines of the Japan Association of Breast and Thyroid Sonology.

Implementation of AS

In the early period of our AS clinical trial, we presented two options (AS and IS) almost equally to the patients who were diagnosed with PTMCs that are suitable for AS. However, with the accumulation of favorable outcomes of AS, we gradually shifted to the recommendation of AS in such cases. At present, we recommend AS as the initial management. Our institution does not use a chest CT scan or other imaging studies to determine whether patients have any distant metastasis. Kawano et al. reported that none of their 1000 consecutive PTMC patients who underwent a chest CT scan before surgery showed metastatic lesions of PTC in the lung [16]. As the sites of PTC metastasis, the lung is the most common site after the cervical lymph nodes; other sites are rare. We thus do not consider a systemic examination for distant metastasis necessary before the initiation of AS.

After their first checkup at our hospital, patients with PTMC who have agreed to undergo AS rather than IS are advised to return 6 months later and at least once a year thereafter [5] for an investigation of whether the size of their tumor(s) had increased and whether new suspicious nodes have appeared. Tumors that have enlarged by ≥3 mm compared to the size at the initiation of AS are regarded as "enlargement," but their AS may be continued until the tumor(s) reach 13 mm in size if the patient prefers to remain under AS. When suspicious nodes appear, a cytological examination with thyroglobulin measurement using the washout of the cytology needles is performed. If the nodes are diagnosed as metastasis, the patient is advised to undergo conversion surgery (CS).

Outcomes of AS in Prospective Studies

Outcomes of Patients Under AS in Japan

Table 6.1 summarizes the outcomes of PTMC patients who underwent AS in representative prospective studies. Retrospective studies of "passive surveillance" performed for patients whose cases are associated with other illnesses precluding immediate surgery are not listed in the table. The first study enrolling 162 patients from Kuma Hospital was published in 2003, reporting that the enlargement rate was 10.2% and the novel node metastasis appearance rate was 1.2% [17]. The second report obtained a 10-year enlargement rate at 15.9% and a 3.4% 10-year node metastasis appearance rate [18]. The most recent study published in 2023 demonstrated much better outcomes: 10- and 20-year enlargement rates at 4.7% and 6.6% and node metastasis appearance rates at 1.0% and 1.6%, respectively [21], which were based on an increased number of enrolled patients.

The Cancer Institute Hospital/Nippon Medical School (CIH/NMS) reported that 7% of PTMCs enlarged and 1% of these cases also showed newly appeared node metastasis [20]. They thereafter published some studies in this subject [22–24]. According to the most recent CIH/NMS report, the 10- and 20-year enlargement rates were 9.9% and 18.0% and the node metastasis appearance rates were 1.4% and 3.9%, respectively [24]. Kuma Hospital reported that one patient who underwent CS (by the patient's preference) after AS and another who chose IS exhibited lung metastasis during postoperative follow-up [21]. However, to date, none of these patients showed distant metastasis during AS or died of thyroid carcinoma.

Outcomes of Patients under AS in Countries Other than Japan

Several institutions in countries other than Japan have performed prospective studies of AS, and their data are favorable overall [25–30] (Table 6.1). However, there are considerable differences in the methods used to evaluate tumor enlargement

Table 6.1 Results of prospective studies of active surveillance (AS) for small papillary thyroid carcinomas (PTCs)

Authors (location) [Ref.]	No. of patients (tumors)	AS period	Definition of enlargement	Enlargement rate	Node metastasis appearance rate	Predictors of tumor enlargement	Predictors of node metastasis appearance
Kuma Hospital (Kobe, Japan) 2003 [17]	162 pts with PTMC	18–113 mos. (avg. 46.5 mos.)	Size increase ≥3 mm	10.2%	1.2%	Not listed	Not listed
Kuma Hospital (Kobe, Japan) 2010 [18]	340 pts with PTMC	18–187 mos. (avg. 74 mos.)	Size increase ≥3 mm	5-yr 6.4% 10-yr 15.9%	5-yr 1.4% 10-yr 3.4%	Not listed	Not listed
Kuma Hospital (Kobe, Japan) 2014 [19]	1235 pts with PTMC	18–227 mos. (avg. 60 mos.)	Size increase ≥3 mm	5-yr 4.9% 10-yr 8.0%	5-yr 1.7% 10-yr 3.9%	Age <40 yrs	Age <40 yrs
Kuma Hospital (Kobe, Japan) 2023 [20]	2705 pts with PTMC	1–15.7 yrs (median 5.5 yrs)	Size increase ≥3 mm	5-yr 3.0% 10-yr 5.5% 15-yr 6.2%	5-yr 0.9% 10-yr 1.1% 15-yr 1.1%	Age <40 yrs, high TSH level, tumor size ≥9 mm	Age <40 yrs, male sex
Kuma Hospital (Kobe, Japan) 2023 [21]	3222 pts with PTMC	1–29.3 yrs (median 7.3 yrs)	Size increase ≥3 mm	10-yr 4.7% 20-yr 6.6%	10-yr 1.0% 20-yr 1.6%	Not listed	Not listed
CIH/NMS (Tokyo) 2010 [22]	300 lesions of asymptomatic PTMC	1–17 yrs (mean 5 yrs)	Max. dia. increased by ≥3 mm	7%	1%	Not listed	Not listed
CIH/NMS (Tokyo) 2016 [23]	384 pts with PTMC (480 tumors)	1–23 yrs (avg. 4.3 yrs)	Max. dia. increased by ≥3 mm	5-yr 6.3% 10-yr 7.3%	0%	Age <50 yrs, No/micro calcification Rich vascularization	Not listed
CIH/NMS (Tokyo) 2021 [24]	571 pts with PTMC (718 tumors)	1–26 yrs (median 7.6 yrs)	Max. dia. increased by ≥3 mm	10-yr 9.9% 20-yr 18.0%	10-yr 1.4% 20-yr 3.9%	Age <40 yrs (either tumor enlargement or node metastasis appearance)	

(continued)

Table 6.1 (continued)

Authors (location) [Ref.]	No. of patients (tumors)	AS period	Definition of enlargement	Enlargement rate	Node metastasis appearance rate	Predictors of tumor enlargement	Predictors of node metastasis appearance
MSKCC (U.S.) 2017 [25]	291 pts with low-risk PTC ≤1.5 cm	6–166 mos. (median 8.2 mos.)	(1) Max. dia. increased by ≥3 mm (2) Tumor volume increased by ≥50%	(1) 2-yr 2.5% 5-yr 12.1% (2) 2-yr 11.5% 5-yr 24.8%	0%	Age <50 yrs	Not listed
MSKCC (U.S.) 2022 [26]	483 pts with low-risk PTC ≤1.5 cm	0.5–17 yrs (median 3.7 yrs)	(1) Tumor volume increased by >72% (2) Max. dia. increased by >3 mm (3) Tumor volume increased by >24%	(1) 59 (12%), 5-yr 15.9% (2) 472 (9%) (3) 64 (15.9%)	7 (1.4%) 5-yr, 1.5%	None	None
Multicenter study (South Korea) 2018 [27]	370 pts with PTMC	23.6–47.0 mos., median 34.1 mos.	(1) Max. dia. increased by ≥3 mm (2) Tumor volume increased by ≥50%	(1) 3-yr 3.2%, 5-yr 6.4% (2) 3-yr 17.3%, 5-yr 36.2%	8.6%	Age <45 yrs	Not listed

University of Antioqula (Colombia) 2020 [28]	102 pts with low-risk PTC ≤1.5 cm	0.2–112 mos. (median 13.9 mos.)	(1) Max. dia. increased by ≥3 mm (2) Tumor volume increased by ≥50%	(1) 2-yr 10.2% (2) 2-yr 23%	0%	Not listed	Not listed
University of Pisa (Italy) 2020 [29]	93 pts with low-risk PTC ≤1.3cm	6–54 mos. (median 19 mos.)	(1) Max. dia. increased by ≥3 mm (2) Tumor volume increased by ≥50%	(1) 2.2% (2) 16% (No time sequence analysis)	(1) 1% (No time sequence analysis)	Not listed	Not listed
Multicenter study (South Korea) 2022 [30]	755 pts with PTMC (Multicenter study)	Median 41.4 mos. (mean 41.4 ± 16.0)	Size increase ≥3 mm in one diameter, ≥2 mm in two dias, or appearance of extrathyroidal extension and node metastasis	2-yr and 5-yr progression rates, 5.3% and 14.2%		Age <30 yrs, male sex, and tumor size ≥6 mm (independent predictors of progression)	Not listed

Cited from Ref. [13] with permission

AS active surveillance, *CIH* Cancer Institute Hospital, *mos* months, *MSKCC* Memorial Sloan Kettering Cancer Center, *NMS* Nippon Medical School, *PTC* papillary thyroid carcinoma, *PTMC* papillary thyroid microcarcinoma, *pts* patients, *yrs* years between Japan and other countries. The first study conducted at Memorial Sloan Kettering Cancer Center (New York) claimed that an evaluation of the tumor volume can be more sensitive for tumor enlargement than the use of the tumor's maximum diameter [25]; the study reported that the 2-year and 5-year tumor volume increase rates (by ≥50%) were 11.5% and 24.8%, respectively, which were much higher than the 2- and 5-year maximum diameter increase rates (by ≥3 mm) at 2.5% and 2.1%, respectively. However, a 7-mm tumor that shows a 1-mm increase corresponds to a 49% increase in the tumor's volume, indicating that (i) an evaluation by the increase in tumor volume is too sensitive and (ii) it is too soon to recommend CS for such tumors.

Nonuniformity of the Tumor Growth Rate

It is an important fact that the tumor enlargement activity of PTMCs is not uniform. Miyauchi et al. investigated the growth rate of 169 PTMCs during AS by determining the tumor volume doubling rate (TV-DR [/year], an inverse of the TV doubling time). Their analyses demonstrated that 3%, 22%, 57%, and 17% of the tumors showed moderate growth (TV-DR >0.5), slow growth (0.1–0.5), stable disease (−0.1 to 0.1), and clear shrinkage, respectively, indicating that spontaneous disease regression (<0.1) can occur in PTMCs during AS [31].

Ito et al. compared the tumor enlargement activity before and after the point of enlargement (PE), defined as a maximal tumor size increase by ≥3 mm (PE-M) and a tumor volume increase by ≥50% (PE-V). Their analyses showed that the tumor doubling rate was significantly decreased in post-PE-M or post-PE-V compared to pre-PE-M or pre-PE-V [32], and they concluded that most PTMCs showed a significant decrease in growth activity after enlargement. Further, Miyauchi et al. calculated the hypothetical TV-DR of PTMCs before presentation based on the assumption that a single carcinoma cell measuring 10 μm was present at the patient's birth and grew at a constant growth rate. As a result, in most cases, the tumor growth activity before presentation was significantly higher than that observed during AS [31]. These findings suggest that the growth activity of PTMCs is generally high at the early phase but becomes significantly lower thereafter, indicating that immediate CS soon after slight enlargement may generally be premature.

Factors Related to PTMC Progression During AS

Young Age

It is well known that old age is a strong prognostic factor for both the disease-free and cause-specific survival of patients with clinical PTC; indeed, age is included in the TNM staging system (tumor size [T], the spread of cancer cells to nearby or distant lymph nodes [N], and the presence of metastasis [M]) issued by the Union for International Cancer Control. However, most of the relevant studies have shown that PTMCs in young patients are more progressive than those in old patients, and reports from two Japanese institutions demonstrated that age <40 years is significantly related to the progression of PTMC [20, 24]. Further, Ito et al. showed that PTCs of young patients (<30 years) were more likely to show recurrence than middle-aged patients [33].

It may thus be likely that immediate surgery without AS is suitable for young patients with PTMC. Miyauchi et al. estimated the lifetime probabilities of PTMC enlargement based on the age decade-specific enlargement rates [34], and they observed that the rates of the lifetime probability of tumor enlargement were 48.6% for patients in their 20s (at presentation), 25.3% for those in their 30s, 20.9% for those in their 40s, 10.3% for those in their 50s, 8.2% for those in their 60s, and 3.5% for those in their 70s. Based on these data, more than half of the PTMC patients in their 20s can avoid undergoing PTMC surgery for the rest of their lives. Conversion surgery for PTMC after enlargement during AS is not technically difficult, and, as described below, the postoperative prognosis and the incidence of surgical complications did not differ from those of the patients who underwent IS. We therefore consider young adults with PTMCs as candidates for AS.

Male Sex

Male sex has prognostic value for clinical PTC, although the value is not high. A single study showed that PTMCs in males are more likely to progress compared to those in females [20].

Serum Thyroid-Stimulating Hormone (TSH) Level

Several investigations have been conducted to resolve the clinical question regarding whether the suppression of thyroid-stimulating hormone (TSH) can prevent the progression of PTMC. At present at least, no prospective studies are available, and the existing findings regarding the effects of TSH suppression on PTMC progression are conflicting [20, 35–38]. However, a 2023 Korean study demonstrated that effective levothyroxine treatment for low time-weighed TSH contributed to a decrease in the progression of PTMC in patients <50 years old [37]. A 2023 study from Kuma Hospital demonstrated that a TSH level higher than the lower normal limit was significantly related to PTMC enlargement in patients <40 years old [20]. Yamamoto et al. revealed that the PTMC growth activity of patients for whom levothyroxine administration was initiated in the mid-course of AS became lower after the administration [38]. Mild TSH suppression by levothyroxine administration may therefore be useful to prevent tumor enlargement in young patients, but prospective studies should be conducted before any conclusion is reached.

Ultrasound Findings

The lack of calcification and rich vascularity on ultrasound were reported to be predictors of PTMC growth [23], but those authors do not exclude such tumors as candidates for AS.

Pregnancy

TSH and human chorionic gonadotropin have structural similarity, indicating the possibility of PTMC growth during pregnancy. However, our institution reported that only 8.0% of PTMCs (in 4 of 50 patients) enlarged during pregnancy [39]. Since none of the four patients showed a dire prognosis (two underwent CS and two continued AS), it is currently concluded that young female patients who are or may become pregnant can be candidates for AS if they desire it.

Comparison Between AS and IS for PTMC

Prognosis

Ito et al. reported an excellent prognosis of PTMC after surgery; the 10-year lymph node, distant recurrence, and carcinoma death rates were 1%, 0%, and 0%, respectively [24]. In an investigation by Miyauchi et al., the 10-year and 20-year node metastasis occurrence/metastasis rates were 1.1% and 1.7% for AS patients and 0.4% and 0.7% for IS patients, respectively [21], indicating that the incidence of node metastasis occurrence rate in the AS group was slightly higher than that of the IS group but the difference was very small, and in the IS group, 10.3% of the patients underwent prophylactic lateral node dissection, which may be one of the reasons for these data. Only 12.3% of patients in that AS group underwent one or more surgeries, and the incidence of the patients who underwent two or more surgeries was significantly higher in the IS group (26/2424; 1.07%) than in the AS group (3/3222; 0.09%) ($p < 0.01$) [21]. Further, Sasaki et al. demonstrated that the overall mortality rate was similar between the AS and IS groups [40]. It has thus been concluded that prognosis of both AS and IS patients is similarly excellent.

Some patients undergo conversion surgery after AS for various reasons, for example, progression of the PTMC or the surgical indication of coexisting thyroid or parathyroid disease, a change in patients' preference, and the treating physician's recommendation. Sasaki et al. showed that at Kuma Hospital the cumulative incidence of CS at 5 years was significantly reduced from 12.3% during the first half-period of their study (February 2002–November 2011) to 4.2% in the study's second half-period (December 2011–June 2017). This result can be expected to be due to the increase in physicians' confidence and patients' trust in AS based on the accumulation of favorable data [40].

Fujishima et al. revealed that although the tumors dissected by CS for disease progression were larger and more often pathological node-positive, and although these tumors showed higher Ki-67 labeling index values than the IS tumors, the postoperative prognosis of the CS and IS patients did not differ [41]. We believe that the high Ki-67 labeling index in the CS tumors in that study indicates that high-risk PTMCs were efficiently selected by active surveillance.

Unfavorable Events

In 2016, Oda et al. reported that permanent vocal cord paralysis and permanent hypoparathyroidism occurred in 0.2% and 1.6% of their patients, respectively [42]. We should focus on the fact that these incidences are the results of surgery by thyroid surgery experts. If the surgeries had been performed by nonexpert surgeons or otolaryngologists, the incidence of unfavorable surgical events would become much higher. Complications such as permanent vocal cord paralysis and permanent hypoparathyroidism could be avoided if patients did not select IS as the management strategy for their PTMCs. More recently, Sasaki et al. reviewed larger cohorts and confirmed that the patients who underwent IS had significantly higher incidences of unfavorable events compared to the patients who chose AS [43], with the following prevalences in those patient groups: levothyroxine administration after diagnosis, 65.2% versus 25.2%; permanent vocal cord paralysis, 0.9% versus 0%; and permanent hypoparathyroidism, 1.4% versus 0.2%.

Another important clinical question is whether the incidence of unfavorable events differs between CS and IS. Sasaki et al. observed that unfavorable events associated with surgery (e.g., vocal cord paralysis, hypoparathyroidism, bleeding) occurred at similar incidences in CS and IS patients [43]. These findings may indirectly support the utility of AS for patients with PTMC.

Medical Costs

The costs of ultrasound and blood examinations, surgery, and medications vary significantly among countries, and studies of the medical costs of IS and AS for patients with PTMC have obtained discrepant results [44–49]. In Japan, clinical practices are usually covered by the national health insurance system, and in 2017 the total cost of immediate surgery and postoperative care for 10 years (including prescription medicines such as L-thyroxine) was US$8437/person, which is 4.1 times the total cost of 10 years of active surveillance ($2052/person) [49].

Quality of Life (QoL)

Several studies from various countries regarding the quality of life (QoL) of patients who undergo AS and those who undergo IS are summarized in Table 6.2 [50–55]. These studies showed essentially that physical complaints such as neck

Table 6.2 Difference in the quality of life (QoL) between patients who underwent active surveillance (AS) and immediate surgery (IS)

Institution (country) [ref.]	Study design	Measurement instrument(s)	Observation period	Summary of the results
University of Ulsan College of Medicine (South Korea) 2019 [50]	QoL was evaluated for 74 and 148 patients who underwent AS and IS (lobectomy), respectively, using the SF-12 and THYCA-QoL	SF-2, THYCA-QoL, and FoP	Median 29.6 mos. for the AS group and 38.0 mos. for IS group	1. SF-12: Physical health, social functioning, and emotional problems scores were lower in the IS group than in the AS group. On multivariate analysis, emotional problems score showed a significant negative linear association between the two groups 2. THYCA-QoL: In the univariate and multivariate analyses, the neuromuscular, throat/mouth, and problems with scar scale scores showed a significant positive association between the groups. The "less interest in sex scale" score showed a significant difference between the groups only in the univariate analysis
Tokyo Women's Medical University (Tokyo) 2020 [51]	Cross-sectional study if 20 and 30 patients who underwent AS or IS, respectively	STAI and originally established system (VAS)	0–8.36 yrs (median 4.1 yrs)	1. Patients in the AS group showed higher scores for both state anxiety and trait anxiety 2. Regardless of whether AS or IS was selected, the trait anxiety score was positively and observation time was negatively associated with the state anxiety score 3. Discomfort in the neck, weak voice, and nervousness about the neck's appearance were less frequent in the AS group than in the IS group

(continued)

Table 6.2 (continued)

Institution (country) [ref.]	Study design	Measurement instrument(s)	Observation period	Summary of the results
Kuma Hospital (Kobe, Japan) 2020 [52]	QoL was evaluated for 298 and 49 patients who underwent AS and operation	THYCA-QoL and HADS	Median 56.5 mos. (32–88 mos.) for the AS group and 84 mos. (64–130 mos.) for the OP group	1. THYCA-QoL: The OP group had more complaints about voice, psychological, problems with scar, and gained weight than the AS group 2. HADS: The AS group had significantly better anxiety, depression, and total scores than the OP group
Multicenter study (South Korea) 2021 [53]	QoL surveys for 674 and 381 patients who chose AS and IS, respectively	A Korean version of a thyroid-specific QoL questionnaire	Median 24.4 mos.	1. Of 817 subjects who completed baseline QoL surveys, the 2-year QoL was good in the order of AS ($n = 500$), IS (hemithyroidectomy) ($n = 238$), and IS (total thyroidectomy) ($n = 79$) groups 2. Among the 101 subjects who underwent CS, the 35 who underwent CS due to disease progression had better QoL than the 66 who showed no disease progression
Nippon Medical School (Tokyo) 2023 [54]	Patients with low-risk PTC (<15 mm) who completed the PRO survey. AS and surgery groups were 249 and 32 patients, respectively	STAI, SF-36v2, VAS	After matching, median 4.0 yrs (0.96–16.1 yrs) for the AS group and 4.0 yrs (0.97–16.1 yrs) for the surgery group	1. After matching, the AS group showed significantly better trait anxiety and MCS than the surgery group 2. The surgery group had better role-social component summary 3. In the AS group, trait anxiety and the time from the onset were significant predictors of state anxiety

(continued)

Table 6.2 (continued)

Institution (country) [ref.]	Study design	Measurement instrument(s)	Observation period	Summary of the results
Multicenter study (Canada) 2024 [55]	Patients who underwent AS ($n = 151$) and IS ($n = 40$) with low-risk PTC <2 cm	The Decision Regret Scale, Fear of Progression Questionnaire, and HADS	Median 14 mos. for the AS group and 16 mos. for the IS group	1. The Decision Regret scale did not differ between the AS and IS groups 2. Fear of progression of disease was higher in the IS group than in the AS group at the baseline, but the difference disappeared at the 1-year follow-up

Cited from Ref. [13] with permission

AS active surveillance, *FoP* fear of progression, *HADS* Hospital Anxiety and Depression Scale, *IS* immediate surgery, *MCS* Mental Component Summary, *mos* months, *PTMC* papillary thyroid microcarcinoma, *SF-12* Short-Form Health Survey Questionnaire, *SF-36v2* Short-Form 36 version 2, *STAI* State-Trait Anxiety Inventory, *THYCA-QoL* Thyroid Cancer-Specific Quality of Life Questionnaire, *VAS* visual analog scale, *yrs* years

discomfort and voice problems were less severe in the AS patients compared to those who underwent IS. The studies' findings regarding the difference in psychological issues such as anxiety and uneasiness between AS and IS patients were conflicting, but this could be significantly affected by the physicians' attitude. If the treating physicians have confidence and belief with adequate knowledge of the evidence for AS, patients would have less worries about their disease. Sawka et al. demonstrated that the level of decision regret did not differ between AS and IS groups, and after a 1-year follow-up, the fear of disease progression was low in both the AS and IS groups [55].

Are There any Markers Predicting PTMC Progression?

A legitimate clinical question is whether any markers can predict the progression of PTMC. Although most PTMCs are indolent, some grow continuously and rather rapidly. In our hospital's patient series, one (0.03%) of the 3222 patients with AS underwent conversion surgery ~2 years after the start of their AS because of the patient's preference; that patient showed lung metastasis 12 years after the PTMC diagnosis, and one (0.04%) of the 2424 patients who underwent IS showed lung recurrence 12 years after surgery [21]. Further, Tuttle et al. reported that the tumor of one of their 482 patients started to show rather rapid growth after AS had been ongoing for >4 years [26]. That patient underwent a CS and was diagnosed with BRAF mutation-positive poorly differentiated carcinoma [26]. If there were any molecular markers predicting the constant and rapid growth of PTMC that are detectable on FNAC specimens, it would be a great help for both physicians and patients. Although *TERT* mutations are known to predict a poor prognosis in PTC patients [56], the mutations were reported to be rare and unrelated to PTMC prognosis [57, 58]. Unfortunately, no molecular markers predicting the prognosis of PTMCs have been identified to date.

Conclusions

If appropriately implemented, active surveillance for PTMC is a safe and quite beneficial management strategy. It is appropriate for active surveillance to be regarded as a first-line management for patients aged ≥20 years.

Disclosure Statement The authors have no disclosures or conflicts of interest.

References

1. Miyauchi A. Clinical trials of active surveillance of papillary microcarcinoma of the thyroid. World J Surg. 2016;40:516–22.
2. Takebe K, Date M, Yamamoto Y. Mass screening for thyroid cancer with ultrasonography. Karkinos. 1994;7:309–17. (In Japanese).
3. Takami H, Ito Y, Okamoto T, Yoshida A. Therapeutic strategy for differentiated thyroid carcinoma in Japan based on a newly established guideline managed by Japanese Society of Thyroid Surgeons and Japanese Association of Endocrine Surgeons. World J Surg. 2011;35:111–21.
4. Ito Y, Onoda N, Okamoto T. The revised clinical practice guidelines on the management of thyroid tumors by the Japan Associations of Endocrine Surgeons: core questions and recommendations for treatments of thyroid cancer. Endocr J. 2020;67:669–717.
5. Japan Association of Endocrine Surgery, eds. Clinical practice guidelines on the management of thyroid tumors 2024. Official Journal of the Japan Association of Endocrine Surgery (2024).
6. Haugen BR, Alexander EK, Bible KC, Doherty GM, Mandel SJ, et al. American Thyroid Association management guidelines for adult patients with thyroid nodules and differentiated thyroid cancer: the American Thyroid Association guidelines task force on thyroid nodules and differentiated thyroid cancer. Thyroid. 2015;26:1–133.
7. Sugitani I, Ito Y, Takeuchi D, Nakayama H, Masaki C, et al. Indications and strategy for active surveillance of adult low-risk papillary thyroid microcarcinoma: consensus statements from the Japan Association of Endocrine Surgery task force on management for papillary thyroid microcarcinoma. Thyroid. 2021;31:183–92.
8. Horiguchi K, Yoshida Y, Iwaku K, Emoto N, Kasahara T, et al. Position paper from the Japan Thyroid Association task force on the management of low-risk papillary thyroid microcarcinoma (T1aN0M0) in adults. Endocr J. 2021;68:763–80.
9. Davies L, Welch HG. Increasing incidence of thyroid cancer in the United States, 1973–2002. JAMA. 2006;595:2164–7.
10. Davies L, Welch HG. Current thyroid cancer trends in the United States. JAMA Otolaryngol Head Neck Surg. 2014;140:317–22.
11. Ahn HS, Kim HJ, Welch HG. Korea's thyroid-cancer "epidemic"—screening and overdiagnosis. N Engl J Med. 2014;371:1765–7.
12. Vaccarella S, Dal Maso L, Laversanne M, Bray F, Plummer M, et al. The impact of diagnostic changes on the rise in thyroid cancer incidence: a population-based study in selected high-resource countries. Thyroid. 2015;25:1127–36.

13. Ito Y, Miyauchi A, Fujishima M, et al. Active surveillance for adult low-risk papillary thyroid microcarcinoma – a review focused on the 30-year experience of Kuma Hospital. Endocr J. 2024;71:7–21.
14. Ito Y, Miyauchi A, Oda H, Kobayashi K, Kihara M, et al. Revisiting low-risk thyroid papillary microcarcinomas resected without observation: was immediate surgery necessary? World J Surg. 2016;40:523–8.
15. Haugen BR, Alexander EK, Bible KC, et al. 2015 American Thyroid Association management guidelines for adult patients with thyroid nodules and differentiated thyroid cancer: the American Thyroid Association guidelines task force on thyroid nodules and differentiated thyroid cancer. Thyroid. 2016;26:1–133.
16. Kawano S, Miyauchi A, Ito Y. Routine chest computed tomography at presentation does not identify distant metastasis in cT1aN0 papillary thyroid carcinoma. Thyroid. 2020;30:1620–4.
17. Ito Y, Uruno T, Nakano K, Takamura Y, Miya A, Kobayashi K, et al. An observation trial without surgical treatment in patients with papillary microcarcinoma of the thyroid. Thyroid. 2003;13:381–7.
18. Ito Y, Miyauchi A, Inoue H, Fukushima M, Kihara M, Higashiiyama T, et al. An observation trial for papillary thyroid microcarcinoma in Japanese patients. World J Surg. 2010;34:28–35.
19. Ito Y, Miyauchi A, Kihara M, Higashiyama T, Kobayashi T, et al. Patient age is significantly related to the progression of papillary microcarcinoma of the thyroid under observation. Thyroid. 2014;24:27–34.
20. Ito Y, Miyauchi A, Fujishima M, Noda T, Sano T, et al. Thyroid-stimulating hormone, age, and tumor size are risk factors for progression during active surveillance of low-risk papillary thyroid microcarcinoma in adults. World J Surg. 2023;47:392–401.
21. Miyauchi A, Ito Y, Fujishima M, Miiya A, Onoda N, Kihara M, et al. Long-term outcomes of active surveillance and immediate surgery for adult patients with low-risk papillary thyroid microcarcinoma: 30-year experience. Thyroid. 2023;33:817–25.
22. Sugitani I, Toda K, Yamada K, Yamamoto N, Ikenaga M, et al. Three distinctly different kinds of papillary thyroid microcarcinoma should be recognized: our treatment strategies and outcomes. World J Surg. 2010;34:1222–31.
23. Fukuoka O, Sugitani I, Ebina A, Toda K, Kawabaya K, et al. Natural history of asymptomatic papillary thyroid microcarcinoma: time-dependent changes in calcification and vascularity during active surveillance. World J Surg. 2016;40:529–37.
24. Nagaoka R, Ebina A, Toda K, Jikuzonoa T, Saitou M, et al. Multifocality and progression of papillary thyroid microcarcinoma during active surveillance. World J Surg. 2021;45:2769–76.
25. Tuttle RM, Fagin JA, Minkowitz G, Wong RJ, Roman B, et al. Natural history and tumor volume kinetics of papillary thyroid cancers during active surveillance. JAMA Otolaryngol Head Neck Surg. 2017;143:1015–20.
26. Tuttle RM, Fagin J, Minkowitz G, Wong R, Roman B, et al. Active surveillance of papillary thyroid cancer: frequency and time course of the six most common tumor volume kinetic patterns. Thyroid. 2022;32:1337–45.
27. Oh HS, Ha J, Kim HI, Kim TH, Kim WG, et al. Active surveillance of low-risk papillary thyroid microcarcinoma: a multi-center cohort study in Korea. Thyroid. 2018;28:1587–94.
28. Sanabria A. Experience with active surveillance of thyroid low-risk carcinoma in a developing country. Thyroid. 2020;7:985–91.
29. Molinaro E, Campopiano MC, Pieruzzi L, Matrone A, Agate L, et al. Active surveillance in papillary thyroid microcarcinomas is feasible and safe: experience at a single Italian center. J Clin Endocrinol Metab. 2020;105:e172–80.
30. Lee EK, Moon JH, Hwangbo Y, Ryu CH, Cho SW, et al. Progression of low-risk papillary thyroid microcarcinoma during active surveillance: interim analysis of a multicenter prospective cohort study of active surveillance on papillary thyroid microcarcinoma in Korea. Thyroid. 2022;32:1328–36.
31. Miyauchi A, Kudo T, Ito Y, Oda H, Yamomoto M, et al. Natural history of papillary thyroid microcarcinoma: kinetic analyses on tumor volume during active surveillance and before presentation. Surgery. 2019;165:25–30.

32. Ito Y, Miyauchi A, Kudo T, Higashiyama T, Masuoka H, et al. Kinetic analysis of growth activity in enlarging papillary thyroid microcarcinomas. Thyroid. 2019;29:1765–73.
33. Ito Y, Miyauchi A, Kihara M, Higashiyama T, Kobayashi K, et al. Prognostic significance of young age in papillary thyroid carcinoma: analysis of 5,733 patients with 150 months' median follow-up. Endocr J. 2014;61:491–197.
34. Miyauchi A, Kudo T, Ito Y, Oda H, Sasai H, et al. Estimation of the lifetime probability of disease progression of papillary microcarcinoma of the thyroid during active surveillance. Surgery. 2018;163:48–52.
35. Kim HI, Jang HW, Ahn HS, Ahn S, Park SY, et al. High serum TSH level is associated with progression of papillary thyroid microcarcinoma during active surveillance. J Clin Endocrinol Metab. 2018;103:446–51.
36. Sugitani I, Fujimoto Y, Yamada K. Association between serum thyrotropin concentration and growth of asymptomatic papillary thyroid microcarcinoma. World J Surg. 2014;38:673–8.
37. Kim HI, Jin M, Ko NG, Oh YL, Shin JH, et al. Effect of TSH levels during active surveillance of PTMC according to age. Endocr Relat Cancer. 2022;29:191–200.
38. Yamamoto M, Miyauchi A, Ito Y, Fujishima M, Sasaki T, et al. Active surveillance outcomes of patients with low-risk papillary thyroid microcarcinoma according to levothyroxine treatment status. Thyroid. 2023;33:1182–9. https://doi.org/10.1089/thy.2023.0046.
39. Ito Y, Miyauchi A, Kudo T, Ota H, Yoshiokia K, et al. Effects of pregnancy on papillary microcarcinomas of the thyroid re-evaluated in the entire patient series at Kuma Hospital. Thyroid. 2016;26:156–60.
40. Sasaki T, Miyauchi A, Ito Y, Kudo T, Kanemura N, et al. Marked decrease over time in conversion surgery after active surveillance of low-risk papillary thyroid microcarcinoma. Thyroid. 2021;31:217–23.
41. Fujishima M, Miiyauchi A, Ito Y, Kudo T, Noda T, et al. Active surveillance is an excellent management technique for identifying patients with progressive low-risk papillary thyroid microcarcinoma requiring surgical treatment. Endocr J. 2023;70:411–8.
42. Oda H, Miyauchi A, Ito Y, Yoshioka K, Nakayama A, et al. Incidence of unfavorable events in the management of low-risk papillary microcarcinoma of the thyroid by active surveillance versus immediate surgery. Thyroid. 2016;26:150–5.
43. Sasaki T, Miyauchi A, Fujishima M, Ito Y, Kudo T, et al. Comparison or postoperative unfavorable events in patients with low-risk papillary thyroid carcinoma: immediate surgery versus conversion surgery following active surveillance. Thyroid. 2023;33:186–91.
44. Lang BH, Wong CK. A cost-effectiveness comparison between early surgery and non-surgical approach for incidental papillary thyroid microcarcinoma. Eur J Endocrinol. 2015;173:347–75.
45. Venkatesh S, Pasternak JD, Beninate T, Drake FT, Kluifthout WP, et al. Cost-effectiveness of active surveillance versus hemithyroidectomy for micropapillary thyroid cancer. Surgery. 2017;161:116–26.
46. Lin JF, Jonker PKC, Cunich M, Sidhu SB, Delbridge LW, et al. Surgery alone for papillary thyroid microcarcinoma is less costly and more effective than long term active surveillance. Surgery. 2020;167:110–6.
47. Youssef MR, Attia AS, Omar M, Aboueisha M, Freeman MN, et al. Thyroid lobectomy as a cost-effective approach in low-risk papillary thyroid cancer versus active surveillance. Surgery. 2022;171:190–6.
48. Kim K, Choi JY, Kim S-J, Lee EK, Lee YK, et al. Active surveillance versus immediate surgery for low-risk papillary thyroid microcarcinoma patients in South Korea: a cost-minimization analysis from the MAeSTro Study. Thyroid. 2022;32:648–56.
49. Oda H, Miyauchi A, Ito Y, Sasai H, Masuoka H, et al. Comparison of the costs of active surveillance and immediate surgery in the management of low-risk papillary microcarcinoma of the thyroid. Endocr J. 2017;64:59–64.
50. Jeon MJ, Lee Y-M, Sung T-Y, Han M, Shin Y-W, et al. Quality of life in patients with papillary thyroid microcarcinoma managed by active surveillance or lobectomy: a cross-sectional study. Thyroid. 2019;29:956–62.

51. Yoshida Y, Horiuchi K, Okamoto T. Patients' view on the management of papillary thyroid microcarcinoma: active surveillance or surgery. Thyroid. 2020;30:681–7.
52. Nakamura T, Miyauchi A, Ito Y, Ito M, Kudo T, et al. Quality of life in patients with low-risk papillary thyroid microcarcinoma: active surveillance versus immediate surgery. Endocr Pract. 2020;26:1451–7.
53. Moon JH, Ryu CH, Cho SW, Choi JY, Chung EJ, et al. Effect of initial treatment choice on 2-year quality of life in patients with low-risk papillary thyroid microcarcinoma. J Clin Endocrinol Metab. 2021;106:724–35.
54. Kazusaka H, Sugitani I, Toda K, Sen M, Saito M, et al. Patient-reported outcomes in patients with low-risk papillary thyroid carcinoma: cross-sectional study to compare active surveillance and immediate surgery. World J Surg. 2022;47:1190–8.
55. Sawka AM, Ghai S, Rotstein L, Irish JC, Pasternak JD, et al. Decision regret following the choice of surgery or active surveillance for small, low-risk papillary thyroid cancer: a prospective cohort study. Thyroid. 2024;34:635–4.
56. Ebina A, Togashi Y, Baba S, Sato Y, Sakata S, et al. *TERT* promoter mutation and extent of thyroidectomy in patients with 1–4 cm intrathyroidal papillary carcinoma. Cancers (Basel). 2020;12:2115.
57. Yabuta T, Matsuse M, Hirokawa M, Yamashita S, Mitsutake N, et al. TERT promoter mutations were not found in papillary thyroid microcarcinomas that showed disease progression on active surveillance. Thyroid. 2017;27:1206–7.
58. De Biase D, Gandolfi G, Ragazzi M, Eszlinger M, Sancisi V, et al. TERT promoter mutations in papillary thyroid microcarcinoma. Thyroid. 2015;25:1013–9.

Surgical Management of Thyroid Cancers

7

Aradhya Nigam and Ashok R Shaha

Editorial
There are many controversies in the surgical management of thyroid carcinomas. First of all, recommendation for the extent of thyroidectomy has been changed; indication of total thyroidectomy has been significantly narrowed. It remains an open question whether and how prophylactic central node dissection for cNO PTC is indicated, and even the significance of prophylactic lateral node dissection for PTC and MTC remains controversial; this is because, even though negative on imaging studies, pathological node metastasis not only in the central but also in the lateral compartment is detected in very high incidences. This chapter details several clinical questions about surgical management, including the extent of initial surgery, and the management of thyroid carcinomas with structural extension to adjacent major organs. The description is easy to understand and very suitable for the study of clinicians and residents.

Yasuhiro Ito

Introduction

As the understanding of the biological underpinnings of thyroid carcinoma has improved, the surgical approach and management of patients have been under constant evolutiont, with changes often met with extensive controversy. Historically,

A. Nigam
Department of Surgery, Memorial Sloan Kettering Cancer Center, New York, NY, USA
e-mail: NigamA@mskcc.org

A. R. Shaha (✉)
Allan H. Selig Chair in Head and Neck Surgery, Memorial Sloan Kettering Cancer Center, Professor of Surgery, Weill-Cornell Medical College, New York, NY, USA
e-mail: shahaa@mskcc.org

P. S. Pai et al. (eds.), *Controversies in Cancer of the Thyroid and Parathyroid Glands*, https://doi.org/10.1007/978-3-032-13130-0_7

universal treatment for patients with thyroid carcinoma aimed to eradicate all residual tumor by recommending treatment with total thyroidectomy and radioactive iodine. Advances in the understanding of thyroid carcinoma have led to improved tumor staging and characterization, with subsequent better recognition of benign, albeit suspicious, nodules misdiagnosed as thyroid cancer. An effort to reduce overtreatment and oversurveillance of these benign nodules in the setting of rising healthcare costs has led to a de-escalation in universal treatment, with management dependent on patient and tumor characteristics. While changes in the treatment approach to thyroid carcinoma patients have been overall progressive, they have been complemented by an extensive amount of controversy over the optimal surgical management of patients. This chapter aims to explore and discuss some of the controversies that are currently evident in the surgical management of patients with thyroid carcinoma. By doing so, we hope to bring to light topics deserving of further investigation that would lead to an improvement in the surgical care of patients and offer the best quality of life.

Trends in the Surgical Approach to Thyroid Carcinoma

Changes in the surgical approach to patients with thyroid carcinoma in the last 15 years have been driven by a better understanding of the disease, reflected in multiple guideline changes. The 2009 American Thyroid Association (ATA) guidelines set the stage for the de-escalation of treatment, stating that omission of postoperative radioactive iodine (RAI) treatment was appropriate for "very-low risk" tumors—defined as well-differentiated thyroid carcinomas less than 1 cm [1]. Further investigation led to a greater de-escalation in the 2015 ATA guidelines where RAI could be omitted for differentiated cancers less than four centimeters, which lends support for hemithyroidectomy as a surgical option for low-risk nodules [2]. These changes were further adopted by the European Society for Medical Oncology [3] guidelines as well as the National Comprehensive Cancer Network (NCCN), which promoted an option between total thyroidectomy or lobectomy for well-differentiated thyroid cancers without extrathyroidal extension or local/distant metastasis. Finally, the changes in the staging system as per the eighth edition of the American Joint Commission of Cancer for patients with differentiated thyroid cancer allowed a more conservative approach for patients less than 55 years old.

The 2009 ATA guidelines introduced a more conservative approach to patients diagnosed with thyroid cancer [4]. This was further cemented over the course of the following decade with a vast reduction in the use of postoperative RAI in low-risk differentiated thyroid carcinomas by half (44–18%) in the period between 2000 and 2018. When evaluated in a single, high-volume institution, Zhu and Yeh found that between 2000 and 2018 there was a substantial increase from 2% to 19% in the use of lobectomy for low-risk thyroid carcinoma, with a concomitant decrease in patients requiring completion thyroidectomy from 73% to 26% over the same time period [5]. These trends in the management of thyroid carcinoma have demonstrated increased adoption of a more conservative approach to thyroid carcinoma in recent years, introducing a more nuanced and individualized treatment approach based on multiple patient and clinical risk factors.

Principles in the Surgical Management of Thyroid Carcinoma

Differentiated Thyroid Carcinomas (Papillary and Follicular Thyroid Carcinoma)

The treatment of differentiated thyroid carcinoma has undergone evolution over the years—with a transition to a more conservative, yet individualized approach to patients [6]. For tumors less than four centimeters, lobectomy remains an option for patients with differentiated carcinomas, particularly in patients without extrathyroidal extension, local or distant metastasis, history of familial syndromes, neck radiation, and no obvious lymph node metastasis. Lobectomy offers the option for select patients to remain off thyroid hormone replacement and reduces surgical morbidity. However, completion thyroidectomy has been recommended for patients whose histopathology reveals high-risk variants, including major angioinvasive follicular thyroid carcinoma (widely invasive), poor differentiation, or based on clinician/patient preference. Total thyroidectomy remains standard of care for tumors greater than four centimeters, presence of nodal or distant metastasis, or presence of extrathyroidal extension.

The trend toward de-escalation treatment in low-risk thyroid carcinoma has now been described as precision treatment. As per the ATA guidelines, the intent of precision treatment aims to "minimize potential harm from overtreatment" of these low-risk tumors, while "appropriately treating and monitoring" higher risk tumors. This shift to a more patient- and risk-based focus of treatment has led to comparable outcomes compared to universal complete resection, but also improved quality of life for patients by avoiding the morbidity involved with total thyroidectomy and potential need for thyroid hormone supplementation.

For patients with preoperatively identified nodal metastasis, complete dissection of the respective cervical nodal compartment is recommended (levels 2–5) over "cherry-picking" of identified nodes to reduce recurrence. However, controversy exists over the advantage of prophylactic central neck dissection and optimal evaluation of the lateral neck, which will be discussed later in this text.

Medullary Thyroid Carcinoma

Surgery currently remains the only treatment option available to achieve therapeutic cure in patients diagnosed with medullary thyroid carcinoma—a rare, but aggressive subtype of thyroid carcinoma that arises from the parafollicular C-cells of the thyroid. Total thyroidectomy with bilateral central neck dissection is supported by ATA guidelines as standard treatment for familial disease. In patients with known inherited genetic disorders, prophylactic total thyroidectomy is advocated based on the risk of disease penetrance. For patients with MEN2A with high-risk RET mutations (Codon 634, Codon 883), current ATA guidelines advocate for prophylactic thyroidectomy around age 5–7 years old. For the highest risk MEN2B RET mutant patients (Codon 918), guidelines call for earlier intervention, with total thyroidectomy recommended by age 2 [7].

Management of the lateral neck in patients with medullary thyroid carcinoma remains more controversial. Similar to differentiated thyroid carcinoma, for preoperatively identified nodal disease, compartment dissection remains the standard of care. Prophylactic dissection, while previously advocated based on familial disease or baseline calcitonin level, has come under extensive recent scrutiny. Further detail into the controversies and optimal management of patients with medullary thyroid carcinoma is reserved for another chapter in this book.

Anaplastic Thyroid Carcinoma

The surgical management of patients with anaplastic thyroid carcinoma is dependent on the extent of disease at presentation. Optimal treatment strategies for the surgical management of patients with anaplastic thyroid carcinoma remain challenging and are discussed in detail in another chapter in this book. Of special note, when an incidental focus of anaplastic thyroid carcinoma is identified within a specimen, optimal management remains controversial. However, the general consensus is to consider total thyroidectomy and external beam radiation [8]. In *BRAF*-mutated patients, dabrafenib and trametinib give excellent response and overall good outcomes. When used in the neoadjuvant setting, combination therapy has the potential to downstage borderline resectable disease.

Thyroid Lobectomy Versus Total Thyroidectomy for Differentiated Thyroid Carcinoma

Historically, total thyroidectomy was advocated for a complete resection of all diseases for all patients with differentiated thyroid carcinoma. Advocates for universal employment of total thyroidectomy further stated that total thyroidectomy would (1) eradicate all potential multifocal and multicentric disease, (2) allow thyroglobulin to be a more accurate marker of residual and recurrent disease, and (3) permit use of RAI for high-risk disease. The 2015 ATA guidelines further cemented the changing perspective of patients with differentiated thyroid carcinomas by advocating for risk stratification of patients based on clinical factors into low-, intermediate-, and high-risk tumors. As a result, providers could consider a more conservative approach to patients without overtreatment of low-risk differentiated carcinomas. Thyroid lobectomy was further advocated as a treatment option for patients with low- to moderate-risk thyroid carcinomas. Lobectomy offered the advantages of (1) reducing bilateral injury to the recurrent laryngeal nerves, (2) preservation of the thyroid function, and (3) no risk of long-term hypoparathyroidism [9]. However, the adoption of thyroid lobectomy in low-risk thyroid carcinoma remains varied [10].

Multiple studies have demonstrated that thyroid lobectomy is an oncologically sound treatment option in select patients, with the option for completion thyroidectomy in higher risk patients (see "Principles of Management" section) [11]. While randomized data evaluating thyroid lobectomy versus total thyroidectomy remain lacking, a large number of studies have supported the use of thyroid lobectomy for low-risk thyroid carcinoma. One of the largest cohort of patients was conducted by Matsuzu et al., evaluating long-term clinical outcomes in patients undergoing thyroid lobectomy at the Ito Hospital between 1985 and 1995 [12]. With a median follow-up time of 17.6 years, the study cohort experienced 25-year thyroid remnant recurrence-free survival of 93%, nodal recurrence-free survival of 90%, and distant metastatic-recurrence-free survival of 93%, demonstrating particularly excellent long-term outcomes in patients less than 45 years old with tumors less than 4 cm without nodal or extrathyroidal invasion. Several follow-up studies, including an evaluation of 61,775 patients by Adam et al and longer-term evaluations after the publication of the 2015 ATA guidelines by Kim et al and Kuba et al, bolstered the argument that thyroid lobectomy was noninferior in terms of patient survival and disease recurrence compared to total thyroidectomy [11, 13, 14]. In their retrospective review of patients at Memorial Sloan Kettering, Nixon and colleagues evaluated T1-T2N0 well-differentiated thyroid carcinoma patients who underwent lobectomy or total thyroidectomy [15]. With a median follow-up of 99 months, they demonstrated that there was no significant difference in local (0% for both) and regional recurrence (0% vs. 0.8%) between both surgical cohorts. Ten-year survival, when compared between lobectomy and total thyroidectomy, was not statistically different in all patient cohorts, including T1 patients (92% vs. 98%; $p = 0.8$), low-risk patients (97% vs. 96%; $p = 0.6$), and even high-risk patients (90% vs. 96%, $p = 0.4$). Furthermore, surgery selected was not associated with worse outcomes on multivariate analysis. Lobectomy also offered improved cost-effectiveness with improved quality-adjusted life-years to patients [16]. However, universal adoption of thyroid lobectomy remains slow.

Several reasons have contributed to the slower-than-expected adoption of thyroid lobectomy for thyroid carcinoma. In 2021, several years after the publication of the 2015 ATA guidelines, Rosko and colleagues conducted a survey study of providers who were provided a clinical vignette of a very low-risk papillary thyroid carcinoma [17]. Among the 264 surgeons surveyed, about half of the surgeons continued to endorse total thyroidectomy with or without central nodal dissection. The most common reasons for recommending complete thyroidal resection remain the ongoing concern for a malignancy present in the contralateral lobe, while other surgeons feel that complete resection would assuage patient anxiety. The concept that total thyroidectomy remains the safe option in patients is further supported by the observation that 30–59% of patients initially classified as low-risk carcinoma are found to contain higher risk features, including extrathyroidal extension or lymph node metastasis. While the clinical significance of these findings remains up for debate, the notion demonstrates the ongoing slow adoption among providers and patients to proceed with a less extensive procedure. The need to reoperate for disease with adverse features remains a concern for the increased operative difficulty to the surgeon, worsened anxiety for the patient, and increased costs associated with a reoperation. It is our opinion that in select patients with low-risk disease, the benefits of proceeding with thyroid lobectomy outweigh the risks as described above. At this point, a frank discussion between the surgeon and the patient will drive the optimal treatment option for the patients. It is important to consider that while many of these decisions are often made by conversation between the surgeon and patient, input from the patient's endocrinologist also has an impact on treatment selection. However, with greater adoption of the ATA guidelines, more recently there has been less interest in the routine use of RAI for well-differentiated thyroid carcinoma.

Role of Central Neck Dissection for Differentiated Thyroid Carcinoma

For patients with preoperatively identified lymph node disease in the central compartment, total thyroidectomy with bilateral central cervical lymphadenectomy remains the standard of care. Furthermore, cervical lymph node metastasis has been reported in approximately 40–60% of patients, reinforcing the notion that a careful preoperative and intraoperative assessment of level VI lymph nodes is required to assess for regional nodal metastasis [18]. The role of prophylactic central neck dissection remains controversial. A randomized trial evaluating the potential therapeutic benefit of central neck dissection has been demonstrated to be too difficult to perform by the ATA [19]. The 2015 ATA guidelines support consideration for prophylactic central neck dissection in patients where nodal staging may impact postoperative clinical course, particularly in patients with T3/T4 disease or with known lateral compartment lymph node disease.

Several arguments have been laid out to support prophylactic central neck dissection. One of the major advantages that prophylactic dissection provides is the ability to evaluate for micrometastatic disease present within the central neck, which would have otherwise not been resected [20–22]. This is supported by reports that have demonstrated lower thyroglobulin levels in patients who have had prophylactic central neck dissection. While the clinical implications of resecting micrometastatic disease are still debated, Hall and colleagues demonstrated no recurrence in the central neck when prophylactic dissection was performed in patients with otherwise no preoperatively identified disease [23]. In addition, proponents have argued that positive nodal disease not previously identified potentially upstages patients, resulting in postoperative radioactive iodine treatment. While the incidence of this occurring has varied, upstaging has been reported in up to one-third of patients greater than 55 years old [24]. Finally, in patients who do not undergo prophylactic central dissection, reoperation in the central neck is technically more difficult than the index surgery.

The clinical significance of prophylactic central neck dissection has been greatly debated as survival benefit has not been shown [25]. In addition, prophylactic central neck dissection has been associated with increased incidence of surgical morbidity with increased transient hypocalcemia and recurrent laryngeal nerve injury. Furthermore, performing central neck dissection does not rule out disease to the lateral neck. While close surveillance has been proposed for patients with micrometastatic disease to the central neck, its clinical significance has remained questioned.

Two noteworthy randomized trials were performed to address the question of prophylactic central neck dissection in attempt to assess the role of prophylactic central neck dissection in differentiated thyroid carcinoma. The first trial by Sippel and colleagues at the University of Wisconsin aimed to evaluate disease outcomes in clinically N0 patients, recruiting 60 patients into the study [26]. At 1 year, they demonstrated no statistically significant difference in short-term outcomes, including rates of hypothyroidism, vocal fold paralysis/changes, or disease outcomes. Although the trial was aborted early due to higher-than-expected rates of hypothyroidism (defined as PTH <10) in the total thyroidectomy cohort, they also demonstrated that quality-of-life measures at 1 year were no different between the two groups. Another randomized trial performed by Viola and colleagues at the University of Pisa randomized 181 clinically N0 patients into total thyroidectomy with and without central dissection cohorts [27]. They demonstrated that while a quarter of patients demonstrated micrometastatic disease, there was no difference in disease recurrence or survival between the two cohorts. However, a greater proportion of prophylactic central neck dissection patients demonstrated permanent hypoparathyroidism (19% vs. 8%; $p = 0.02$), suggesting greater surgical morbidity in this cohort of patients. Ultimately, with no difference in disease outcomes in the setting of increased surgical morbidity, prophylactic central neck dissection did not demonstrate clinical utility.

Many have advocated for prophylactic central neck dissection in patients with differentiated carcinomas who were less than 45 years old, had extrathyroidal extension, BRAF mutation, or had multifocal disease [20, 28]. However, our practice at our institution is to not perform prophylactic central neck dissection but rather advocate for close evaluation of the central neck at the time of operation. Central neck dissection is reserved for known or suspicious central neck disease. Increasing studies have evaluated the implication of molecular profiling on disease aggressiveness and subsequent prophylactic central neck dissection. While data for high-risk genetic disease is encouraging, change in practice patterns is still pending further study and societal guideline adoption. We generally use a frozen section of the lymph nodes to tailor the extent of surgery.

Evaluation and Management of the Lateral Neck in Differentiated Thyroid Carcinoma

Occult metastatic disease in the lateral neck is identified in 30–60% of patients with differentiated thyroid carcinoma. Metastasis to the central neck represents one of the greatest predictors of metastasis to the lateral neck, with central neck metastasis significantly increasing the risk of lateral neck disease. Similar to central neck disease, compartmental dissection is recommended in all patients with preoperatively identified metastatic disease. Opposed to central neck disease, disease identified in the lateral neck typically leads to resection of cervical compartment levels II, III, and IV along the sternocleidomastoid, with levels I and V reserved for patients with identified disease in the respective compartment.

Assessment of the lateral neck typically involves physical examination of the neck with ultrasound of the lateral compartments. Findings seen on ultrasound, including size greater than 10 mm, loss of a fatty hilum, peripheral hypervascularity, taller than wide morphology, and calcifications clue providers into performing an FNA biopsy of the suspicious lesion and thyroglobulin wash. CT imaging has been demonstrated to be useful for the evaluation of extent of disease and its relation to other critical cervical structures. "Skip metastases" of thyroid carcinoma to the lateral neck bypassing the central and Delphian lymph nodes have been described primarily for the upper pole nodules [29].

Lateral neck dissection has typically been reserved for patients with known, biopsy-proven disease in the lateral neck. Formal dissection of the respective compartment has been demonstrated to be oncologically superior to "berry picking," demonstrating improved local control, although having no effect on overall survival. Prophylactic lateral neck dissection has remained controversial. For papillary and follicular thyroid carcinomas, prophylactic ipsilateral lateral dissection is generally not recommended. Recently, however, prophylactic ipsilateral dissection has been considered for patients with concern for suspicious disease not otherwise clinically apparent, particularly in larger tumors [30]. This has been particularly considered in patients with extensive central nodal disease, upper pole lesions, and carcinomas with extensive extrathyroidal extension or lymphovascular invasion. Similarly, prophylactic contralateral lateral neck, while generally not recommended, has been considered for patients with extensive ipsilateral lateral disease.

For medullary thyroid carcinoma, prophylactic lateral neck dissection has been indicated, but remains controversial [31, 32]. The risk of lateral neck metastasis has been directly associated with calcitonin levels, size of the tumor, and RET mutation status. Even the ATA guidelines for medullary thyroid carcinoma have stated that consideration for lateral neck dissection should be made for elevated calcitonin levels greater than 200 pg/mL. Other studies have indicated lower thresholds for ipsilateral lateral neck dissection when calcitonin levels are greater than 20 pg/mL and bilateral neck dissection when greater than 200 pg/mL. Adoption of this practice remains varied by institution as more recent studies have demonstrated no differences in disease-specific outcomes with prophylactic lateral neck dissection. At our institution, prophylactic dissection is dependent on the patient's preoperative calcitonin and size of the primary tumor but is generally not recommended in the absence of known metastatic disease. Further studies will help to delineate which patients would be served best with more extensive resection.

Management of Microcarcinomas

The rising incidence of thyroid carcinoma has largely been attributed to the increased identification of papillary thyroid microcarcinomas. These carcinomas—designated as carcinomas measuring less than 1 cm—have been estimated to represent approximately 20–40% of all thyroid carcinomas [33]. The optimal management of patients with papillary thyroid microcarcinomas has recently focused on active surveillance of patients [34]. Long-term evaluation of patients with microcarcinomas by Miyauchi and Ito in the Kuma Hospital demonstrated a low incidence of patients who developed interval growth of nodules requiring surgery, with the incidence of long-term recurrence being exceedingly rare [35]. Based on similar observations as the Kuma Hospital experience, recent ATA guidelines have advocated for no FNA biopsy for patients with suspicious thyroid nodules less than 1 cm, except where clinically indicated. While further evaluation of the management of patients with microcarcinomas is discussed in another chapter of this book, it has been shown that the adoption of active surveillance has been accepted for a variety of reasons. At our institution, owing to the work of Tuttle and colleagues, patients are risk stratified into ideal, appropriate, or inappropriate patient cohorts for active surveillance based on patient and tumor factors [36, 37]. We believe that stratification of patients enables acknowledgment of risk factors for disease progression and helps guide surveillance protocols, but also demonstrates active surveillance as a safe management strategy.

In addition to active surveillance of microcarcinomas, nonsurgical treatment approaches have recently been proposed for the management of low-risk thyroid carcinomas in lieu of active surveillance. Ultrasound-guided percutaneous ethanol ablation has demonstrated increased promise as an alternative treatment option [38]. Ethanol ablation has been demonstrated to be a safe and feasible option, while being a cheaper alternative to surgical intervention for patients with microcarcinomas, and has previously demonstrated utility in papillary thyroid metastasis with reasonably demonstrated observational outcomes. While its clinical utility is still pending further study, it has demonstrated benefit in a subset of small cohort studies. Other treatment options that have been studied included radiofrequency and laser ablation but remain less studied, with benefits demonstrated in low-cohort studies [39, 40]. While the experience with these alternative treatment strategies remains controversial, we believe that familiarity with these nonsurgical options is important and should remain as part of the surgeon's armamentarium.

Management of Patients with Locally Advanced Thyroid Carcinomas

The incidence of local invasion of well-differentiated thyroid carcinoma has been demonstrated in 13–22% of patients. Preoperative suspicion of locally advanced disease as defined by the presence of voice changes, dysphagia, hemoptysis, or tumor enlargement should prompt axial imaging with a CT of the neck and chest, as well as consideration for flexible laryngoscopy. Historically, locally advanced thyroid carcinoma was broadly defined and often provider dependent. Recently, consensus by the American Head and Neck Society (AHNS) and International Thyroid Oncology group aimed to define locally [41]advanced thyroid carcinoma into four groups: (1) structurally or surgically advanced tumors with local or distant spread; (2) biochemically advanced tumors refractory to RAI or TSH suppression; (3) histologically or molecularly advanced tumors with poorly differentiated pathologic features; and (4) clinically advanced tumors based on provider assessment [41]. Advanced tumors, whether in the preoperative or postoperative setting, require multidisciplinary discussion between providers and patients to determine optimal treatment strategies and goals. While a more in-depth discussion of locally advanced tumors is discussed in another chapter, surgical resection remains the mainstay of treatment for tumors with advanced disease on initial presentation or as a recurrence.

Controversy exists over the best treatment for patients with structurally advanced thyroid carcinoma. For patients with recurrent laryngeal nerve involvement, attempts at separating the nerve and tumors should be made. Particularly in patients with intact phonation, "shaving" of the tumors has demonstrated no difference in disease-specific outcomes compared to resection of the nerve. In cases where the nerve has been grossly involved, resection with reconstruction has been advised. Reconstruction involves entire primary repair (in short segment disease) to utilization of vascular grafts (in larger defects) have been used with the ansa cervicalis or autologous nerve grafts. Other options utilizing collagen fibers and silicon tubes remain more experimental.

Vascular involvement has been described in up to 13% of patients with advanced thyroid carcinoma. More commonly, vascular invasion has involved venous structures, including the internal jugular vein, subclavian vein, and innominate vein, while invasion of arterial structures has remained rarer. Concerns over sequela from increased intracranial pressure remain less common in patients who have unilateral ligation; however, they are more prevalent in patients requiring bilateral ligation. Selection of which patients undergo venous reconstruction remains surgeon-dependent and dependent on the risk of developing symptoms. The described options for reconstruction have included internal to external jugular vein anastomosis, internal jugular-internal jugular venous bypass, and internal jugular-external jugular venous bypass with good outcomes. For arterial involvement, shaving of the adventitial layer has been described to remove the tumor with negative margins. For grossly involved arterial disease, resection and reconstruction with autologous or synthetic grafts have been described, although the incidence of mortality or neuromorbidity has been reported to occur in 10% of patients.

Management of Tracheal and Esophageal Involvement

Tracheal invasion has been documented to be a poor prognostic factor in patients with thyroid carcinoma. Similar to locally advanced thyroid carcinoma, complete resection remains the standard of care where possible. However, selection of surgical resection remains dependent on the extent of invasion and location of the disease [42]. The two major staging systems that have been proposed to drive surgical management of thyroid carcinoma invasion into the trachea have included the McCaffrey [43] staging system, which evaluates the extent of invasion, and Shin staging system [44], which describes the pathologic extent of invasion. Regardless of the staging system used, both describe surgical selection to be based on obtaining negative margins. For tumors abutting the trachea, "shaving" off the tumor is oncologically adequate for resection. For more involved and invasive diseases, both staging systems advocate for total/partial tracheal resection. Maximal tracheal resection has been described to be about 5–6 cm or up to 8 tracheal rings. Regardless, optimal management of patients with tracheal involvement remains a challenge for the surgeon, with surgical selection dependent on surgical experience and attempt to control future disease morbidity.

Patients with esophageal involvement also pose a challenge to the surgeon as patients with tumor invasion to this depth often present with concomitant tracheal involvement. Management of esophageal invasion, similar to tracheal invasion, depends on the extent of involvement. Resection of the esophagus can be performed with resection of the adventitia and muscularis layers without additional repair. For full-thickness involvement or tumors that encase the esophagus, resection with primary repair with buttress or segmental resection can be performed. The described flap options have included the forearm-free flap, gastric conduit, or jejunal interposition.

Surgical Management of Recurrent Thyroid Carcinoma

Thyroid carcinoma recurrence, according to the ATA risk stratification system, has described tumor recurrence rates to be between 1% in low-risk carcinomas to about 50% in patients with high-risk carcinomas [45]. Surgery with negative margins remains the best way to avoid recurrence; however, factors associated with recurrence have included extrathyroidal extension, poorly differentiated histology, cervical lymph node metastasis, lymphovascular invasion, and elevated post-resection thyroglobulin levels. Diagnostic evaluation with ultrasound or CT scan with FNA biopsy remains the standard mode of diagnosing recurrence. Surgery is currently described as the mainstay of treatment for recurrence of disease [46]. As per the ATA, surveillance may be considered for patients with asymptomatic, low-volume disease. For patients with unresectable disease or suspicion of residual disease after tumor recurrence resection, external beam radiation therapy or adjuvant RAI therapy may be considered. Targeted therapy has been proposed as an option for unresectable disease but remains dependent on the genetic signature of the tumor. Similar to advanced tumors, management of patients with thyroid carcinoma recurrence remains dependent on a multidisciplinary discussion.

Conclusion

The management of patients with thyroid carcinoma has undergone an extensive amount of change over the years that has been reflected with every new edition of the ATA guidelines. Surgery currently remains the only treatment modality to achieve cure; however, aspects surrounding the extent of resection remain controversial. Ultimately, debate surrounding indications to perform a prophylactic central or lateral neck dissection for well-differentiated cancer, surveillance of microcarcinomas, and optimal resection of locally advanced disease is subject to patient preference and surgeon experience. A better understanding of the biology of the particular thyroid carcinoma remains a pervasive component of the tumor aggressiveness that can drive disease outcomes and improved control of the carcinoma. Regardless, ongoing advances and better understanding of the reports that alter societal guidelines will hopefully improve the surgical management of patients with thyroid carcinoma. Minimizing complications and ensuring better quality of life should be the main oncologic principle, with the understanding that in thyroid cancer biology, generally "less is more."

Disclosure Statement The authors have no disclosures or conflicts of interest.

References

1. American Thyroid Association Guidelines Taskforce on Thyroid N, Differentiated Thyroid C, Cooper DS, et al. Revised American Thyroid Association management guidelines for patients with thyroid nodules and differentiated thyroid cancer. Thyroid. 2009;19(11):1167–214. https://doi.org/10.1089/thy.2009.0110.
2. Haugen BR, Alexander EK, Bible KC, et al. 2015 American Thyroid Association management guidelines for adult patients with thyroid nodules and differentiated thyroid cancer: the American Thyroid Association guidelines task force on thyroid nodules and differentiated thyroid cancer. Thyroid. 2016;26(1):1–133. https://doi.org/10.1089/thy.2015.0020.
3. Filetti S, Durante C, Hartl D, et al. Thyroid cancer: ESMO clinical practice guidelines for diagnosis, treatment and follow-updagger. Ann Oncol. 2019;30(12):1856–83. https://doi.org/10.1093/annonc/mdz400.
4. Lohia S, Morris LGT, Roman BR. Association between implementation of the 2009 American Thyroid Association guidelines and De-escalation of treatment for low-risk papillary thyroid carcinoma. JAMA Otolaryngol Head Neck Surg. 2020;146(11):1081–2. https://doi.org/10.1001/jamaoto.2020.3024.
5. Zhu CY, Sha SW, Tseng CH, et al. Trends in the surgical management of known or suspected differentiated thyroid cancer at a single institution, 2010–2018. Thyroid. 2020;30(11):1639–45. https://doi.org/10.1089/thy.2019.0783.
6. Shaha A. Selective surgical management of well-differentiated thyroid cancer. Ann N Y Acad Sci. 2008;1138:58–64. https://doi.org/10.1196/annals.1414.010.
7. Accardo G, Conzo G, Esposito D, et al. Genetics of medullary thyroid cancer: an overview. Int J Surg. 2017;41(Suppl 1):S2–6. https://doi.org/10.1016/j.ijsu.2017.02.064.
8. Keutgen XM, Sadowski SM, Kebebew E. Management of anaplastic thyroid cancer. Gland Surg. 2015;4(1):44–51. https://doi.org/10.3978/j.issn.2227-684X.2014.12.02.
9. Hartl DM, Guerlain J, Breuskin I, et al. Thyroid lobectomy for low to intermediate risk differentiated thyroid cancer. Cancers (Basel). 2020;12(11) https://doi.org/10.3390/cancers12113282.

10. Gordon AJ, Dublin JC, Patel E, et al. American Thyroid Association guidelines and national trends in management of papillary thyroid carcinoma. JAMA Otolaryngol Head Neck Surg. 2022;148(12):1156–63. https://doi.org/10.1001/jamaoto.2022.3360.
11. Kuba S, Yamanouchi K, Hayashida N, et al. Total thyroidectomy versus thyroid lobectomy for papillary thyroid cancer: comparative analysis after propensity score matching: a multicenter study. Int J Surg. 2017;38:143–8. https://doi.org/10.1016/j.ijsu.2016.09.083.
12. Matsuzu K, Sugino K, Masudo K, et al. Thyroid lobectomy for papillary thyroid cancer: long-term follow-up study of 1,088 cases. World J Surg. 2014;38(1):68–79. https://doi.org/10.1007/s00268-013-2224-1.
13. Adam MA, Pura J, Gu L, et al. Extent of surgery for papillary thyroid cancer is not associated with survival: an analysis of 61,775 patients. Ann Surg. 2014;260(4):601–5; discussion 605–7. https://doi.org/10.1097/SLA.0000000000000925.
14. Kim SK, Park I, Woo JW, et al. Total thyroidectomy versus lobectomy in conventional papillary thyroid microcarcinoma: analysis of 8,676 patients at a single institution. Surgery. 2017;161(2):485–92. https://doi.org/10.1016/j.surg.2016.07.037.
15. Nixon IJ, Ganly I, Patel SG, et al. Thyroid lobectomy for treatment of well differentiated intra-thyroid malignancy. Surgery. 2012;151(4):571–9. https://doi.org/10.1016/j.surg.2011.08.016.
16. Lang BH, Wong CKH. Lobectomy is a more cost-effective option than total thyroidectomy for 1 to 4 cm papillary thyroid carcinoma that do not possess clinically recognizable high-risk features. Ann Surg Oncol. 2016;23(11):3641–52. https://doi.org/10.1245/s10434-016-5280-6.
17. Rosko AJ, Gay BL, Reyes-Gastelum D, Hamilton AS, Ward KC, Haymart MR. Surgeons' attitudes on total thyroidectomy vs lobectomy for management of papillary thyroid microcarcinoma. JAMA Otolaryngol Head Neck Surg. 2021;147(7):667–9. https://doi.org/10.1001/jamaoto.2021.0525.
18. Iyer NG, Shaha AR. Management of thyroid nodules and surgery for differentiated thyroid cancer. Clin Oncol (R Coll Radiol). 2010;22(6):405–12. https://doi.org/10.1016/j.clon.2010.03.009.
19. Carling T, Carty SE, Ciarleglio MM, et al. American Thyroid Association design and feasibility of a prospective randomized controlled trial of prophylactic central lymph node dissection for papillary thyroid carcinoma. Thyroid. 2012;22(3):237–44. https://doi.org/10.1089/thy.2011.0317.
20. Grsic K, Bumber B, Curic Radivojevic R, Leovic D. Prophylactic central neck dissection in well-differentiated thyroid cancer. Acta Clin Croat. 2020;59(Suppl 1):87–95. https://doi.org/10.20471/acc.2020.59.s1.11.
21. Kwon O, Lee S, Bae JS. The role of prophylactic central compartment neck dissection in patients with T1-T2 cN0 papillary thyroid carcinoma. Gland Surg. 2023;12(3):344–53. https://doi.org/10.21037/gs-22-550.
22. Shirley LA, Jones NB, Phay JE. The role of central neck lymph node dissection in the management of papillary thyroid cancer. Front Oncol. 2017;7:122. https://doi.org/10.3389/fonc.2017.00122.
23. Hall CM, Snyder SK, Maldonado YM, Lairmore TC. Routine central lymph node dissection with total thyroidectomy for papillary thyroid cancer potentially minimizes level VI recurrence. Surgery. 2016;160(4):1049–58. https://doi.org/10.1016/j.surg.2016.06.042.
24. Giordano D, Valcavi R, Thompson GB, et al. Complications of central neck dissection in patients with papillary thyroid carcinoma: results of a study on 1087 patients and review of the literature. Thyroid. 2012;22(9):911–7. https://doi.org/10.1089/thy.2012.0011.
25. Patel KN. The year in thyroidology: surgical science. Thyroid. 2023;33(1):21–3. https://doi.org/10.1089/thy.2022.0659.
26. Sippel RS, Robbins SE, Poehls JL, et al. A randomized controlled clinical trial: no clear benefit to prophylactic central neck dissection in patients with clinically node negative papillary thyroid cancer. Ann Surg. 2020;272(3):496–503. https://doi.org/10.1097/SLA.0000000000004345.
27. Viola D, Materazzi G, Valerio L, et al. Prophylactic central compartment lymph node dissection in papillary thyroid carcinoma: clinical implications derived from the first prospective randomized controlled single institution study. J Clin Endocrinol Metab. 2015;100(4):1316–24. https://doi.org/10.1210/jc.2014-3825.

28. Haymart MR, Esfandiari NH, Stang MT, Sosa JA. Controversies in the management of low-risk differentiated thyroid cancer. Endocr Rev. 2017;38(4):351–78. https://doi.org/10.1210/er.2017-00067.
29. Asimakopoulos P, Shaha AR, Nixon IJ, et al. Management of the neck in well-differentiated thyroid cancer. Curr Oncol Rep. 2020;23(1):1. https://doi.org/10.1007/s11912-020-00997-6.
30. Fujishima M, Miyauchi A, Ito Y, Kudo T, Kihara M, Miya A. Selective prophylactic lateral node dissection improves the ipsilateral lateral node recurrence-free survival: a retrospective single-center cohort study. Ann Med Surg (Lond). 2020;57:190–5. https://doi.org/10.1016/j.amsu.2020.07.046.
31. Shaghaghi A, Salari A, Jalaeefar A, Shirkhoda M. Management of lymph nodes in medullary thyroid carcinoma: a review. Ann Med Surg (Lond). 2022;81:104538. https://doi.org/10.1016/j.amsu.2022.104538.
32. Spanheimer PM, Ganly I, Chou JF, et al. Prophylactic lateral neck dissection for medullary thyroid carcinoma is not associated with improved survival. Ann Surg Oncol. 2021;28(11):6572–9. https://doi.org/10.1245/s10434-021-09683-8.
33. Lin JD. Increased incidence of papillary thyroid microcarcinoma with decreased tumor size of thyroid cancer. Med Oncol. 2010;27(2):510–8. https://doi.org/10.1007/s12032-009-9242-8.
34. Brito JP, Hay ID. Management of papillary thyroid microcarcinoma. Endocrinol Metab Clin N Am. 2019;48(1):199–213. https://doi.org/10.1016/j.ecl.2018.10.006.
35. Miyauchi A, Ito Y. Conservative surveillance management of low-risk papillary thyroid microcarcinoma. Endocrinol Metab Clin N Am. 2019;48(1):215–26. https://doi.org/10.1016/j.ecl.2018.10.007.
36. Shaha AR, Tuttle RM. Active surveillance for micropapillary thyroid carcinoma: a clinical review. Gland Surg. 2024;13(1):100–7. https://doi.org/10.21037/gs-22-558.
37. Shaha AR, Tuttle RM. Nuances in the surgical management of thyroid cancer. Indian J Surg Oncol. 2022;13(1):1–6. https://doi.org/10.1007/s13193-021-01362-0.
38. Hay ID, Lee RA, Kaggal S, et al. Long-term results of treating with ethanol ablation 15 adult patients with cT1aN0 papillary thyroid microcarcinoma. J Endocr Soc. 2020;4(11):bvaa135. https://doi.org/10.1210/jendso/bvaa135.
39. Zhang M, Luo Y, Zhang Y, Tang J. Efficacy and safety of ultrasound-guided radiofrequency ablation for treating low-risk papillary thyroid microcarcinoma: a prospective study. Thyroid. 2016;26(11):1581–7. https://doi.org/10.1089/thy.2015.0471.
40. Zhou W, Jiang S, Zhan W, Zhou J, Xu S, Zhang L. Ultrasound-guided percutaneous laser ablation of unifocal T1N0M0 papillary thyroid microcarcinoma: preliminary results. Eur Radiol. 2017;27(7):2934–40. https://doi.org/10.1007/s00330-016-4610-1.
41. Shonka DC Jr, Ho A, Chintakuntlawar AV, et al. American head and neck society endocrine surgery section and international thyroid oncology group consensus statement on mutational testing in thyroid cancer: defining advanced thyroid cancer and its targeted treatment. Head Neck. 2022;44(6):1277–300. https://doi.org/10.1002/hed.27025.
42. Chernichenko N, Shaha AR. Role of tracheal resection in thyroid cancer. Curr Opin Oncol. 2012;24(1):29–34. https://doi.org/10.1097/CCO.0b013e32834d6dd7.
43. McCaffrey TV. Classification of laryngotracheal stenosis. Laryngoscope. 1992;102(12 Pt 1):1335–40. https://doi.org/10.1288/00005537-199212000-00004.
44. Shin DH, Mark EJ, Suen HC, Grillo HC. Pathologic staging of papillary carcinoma of the thyroid with airway invasion based on the anatomic manner of extension to the trachea: a clinicopathologic study based on 22 patients who underwent thyroidectomy and airway resection. Hum Pathol. 1993;24(8):866–70. https://doi.org/10.1016/0046-8177(93)90136-5.
45. Cavalheiro BG, Shah JP, Randolph GW, et al. Management of recurrent well-differentiated thyroid carcinoma in the neck: a comprehensive review. Cancers (Basel). 2023;15(3) https://doi.org/10.3390/cancers15030923.
46. Coca-Pelaz A, Rodrigo JP, Shah JP, et al. Recurrent differentiated thyroid cancer: the current treatment options. Cancers (Basel). 2023;15(10) https://doi.org/10.3390/cancers15102692.

Management of Retrosternal Goiter

8

Madan Kapre, Neeti Kapre Gupta, Sonam Khokhar, Sanjog Singh, and Swapnil Deshpande

Editorial

Kapre and colleagues have reviewed their experience and expertise in the management of retrosternal goiter. They have discussed the definition of substernal goiter and adopted a substernal goiter classification. The indications for surgery are well discussed, along with a surgical approach. Most of the substernal goiters can be easily removed through the neck, and only a small percentage will require a transthoracic approach. The risks and complications are well-described by the authors. They have also discussed the indications for sternal split. The surgical steps are well-described, and intraoperative problems and complications need special attention. This is a common surgical problem in goiter surgery, and the operating surgeon should be familiar with retrieving the substernal portion of the goiter and avoiding major thoracic complications, especially bleeding from the inferior thyroid veins. Intraoperative nerve monitoring is quite helpful.

The extent of thyroidectomy should be guided primarily by the extent of disease observed on CT imaging. It may be appropriate to consider unilateral thyroidectomy if the contralateral lobe is small or with minimal nodularity. Whether there is a need for radiofrequency ablation (RFA) remains unclear at this time but may be a new consideration in high-risk individuals. The goal of the surgery should be to relieve the compression symptoms, and the decision to perform surgery should be based on patient symptomatology rather than tracheal displacement alone. Due consideration should be given to high-risk complications in these individuals.

Ashok R. Shaha

M. Kapre · N. K. Gupta (✉) · S. Khokhar · S. Singh
Department of ENT & Head & Neck Surgery, Neeti Clinics Pvt Ltd, Nagpur, India

S. Deshpande
Department of Cardiothoracic Surgery, Dr K.G Deshpande Memorial Hospital, Nagpur, India

P. S. Pai et al. (eds.), *Controversies in Cancer of the Thyroid and Parathyroid Glands*, https://doi.org/10.1007/978-3-032-13130-0_8

Introduction

Retrosternal goiters constitute roughly 1–3% of all goiters [1], with incidence rates typically increasing with age and the majority present in the fifth to sixth decades of life [2]. If we consider the incidence as a percentage of all patients undergoing thyroidectomy, rates can vary anywhere between 1% and 20% [3–5]. This is essentially because the definitions of retrosternality are extremely variable. Lahey and Swinton [4] defined substernal goiter as a "gland in which the greatest diameter of the intrathoracic component by x-ray was well below the upper aperture of the thoracic inlet," whereas Katlic, Grillo, and Wang [3] described substernal goiter as when greater than 50% of the goiter is present substernally. Numerous classifications are also in practice to categorize the extent of retrosternality. Higgins [6] based his classification scheme on the percentage of goiter in the neck versus the percentage of goiter in the chest as follows:

1. >50% in the neck being described as substernal
2. >50% in the chest as partially intrathoracic
3. >80% in the chest as completely intrathoracic.

The grading system described by Cho and Cohen [7] classifies grade I as 0–25% of the goiter within the chest, grade II as 26–50%, grade III as 51–75%, and grade IV as greater than 75%. The authors of this text find the anatomical classification given by Randolph et al. [8] to be the most helpful and clinically relevant (Table 8.1).

Anterior mediastinal extension is significantly more common (85%) than posterior (15%) [9, 10]. Type III, which is isolated mediastinal goiter, constitutes only 0.2–2% of all goiters requiring surgical treatment [3, 6].

In the anterior descent, the goiter remains anterior to subclavian and innominate vessels and the recurrent laryngeal nerve lies deep to it. This is a normal orientation of the gland to nerve as in cervical goiter surgery. However, in posterior mediastinal extensions, the nerve lies superficial to the gland. Surgeons need to be extremely careful regarding this altered surgical anatomy since the nerve being anteriorly placed is at particular peril, most severely in type IIB2 retrosternal goiters (contralateral posterior mediastinal extension between the trachea and the esophagus). Thus, this classification helps us to understand the planar orientation of the recurrent laryngeal nerve and in turn predicts the surgical difficulty. This aids greatly in preoperative counseling of the patients about the anticipated risks of neural damage. The vascular supply also differs according to the type of retrosternal goiter. Both type I and II goiters derive the majority of their blood supply from cervical blood vessels, namely the inferior thyroid artery and thyrocervical trunk. However, isolated mediastinal or type III retrosternal goiters can derive their blood supply from the aorta, subclavian, internal mammary, thyrocervical trunk, thyroidea ima, or innominate arteries [8]. This knowledge is of paramount importance while planning their surgical resection.

Table 8.1 Substernal goiter classification (Randolph et al.)

Type	Location	Anatomy	Prevalence	Approach, comment
I	Anterior mediastinum	Anterior to great vessels, trachea, RLN	85%	Transcervical (sternotomy, only if intrathoracic goiter diameter > thoracic inlet diameter)
II	Posterior mediastinum	Posterior to great vessels, trachea, RLN	15%	As above; also consider sternotomy or right posterolateral thoracotomy if type IIB
IIA	Ipsilateral extension			
IIB	Contralateral extension			
B1	Extension posterior to both the trachea and the esophagus			
B2	Extension between the trachea and the esophagus			
III	Isolated mediastinal goiter	No connection to orthotopic gland; may have mediastinal blood supply	<1%	More likely to require sternotomy

Pathophysiology

There are several theories proposed for retrosternal extension of goiters, a prominent few being embryological fragmentation of the thyroid anlagen [8], an embryological cell rest from the thyroid has migrated caudally with progressive attenuation of the connecting stalk with the thyroid [11], or implantation from a previous surgery. Similarly, the descent into the chest has been attributed to gravitational migration, anatomical constraints offered by strap muscles anteriorly, trachea medially, and vertebrae posteriorly. This, in addition to repetitive movements of deglutition and negative intrathoracic pressure, is said to facilitate inferior growth of the nodular goiter along the facilitatory cervical and mediastinal fascial planes. However, Professor Lahey from Mayo Clinic emphatically states that all retrosternal goiters have their origin from the cervical gland counterpart [4].

Symptomatology and Clinical Examination

Retrosternal goiters are significantly more common in females, and typical age at presentation is the fifth or sixth decade of life. Eliciting a thorough family history is important.

These goiters may be entirely asymptomatic in a small number of patients (roughly 20%) [12, 13]. The majority, however, present with a painless anterior neck swelling of a long-standing duration that seems to be progressively increasing in size. A rapid increase in size and development of pain are warning signs. This could be simply due to intranodular hemorrhage or rarely caused by malignant transformation. Compressive symptoms may include difficulty in breathing, swallowing, or simply a choking sensation in the neck or throat. Symptoms generally worsen when lying down or in the supine position. Due to these vague symptoms, predominantly retrosternal goiters with a small cervical component are often misdiagnosed as chronic obstructive airway diseases such as COPD and asthma. They are under the care of pulmonologists often for prolonged periods of time before a diagnosis of retrosternal goiter is established on imaging. An acute respiratory distress may sometimes directly be the presenting symptom (5–10%) [13]. Other dangerous implications may be flushing of the face and breathing difficulty on raising arms above the level of the shoulders. This occurs due to thoracic inlet obstruction and subsequent venous congestion due to compression on the superior vena cava. Rarely, the goiter may press upon the cervical sympathetic trunk, producing drooping of eyelids (ptosis), constriction of the pupils of eyeballs (miosis), or sunken eyeballs (enophthalmos). Similarly, very rarely compression on the esophagus and retrograde pressure may lead to the formation of esophageal varices and hematemesis.

Examination of the retrosternal goiter should be done standing behind the patient and palpating the swelling with the tips of the phalanges. Mobility of the swelling with swallowing movements, consistency, and nodularity must be reported. An assessment of the tracheal shift by palpation just above the sternal notch is important. It is also of importance to note whether in neck extension position the clinician is able to insinuate his fingertips between the lower limit of the swelling and the suprasternal notch. This helps in determining the true retrosternal nature of the swelling and decide whether or not a transcervical delivery is possible. One more method to ascertain this is to request the patient to lie supine on the examination table and administer a shoulder bag just as is anticipated during the surgical procedure. If upon this maneuver getting below the swelling becomes possible, it is more likely that a transcervical approach will be sufficient (Fig. 8.1). Pemberton's sign, which is facial congestion and plethora with respiratory difficulty upon raising upper limbs as described above, is a classically described sign of a significant mediastinal extension of the goiter [14].

A preoperative laryngoscopy and documentation of vocal status are absolutely necessary as part of the assessment and from a medico-legal standpoint. It is also important to share with the anesthesia team degree of skewing of the larynx or distortion of the laryngeal inlet since this may be relevant information for them to plan their strategies for intubation.

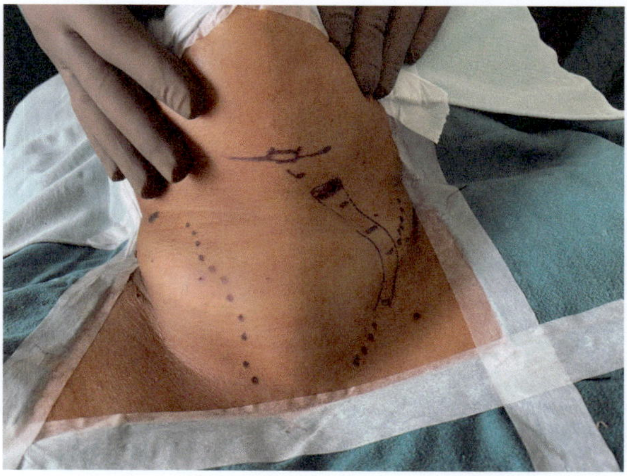

Fig. 8.1 Assessment of retrosternal extension and tracheal deviation by the goiter

Investigations

It is mandatory to establish the histology of these goiters. Therefore, a fine-needle aspiration cytology, preferably under the guidance of ultrasound to target the most representative nodule, is recommended. Similarly, the thyroid function should be recorded by way of estimation of thyroid hormones T3, T4, and TSH levels.

Although ultrasound remains the workhorse for thyroid imaging, its utility in retrosternal goiters is limited. An axial contrast-enhanced CT scan is the bare minimum imaging modality to be employed for these goiters. CT scan allows the exact delineation of the inferior extent of the gland. It gives meaningful information regarding the relationships with the trachea, the esophagus, and great vessels, especially the innominate artery and vein and the aortic arch [15, 16] (Figs. 8.2 and 8.3). By assessment of the disease involving tracheo-esophageal groove, it provides a good risk estimate of nerve injury. It can accurately estimate the tracheal luminal narrowing and provides objective records of the degree of airway compromise. Therefore, it is actually advisable to discuss the radiology scans with anesthesia team preoperatively to help them prepare for this difficult airway situation. CT scan also aids in cervical node detection and mapping. CT characteristics of infiltrative or irregular margins, micro-calcifications, and nodal metastases are indicators of a potential malignancy.

An MRI scan may occasionally be considered in suspected vascular or visceral involvement for additional information on the degree of invasion into the soft tissues.

Barium swallow studies may be seldom helpful in posterior mediastinal extensions, but generally esophageal compression correlates to the clinical symptom of dysphagia reasonably well. Therefore, we need not recommend barium swallow studies routinely for nonsymptomatic retrosternal goiter patients [8].

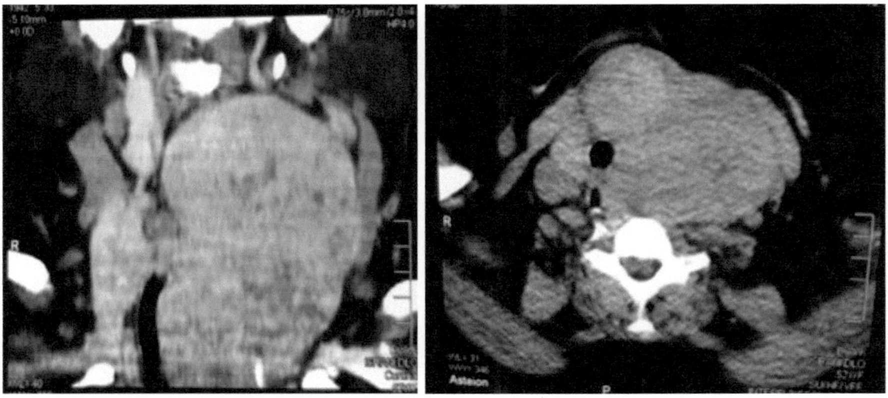

Figs. 8.2 and 8.3 A coronal and axial CT image of retrosternal goiter with luminal compromise

Flow volume loop analysis was routinely practiced to diagnose or even monitor patients (who were not willing to undergo surgical removal) with retrosternal goiters. However, the concordance of flow volume loop results and tracheal caliber is modest [8]. Often, mild narrowing of airways is missed by them and flow volume loop studies can detect tracheal stenosis only when the tracheal diameter reduces to less than 5 mm [8].

Surgical Treatment

Retrosternal extension of the goiter itself is an indication for surgical intervention [8]. Needless to say, other compressive symptoms such as breathlessness, especially on lying down, and difficulty in swallowing are clear indications as well. Sudden-onset rapid increase in size and appearance of pain may indicate intralesional hemorrhage and warrant reasonably urgent intervention. Malignancy detected on cytopathology deserves treatment on merit of differentiated thyroid cancers, with special attention to level VI clearance, that is, removal of superior mediastinal lymph nodes [17].

After due diligence to the interpretation of imaging and cytopathology, ensuring the general medical fitness of the patient to undergo the said surgical procedure, a detailed discussion with the anesthesia team is important to plan strategies for intubation. Often, utilization of video laryngoscope and technique of fiber-optic intubation is helpful. Similarly, a cardiothoracic surgical team should always be on board during the planning and execution of the surgery. Detailed informed counseling of the patient and relatives is of paramount importance. Possible approaches under consideration, including the plan for and extent of sternotomy, should be discussed beforehand. A reliable estimate of complications, namely bleeding, risk of neural injury, and hypoparathyroidism, should be explained. As was alluded to previously, chances of the above will vary depending on the type of retrosternal extension, which can be predicted based on imaging. The surgical team may decide to employ

Table 8.2 Classification and approach for retrosternal goiters (Tolley et al)

Grade	Anatomical location	Approach
1	Above aortic arch (above T4)	Cervical
2	Aortic arch to pericardium	Manubriotomy
3	Below right atrium	Full sternotomy

surgical adjuncts such as a harmonic scalpel, intraoperative nerve monitoring and parathyroid imaging.

Most, if not all goiters with extension into the superior mediastinum, can be delivered through the neck. Probably the reason is in their descent itself, because as they slowly grow toward the mediastinum, they also make way for their exit through the cervical route. The guiding principles for the possibility of the removal through the neck are as follows: the benign lesions carry their blood supply as they descend into the superior mediastinum. Hence, it is relatively bloodless, and the planes are easily dissected. The goiter that are in the transverse diameter lesser than the exit of the mediastinum are similarly accessible through the neck.

The goiter, which descends up to the arch, generally classified as perivascular, is again usually removable through a cervical approach.

However, the malignant lesions do not respect the planes and are infiltrative. These lesions have acquired blood supply by collateral vessels in the superior mediastinum, and the management of their vasculature can be quite challenging.

We recommend that if there is any doubt about the accessibility of these goiters, then the surgery should be performed, preferably where the infrastructure facilities allow intervention by a thoracic surgeon.

There are certain operative tips that help in the delivery of these lesions—head-down position, gentle traction, and strictly adhering to the planes. The structure at risk is the inferior parathyroid, and, as such, it is imperative that the superior parathyroids are protected and confirmed to be functional before proceeding with inferior pole dissection.

While determining the approach—transcervical or sternotomy—the authors find the classification given by Tolley et al. [18] very useful (Table 8.2).

In the literature, about 1% of nonmalignant retrosternal goiters and 3% of malignant ones require a sternotomy [19].

Definite indications of sternotomy are as follows:

1. Posterior mediastinal goiter with contralateral extension (type II B)
2. Superior vena cava syndrome
3. Isolated type III mediastinal goiter
4. Recurrent retrosternal goiter

The approach for retrosternal extension can also be achieved using median 1/3rd cleidotomy to extend the thoracic outlet. This approach is useful in case of adhesions present due to a previous surgery or malignancy, but the extent is only up to the anterior mediastinum [20].

Sternotomy Approach

1. Upper partial sternotomy: midline incision of the manubrium, upper body of sternum extending up to the fourth or fifth intercostal space and then cutting the body of sternum transversely into the intercostal space.
2. Complete median sternotomy: midline incision cutting the whole of sternum (manubrium, body of sternum, and xiphoid process).

Upper Partial Sternotomy

Indications

Anterior mediastinal extension of retrosternal goiter requiring sternal approach (Fig. 8.4).

Surgical Steps (Fig. 8.5)

Skin incision begins from the midpoint of the neck and extends over the manubrium and body of sternum up to the third/fourth/fifth space in the midline. The suprasternal ligament is divided with diathermy or scissors. A saw is then used to perform median sternotomy up to the appropriate space. Then, the saw is turned

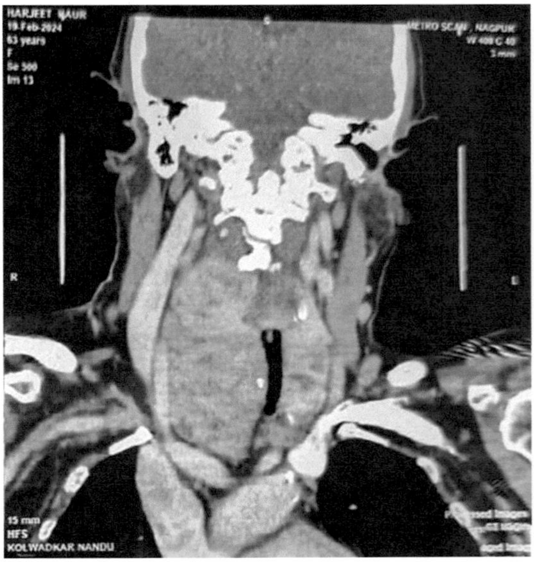

Fig. 8.4 Multinodular goiter extending up to the anterior mediastinum in CT neck and chest. These cases can be done by upper partial sternotomy if the thyroid mass cannot be removed by neck incision

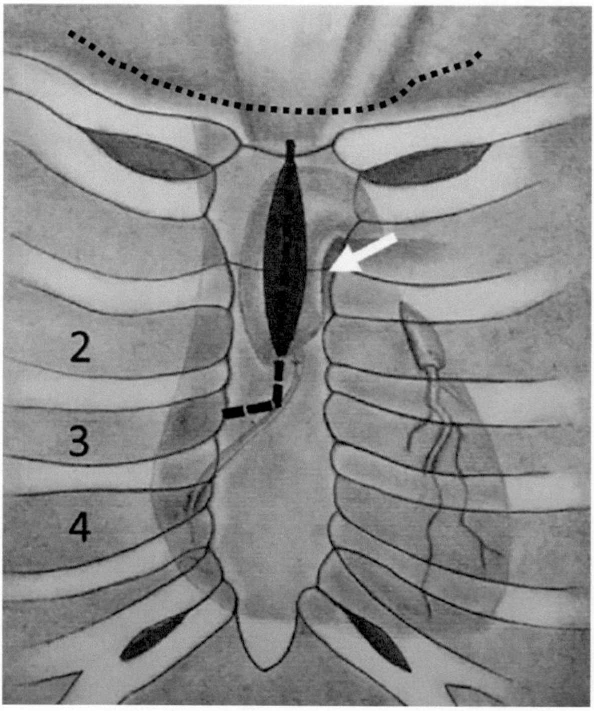

Fig. 8.5 Upper partial sternotomy

90° and the intercostal space is entered to divide the sternum. Care has to be taken to preserve the right internal mammary artery and if injured has to be clipped promptly both proximally and distally. The opening of the right pleura has to be accounted for with an additional pleural underwater drain. Once the sternotomy is complete, hemostasis is achieved and the sternum is retracted. The prepericardial fat is dissected, and innominate vein is identified. The mobilized thyroid mass present in the neck is then traced to mediastinum in relation to the innominate vein and right brachiocephalic trunk. Rarely, thyroid mass with just anterior mediastinal extension does not derive any major blood supply from mediastinum. Therefore, mobilization from the surrounding adhesions taking care of the blood vessels usually delivers the mass to the neck. At times, the innominate vein has to be taped as the mass goes posterior to the vein and anterior to the aortic arch. Careful examination to ensure the integrity of the pericardium is mandatory. Underwater pleural drain is inserted substernally and in right pleural cavity if needed and then the sternum is closed. The subcutaneous tissue is approximated from the body to the manubrium up to the neck incision. Skin is finally sutured with due care to avoid dogearing at the tripointer junction of the neck and sternal wound.

Complete Sternotomy

Indications

1. Recurrent retrosternal goiter (Fig. 8.6)
2. Type III retrosternal goiter
3. Malignant retrosternal goiter requiring mediastinal lymph node clearance

Steps

Skin markings are first made two fingers below the xiphoid process (Fig. 8.7). After the skin incision, the suprasternal ligament is divided. The anterior rectus sheath attached to the xiphoid process is divided into two halves. The manubrium, body, and xiphoid are then divided by sternal saw. The prepericardial fat is dissected and innominate vein identified. The thyroid mass is dissected from the neck, and the lower end is delineated from the relevant structures, namely the innominate vein, aortic arch, and arch vessels. Only in case of posterior mediastinum extension the arch vessels have to be looped and thyroid mass needs to be mobilized between the arch of the aorta and tracheal bifurcations. In type III retrosternal goiter, the blood supply is almost inevitably entirely mediastinal. Therefore, these feeding vessels need to be meticulously identified and divided before mobilizing the gland. Mediastinal lymph node clearance, when indicated, can be achieved by opening the pleural cavity and approaching the lung hilum. Even in very deep mediastinal thyroid extensions, opening of the pericardium is mostly not needed unless there is pericardial involvement in thyroid malignancy. After the completion of the procedure, hemostasis is achieved, mediastinal and pleural underwater seal drains are

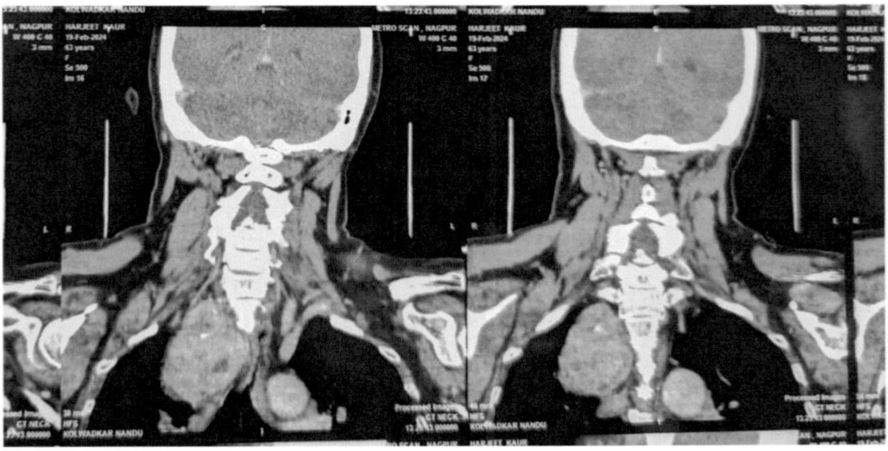

Fig. 8.6 A coronal CT scan showing Multinodular goiter extending deep into the mediastinum

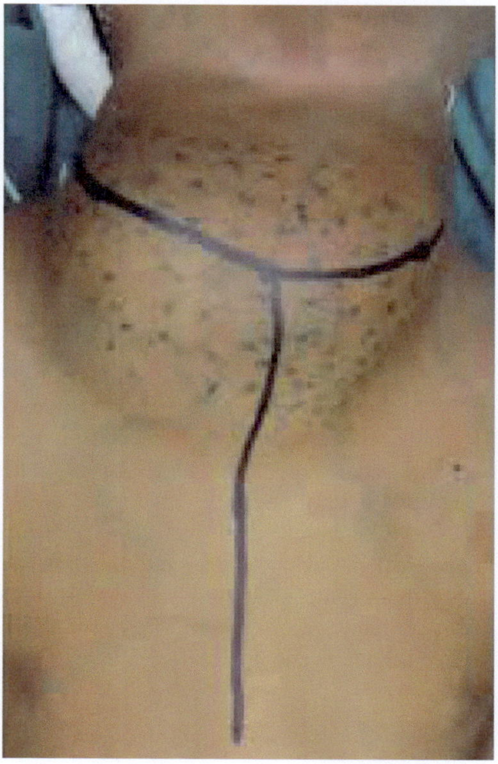

Fig. 8.7 Preoperative marking of neck and sternal incision

inserted, and the sternum is closed. The subcutaneous tissues are then approximated from rectus sheath and over the xiphoid process up to the midline of neck incision. Finally, the skin incision is sutured.

Complications

There are complications that are inherent to any thyroid surgery, but there are certain additional risks involved.

The Recurrent Laryngeal Nerve

As discussed previously, the nerve may actually be ventral or superficial to the thyroid and requires thorough knowledge of anatomy and a skillful surgeon to navigate the nerve and preserve it in this scenario. Nerve monitor is immensely useful to identify and safeguard the functional continuity of the nerve. The nerve may similarly be displaced laterally. It needs to be dissected diligently, strictly adhering to the thyroid swelling and preferably by blunt dissection.

The Inferior Parathyroid Gland

These may not be easily identified and their blood supply probably will be compromised because of unpredictability of the level of ligation of the inferior thyroid artery. The imaging basedd parathyroid recognition techniques either by probe or by a camera are helpful. Similarly, additional injection of indocyanine green is a useful adjunct as it also provides confirmatory information regarding the vascularity and viability of the preserved parathyroid glands.

Other Complications

Injury to the great vessels, such as the innominate artery or vein, is easily avoidable by gentle section into the right plane. Such complication always needs help from a vascular surgeon. Meticulous dissection, anastomosis or grafting is done as warranted by the intra-operative situation.

Injury to the chyle duct, particularly on the left side, is more troublesome; it may not be evident during surgery and may present late in the postoperative period. This can be managed conservatively in case of low volume leaks. In case of high-volume leaks, surgical exploration may be warranted. Other approaches are embolization by interventional radiological techniques or a ligation via endoscope-assisted thoracoscopy.

Complications Specific to Sternotomy Procedure may be as Follows

A. Sternal retraction in the upper partial sternotomy is difficult, and excessive retraction causes sternal fracture and costochondral junction fracture, causing significant postoperative pain.
B. Innominate vein injury.
C. Phrenic nerve injury while doing mediastinal lymph node clearance.
D. Right innominate artery injury for type II B retrosternal goiter.
E. Bleeding, especially in type III retrosternal goiter.
F. Sternal wound infection (superficial and deep).

Summary

The incidence of retrosternal goiter is quite rare. They are often misdiagnosed to begin with and are often detected on imaging. Since most of the CT scans are performed in a supine position, there is a word of caution for overestimation of retrosternal extension. Clinical examination, particularly the ability to insinuate your finger between the thyroid and suprasternal notch in a hyperextended neck, will reassure the delivery by cervical route. The involvement of a cardiothoracic surgeon, although not required in most cases, is certainly desirable to plan these surgeries where a team and infrastructure are available, especially when we suspect malignancy or extension of the thyroid in the perivisceral plane that is between the esophagus and the trachea.

References

1. Kapre M. Thyroid surgery: principles and practice. CRC Press; 2020.
2. Cullinane C, Evoy D, McDermott E, Prichard R. The surgical management of retrosternal goiter; an ongoing controversy. World J Surg Surg Res. 2021;4:1328.
3. Katlic MR, Wang CA, Grillo HC. Substernal goiter. Ann thoracic Surg. 1985;39(4):391–9.
4. Lahey FH, Swinton NW. Intra-thoracic goiter. Surg Gynecol Obstet. 1934;59:627–37.
5. Testini M, Gurrado A, Avenia N, Bellantone R, Biondi A, Brazzarola P, Calzolari F, Cavallaro G, De Toma G, Guida P, Lissidini G. Does mediastinal extension of the goiter increase morbidity of total thyroidectomy? A multicenter study of 19,662 patients. Ann Surg Oncol. 2011;18:2251–9.
6. Higgins CC. Intrathoracic goiter. Arch Surg. 1927;15:895–912.
7. Cohen JP, Cho HT. Surgery for substernal goiters. Oper Techn Otolaryngol Head Neck Surg. 1994;5(2):118–25.
8. Randolph GW. Surgery of the thyroid and parathyroid glands. 2nd ed. Elsevier; 2013. p. 736.
9. Newman E, Shaha AR. Substernal goiter. J Surg Oncol. 1995;60(3):207–12.
10. Kacprzak G, Karas J, Rzechonek A, Blasiak P. Retrosternal goiter located in the mediastinum: surgical approach and operative difficulties. Interact Cardiovasc Thorac Surg. 2012;15(5):935–7.
11. Sackett WR, Reeve TS, Barraclough B, Delbridge L. Thyrothymic thyroid rests: incidence and relationship to the thyroid gland. J Am Coll Surg. 2002;195(5):635–40.
12. Netterville JL, Coleman SC, Smith JC, Smith MM, Day TA, Burkey BB. Management of substernal goiter. Laryngoscope. 1998;108(11):1611–7.
13. Mackle T, Meaney J, Timon C. Tracheoesophageal compression associated with substernal goiter. Correlation of symptoms with cross-sectional imaging findings. J Laryngol Otol. 2007;121:358–61.
14. Giulea C, Enciu O, Nadragea M, Badiu C, Miron A. Pemberton's sign and intense facial edema in superior vena cava syndrome due to retrosternal goiter. Acta Endocrinologica (Bucharest). 2016;12(2):227.116.
15. Mercante G, Gabrielli E, Pedroni C, Formisano D, Bertolini L, Nicoli F, Valcavi R, Barbieri V. CT cross-sectional imaging classification system for substernal goiter based on risk factors for an extracervical surgical approach. Head Neck. 2011;33(6):792–9.
16. Riffat F, Del Pero MM, Fish B, Jani P. Radiologically predicting when a sternotomy may be required in the management of retrosternal goiters. Ann Otol Rhinol Laryngol. 2013;122(1):15–9.
17. Haugen BR, Alexander EK, Bible KC, Doherty GM, Mandel SJ, Nikiforov YE, Pacini F, Randolph GW, Sawka AM, Schlumberger M, Schuff KG. 2015 American Thyroid Association management guidelines for adult patients with thyroid nodules and differentiated thyroid cancer: the American Thyroid Association guidelines task force on thyroid nodules and differentiated thyroid cancer. Thyroid. 2016;26(1):1–33.
18. Huins CT, Georgalas C, Mehrzad H, Tolley NS. A new classification system for retrosternal goiter based on a systematic review of its complications and management. Int J Surg. 2008;6(1):71–6.
19. Lahey FH. The surgical management of intrathoracic goiter. Surg Gynecol Obstet. 1931;53:346–54.
20. Dagan E, Kleid S. Obviating the need for sternotomy: safety and effectiveness of microdebrider use for retrosternal goiter. Head Neck. 2018;40:837–41. https://doi.org/10.1002/hed.25070.

9 Surgical Management of Locally Advanced Thyroid Cancers

Sueyoshi Moritani

Editorial

The author Sueyoshi Moritani has extensively described the surgical management for advanced thyroid cancer extending to the adjacent organs. Although not often, thyroid carcinoma, especially papillary and anaplastic carcinomas, can extend to adjacent organs and the management of these involvements are critical. The recurrent laryngeal nerve (RLN) invasion can be addressed by shave resection or resection and reconstruction which helps to maintain the vocal cord bulk. This is an important and effective technique which is not yet performed in many institutions. The trachea is the other more commonly involved organ, the managed either by shave resection or resection and anastomosis which has been nicely detailed. Other than these, management of extension to other adjacent organs like larynx and oesophagus and involvement of lymph nodes located in parapharyngeal space and the mediastinum, are comprehensively described. The accompanying images are illustrative and greatly help the reader understand the indication and techniques of extensive surgery for invasive thyroid carcinoma.

Yasuhiro Ito

Introduction

The thyroid gland is located at the tracheal–laryngeal transition and is in close proximity to the aerodigestive tract, including the recurrent laryngeal nerve (RLN). Consequently, invasion of adjacent organs by thyroid cancer can impair phonation,

S. Moritani (✉)
Omi Medical Center, Center for Otolaryngology, Head and Neck Thyroid Surgery, Kusatsu, Shiga, Japan

P. S. Pai et al. (eds.), *Controversies in Cancer of the Thyroid and Parathyroid Glands*, https://doi.org/10.1007/978-3-032-13130-0_9

respiration, and swallowing, significantly impacting both prognosis and quality of life (QOL). Invasion typically begins at the outer surface of the aerodigestive tract and progresses toward the luminal structures. Differentiated thyroid carcinoma (DTC) is a slow-growing malignancy often detected as a superficial invasion of the aerodigestive tract surface. However, due to its slow progression, symptoms are typically absent; when symptoms do appear, the disease is often advanced, with extensive infiltration involving multiple organs, making it unresectable in some cases. Airway obstruction and bleeding are common complications of unresectable, locally advanced DTC and are among the leading causes of mortality in these cases [1]. Surgical intervention is therefore recommended to achieve local disease control.

The primary sites of invasion in thyroid cancer are the aerodigestive tract, including the RLN, with a prevalence of 1–8% among all patients with thyroid cancer, increasing to 10–20% in cases of local recurrence. Since invasion typically begins at the outer surface of these organs, cases where the invasion extends into the lumen are relatively rare, with a reported prevalence of approximately 25% [2]. Although no definitive consensus exists regarding the resection of surrounding organs, such as the aerodigestive tract and major blood vessels in DTC, many support functional preservation surgeries. These include shaving for superficial invasion and combined resection with reconstruction for intraluminal invasion [3, 4]. Shaving procedures for superficial invasion are widely supported, with several reports indicating that microscopic residual disease does not significantly affect prognosis or recurrence, making it an acceptable approach.

Invasion of the aerodigestive tract or major blood vessels can occur not only directly from thyroid cancer but also through metastatic lymph nodes. Such invasion often involves multiple organs, necessitating extensive surgical procedures [5]. Although surgical resection is the primary treatment option, the decision to proceed with surgery should be determined by an experienced multidisciplinary team. This decision should be based on a comprehensive assessment of the tumor's extent, the potential risks of surgical complications, the expected postoperative impact on QOL, including swallowing and phonation, and the patient's overall prognosis.

Recurrent Laryngeal Nerve (RLN) Invasion

The prognosis for patients with RLN involvement alone is better than that for patients with aerodigestive invasion by DTC. However, from a functional perspective, unilateral vocal fold palsy results in hoarseness and dysphagia, while bilateral palsy causes dyspnea and significantly reduces QOL [6–9]. The RLN is a motor nerve responsible for vocal fold movement. In cases of RLN involvement accompanied by preoperative vocal cord palsy, the degree of infiltration is often severe, and combined RLN resection is generally recommended [10]. Conversely, even in the absence of preoperative vocal cord palsy, intraoperative findings frequently reveal RLN involvement [11]. In such cases without vocal cord palsy, infiltration is often superficial or partial. For patients with superficial (epineurial) invasion of the RLN, shave excision is recommended to preserve the RLN. This approach uses sharp dissection to minimize residual tumors while preserving vocal cord function [12].

1. Shave Excision for Cases with RLN Invasion and Without Preoperative Vocal Cord Palsy

   Tumor recurrence at the shaved site occurs in approximately 5% of patients whose extrathyroidal extension of DTC is confined to the RLN. Shave excision may result in permanent vocal cord paralysis in 8–25% of patients without preoperative RLN palsy, with recovery of vocal cord mobility typically occurring within 6 months [6, 13–17]. However, shave excision for advanced infiltration beyond the epineurium and into the perineurium, even in the absence of preoperative vocal cord palsy, almost always results in microscopic residuals. Therefore, intraoperative management should be tailored to the extent of RLN involvement. Electromyographic potentials from RLN stimulation at the proximal end of the infiltrate can aid in determining whether RLN resection is necessary [18]. Additionally, the patient's performance status and swallowing function should be carefully evaluated when deciding between shaving or excising the RLN. RLN palsy increases the risk of aspiration, particularly in older patients with swallowing dysfunction, which can lead to aspiration pneumonia (Fig. 9.1).

2. RLN Resection and Reconstruction for Cases with Severe RLN Invasion

   RLN resection for unilateral RLN infiltration results in the affected vocal fold being fixed in a paramedian position. Atrophy of the intralaryngeal muscles sub-

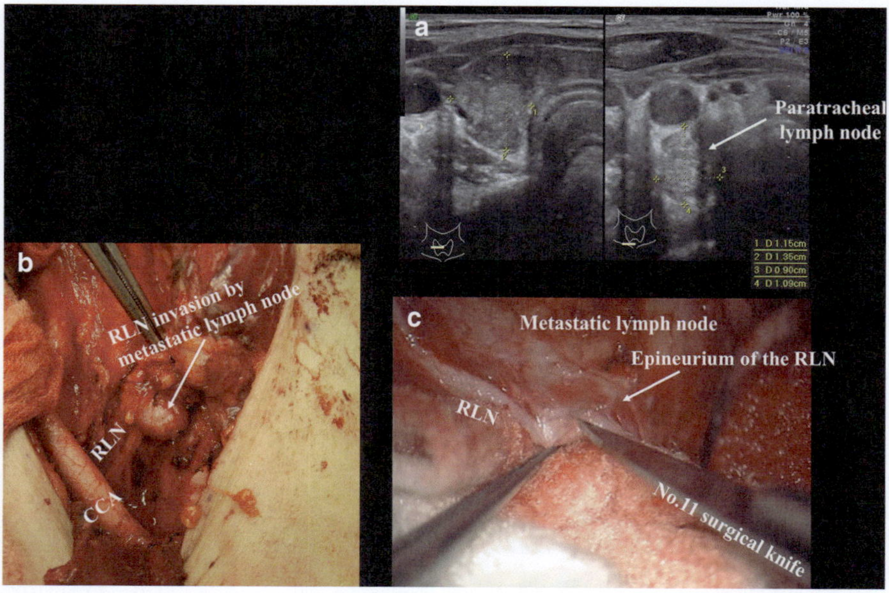

Fig. 9.1 Shave excision for superficial invasion of the RLN. PTC (T3N1aM0) with RLN invasion caused by paratracheal lymph node metastasis in a female patient in her late 30s. The preoperative US revealed lymph node metastasis in the right paratracheal region (**a**). No right vocal cord palsy was observed preoperatively. A total thyroidectomy and bilateral central compartment dissection were performed. Paratracheal lymph node metastasis invading the right RLN was identified. Sharp excision of the right RLN was performed under surgical microscope guidance (**b**, **c**). This patient experienced transient right vocal cord palsy, with vocal cord movement improved 1 month after surgery. PTC papillary thyroid carcinoma, US ultrasonography, RLN recurrent laryngeal nerve

sequently enlarges the glottic gap, further exacerbating hoarseness and dysphagia. While RLN reconstruction does not restore vocal cord movement due to misdirected nerve regeneration, it often improves phonatory function by stabilizing the vocal cords in the median position and preventing intralaryngeal muscle atrophy. Although this process typically takes several months, RLN reconstruction can significantly enhance phonatory outcomes. Therefore, simultaneous RLN reconstruction is recommended for patients undergoing nerve resection to optimize functional recovery.

The literature on RLN reconstruction is largely retrospective. With immediate RLN reconstruction, phonatory function typically recovers within 1 year [19–21]. While the recovery process is slower compared to two-stage phonatory reconstruction methods like type I thyroplasty or arytenoid internalization, the improvement in speech function is often similar or even better [22, 23].

Surgical techniques for RLN reconstruction include end-to-end anastomosis, free nerve grafting, anastomosis of the cervical nerves with the RLN, and anastomosis of the vagus nerve with the RLN [19]. All reconstruction methods aim to improve phonatory function and should be selected based on intraoperative findings (Fig. 9.2). In cases where RLN involvement occurs at the ligament of Berry, identifying the distal portion of the nerve after resection can be challenging. The

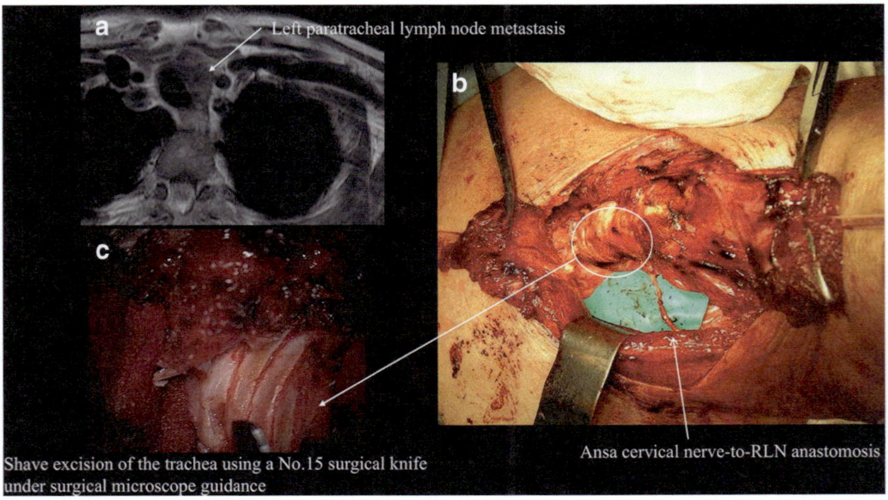

Fig. 9.2 RLN resection and immediate reconstruction for gross invasion of the RLN. PTC (T1aN1aM0) with RLN and superficial tracheal invasion caused by paratracheal lymph node metastasis in a male patient in his early 70s. Preoperative MRI imaging indicated tracheal invasion by left paratracheal lymph node metastasis (**a**). Left-sided vocal cord paralysis was also observed preoperatively. A total thyroidectomy and bilateral central compartment dissection were performed. Paratracheal lymph node metastasis was found to invade the left RLN and the left side of the trachea. Left RLN resection and immediate reconstruction using the ansa cervical nerve were conducted, along with shave excision of the trachea from the first to the fourth tracheal cartilage (**b**, **c**). PTC papillary thyroid carcinoma, MRI magnetic resonance imaging, RLN recurrent laryngeal nerve

laryngeal approach, which involves dividing the inferior pharyngeal constrictor muscle along the lateral edge of the thyroid cartilage to locate the nerve beneath the muscle or behind the thyroid cartilage, is particularly helpful for RLN reconstruction in these scenarios [24, 25].

Tracheal Invasion

1. Two Types of Tracheal Resection for Tracheal Invasion

   Surgical resection is crucial in managing airway invasion by DTC, as it addresses airway narrowing and dysphagia. However, the trachea is a vital organ involved in breathing, speech, and swallowing, raising concerns that tracheal resection may negatively affect postoperative QOL. The decision to perform tracheal resection requires a careful balance between the reduction in QOL and the anticipated postoperative prognosis.

   Thyroid cancer typically invades the airway by progressing from the outer membrane toward the lumen. Deep invasions extending into the lumen require combined airway resection. In cases of superficial tracheal invasion, one surgical approach is shave excision, which involves sharply excising the superficial tracheal invasion while preserving the tracheal tubular structure. Combined airway resection for superficial tracheal invasion is curative but requires primary reconstruction, tracheal stoma formation, and staged closure. In contrast, shave excision avoids tracheal reconstruction and tracheocutaneous fistula closure but carries a higher risk of recurrence due to residual tumor at the resection margins. This is particularly true for shave excisions involving invasion beyond the tracheal cartilage, across multiple tracheal cartilages, or involving the membranous portion of the trachea, where the likelihood of tumor remnants at resection margins is significant [26].

   Reports on combined airway resection for tracheal invasion are limited to retrospective studies from single centers with small case numbers. While a bias exists as the degree of invasion is generally more substantial in cases of non- or incomplete resection with gross residual disease, comparison between complete resection and non- or incomplete resection group consistently shows worse prognoses for the latter [27–30].

2. Shave Excision for Cases with Superficial Tracheal Invasion

   No study has directly compared the outcomes of tracheal resection versus shave excision for superficial tracheal invasion. However, most reports recommend shave excision for superficial invasion, citing a reasonable local control rate (71.9–95.0%) [31–34] and favorable prognosis [31, 32, 35, 36]. Several of these studies also report microscopic residuals at the resection site [31, 33, 37]. For instance, Ito et al. found that approximately half of the patients undergo shave excision for superficial tracheal invasion by PTC, with intraoperative findings confirming macroscopic curative resection exhibited microscopic residuals at the cut surface. Despite this, the local control rate in these patients remained high, suggesting that microscopic residuals have a minimal impact on local recurrence [31]. Conversely, some studies advocate tracheal resection over shave excision [38, 39]. Tsai et al. reported on 16 cases of superficial tracheal invasion treated with shave excision, with adjuvant therapy administered in 15 cases. Local recurrence was observed in eight cases, and three patients died from airway recurrence. Although the details of local recurrence and tumor residuals were not fully described, gross residuals were present in seven cases, suggesting a strong association between gross residuals and poor local control [39].

Shave excision may be a viable treatment option for superficial tracheal invasion, as local control is excellent in most cases where macroscopic curative resection is achieved, even in the presence of microscopic residuals. However, outcomes are poor in cases of gross residual disease. Therefore, it is essential to thoroughly evaluate the extent of tracheal invasion, including the degree of progression, and consider the expertise of the treatment team when selecting a surgical approach (Fig. 9.3).

3. Complete Resection and Reconstruction of the Trachea for Cases with Intraluminal Invasion

Tracheal resection is required when DTC invades the tracheal lumen. Surgical options for addressing such lesions include sleeve or partial resections (wedge or window resections). Sleeve resection involves removing the trachea in the infil-

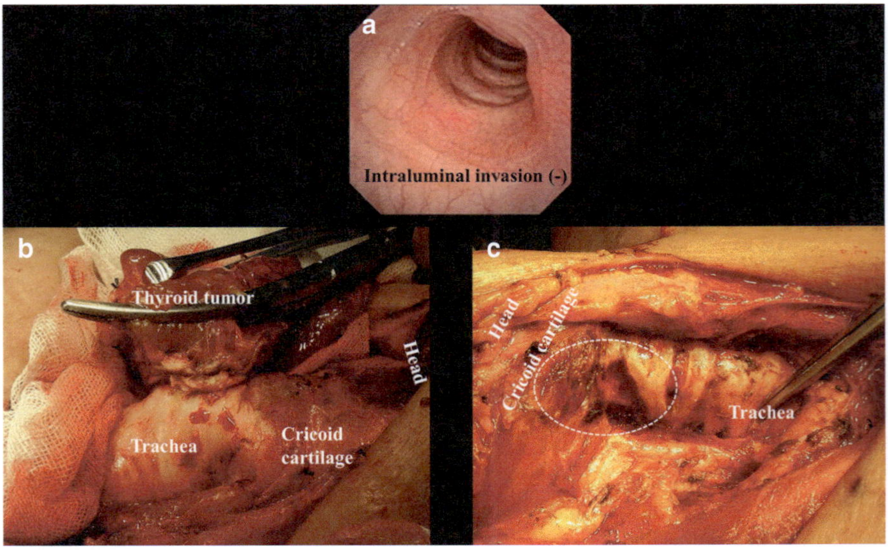

Fig. 9.3 Shave excision for superficial tracheal invasion. PTC (T4aN0M0) with superficial tracheal invasion in a female patient in her early 80s. The preoperative endotracheal evaluation showed no evidence of intraluminal tracheal invasion (**a**). A right thyroid lobectomy and central compartment dissection were performed. Superficial invasion of the cricoid cartilage and trachea by the primary tumor was identified. Shave excision was carried out from the right side of the cricoid cartilage to the third tracheal cartilage. The infiltrated tracheal area was resected along with the tracheal cartilage, preserving only the tracheal mucosal layer. A tracheostomy was not performed (**b**, **c**). PTC papillary thyroid carcinoma

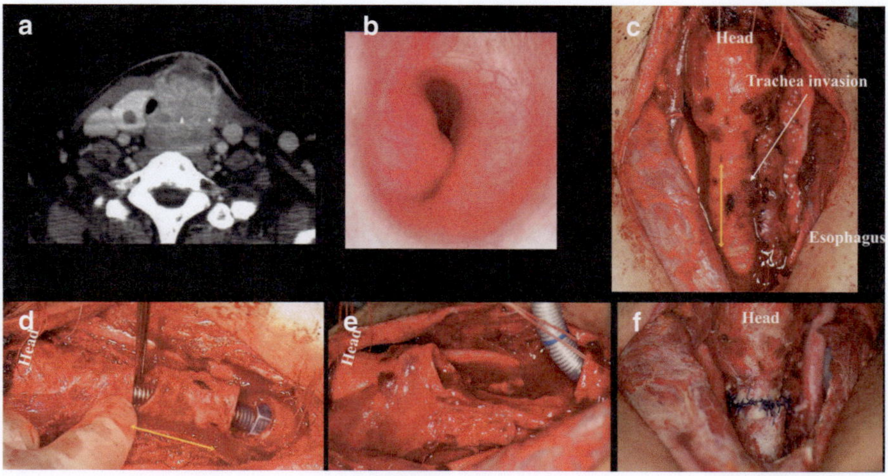

Fig. 9.4 Sleeve resection and end-to-end anastomosis for intraluminal tracheal invasion. PTC with aerodigestive tract and cervical skin invasion in a female patient in her 60s. Preoperative CT and endotracheal evaluation revealed significant tracheal invasion from the left thyroid lobe, with suspected esophageal invasion (**a**, **b**). The airway was secured using PCPS, followed by a total thyroidectomy. Resections included the RLN and the muscle layer of the esophagus. The invaded portion of the trachea, measuring six rings (3 cm in length), was resected (**c**, **d**: yellow double-headed arrow), and an end-to-end tracheal anastomosis was performed (**e**, **f**). Photographs of this case were kindly provided by Professor Hidemitsu Tsutsui. PTC papillary thyroid carcinoma, CT computed tomography, RLN recurrent laryngeal nerve, PCPS percutaneous cardiopulmonary support

trated area in a tubular segment, followed by one-stage closure using end-to-end anastomosis (Fig. 9.4). Partial tracheal resection involves resecting the infiltrated portion of the trachea with a safety margin, often requiring the creation of a stoma to address the tracheal defect. Tracheal stoma closure is typically achieved in two stages (Fig. 9.5). When tracheal invasion reaches the submucosa, it tends to spread circumferentially rather than longitudinally [40, 41]. Because partial tracheal resection increases the likelihood of residual tumor at the resection margins and complicates tracheal stomal closure, several reports recommend sleeve resection with concurrent end-to-end anastomosis as the preferred approach (Fig. 9.6).

A systematic review of sleeve resection reported 5- and 10-year disease-specific survival rates of 75.8–90% and 54.5–69.2%, respectively. Postoperative complications occurred in 27% of cases (95% CI: 20.0–36.0), and perioperative mortality was reported at 2.0% (95% CI: 1.0–4.0). Permanent tracheal stomas were required in 4% of patients (95% CI: 2.0–8.0) after sleeve resection [42]. In contrast, a systematic review comparing sleeve and window resections showed postoperative complication rates of 14.1% (95% CI: 8.3–19.9) for sleeve resection and 19.8% (95% CI: 6.9–32.8) for window resection. Anastomotic failure after sleeve resection was observed in cases with 2.2% (95% CI: 1.2–3.1). Sleeve resection with end-to-end anastomosis is generally limited to seven tracheal rings

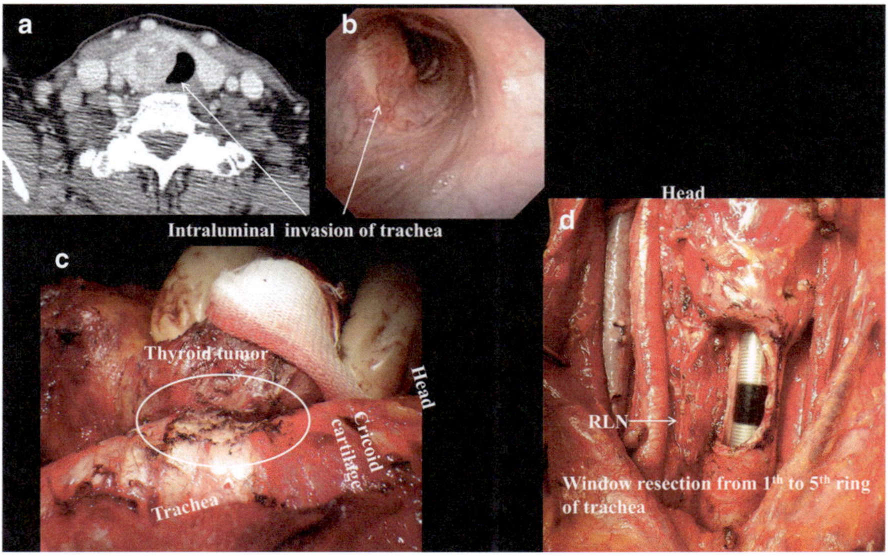

Fig. 9.5 Window resection for intraluminal tracheal invasion. PTC (T4aN1bM0) with intraluminal tracheal invasion in a female patient in her early 60s. Preoperative CT indicated gross tracheal invasion by the thyroid tumor, and laryngotracheal examination confirmed intraluminal tracheal invasion (**a**, **b**). A total thyroidectomy and right lateral neck dissection were performed. From the first to fifth rings, the circumferential resection of 50% of the trachea was performed to address the intraluminal invasion (**c**, **d**). The tracheal stoma was successfully closed using a cervical hinge flap 3 months post-surgery. PTC papillary thyroid carcinoma, CT computed tomography

(5–6 cm), with the resection of 2–3 rings being the most common scenario [43]. Reports including over 40 window resections reveal pathological residuals at the resection margins in 35% of cases according to Ito et al. [44] and 65.8% according to Ebihara et al. [45] Despite the presence of residuals, no significant differences in local recurrence rates were observed between patients with positive versus negative margins in either study. The recurrence rates at tracheal invasive sites following window resection ranged from 4–17.1%, with disease-specific survival rates of 78.9–94.0% at 5 years and 60.8–92.0% at 10 years [44–46]. In comparison, the recurrence rates at tracheal invasive sites following sleeve resection ranged from 0.0% to 12.3% [39, 40, 42, 47].

Approximately 16.5–61.0% of patients require a permanent tracheal stoma after window resection. Moritani et al. reported that window resection in 76 cases resulted in a permanent tracheal stoma in 61% of patients, with a higher likelihood observed in those undergoing resection of more than half the tracheal circumference [46]. Ebihara et al. reported that although tracheal stoma closure is staged, this approach is effective in older patients due to fewer complications and the absence of a need for cervical fixation [45].

Sleeve resection with concurrent end-to-end anastomosis for intraluminal tracheal invasion offers significant advantages, including no residual tumor at the

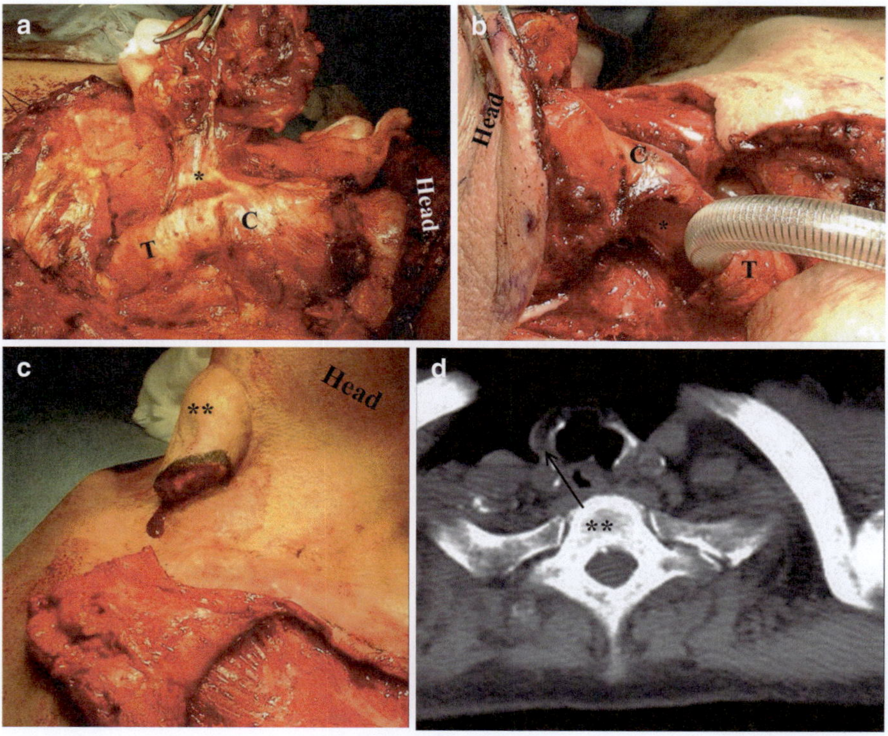

Fig. 9.6 Window resection and staged tracheal stomal closure using a D-P flap combined with nasal septal cartilage for intraluminal tracheal invasion. PTC (T4aN1bM0) with intraluminal tracheal invasion in a male patient in his late 70s. A total thyroidectomy and right lateral neck dissection were performed. Intraoperatively, intraluminal cricoid-trachea invasion, superficial esophageal invasion, and right RLN invasion by the primary thyroid tumor were observed. Circumferential resection of more than 50% of the cricotracheal segment and resection of the membranous portion of the trachea were performed for intraluminal invasion (**a**, **b**: *). A longitudinal resection was performed from the cricoid cartilage to the fourth tracheal ring. The resulting cricotracheal defect was reconstructed using a D-P flap combined with nasal septal cartilage (**c**, **d**: **). The cricotacheal stoma was closed after staged reconstructive surgery. Computed tomography revealed that the reconstructed area of the cricotracheal extended from the tracheal cartilage beyond the midline to the membranous portion (**d**: **). PTC papillary thyroid carcinoma, RLN recurrent laryngeal nerve, C cricoid cartilage, T trachea, D–P deltopectoral

resection margins, improved prognosis, fewer fatal postoperative complications, and superior functional reconstruction. Conversely, while less commonly reported, window resection provides a favorable prognosis, avoids the need for cervical fixation, and is particularly beneficial for older patients. Selecting a surgical approach requires a comprehensive evaluation of the extent of tracheal invasion, including the degree of progression, as well as consideration of the expertise and capabilities of the surgical team. Careful assessment of the patient's condition and the team's skills is essential to determine the most appropriate surgical strategy.

Laryngeal Invasion

Laryngeal invasion by thyroid carcinoma occurs directly through the thyroid and cricoid cartilage into the paraglottic space via an anterior route or through posterior extension around the thyroid cartilage into the paraglottic space. The pharynx may also be invaded by the posterior extension of the tumor around the thyroid cartilage into the pyriform sinus [48]. Intraluminal invasion of the larynx by DTC is uncommon; however, when it occurs, it can cause significant morbidity and, in some cases, mortality due to airway obstruction [49]. For tracheal invasion involving the cricoid cartilage, postoperative functional outcomes can often be predicted based on the extent of airway resection and RLN involvement. However, predicting postoperative functional outcomes becomes more challenging when the invasion involves the thyroid cartilage or intralaryngeal space. Laryngeal framework resection, including shave excision, is often performed to address superficial thyroid cartilage invasion. Laryngeal function is typically preserved if the resection is limited to the unilateral thyroid cartilage lamina (Fig. 9.7). Though infrequent, involvement of the

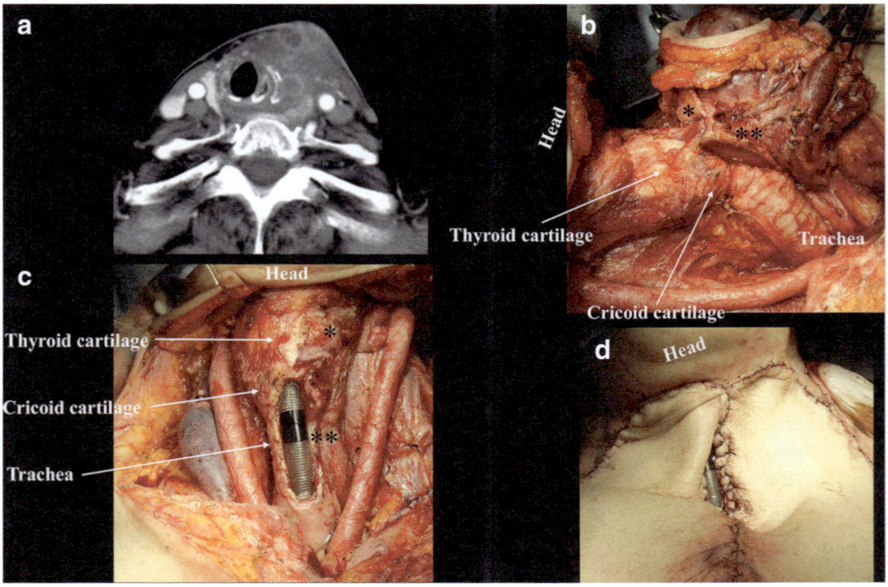

Fig. 9.7 Laryngeal framework resection of the thyroid cartilage and window resection of the cricoid-trachea for aerodigestive tract invasion. PTC (T4aN1bM0) with aerodigestive tract and cervical skin invasion in a female patient in her late 70s. Preoperative CT showing revealed an aerodigestive tract, including the larynx and esophagus, cervical skin invasion, and suspected CCA invasion by the primary thyroid tumor (**a**). The surgical approach included a total thyroidectomy combined with a left lateral neck dissection. A laryngeal framework resection was performed for superficial laryngeal invasion (**b**, **c**: *), and a window resection from the cricoid cartilage to the sixth tracheal ring was carried out for intraluminal invasion (**b**, **c**: **). The esophageal muscle layer was resected for superficial invasion. The cervical skin and surrounding muscles were excised along with the tumor, and the defect was reconstructed using bilateral D-P flaps (**d**). The primary thyroid tumor also invaded the left RLN and vagal nerve, both of which were resected. Unilateral thyroid cartilage lamina was removed for laryngeal infiltration. The cricoid-tracheal stoma was closed 3 months after surgery. PTC papillary thyroid carcinoma, CT computed tomography, CCA common carotid artery, RLN recurrent laryngeal nerve, D-P deltopectoral

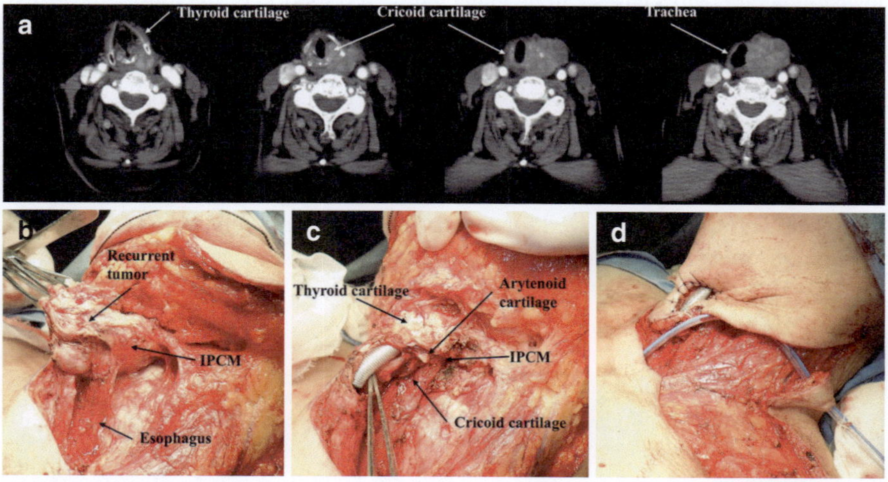

Fig. 9.8 Partial laryngectomy for intraluminal invasion of the larynx and trachea. FTC recurrence with aerodigestive tract and cervical skin invasion in a female patient in her late 60s. Preoperative CT showed aerodigestive tract invasion, including the larynx-trachea and pharynx-esophagus, as well as cervical skin invasion by the primary thyroid tumor. The recurrent tumor extended directly into the paraglottic space around the posterior border of the thyroid cartilage (**a**). The surgical approach included resection of the pharyngeal and esophageal muscle layers (**b**), partial laryngectomy for intraluminal laryngeal invasion, and a window resection from the cricoid cartilage to the fourth tracheal ring for intraluminal tracheal invasion (**c**). The cervical skin overlying the tumor was excised. During the partial laryngectomy, the laryngeal structures immediately below the left vocal cord, including the left side of the cricoid and thyroid cartilage, were resected (**b**). The laryngotracheal stoma and cervical skin defects were reconstructed using a D-P flap (**d**). FTC follicular thyroid carcinoma, CT computed tomography, IMPC inferior pharyngeal constrictor muscle, D-P deltopectoral flap

paraglottic or intralaryngeal space requires intralaryngeal resection depending on the degree of invasion [50, 51] (Fig. 9.8). Surgical options such as partial laryngectomy or vertical hemi-laryngectomy may serve as useful references for these cases [52, 53].

In cases of extensive invasion, preserving laryngeal function becomes increasingly difficult, making total laryngectomy a more viable treatment option [54]. However, since laryngeal invasion by DTC is often confined to one side of the larynx and resection offers a favorable long-term prognosis, total laryngectomy should be considered only when necessary.

Esophageal/Pharyngeal Invasion

Esophageal and pharyngeal musculature can become involved through direct tumor or extracapsular extension from affected paratracheal lymph nodes. The esophageal mucosa serves as a robust barrier against tumor penetration, and luminal surface invasion is rare. Most cases can be managed with resection of the muscle layer [5]. The esophageal muscular layer comprises internal circular and lateral longitudinal muscles. Resection of the lateral muscle layer generally allows for early postoperative oral intake. Even when the muscular layer is partially exposed following muscular layer resection, esophageal reconstruction is not required as long as the tubular structure is preserved (Figs. 9.9 and 9.10). In cases requiring total cervical esophagectomy with laryngectomy, autografts of luminal organs, such as free jejunal grafts, are commonly employed for reconstruction. Conversely, partial esophagectomies are often reconstructed using thin skin flaps, such as free forearm flaps (Fig. 9.11).

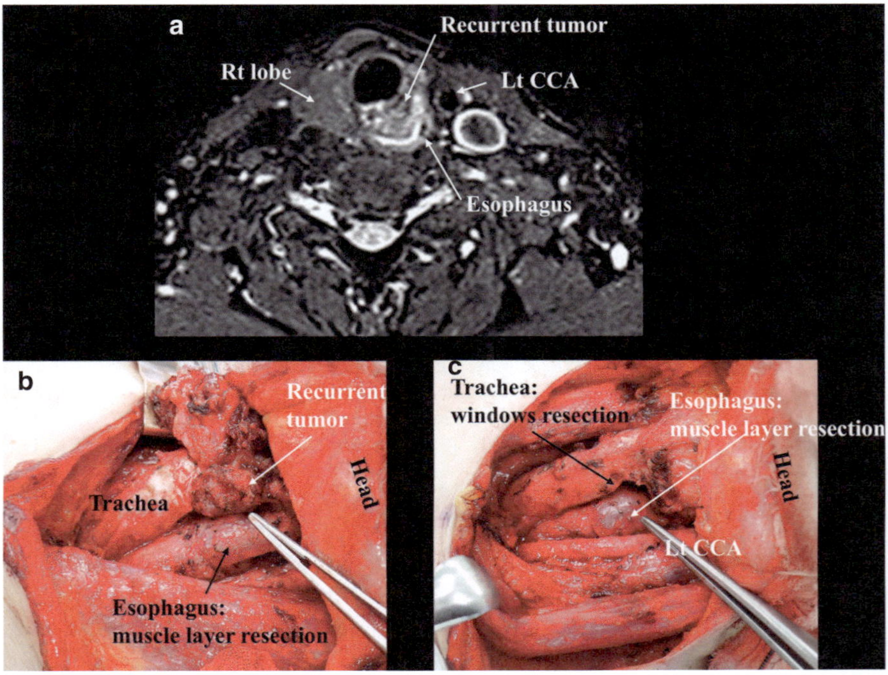

Fig. 9.9 Muscle layer resection of the esophagus and window resection of the trachea for aerodigestive tract invasion. Recurrent PTC with aerodigestive tract invasion in a female patient in her late 50s. The recurrent tumor extended between the trachea and esophagus in the left paratracheal region. MRI indicated no involvement of the CCA, but tracheal and esophageal invasion was suspected (**a**). A right thyroid lobectomy and removal of the recurrent tumor in the left paratracheal region were performed. The recurrent tumor was found to invade both the trachea and esophagus. Window resection was performed to remove part of the tracheal cartilage and membranous portion, extending from the left side of the cricoid cartilage to the third tracheal ring. Additionally, a 4-cm segment of the esophageal muscular layer was resected from the left side of the hypopharynx to the cervical esophagus, preserving the mucosal layer. The esophageal lumen remained intact (**b**, **c**). A tracheocutaneous fistula was created and successfully closed 3 months after the tracheostomy. PTC papillary thyroid carcinoma, CCA common carotid artery

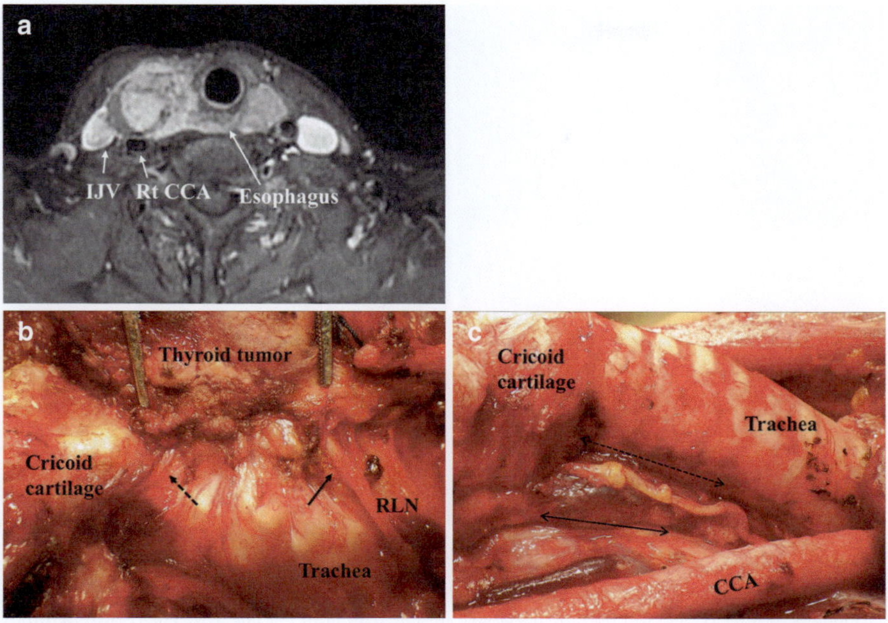

Fig. 9.10 Muscle layer resection of the esophagus and RLN resection with immediate reconstruction for esophageal and RLN invasion. PTC (T4aN1bM0) with esophageal and RLN invasion in a female patient in her late 60s. Preoperative MRI suggested hypopharyngeal and cervical esophageal involvement. Preoperative right-sided vocal cord paralysis was observed (**a**). A total thyroidectomy and bilateral lateral neck dissection were performed. The right RLN was found to be involved by the primary thyroid tumor (arrow: proximal portion of the RLN; dotted arrow: distal portion of the RLN, **b**). A 3-cm muscle layer resection was performed from the hypopharynx to the cervical esophagus, preserving only the mucosal layer (double-headed arrow). The RLN was resected and reconstructed with free nerve grafting using the greater auricular nerve (dotted double-headed arrow, **c**). PTC papillary thyroid carcinoma, RLN recurrent laryngeal nerve, MRI magnetic resonance imaging

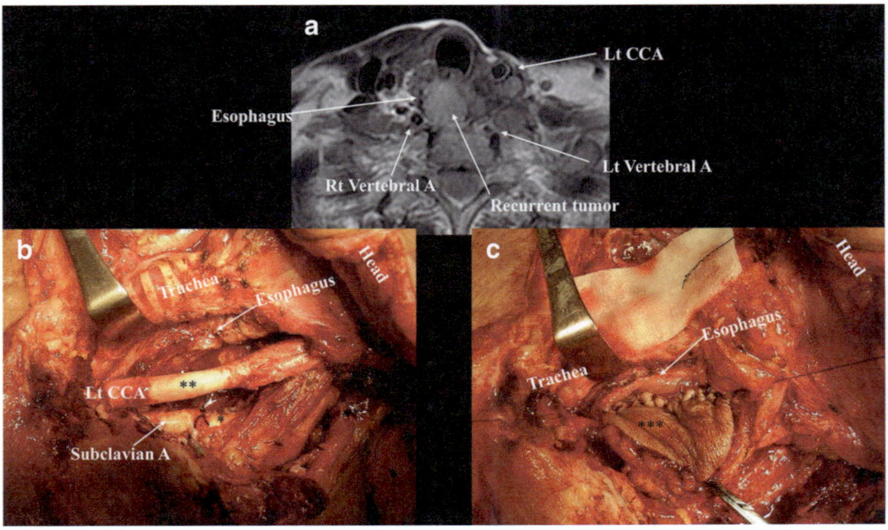

Fig. 9.11 Partial esophagectomy and reconstruction of the esophagus using a free forearm flap for intraluminal invasion of the esophagus. Recurrent PTC with invasion of the CCA, vertebral artery, esophagus, left RLN, and left phrenic nerve in a female patient in her late 70s. The recurrent tumor extended between the trachea and esophagus in the left paratracheal region. MRI suggested involvement of the CCA, vertebral artery, esophagus, and prevertebral fascia (**a**). Preoperative left-sided vocal cord paralysis was also observed. A subadventitial resection of the left CCA was performed, while the left vertebral artery, RLN, and phrenic nerve were resected, along with a partial esophagectomy. The cervical esophagus was reconstructed using a free forearm flap (**b**, **c**). *Resection of the left vertebral artery; **subadventital resection of the left CCA; ***reconstruction of the cervical esophagus using free forearm flap. PTC papillary thyroid carcinoma, MRI magnetic resonance imaging, RLN recurrent laryngeal nerve, PTC papillary thyroid carcinoma, CCA common carotid artery, RLN recurrent laryngeal nerve, MRI magnetic resonance imaging

Great Vessel Invasion

The carotid artery is elastic and consists of three layers: the intima, tunica media, and adventitia. Resection confined to the adventitia carries a low risk of arterial rupture or aneurysm formation. However, resection extending into the tunica media necessitates arterial reconstruction. Preoperative imaging often makes it challenging to diagnose great vessel invasion definitively. Therefore, surgeries involving suspected carotid artery invasion require preparation for arterial reconstruction. Although carotid reconstruction reduces complications (15–20%) and mortality (16–20%), postoperative complication rates for carotid artery invasion in head and neck squamous cell carcinoma (HNSCC) remain high [55, 56]. Circumferential involvement exceeding 180° on enhanced computed tomography or 270° on enhanced magnetic resonance imaging has been identified as a predictive factor for great vessel invasion [57, 58].

Although several studies have focused on carotid artery invasion in HNSCC, there are fewer reports on great vessel invasion by DTC. Moritani et al. evaluated 49 patients with carotid artery invasion by PTC, of whom 47 underwent sub-adventitial resection, and 2 underwent carotid artery resection and reconstruction. Among 20 patients treated initially with sub-adventitial resection, the 10-year disease-specific survival rate was 69.3%. Local or regional recurrence occurred in 14 patients (29%), but recurrence at the site of carotid artery invasion area was only 2%. The treatment outcomes for carotid artery invasion in PTC compared favorably with those in HNSCC, likely due to the lower biological aggressiveness of PTC [59]. Great vessels remain highly vulnerable to external forces or infection after sub-adventitial resection. Locally advanced DCT with carotid artery invasion often involves multiple organs, necessitating careful attention to infection control, particularly during intraluminal resection of the aerodigestive tract (Figs. 9.12 and 9.13).

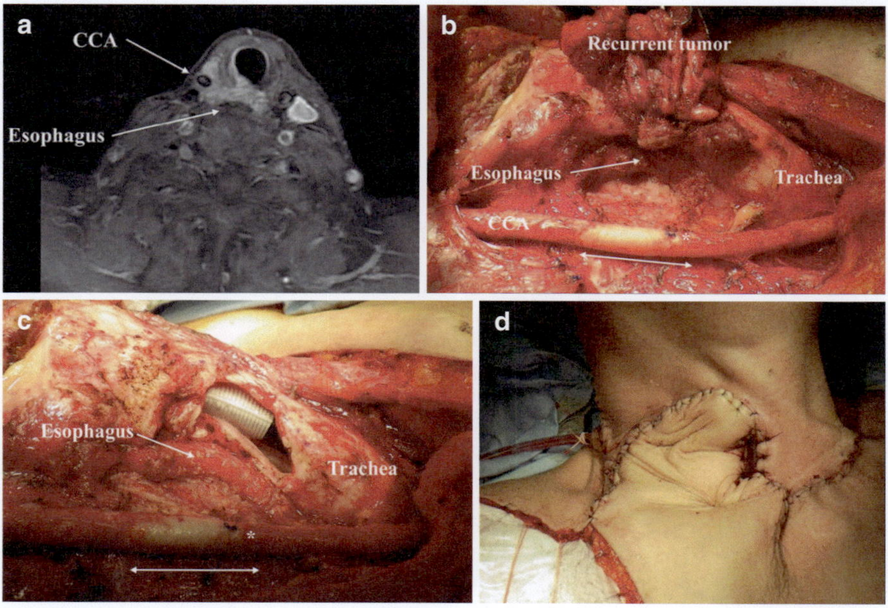

Fig. 9.12 Subadventitial resection for carotid artery invasion. Recurrent PTC with CCA and aerodigestive tract invasion in a female patient in her early 70s. Preoperative MRI showed circumferential encasement of over 180° of the right CCA and suspected tracheoesophageal invasion by the recurrent tumor (**a**). Subadventitial resection and suture repair of the CCA was performed (**b**, **c**: double-headed arrow, *), along with window resection of the tracheal wall from the first to sixth rings and the esophagus muscle layer resection. The right carotid artery was covered using a D-P flap to separate it from the tracheocutaneous fistula (**d**). The tracheocutaneous fistula was successfully closed 2 months after surgery. PTC papillary thyroid carcinoma, MRI magnetic resonance imaging, CCA common carotid artery, RLN recurrent laryngeal nerve, D-P deltopectoral

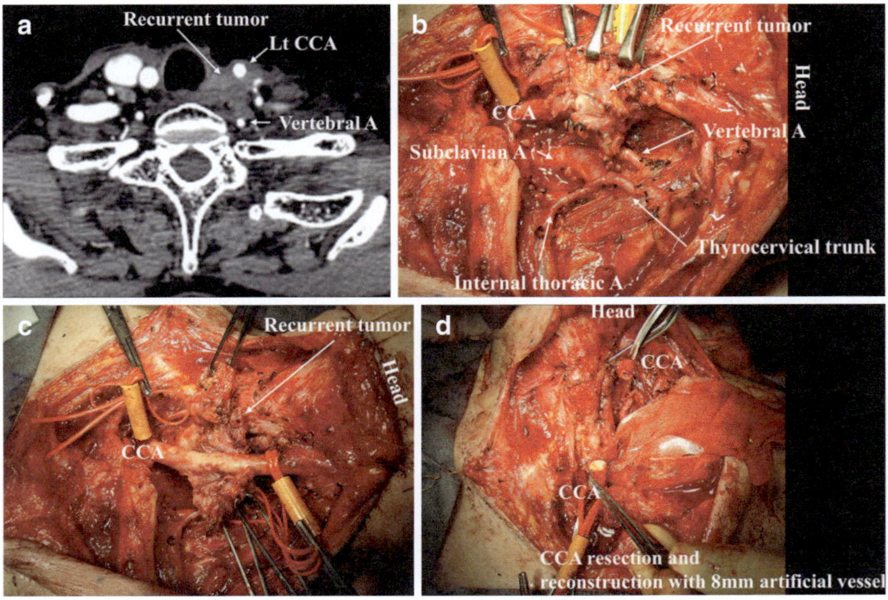

Fig. 9.13 Carotid artery resection and reconstruction for gross carotid artery invasion. Recurrent PTC with CCA and aerodigestive tract invasion in a female patient in her early 70s. Preoperative CT showed circumferential encasement of the left CCA and suspected tracheoesophageal and prevertebral invasion by the recurrent tumor. Extensive infiltration of the left CCA was particularly noted (**a**). The recurrent tumor was resected following vascular reconstruction to address carotid artery invasion. The left vertebral artery was preserved, but the left CCA was resected and reconstructed using an artificial vessel due to tumor invasion extending beyond the tunica media (**b**–**d**). Shave excision was performed for tracheal-infiltrated areas, and muscle layer resection was performed for esophageal invasion. The left vagal nerve was also resected. PTC papillary thyroid carcinoma, CCA common carotid artery, CT computed tomography

Lymph Node Metastasis in the Parapharyngeal Space (PPS)

The PPS is anatomically described as an inverted pyramid, with its base at the skull base and its apex at the greater cornu of the hyoid bone. The posterior portion of the PPS houses critical structures, including the internal carotid arteries, internal jugular veins, lower cranial nerves (CN IX–XII), and sympathetic nerves. PPS tumors are uncommon, comprising only 0.5% of all head and neck tumors. Approximately 80% of PPS tumors are benign, with salivary gland tumors accounting for 40% and neural tumors for 30% [60, 61]. Most salivary tumors originate in the deep lobes of the parotid gland and are typically located in the anterior part of the PPS. In contrast, metastatic tumors, which account for the remaining 20% of cases, are primarily located in the posterior PPS, where the internal carotid artery, internal jugular vein, and lower cranial nerves are densely distributed. The anatomical characteristics of the PPS, including the surgical barrier posed by the mandible and the late-onset symptoms as the tumor grows, make surgical access challenging. Parapharyngeal metastases are often deemed unresectable upon detection. Even when resectable, these metastases are likely to result in functional impairment due to deficits in the lower cranial nerves [62].

Parapharyngeal metastases from thyroid cancer frequently recur. However, metastases to the PPS are rare, even in cases involving initial treatment, as direct lymphatic drainage from the superior pole of the thyroid gland to the PPS occurs in only approximately 20% of cases [63]. In recurrent cases, neck dissection and/or removal of metastatic cervical lymph nodes may alter lymphatic drainage pathways, leading to retrograde flow and atypical metastasis to the PPS lymph nodes [64]. Surgical approaches to the PPS include transoral, transcervical, or transcervical-trans-parotid techniques, with or without several mandibulotomies. The transcervical approach is commonly reported for PPS tumor removal. Regardless of the chosen approach, accurately identifying the location of major structures and parapharyngeal metastases is critical to securing a safe operative field. Tumor invasion and excision pose risks to lower cranial nerves, making them susceptible to damage. Postoperative complications such as upper airway obstruction or dysphagia due to pharyngeal swelling are also noted [65] (Figs. 9.14 and 9.15).

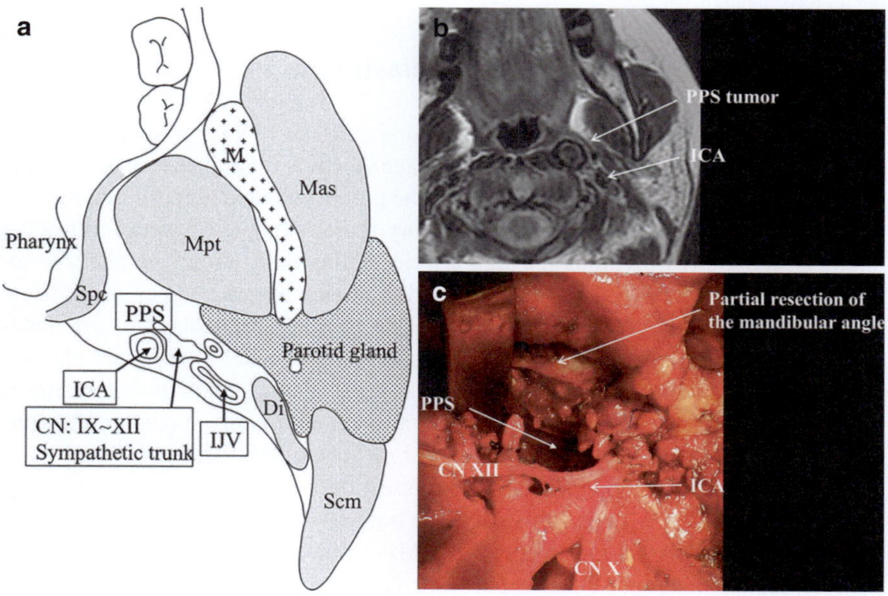

Fig. 9.14 PPS metastasis of recurrent PTC. Recurrent PTC involving the left cervical and parapharyngeal spaces (PPS) in a female patient in her early 60s. The PPS is anatomically shaped like an inverted pyramid, with its base at the skull base and its apex at the greater horn of the hyoid bone (**a**). Preoperative MRI revealed a PPS tumor adjacent to the pharyngeal constrictor muscle on the medial side of the left ICA (**b**). A left radical neck dissection, including resection of the SCM, IJV, and spinal accessory nerve, was performed due to gross extranodal invasion at level II. Extirpation of the PPS metastasis was also carried out (**c**). Partial resection of the PPS invaded the left hypoglossal nerve and sympathetic trunk, which were partially resected due to tumor invasion. Partial resection of the mandibular angle proved effective in securing the surgical field for PPS surgery. PTC papillary thyroid carcinoma, MRI magnetic resonance imaging, CN IX glossopharyngeal nerve, CN X vagal nerve, CN XI accessory nerve, CN XII hypoglossal nerve, Di digastric muscle, ICA internal carotid artery, IJV internal jugular vein, M mandible, Mas masseter muscle, Mpt medial pterygoid muscle, PPS parapharyngeal space, Scm sternocleidomastoid muscle, Spc superior pharyngeal constrictor

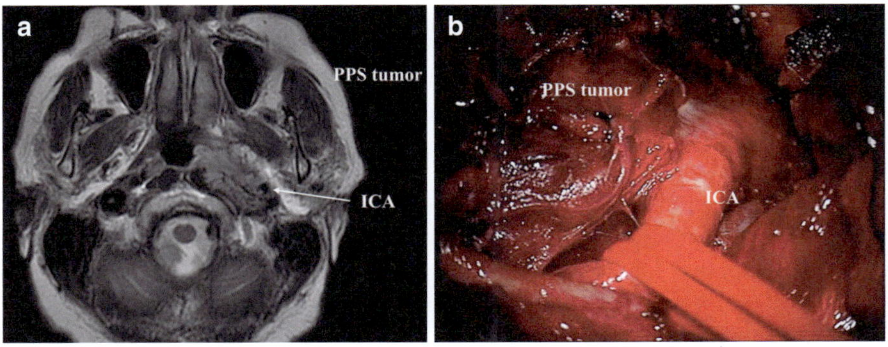

Fig. 9.15 PPS metastasis of recurrent PTC (unresectable). Recurrent PTC involving the left PPS in a female patient in her early 70s. Preoperative MRI revealed a left PPS tumor suspected to involve the left internal carotid artery and prevertebral fascia (**a**). The prevertebral muscles were resected en bloc with the PPS tumor; however, a portion of the tumor remained at the site of internal carotid artery invasion (**b**). PTC papillary thyroid carcinoma, MRI magnetic resonance imaging, PPS parapharyngeal space

Lymph Node Metastasis in the Mediastinum

The perithyroid glandular lymphatic network consists of two primary drainage pathways. The primary lymph drainage system includes lymphatic vessels in the central compartment, which descend along the pretracheal and paratracheal regions to the upper mediastinal nodes. The secondary lymph drainage system follows the lateral lymphatic vessels along the jugular vein. Additionally, direct lymphatic communication exists between the lateral cervical nodes and the upper mediastinal nodes via the central compartment nodes. Due to this lymphatic flow, the upper mediastinum is a common site of metastasis in thyroid cancer [66]. Upper paratracheal metastases along the RLN are particularly prevalent. Lymph node metastases in the pretracheal, paraesophageal, and lateral cervical regions, including the contralateral neck, are considered risk factors for mediastinal metastases [67].

Most studies on the upper mediastinal dissection (UMD) in DTC have focused on the outcomes of UMD performed via the transcervical approach in conjunction with central neck dissection. Reports on UMD using sternotomy are limited. The transcervical approach for UMD is performed as an extension of central dissection, which is less invasive and safer. It should be considered for patients at risk of upper mediastinal metastases that can be addressed through this approach [68]. Conversely, mediastinal dissection by sternotomy is not recommended unless mediastinal metastases are suspected on preoperative imaging [69].

Two surgical approaches are commonly used for mediastinal dissection: partial sternoclavicular joint and manubrium resection and sternotomy. Sternotomy can involve various incisions, including L-shaped, inverted L, inverted T, and longitudinal incisions. Securing the surgical field and performing careful surgical manipulation are essential in both approaches. Partial sternoclavicular joint and manubrium resections can provide almost the same surgical exposure as partial sternotomy when wide-bone resection is performed. However, due to potential negative outcomes such as joint deformity, restricted motion around the sternoclavicular joint, arthritis, and complications arising from dead space caused by bone resection, this approach is generally reserved for mediastinal surgeries with relatively limited operative fields.

Moritani et al. reported a 10-year survival rate of 60% in 58 patients with PTC who underwent UMD. They concluded that UMD is an effective treatment for improving prognosis in patients with upper mediastinal metastases that cannot be fully resected via the transcervical approach [70]. While the surgical indication should consider tumor extent, operative stress, and the patient's overall condition, UMD for patients with upper mediastinal metastases remains a viable treatment option, offering the potential for long-term prognosis in several cases (Figs. 9.16 and 9.17).

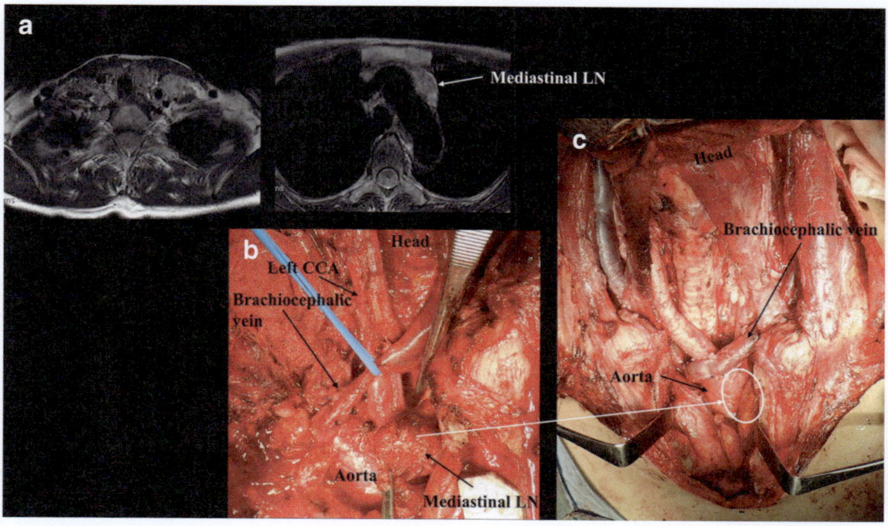

Fig. 9.16 Upper mediastinal dissection through a reverse T-incision of the sternum. PTC (T4aN1bM0) in a female patient in her early 50s. Preoperative MRI indicated extrathyroidal extension, bilateral cervical metastases, and multiple mediastinal metastases involving the pre-vascular, upper, and lower paratracheal nodes (**a**). Normal vocal cord movement was observed preoperatively. A total thyroidectomy, bilateral neck dissection, and superior mediastinal dissection were performed through a reverse T-incision of the sternum. The left RLN was resected and reconstructed due to the extrathyroidal extension, and shave excision of the trachea and esophagus was performed. Superior mediastinal metastases were identified in the pre-vascular node and the upper and lower RLN nodes in the mediastinum (**b**, **c**). PTC papillary thyroid carcinoma, MRI magnetic resonance imaging, RLN recurrent laryngeal nerve

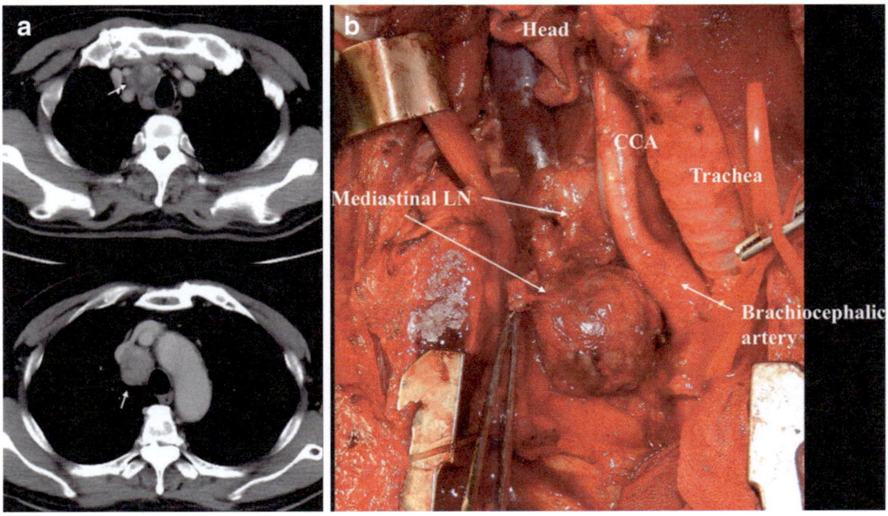

Fig. 9.17 Upper mediastinal dissection through a reverse T-incision of the sternum. PTC (T3N1bM0) in a male patient in his early 60s. Preoperative CT revealed consecutive lymph node enlargements extending from the neck to the upper mediastinum in the paratracheal region (**a**). A total thyroidectomy, right neck dissection, and superior mediastinal dissection were performed through a reverse T-incision in the sternum (**b**). PTC papillary thyroid carcinoma, CT computed tomography

Declaration of Interest The author has no conflicts of interest to disclose.

Funding This research received no specific grant from any funding agency in the public, commercial, or not-for-profit sectors.

References

1. McConahey WM, Hay ID, Woolner LB, van Heerden JA, Taylor WF. Papillary thyroid cancer treated at the Mayo Clinc, 1946 through 1970: initial manifestations, pathologic findings, therapy, and outcome. Mayo Clin Proc. 1986;61(12):978–96.
2. Brauckhoff M. Classification of aerodigestive tract invasion from thyroid cancer. Langenbeck's Arch Surg. 2014 Feb;399(2):209–16.
3. Su SY, Milas ZL, Bhatt N, Roberts D, Clayman GL. Well-differentiated thyroid cancer with aerodigestive tract invasion: long-term control and functional outcomes. Head Neck. 2016;38(1):72–8.
4. Shadmehr MB, Farzanegan R, Zangi M, Mohammadzadeh A, Sheikhy K, et al. Thyroid cancers with laryngotracheal invasion. Eur J Cardiothorac Surg. 2012;41(3):635–40.
5. McCaffrey JC. Aerodigestive tract invasion by well differentiated thyroid carcinoma: diagnosis, management, prognosis, and biology. Laryngoscope. 2006;116(1):1–11.
6. Lang BH, Lo CY, Wong KP, Wan KY. Should an involved but functioning recurrent laryngeal nerve be shaved or resected in a locally advanced papillary thyroid carcinoma? Ann Surg Oncol. 2013;20(9):2951–7.

7. Ito Y, Kihara M, Takamura Y, Kobayashi K, Miya A, et al. Prognosis and prognostic factors of patients with papillary thyroid carcinoma requiring resection of recurrent laryngeal nerve due to carcinoma extension. Endocr J. 2012;59(3):247–52.
8. Brooks JA, Abdelhamid Ahmed AH, Al-Qurayshi Z, Kamani D, Kyriazidis N, et al. Recurrent laryngeal nerve invasion by thyroid cancer: laryngeal function and survival outcomes. Laryngoscope. 2022;132(11):2285–92.
9. Moritani S. Impact of gross extrathyroidal extension into major neck structures on the prognosis of papillary thyroid carcinoma according to the American Joint Committee on Cancer eighth edition. Endocr J. 2020;67(9):941–8.
10. Fundakowski CE, Hales NW, Agrawal N, Barczyński M, Camacho PM, et al. Surgical management of the recurrent laryngeal nerve in thyroidectomy: American Head and Neck Society Consensus Statement. Head Neck. 2018;40(4):663–75.
11. Kumai Y, Kodama N, Murakami D, Yumoto E. Comparison of vocal outcome following two different procedures for immediate RLN reconstruction. Eur Arch Otorrinolaringol. 2016;273(4):967–72.
12. Wu CW, Dionigi G, Barczynski M, Chiang FY, Dralle H, et al. International neuromonitoring study group guidelines 2018: Part II: optimal recurrent laryngeal nerve management for invasive thyroid cancer-incorporation of surgical, laryngeal, and neural electrophysiologic data. Laryngoscope. 2018;128(Suppl 3):S18–27.
13. Kihara M, Miyauchi A, Yabuta T, Higashiyama T, Fukushima M, et al. Outcome of vocal cord function after partial layer resection of recurrent laryngeal nerve in patients with papillary thyroid cancer. Surgery. 2014;155(1):184–9.
14. Lee HS, Kim SW, Park T, Nam GY, Hong JC, et al. Papillary thyroid carcinoma with exclusive involvement of a functioning recurrent laryngeal nerve may be treated with shaving technique. World J Surg. 2015;39(4):969–74.
15. Moritani S, Takenobu M, Yoshioka K, Kawamoto K, Fujii T, et al. Novel surgical methods for reconstruction of the recurrent laryngeal nerve: microscope-guided partial layer resection and intralaryngeal reconstruction of the recurrent laryngeal nerve. Surgery. 2021;169(5):1124–30.
16. Nishida T, Nakao K, Hamaji M, Kamiike W, Kurozumi K, et al. Preservation of recurrent laryngeal nerve invaded by differentiated thyroid cancer. Ann Surg. 1997;226(1):85–91.
17. Miyamaru S, Kumai Y, Murakami D, Kodama N, Miyamoto T, et al. Phonatory function in patients with well-differentiated thyroid carcinoma following meticulous resection of tumors adhering to the recurrent laryngeal nerve. Int J Clin Oncol. 2019;24(12):1536–42.
18. Kamani D, Darr EA, Randolph GW. Electrophysiologic monitoring characteristics of the recurrent laryngeal nerve preoperatively paralyzed or invades with malignancy. Otolaryngol Head Neck Surg. 2013;149(5):682–8.
19. Miyauchi A, Matsusaka K, Kihara M, Matsuzuka F, Hirai K, et al. The role of Ansa-to-recurrent-laryngeal nerve anastomosis in operations for thyroid cancer. Eur J Surg. 1998;164(12):927–33.
20. Wang W, Liu F, Zhang C, Li M, Chen S, et al. Immediate Ansa Cervicalis-to-recurrent laryngeal nerve anastomosis for the Management of Recurrent Laryngeal Nerve Infiltration by a Differentiated Thyroid Carcinoma. ORL J Otorhinolaryngol Relat Spec. 2020;82(2):93–105.
21. Iwaki S, Maeda T, Saito M, Otsuki N, Takahashi M, et al. Role of immediate recurrent laryngeal nerve reconstruction in surgery for thyroid cancers with fixed vocal cords. Head Neck. 2017;39(3):427–31.
22. Yumoto E, Sanuki T, Kumai Y. Immediate recurrent laryngeal nerve reconstruction and vocal outcome. Laryngoscope. 2006;116(9):1657–61.
23. Sanuki T, Yumoto E, Minoda R, Kodama N. The role of immediate recurrent laryngeal nerve reconstruction for thyroid cancer surgery. J Oncol. 2010;2010:846235.
24. Miyauchi A, Ito Y, Miya A, Higashiyama T, Tomoda C, et al. Lateral mobilization of the recurrent laryngeal nerve to facilitate tracheal surgery in patients with thyroid cancer invading the trachea near Berry's ligament. World J Surg. 2007;31(11):2081–4.
25. Miyauchi A, Masuoka H, Tomoda C, Takamura Y, Ito Y, et al. Laryngeal approach to the recurrent laryngeal nerve involved by thyroid cancer at the ligament of berry. Surgery. 2012;152(1):57–60.

26. Shindo ML, Caruana SM, Kandil E, McCaffrey JC, Orloff LA, et al. Management of invasive well-differentiated thyroid cancer: an American Head and Neck Society consensus statement. AHNS consensus statement. Head Neck. 2014;36(10):1379–90.
27. Brauckhoff M, Machens A, Thanh PN, Lorenz K, Schmeil A, et al. Impact of extent of resection for thyroid cancer invading the aerodigestive tract on surgical morbidity, local recurrence, and cancer-specific survival. Surgery. 2010;148(6):1257–66.
28. Hartl DM, Zago S, Leboulleux S, Mirghani H, Déandreis D, et al. Resection margins and prognosis in locally invasive thyroid cancer. Head Neck. 2014;36(7):1034–8.
29. Avenia N, Vannucci J, Monacelli M, Lucchini R, Polistena A, et al. Thyroid cancer invading the airway: diagnosis and management. Int J Surg. 2016;28(Suppl 1):S75–8.
30. Wada N, Nakayama H, Masudo Y, Suganuma N, Rino Y. Clinical outcome of different modes of resection in papillary thyroid carcinomas with laryngotracheal invasion. Langenbeck's Arch Surg. 2006;391(6):545–9.
31. Ito Y, Fukushima M, Yabuta T, Tomoda C, Inoue H, et al. Local prognosis of patients with papillary thyroid carcinoma who were intra- operatively diagnosed as having minimal invasion of the trachea: a 17-year experience in a single institute. Asian J Surg. 2009;32(2):102–8.
32. Moritani S. Surgical management of cricotracheal invasion by papillary thyroid carcinoma. Ann Surg Oncol. 2015;22(12):4002–7.
33. McCarty TM, Kuhn JA, Williams WL Jr, Ellenhorn JD, O'Brien JC, et al. Surgical management of thyroid cancer invading the airway. Ann Surg Oncol. 1997;4(5):403–8.
34. Tsukahara K, Sugitani I, Kawabata K. Surgical management of tracheal shaving for papillary thyroid carcinoma with tracheal invasion. Acta Otolaryngol. 2009;129(12):1498–502.
35. Peng A, Li Y, Yang X, Xiao Z, Tang Q, et al. A review of the management and prognosis of thyroid carcinoma with tracheal invasion. Eur Arch Otorrinolaringol. 2015;272(8):1833–43.
36. Kim H, Jung HJ, Lee SY, Kwon TK, Kim KH, et al. Prognostic factors of locally invasive well-differentiated thyroid carcinoma involving the trachea. Eur Arch Otorrinolaringol. 2016;273(7):1919–26.
37. Czaja JM, McCaffrey TV. The surgical management of laryngotracheal invasion by well-differentiated papillary thyroid carcinoma. Arch Otolaryngol Head Neck Surg. 1997;123(5):484–90.
38. Park CS, Suh KW, Min JS. Cartilage-shaving procedure for the control of tracheal cartilage invasion by thyroid carcinoma. Head Neck. 1993;15(4):289–91.
39. Tsai YF, Tseng YL, Wu MH, Hung CJ, Lai WW, et al. Aggressive resection of the airway invaded by thyroid carcinoma. Br J Surg. 2005;92(11):1382–7.
40. Ozaki O, Sugino K, Mimura T, Ito K. Surgery for patients with thyroid carcinoma invading the trachea: circumferential sleeve resection followed by end-to-end anastomosis. Surgery. 1995;117(3):268–71.
41. Shin DH, Mark EJ, Suen HC, Grillo HC. Pathologic staging of papillary carcinoma of the thyroid with airway invasion based on the anatomic manner of extension to the trachea: a clinicopathologic study based on 22 patients who underwent thyroidectomy and airway resection. Hum Pathol. 1993;24(8):866–70.
42. Piazza C, Lancini D, Tomasoni M, D'Cruz A, Hartl DM, Kowalski LP, et al. Tracheal and Cricotracheal resection with end-to-end anastomosis for locally advanced thyroid cancer: a systematic review of the literature on 656 patients. Front Endocrinol (Lausanne). 2021;12:779999.
43. Allen M, Spillinger A, Arianpour K, Johnson J, Johnson AP, et al. Tracheal resection in the Management of Thyroid Cancer: an evidence-based approach. Laryngoscope. 2021;131(4):932–46.
44. Ito Y, Miyauchi A, Kihara M, Higashiyama T, Kobayashi K, et al. Airtight tracheocutaneostomy after window resection of the trachea for invasive papillary thyroid carcinoma: experience of 109 cases. World J Surg. 2014;38(3):660–6.
45. Ebihara M, Kishimoto S, Hayashi R, Miyazaki M, Shinozaki T, et al. Window resection of the trachea and secondary reconstruction for invasion by differentiated thyroid carcinoma. Auris Nasus Larynx. 2011;38(2):271–5.
46. Moritani S. Window resection for intraluminal Cricotracheal invasion by papillary thyroid carcinoma. World J Surg. 2017;41(7):1812–9.

47. Gaissert HA, Honings J, Grillo HC, Donahue DM, Wain JC, et al. Segmental laryngotracheal and tracheal resection for invasive thyroid carcinoma. Ann Thorac Surg. 2007;83(6):1952–9.
48. McCaffrey TV, Bergstralh EJ, Hay ID. Locally invasive papillary thyroid carcinoma: 1940–1990. Head Neck. 1994;16(2):165–72.
49. Carter N, Milroy CM. Thyroid carcinoma causing fatal laryngeal occlusion. J Laryngol Otol. 1996;110:1176–8.
50. Bayles SW, Kingdom TT, Carlson GW. Management of thyroid carcinoma invading the aerodigestive tract. Laryngoscope. 1998;108:1402–7.
51. Moritani S. Surgical management of laryngeal invasion by papillary thyroid carcinoma: a retrospective analysis. Thyroid. 2015;25:528–33.
52. Giovanni A, Guelfucci B, Gras R, Yu P, Zanaret M. Partial front lateral laryngectomy with epiglottic reconstruction for management of early-stage glottic carcinoma. Laryngoscope. 2001;111(4 Pt 1):663–8.
53. Biller HF, Ogura JH, Pratt LL. Hemilaryngectomy for T2 glottic cancers. Arch Otolaryngol. 1971;93(3):238–43.
54. Price DL, Wong RJ, Randolph GW. Invasive thyroid cancer: management of the trachea and esophagus. Otolaryngol Clin N Am. 2008;41(6):1155–68.
55. Snyderman CH, D'Amico F. Outcome of carotid artery resection for neoplastic disease: a meta-analysis. Am J Otolaryngol. 1992;13(6):373–80.
56. Ozer E, Agrawal A, Ozer HG, Schuller DE. The impact of surgery in the management of the head and neck carcinoma involving the carotid artery. Laryngoscope. 2008;118(10):1771–4.
57. Yu Q, Wang P, Shi H, Luo J. Carotid artery and jugular vein invasion of oral-maxillofacial and neck malignant tumors: diagnostic value of computed tomography. Oral Surg Oral Med Oral Pathol Oral Radiol Endod. 2003;96(3):368–72.
58. Yousem DM, Hatabu H, Hurst RW, Seigerman HM, Montone KT, et al. Carotid artery invasion by head and neck masses: prediction with MR imaging. Radiology. 1995;195(3):715–20.
59. Moritani S. Appropriateness of subadventitial resection for invasion of the carotid artery by papillary thyroid carcinoma. World J Surg. 2019;43(2):519–26.
60. Khafif A, Segev Y, Kaplan DM, et al. Surgical management of parapharyngeal space tumors: a 10-year review. Otolaryngol Head Neck Surg. 2005;132:401–6.
61. Cohen SM, Burkey BB, Netterville JL. Surgical management of parapharyngeal space masses. Head Neck. 2005;27:669–75.
62. Eisele DW, Richmon JD. Contemporary evaluation and management of parapharyngeal space neoplasms. J Laryngol Otol. 2013;127(6):550–5.
63. Rouvier H. Anatomie Humaine, et Topograhique. 10th ed. Paris: Masson et Cie; 1967. p. 506.
64. McCormack KR, Sheline GE. Retropharyngeal spread of carcinoma of the thyroid. Cancer. 1970;26(6):1366–9.
65. Moritani S. Parapharyngeal metastasis of papillary thyroid carcinoma. World J Surg. 2016;40(2):350–5.
66. Chouke KS, Whitehead RW, Parker AE. Is there a closed lymphatic system connecting the thyroid and thymus gland? Surg Gynecol Obstet. 1952;54:865–71.
67. Zhang TT, Qu N, Hu JQ, Shi RL, Wen D, et al. Mediastinal lymph node metastases in thyroid cancer: characteristics, predictive factors, and prognosis. Int J Endocrinol. 2017;2017:1868165.
68. Woo JH, Park KN, Lee JY, Lee SW. Predictive factors of superior mediastinal nodal metastasis from papillary thyroid carcinoma—a prospective observational study. PLoS One. 2016;11(2):e0148420.
69. Ito Y, Miyauchi A. Lateral and mediastinal lymph node dissection in differentiated thyroid carcinoma: indications, benefit, and risks. World J Surg. 2007;31(5):905–15.
70. Moritani S, Takenobu M, Yasunaga M, Kawamoto K, Fujii T, et al. Surgical indications for upper mediastinal dissection by sternotomy in patients with papillary thyroid carcinoma. Endocr J. 2022;69(10):1245–51.

Remote-Access Robotic and Endoscopic Thyroidectomy

10

Kyung Tae

Editorial

Thyroid surgery has become safer, and the morbidity is extremely low. Adjuncts of thyroid surgery have improved hemostasis and preservation of superior and recurrent laryngeal nerve, as well as the parathyroid glands. The only factor heretofore not addressed was the surgical scar. Remote-access thyroidectomy addresses the issue of cosmesis while maintaining the low morbidity in thyroid surgery. It is done using either the endoscope or the robot various approaches via the axilla or periareolar port either singly or in combination, the retro-aural or transoral route. Transoral thyroidectomy can be heralded as the true scarless surgery.

Based on the premise of being cosmetic, remote-access thyroidectomy requires careful patient selection, transcending cultural preferences, crossing financial barriers, based on personal expertise, and overcoming a steep learning curve. Expertise is not ubiquitous as the number of surgeries required to reach the finesse of a traditional open thyroidectomy takes a while.

The question then arises—is there a need for remote-access thyroidectomy? The patient preference is more a reflection of the counseling and information that the patient garners from "Google and AI tools." The morbidity (embolism, tracheal and esophageal injury, nerve injury, paresthesia, and scarring), cost, and duration of surgery might make one reconsider this approach. However, for a carefully selected patient, remote-access thyroidectomy by an expert offers a viable alternative, with the significant benefit of no visible neck scar. Its necessity is driven by a patient's desire for improved cosmetic results, rather than a clinical requirement for most cases.

Prathamesh S. Pai

K. Tae (✉)
Department of Otolaryngology-Head and Neck Surgery, College of Medicine, Hanyang University, Seoul, Republic of Korea
e-mail: kytae@hanyang.ac.kr

P. S. Pai et al. (eds.), *Controversies in Cancer of the Thyroid and Parathyroid Glands*, https://doi.org/10.1007/978-3-032-13130-0_10

Introduction

Conventional transcervical thyroidectomy is a well-established surgical standard. However, it leaves a visible scar on the central neck, which is a significant concern, particularly among women—a demographic in which thyroid cancer is prevalent. Over the past 25 years, efforts to address this issue have driven the development of remote-access thyroidectomy techniques utilizing endoscopy or robotic systems to minimize visible scarring [1]. Remote-access thyroidectomy, employing approaches such as cervical, axillary, anterior chest, breast, postauricular, or transoral routes, has gained global traction due to its excellent cosmetic outcomes [2–36]. Despite its advantages, remote-access thyroidectomy faces several challenges, including appropriate patient selection, cultural preferences, financial barriers, variability in healthcare systems, technical complexity, steep learning curves, and competition from emerging minimally invasive treatments, such as thermal ablation or active surveillance. This chapter reviews the historical evolution of remote-access thyroidectomy, discusses patient selection criteria, evaluates surgical outcomes, highlights the advantages and limitations of various approaches, and addresses contemporary controversies surrounding its role in thyroid surgery.

History and Evolution of Remote-Access Thyroidectomy

The first endoscopic thyroidectomy was performed in 1997 by Huscher et al. via a cervical approach in Italy [2]. This method involved 3–4 small ports, including a 12 mm endoscopic port and 2–3 operating instrument ports positioned in the anterior and lateral neck. The working space was maintained using low-pressure CO_2 insufflation.

In 1999, Miccoli et al. introduced a direct-access technique termed minimally invasive video-assisted thyroidectomy (MIVAT). This method utilized a 1.5–2 cm central neck incision and did not require CO_2 insufflation, thereby reducing the risk of CO_2-related complications [3]. The primary advantage of MIVAT lies in its minimally invasive nature, rather than in improved cosmesis, as the procedure still results in a neck scar, albeit smaller than that left by conventional methods [1]. Numerous studies have reported that MIVAT is associated with reduced postoperative pain and superior cosmetic outcomes compared to conventional thyroidectomy [4].

Subsequently, various remote-access thyroidectomy techniques extending beyond the neck were developed. These included approaches via the anterior chest, axillary, breast, retroauricular, and transoral routes (Table 10.1).

Table 10.1 History and evolution of remote-access thyroidectomy

Year	Authors	Approaches
1997	Hüscher et al.	Cervical approach with CO_2 insufflations
1999	Miccoli et al.	Minimally invasive video-assisted thyroidectomy (MIVAT)
2000	Ikeda et al.	Axillary approach with CO_2 insufflations
2000	Ogami et al.	Breast approach with CO_2 insufflations
2001	Kitano et al.	Cervical lifting approach without CO_2 insufflations
2002	Shimizu et al.	Video-assisted neck surgery (VANS) without CO_2 insufflations
2002	Ikeda et al.	Ant. chest approach with CO_2 insufflations
2003	Shimazu et al.	Axillo-bilateral breast approach (ABBA) with CO_2 insufflations
2006	Chung et al.	Gasless transaxillary approach with anterior chest port
2007	Youn et al.	Bilateral axillo-breast approach (BABA) with CO_2 insufflations
2011	Tae et al.	Gasless unilateral axillary (GUA)/axillo-breast (GUAB) approaches
2011	Terris et al.	Gasless robotic facelift (retroauricular) approach
2011	Wilhelm et al.	Transoral approach using sublingual and vestibular incisions
2013	Nakajo et al.	Gasless transoral endoscopic approach
2014	Wang et al.	Transoral endoscopic vestibular approach with CO_2 insufflations
2016	Anuwung et al.	Transoral endoscopic thyroidectomy vestibular approach (TOETVA) with CO_2 insufflations
2018	Kim et al.	Transoral robotic thyroidectomy with CO_2 insufflations

Anterior Chest Approach

The anterior chest approach using CO_2 insufflation was first reported in 2002 [5]. This procedure employs three small ports on the anterior chest wall, consisting of a 12 mm endoscopic port and two 5 mm ports for operating instruments. A gasless anterior chest approach was also introduced in the same year, utilizing three ports on the anterior chest wall and a cervical region-lifting device to maintain the working space without CO_2 insufflation [6].

Additionally, a gasless infraclavicular approach termed "video-assisted neck surgery (VANS)" was developed by Shimizu et al. in 2002 [7]. This technique involves a 3–4 cm incision in the anterior chest wall below the clavicle, along with a 5 mm lateral neck incision for inserting a 5 mm endoscope. After the skin flap is dissected, two Kirschner wires are used to sustain the cervical working space without the need for CO_2 insufflation.

Transaxillary Approach

The endoscopic axillary approach utilizing three axillary trocars with CO_2 insufflation was first introduced by Ikeda et al. in 2000 [8]. Subsequently, a gasless endoscopic transaxillary approach was developed by Chung et al. in 2006 [9]. With advancements in robotic surgical technologies, the gasless robotic transaxillary approach was performed using the da Vinci surgical robot (Intuitive Surgical, Inc., Sunnyvale, CA) in 2009, which has since gained widespread adoption [10]. Initially, the gasless transaxillary approach involved a 6 cm axillary incision supplemented with a small anterior chest port; however, this technique has evolved to employ a single axillary incision, eliminating the need for an anterior chest port [11]. Further modifications have included the development of the gasless unilateral axillo-breast (GUAB) approach and the gasless unilateral axillary (GUA) approach by Tae et al. [12–15] The GUAB approach incorporates an 8 mm breast port located at the areola margin, in addition to the axillary incision [14, 15]. The breast port allows a wider angular range between the robotic or endoscopic instruments, facilitating instrument manipulation and reducing the risk of collisions. To avoid the circumareolar incision for cosmetic considerations, Tae et al. later introduced an 8 mm auxiliary incision positioned just below the primary axillary incision for trocar insertion [14, 15]. This axillary incision minimizes the size of the primary axillary incision while maintaining optimal surgical access.

Breast Approach

The breast approach with a chest port was initially developed by Ogami et al. in 2000 [16]. This technique employs two breast ports and a parasternal port with CO_2 insufflation. However, the parasternal incision is prone to hypertrophic scarring, prompting the development of various modifications to avoid this incision. One such modification is the axillo-bilateral breast approach (ABBA), introduced by Shimazu et al. in 2003, which utilizes two breast ports and one axillary port [17]. Another is the bilateral axillo-breast approach (BABA), developed and popularized by Youn et al. in 2007 [18]. BABA represents a refinement of ABBA, incorporating an additional axillary port for enhanced flexibility. This technique requires four incision sites: two circumareolar incisions and one in each axillary area. Additionally, the unilateral or bilateral axillo-breast approaches with CO_2 insufflation employ one breast port and two axillary ports on one or both sides, offering further variations tailored to patient-specific and procedural requirements [19].

Retroauricular (Facelift) Approach

The retroauricular (facelift) thyroidectomy technique was initially developed in the United States by Terris et al. in 2011 using a surgical robot [20, 21]. However, this procedure gained wider recognition and adoption primarily through the efforts of Korean surgeons [22, 23]. The retroauricular approach utilizes incisions made in the postauricular and occipital hairline regions, a technique familiar to head and neck surgeons due to its established use in parotidectomy procedures. This method offers several advantages, including a smaller area of dissection and a shorter distance from the incision site to the thyroid gland compared to the transaxillary approach and BABA [21].

Transoral Approach

The transoral approach was first explored in 2008 by Witzel et al., who conducted trials using a central sublingual route on cadaveric and pig models [24]. Their technique involved a 15-mm central sublingual incision to place an axilloscope, along with two small lateral incisions on the external neck skin for endoscopic instruments. In 2009, Karakas et al. introduced a lateral sublingual approach on cadaveric and pig models, creating a 2-cm incision on the lateral floor of the mouth to access the thyroid glands in an oblique, lateral-to-medial direction [25]. However, this approach proved more suitable for parathyroidectomy than thyroidectomy and was subsequently trialed in two human patients. The technique was limited by a narrow working space and a high risk of hypoglossal nerve injury.

The first transoral approach in humans was conducted by Wilhelm et al. in 2010 using a combination of one sublingual and two vestibular ports [26]. While initially promising, this technique did not achieve widespread adoption and was performed only in select centers.

In 2011, Richmon described the use of tri-vestibular incisions in a cadaveric model with the da Vinci robot [27], laying the foundation for the modern transoral vestibular approach. The first human application of the transoral vestibular approach using a gasless method with a premandibular incision occurred in Japan in 2013 [28]. This technique employed an external retraction system to maintain the working space but resulted in a high incidence of mental nerve injuries due to the extensive 3-cm incision at the oral vestibule.

In 2014, the first human transoral tri-vestibular endoscopic thyroidectomy with CO_2 insufflation was reported in China [29]. The tri-vestibular approach gained significant traction following Anuwong's 2016 study involving 60 patients, which introduced the term "transoral endoscopic thyroidectomy vestibular approach (TOETVA)." [30] Subsequently, the robotic tri-vestibular approach incorporating an axillary port was reported in 2018 [31–33]. Currently, the transoral tri-vestibular approach with CO_2 insufflation—using either endoscopy or a surgical robot—represents the most widely practiced technique for transoral thyroidectomy.

A gasless transoral tri-vestibular approach was introduced in 2019 [34]. This method avoids complications associated with CO_2 insufflation by using an external retractor to maintain the working space. However, the gasless technique offers inferior surgical visualization and space maintenance compared to CO_2 insufflation.

In the same year, a gasless transoral thyroidectomy technique using the da Vinci single port (SP) system was introduced [35]. This method involves a 3-cm central vestibular incision, but the extensive oral dissection and large incision increase the risk of mental nerve injury. Additionally, the single central oral incision allows for the use of only two robotic instruments, limiting its utility.

A hybrid transoral and submental thyroidectomy technique was also introduced in 2018 [36]. This approach addresses some limitations of the tri-vestibular method, such as challenges in extracting large tumors and reducing the risk of mental nerve injury. However, the presence of a submental scar may be unacceptable to some patients.

Classification of Remote-Access Thyroidectomy

The classification of remote-access thyroidectomy is determined by the location of the remote incision, the use of surgical robotics or endoscopy, and the application of CO_2 insufflation versus gasless techniques (Table 10.2). Remote-access thyroidectomy has been performed through incisions in the infraclavicular region, anterior chest, breast, axillary region, retroauricular area, and vestibular space [1].

Robotic techniques are predominantly employed for the transaxillary, BABA, and retroauricular methods, whereas endoscopic techniques are primarily used for the infraclavicular and breast approaches. The transoral approach can be performed using either endoscopic or robotic methods.

Endoscopic procedures offer several advantages, including lower cost, ease of use, familiarity with laparoscopic systems and instruments, and potential reductions in operative time [1, 37, 38]. Conversely, robotic procedures provide notable benefits, such as a three-dimensional magnified view, fine motion scaling, tremor filtration, advanced instrumentation with enhanced range of motion, and improved opportunities for surgical education. Additionally, the ability to utilize three robotic instruments simultaneously enhances countertraction, facilitates dissection, and improves surgical dexterity and ergonomics. However, robotic techniques have notable drawbacks, including high costs, longer operative times, and greater technical complexity.

Table 10.2 Classification of remote-access thyroidectomy

Based on the site of incisions	Minimally invasive video-assisted thyroidectomy (MIVAT)
	Chest approach
	  Anterior chest approach using 3 ports
	  Gasless infraclavicular approach; video-assisted neck surgery (VANS)
	Breast approach
	  Breast approach with parasternal port
	  Axillo-bilateral breast approach (ABBA)
	  Bilateral axillo-breast approach (BABA)
	  Unilateral/bilateral axillo-breast approach
	Axillary approach
	  Axillary approach using 3 ports
	  Gasless axillary approach with anterior chest port
	  Gasless single incision axillary approach
	  Gasless unilateral axillo-breast (GUAB) or axillary (GUA) approach
	Retroauricular (facelift) approach
	Transoral approach
	  Vestibular approach
	  Sublingual approach
	  Transoral approach with submental incision

Based on the use of CO_2	CO_2 insufflations method Gasless method
Based on the surgical system	Robotic procedure Endoscopic procedure

Regarding CO_2 insufflation, the infraclavicular, transaxillary, and retroauricular approaches are typically performed using gasless techniques, while various breast–chest or axillo-breast approaches—including ABBA, BABA, and unilateral or bilateral axillo-breast approaches—and the transoral approach commonly employ CO_2 insufflation.

Although CO_2 insufflation carries a low risk when pressure levels are maintained at 4–6 mmHg, it can result in complications such as subcutaneous emphysema, hypercapnia, respiratory acidosis, cerebral edema, and CO_2 embolism [39]. In contrast, gasless techniques provide several advantages, including the elimination of CO_2-related complications and a clear surgical view without gas fumes. These methods also allow surgeons to use conventional instruments commonly employed in traditional thyroidectomy for skin flap dissection and bleeding control [1].

Eligibility and Contraindications of Remote-Access Thyroidectomy

Remote-access thyroidectomy is a viable option for patients seeking a scarless neck surgery, provided they meet specific eligibility criteria [40]. Indications include benign thyroid nodules measuring less than 6–8 cm in diameter and follicular neoplasms and nodules with an intermediate risk profile that are less than 4 cm [1, 33, 38]. Additionally, differentiated thyroid carcinomas measuring less than 2–4 cm in maximal dimension, including cases with minimal extrathyroidal extension or invasion of strap muscles, are potential candidates. Even differentiated thyroid carcinoma with metastasis to the central or lateral compartment lymph nodes can be included in the indications for this procedure [14, 15, 33]. Patients with multinodular or toxic diffuse goiters may also be suitable, provided the size of the unilateral thyroid lobe does not exceed 8–10 cm.

Exclusion criteria for remote-access thyroidectomy encompass gross extrathyroidal extension, large conglomerated metastatic lymph nodes invading surrounding structures, large substernal goiters, and any history of prior neck surgery or irradiation [14, 15, 33]. Relative contraindications should also be carefully considered, particularly in the context of patient or disease characteristics, such as extreme morbid obesity or large goiters associated with Graves' disease or Hashimoto's thyroiditis. Large goiters can increase intraoperative bleeding risk and compromise thyroid tissue integrity [1].

It is important to note that the specific indications and contraindications for remote-access thyroidectomy may vary depending on the approach employed, as each technique offers unique advantages and limitations. Furthermore, eligibility criteria can be extended based on the surgeon's expertise and experience. With continuous advancements in remote-access techniques, the procedural capabilities and boundaries are expected to evolve, broadening the spectrum of feasible applications.

Four Common Remote-Access Thyroidectomy

Among the various remote-access thyroidectomy techniques, the gasless robotic transaxillary approach, robotic BABA, gasless robotic retroauricular approach, and the vestibular approach employing either endoscopy or a surgical robot are the most widely adopted methods in current practice [1]. Each of these approaches offers distinct advantages and presents specific limitations, necessitating that surgeons comprehensively understand the benefits and constraints associated with each technique.

Robotic Gasless Unilateral Axillary (GUA) Approach

Surgical Procedure

The GUA approach begins with the patient positioned supine, the neck slightly extended, and the arm on the lesion side elevated to expose the axillary fossa. A 5- to 6-cm skin incision is made in the axillary fossa (Fig. 10.1a) [14, 15], and a skin flap is elevated under direct vision within the subplatysmal plane over the pectoralis major muscle, extending from the axilla to the anterior neck region (Fig. 10.1b). Dissection continues through the interval between the two heads of the sternocleidomastoid (SCM) muscle and beneath the sternothyroid muscle to expose the thyroid gland. An external retractor is then placed to establish adequate working space without the need for CO_2 insufflation. A secondary 0.8-cm skin incision is made just inferior to the main axillary incision to allow the insertion of a robotic trocar, reducing the required length of the primary axillary incision. Three robotic arms, comprising a robotic endoscope and two instruments, are introduced via the main

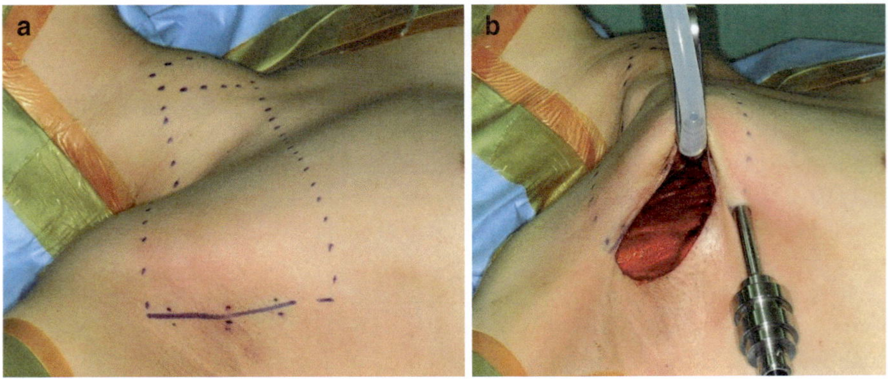

Fig. 10.1 The gasless transaxillary approach. (**a**) A 5–6 cm skin incision is made in the axillary fossa, and a second 0.8 cm skin incision is made inferior to the axillary incision. (**b**) A skin flap is elevated under direct vision within the subplatysmal plane over the pectoralis major muscle, extending from the axilla to the anterior neck region. An external retractor is then placed to establish adequate working space without the need for CO_2 insufflation

axillary incision port, while a third robotic instrument is inserted through the secondary axillary incision [1].

The superior thyroid vessels are divided individually, close to the thyroid gland, using Harmonic curved shears to preserve the external branch of the superior laryngeal nerve. The superior parathyroid gland is meticulously identified and preserved with its vascular supply intact. The thyroid gland is subsequently retracted medially to enable dissection of the paratracheal lymph nodes and perithyroidal soft tissue while maintaining the integrity of the recurrent laryngeal nerve (RLN) along its entire course. The isthmus is divided, completing the ipsilateral lobectomy and central neck dissection. Finally, a suction drain is placed, and the surgical wound is closed.

Advantages and Limitations

The feasibility of the robotic gasless transaxillary approach has been supported by evidence from multiple studies [10, 11, 15]. This gasless technique offers notable advantages, including the maintenance of a clear surgical field without gas fumes and the elimination of complications associated with carbon dioxide insufflation. Moreover, this approach allows the use of conventional instruments typically employed in standard thyroidectomy to dissect skin flaps and achieve hemostasis. The gasless transaxillary approach facilitates an adequate surgical view of the thyroid and lateral neck compartment, as well as access for three robotic instruments. When performed by experienced surgeons, this technique enables total thyroidectomy and lateral neck dissection. However, the approach presents specific limitations. The unilateral incision can pose challenges in accessing the contralateral thyroid gland and complicates dissection of the level IIb lymph node region [41, 42]. Consequently, the surgical completeness of total thyroidectomy and lymph node yield may be inferior compared to conventional techniques. A meta-analysis reported that the proportion of patients achieving stimulated thyroglobulin levels below 1.0 ng/mL was significantly lower with the gasless transaxillary approach compared to conventional, BABA, and transoral methods [43]. Additionally, the extensive dissection required to create the working space has been associated with increased surgical morbidity. Recent advancements, including the development of the da Vinci SP surgical robot system, have addressed some of these limitations. The reduced dissection area required for the SP system has been associated with decreased surgical morbidity, enhancing the safety profile of the gasless transaxillary approach [44].

Robotic Bilateral Axillo-Breast Approach

Surgical Procedure

The patient is positioned supine on the operating table, with the neck extended to optimize surgical exposure, supported by a pillow placed beneath the shoulders. To ensure access to the axillae, the arms are abducted. An elastic bandage supports the lower portion of the breast, elevating the areolar area to improve visualization of the

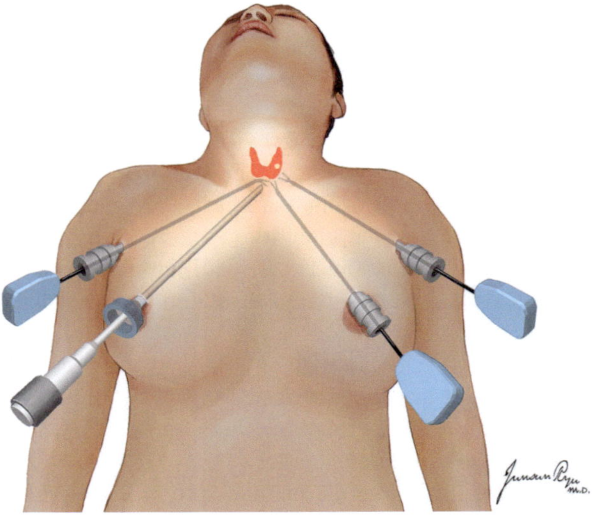

Fig. 10.2 The bilateral axillo-breast approach (BABA) with CO_2 insufflation. Four skin incisions are made: a 12 mm incision above the right areola for the robotic endoscope, an 8 mm incision above the left areola, and two additional 8 mm incisions in the bilateral axillary regions. (Reproduced from Tae et al. [1])

lower neck region and eliminate blind spots. A diluted epinephrine solution is injected into the subcutaneous space in both the chest and neck to minimize bleeding during dissection. Four incisions are created: a 12-mm incision above the right areola for the robotic endoscope, an 8-mm incision above the left areola, and two 8-mm incisions in the bilateral axillary regions (Fig. 10.2) [18, 45]. Blunt dissection is performed using a vascular tunneler, and the working space is extended to the level of the thyroid cartilage superiorly and the medial border of the sternocleidomastoid muscle laterally. This space is maintained using CO_2 insufflation at a pressure of 5–6 mmHg. Following docking of the robotic system, the midline fascia between the strap muscles is divided, and the isthmus is dissected. The thyroid gland is then resected while preserving the parathyroid glands and RLNs. The excised specimen is retrieved in a plastic bag through the 12-mm breast port. Finally, the midline of the strap muscles is reapproximated, a suction drain is inserted, and the skin is closed [1].

Advantages and Limitations

The BABA technique offers several advantages, including a symmetrical bilateral view of anatomical structures, which many surgeons find familiar and straightforward to adapt to. This approach facilitates access to both thyroid lobes and lateral neck compartments [1, 38]. Total thyroidectomy and bilateral lateral neck dissection are feasible through these incisions. However, the surgical invasiveness required to create the working space is greater than that of other remote-access approaches. Additionally, performing central neck dissection can be challenging due to limited access to the central neck compartment, as the clavicle and manubrium may obstruct the downward view. This limitation can be mitigated by employing an elastic band to elevate the areolar region, thereby enhancing visualization of the lower neck area [46]. While postoperative cosmetic outcomes are generally favorable, some patients may find the areolar incisions less acceptable.

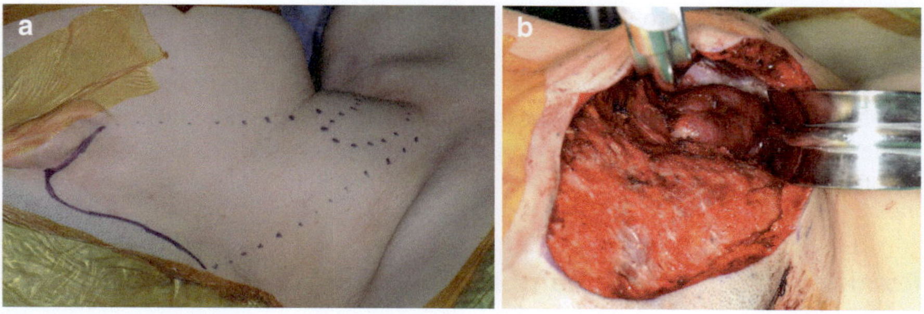

Fig. 10.3 The gasless retroauricular approach. (**a**) A skin incision is initiated within the postauricular sulcus, curving posteriorly at the upper third of the auricle, and extending along the occipital hairline. (**b**) After elevating the skin flap, the strap muscles are dissected and retracted superiorly to expose the thyroid gland

Robotic Gasless Retroauricular (Facelift) Approach

Surgical Procedure

A skin incision is initiated within the postauricular sulcus, curving posteriorly at the upper third of the auricle, and extending along the occipital hairline (Fig. 10.3a) [1, 21–23]. The skin flap is elevated in the subplatysmal plane over the SCM muscle under direct visualization. Elevation extends posteriorly to the posterior border of the SCM, superiorly to the lower border of the mandible, and inferiorly to the sternal notch. During this process, the great auricular nerve and the external jugular vein are meticulously identified and preserved. The omohyoid, sternohyoid, and sternothyroid muscles are subsequently dissected and retracted superiorly to expose the thyroid gland, after which an external retractor is deployed to maintain the working space (Fig. 10.3b). A 30-degree face-down endoscope and three robotic instruments—Maryland dissectors, Prograsp forceps, and Harmonic curved shears—are introduced through the postauricular incision. In most cases, a self-retaining retractor or assistance is required to laterally retract the SCM and skin flap, ensuring adequate working space. Key anatomical structures, including the parathyroid glands and the RLN in the tracheoesophageal groove, are identified and preserved. The Berry's ligament and thyroid isthmus are carefully dissected to complete the lobectomy (Fig. 10.3b). Finally, a suction drain is positioned, and the surgical wound is closed in a layered manner.

Advantages and Limitations

The retroauricular approach necessitates a smaller dissection area compared to the BABA and transaxillary approach. Moreover, the absence of CO_2 insufflation eliminates complications associated with gas insufflation. This technique provides excellent visualization and access to the lateral neck compartment, facilitating comprehensive lateral neck dissection, including levels II, III, IV, and V [1]. However, the approach is constrained by a relatively narrow working space and limited accessibility to the contralateral thyroid lobe when using a unilateral incision. In cases where contralateral lobe access proves insufficient, a separate retroauricular incision may be required. Therefore, this method is most suitable for isolated thyroid lobectomy, with or without concurrent lateral neck dissection. Cosmetic outcomes are generally favorable, although the postauricular scar demonstrates a greater tendency for hypertrophic changes compared to scars from conventional thyroidectomy [47].

Robotic and Endoscopic Transoral Approach

Surgical Procedure

The patient is positioned supine with a shoulder pillow to facilitate optimal neck extension, and general anesthesia is administered via oral or nasal intubation [1]. The endoscopic transoral approach utilizes a three-port technique within the vestibule. A horizontal central incision, approximately 1.5 cm in length, is made at the base of the lower lip frenulum, accompanied by 5-mm lateral incisions near the oral commissures, ensuring careful preservation of the mental nerve (Fig. 10.4a) [30, 33]. The working space is developed through hydrodissection using an epinephrine solution, followed by blunt dissection with dilators extending inferiorly to the sternal notch and bilaterally to the SCM muscle. Trocars are then inserted, and CO_2 insufflation is maintained at a pressure of 5–6 mmHg.

In the transoral robotic approach, blunt dissection is initially performed in the submental region, with the working space established within the subplatysmal layer inferior to the thyroid notch, allowing sufficient room for robotic instrument placement. Following the creation of the initial working space, robotic arms are docked. The skin flap is subsequently extended inferiorly to the sternal notch and laterally to the lateral border of the SCM using robotic instrumentation. An additional axillary port is created at the right axillary fossa to accommodate a third robotic instrument, such as ProGrasp or Cardinal forceps (Fig. 10.4b). This additional instrument provides countertraction similar to conventional thyroidectomy, facilitates specimen removal, and enables drainage placement.

For thyroidectomy, the midline fascia between the strap muscles is divided, and the sternohyoid and sternothyroid muscles are dissected to expose the thyroid gland. Retraction of the strap muscles laterally is achieved with an external stitch to enhance the surgical field visibility during the endoscopic procedure. The procedure begins with dissection and division of the isthmus, followed by thyroidectomy, ensuring preservation of the RLN and parathyroid glands (Fig. 10.4c). Special attention is required to identify and preserve the RLN, particularly during dissection of Berry's ligament. Specimen removal is achieved using a plastic retrieval bag via the central oral incision in the endoscopic approach or through the axillary port in the robotic approach. The strap muscles are re-approximated, and the vestibular surgical wound is closed with absorbable sutures; typically, drainage placement is unnecessary.

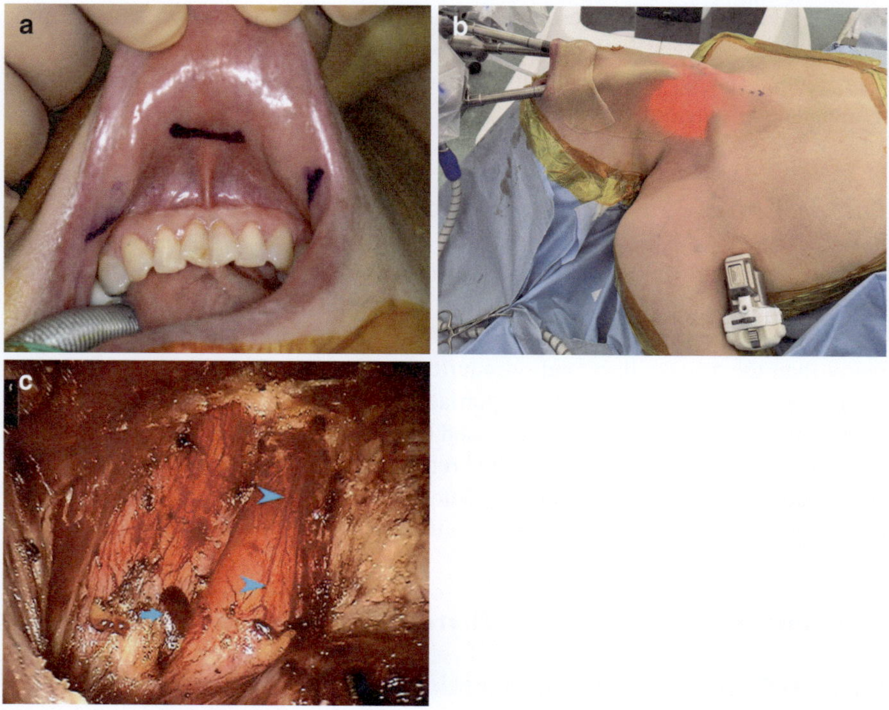

Fig. 10.4 The transoral approach with CO_2 insufflation. (**a**) A central incision measuring 1.5 cm is made at the base of the lower lip frenulum, with lateral incisions placed near the oral commissure, avoiding injury to the mental nerve. (**b**) In the robotic transoral procedure, an additional axillary port is created in the axillary fossa to accommodate a third robotic instrument. (**c**) Surgical view following lobectomy while preserving the recurrent laryngeal nerve and parathyroid glands. Arrow indicates the superior parathyroid gland; arrowheads indicate the recurrent laryngeal nerve

Advantages and Limitations

A significant advantage of the transoral approach is its superior cosmetic outcome, as it eliminates the need for visible cutaneous skin incisions, apart from a small axillary incision in the transoral robotic procedure [48]. This method is also less invasive compared to other remote-access thyroidectomy techniques in terms of creating a working space. The midline approach with a top-down view offers bilateral visualization of the thyroid glands and the central neck compartment [1, 38], enabling comprehensive procedures such as total thyroidectomy and central neck dissection, including up to level VII. Additionally, this approach allows for effective dissection of lymph nodes in levels III and IV [49, 50]. However, dissection of level II lymph nodes remains challenging due to the limited surgical axis, suboptimal visualization, and restricted instrument reach.

In robotic procedures, although the technical advantages are notable, the initial creation of the working space relies on endoscopic techniques. Consequently, this dual requirement for endoscopic and robotic system equipment can increase procedural complexity and resource demands. The transoral approach also carries specific disadvantages, including risks of skin flap injury or perforation, complications related to CO_2 insufflation, mental nerve injury, and potential infection risks associated with the oral cavity flora [51].

Comparison of Four Common Remote-Access Thyroidectomies

The degree of surgical invasiveness related to skin flap elevation is greatest in the BABA and transaxillary approach, while it is minimal in the transoral approach. Both the BABA and transoral approaches facilitate total thyroidectomy more effectively than the transaxillary and retroauricular approaches. Although central neck dissection is feasible with all four approaches, it is relatively more challenging in BABA due to limited visualization caused by the obstruction of the manubrium and clavicle. For lateral neck dissection, the retroauricular approach is superior to other techniques. Postoperative cosmetic outcomes are optimal with the transoral approach, although all four procedures achieve satisfactory cosmetic results.

Outcomes of Remote-Access Thyroidectomy

Surgical Outcomes and Complications

The surgical outcomes and complication rates associated with remote-access thyroidectomy have been reported to be comparable to those of conventional transcervical thyroidectomy in several meta-analyses [37, 43, 52, 53]. However, some studies have noted discrepancies in these findings. These data suggest that remote-access thyroid surgery is, at a minimum, not inferior to the conventional approach when performed by experienced surgeons.

Nevertheless, complication rates may be elevated during the learning curve, particularly for low-volume surgeons. Certain meta-analyses have demonstrated a higher transient RLN palsy rate in some remote-access techniques compared to the conventional approach [54]. Conversely, rates of hematoma, seroma, and permanent hypoparathyroidism appear comparable between traditional and remote-access methods. However, serious complications—including esophageal and tracheal injury, airway compromise from hematomas, and, in rare cases, CO_2 embolism—can occur. To optimize surgical outcomes, strict patient selection criteria and prioritization of patient safety are essential, particularly during the steep learning curve. Furthermore, comprehensive training programs for surgeons are imperative, and the possibility of conversion to an open procedure, which occurs in approximately 1% of cases, should be clearly communicated to patients preoperatively [55].

Intraoperative neural monitoring (IONM) has been proposed to reduce the incidence of RLN palsy during remote-access thyroid surgery. However, IONM faces limitations in this context, including higher failure rates, deviations from standard protocols, and challenges in troubleshooting during surgery [56].

Preservation of the parathyroid glands remains challenging in both traditional and remote-access thyroid surgeries. The use of near-infrared autofluorescence (NIRAF) detection and indocyanine green (ICG) angiography may facilitate the identification of parathyroid glands, reduce rates of temporary hypoparathyroidism, and predict postoperative parathyroid function [57].

Remote-access techniques are associated with unique complications. For instance, transient brachial plexus injury has been reported in robotic transaxillary approaches, though proper arm and shoulder positioning can mitigate this risk. In the retroauricular approach, marginal branch facial nerve injury can result from robotic instrument compression at the postauricular port [23]. Mental nerve injury is another concern in the transoral approach. To minimize this risk, central vestibular incisions should be confined to the central safety triangle zone, and lateral incisions should be placed near the oral commissure. Additionally, chin and central vestibular area dissection should be minimized [51, 58].

CO_2-related complications—including embolism, subcutaneous emphysema, and hypercapnia—may arise during transoral and BABA thyroidectomy due to CO_2 insufflation. Although the incidence of CO_2 embolism in transoral and BABA thyroidectomy is reported to be very low [39, 51], fewer than 20 cases have been documented in the literature. The actual incidence may be underreported or underestimated.

Infection is a potential risk in all approaches, with the transoral method theoretically carrying a higher risk [51]. Preventive measures include antiseptic treatment of the surgical space, thorough saline irrigation to remove blood clots and debris, and appropriate perioperative antibiotic administration.

Rarely, recurrence along the operative tract may occur after remote-access thyroidectomy. This complication, typically attributed to tumor rupture and spillage during the procedure, is more common during the learning curve. It has been observed in thyroidectomy for benign tumors and conventional thyroidectomy. Adequate surgeon experience, proper patient selection, sufficient operative workspace creation, and careful handling of the tumor capsule are critical to minimizing this risk. Sharp instruments should not be used to hold the tumor capsule, and all suspicious tumor tissue should be meticulously removed from the operative field.

Surgical Completeness for Total Thyroidectomy

Achieving surgical completeness in total thyroidectomy through unilateral gasless transaxillary and retroauricular approaches presents inherent challenges due to limited visualization and restricted access to the contralateral lobe. Consequently, surgical completeness is a pertinent concern in remote-access thyroidectomy. Surrogate markers such as thyrotropin (TSH)-stimulated thyroglobulin levels and radioactive iodine (RAI) uptake are commonly utilized to evaluate the adequacy of total thyroidectomy. A meta-analysis has demonstrated that the rate of achieving stimulated thyroglobulin <1.0 ng/mL at postoperative RAI ablation is generally higher with the gasless transaxillary approach compared to the BABA, transoral, and conventional methods [43]. However, the outcomes among BABA, transoral, and conventional approaches were found to be comparable.

Operative Time

The operative duration for remote-access thyroidectomy is significantly prolonged compared to conventional approaches, primarily due to the extended time required for flap dissection and robotic docking [1, 59]. Studies indicate that the surgical time for remote-access techniques increases by 30–50% relative to conventional methods. This increase arises from the additional time required to elevate the skin flap to access the thyroid gland, dock the robotic system, and exchange instruments between robotic and endoscopic platforms. Nonetheless, with increased surgical experience, the operative time associated with remote-access thyroidectomy has been observed to decrease.

Learning Curves

Remote-access thyroid surgery is a technically demanding procedure, necessitating an extensive learning curve to achieve proficiency. Accelerating this learning curve is crucial to minimizing complications. Reported case volumes required to overcome the learning curve vary by approach, with estimates of 10–60 cases for the gasless transaxillary approach, 33–50 cases for the BABA approach, and 11–58 cases for the transoral approach [60]. Proficiency in remote-access thyroidectomy is multifaceted and cannot be solely defined by operative time or case volume. Metrics such as complication rates, reoperation rates, mortality rates, and patient satisfaction must be taken into account. Additionally, mastery of individual steps within a procedure does not necessarily equate to proficiency in the technique as a whole.

Oncologic Outcomes for Thyroid Cancer

Oncologic outcomes are a critical consideration in the treatment of thyroid cancer and should not be overshadowed by a focus on cosmetic or functional outcomes when evaluating the remote-access approach. A meta-analysis demonstrated recurrence rates after thyroidectomy for papillary thyroid carcinoma (PTC) of 1.31% with the conventional method, 0.89% for the gasless transaxillary approach, 0.62% for the BABA, and 0% for the transoral approach. These differences were not statistically significant when adjusted for follow-up duration [43]. Remote-access thyroidectomy is generally indicated for small, low-risk PTCs, which have an excellent prognosis regardless of surgical approach or extent of surgery. Thus, the oncologic safety of remote-access thyroidectomy appears to be acceptable for low-risk PTC, though its long-term outcomes require further validation.

Nevertheless, evidence regarding oncologic outcomes such as locoregional recurrence and survival following remote-access thyroidectomy remains limited. Additional studies with extended follow-up periods and larger patient cohorts are essential to evaluate the long-term oncologic safety of these approaches comprehensively.

Cosmesis and Quality of Life (QOL)

The primary advantage of remote-access thyroidectomy is its superior cosmetic outcomes compared to the conventional transcervical approach [47, 48, 61]. Most studies have reported excellent postoperative cosmetic results associated with remote-access thyroid surgery. Techniques employing CO_2 insufflation, such as the transoral and BABA approaches, rely on small incisions in remote-access sites, resulting in better cosmesis compared to gasless methods, which require longer incisions at remote sites. Among the remote-access techniques, the transoral approach offers the greatest cosmetic benefits, followed by the transaxillary and retroauricular methods [47, 48]. Moreover, long-term cosmetic satisfaction after scar maturation is significantly higher with the transaxillary approach than with conventional thyroidectomy [62].

QOL following remote-access thyroidectomy is comparable to or better than that of the conventional approach. Improved QOL is often attributed to higher scores for appearance satisfaction. A cohort study demonstrated that the physical composite score of the remote-access approach, including the postauricular and transaxillary methods, was significantly better than that of the conventional approach, with benefits persisting up to 5 years postoperatively [63].

Voice and Swallowing Outcomes

Voice quality outcomes following remote-access thyroidectomy are reported to be comparable or superior to those observed with the conventional approach. Several studies have demonstrated similar Voice Handicap Index scores and overall voice quality between remote-access and conventional techniques. Conversely, other investigations have indicated improved voice outcomes with remote-access thyroidectomy, particularly with transaxillary, retroauricular, and transoral approaches. Notably, remote-access methods have shown significantly better preservation of the highest vocal frequency [64–66]. Nonetheless, further research is required to confirm and delineate the impact of remote-access thyroidectomy on voice function.

Regarding swallowing function, postoperative changes appear similar between remote-access and conventional approaches [67]. However, the evidence on swallowing outcomes after remote-access thyroidectomy remains limited and inconclusive. While some studies have suggested that robotic thyroidectomy offers advantages in preserving postoperative swallowing function, others have reported equivalent outcomes between robotic and conventional methods. A specific study on gasless transaxillary thyroidectomy reported superior postoperative swallowing outcomes compared to the conventional technique [68].

Remote-Access Lateral Neck Dissection

The application of remote-access robotic and endoscopic thyroid surgery has been extended to lateral neck dissection in cases of thyroid cancer with lateral compartment lymph node metastases. Remote-access lateral neck dissection has been successfully performed using various approaches, including the gasless axillary, breast–chest, infraclavicular, BABA, gasless retroauricular, and transoral methods, as well as combinations of these techniques [69]. However, patients with bulky or multilevel nodal metastases in the lateral neck compartment are generally contraindicated for this approach. The extent of lateral neck dissection achievable through remote-access techniques is comparable to that of conventional approaches, encompassing levels IIa, III, IV, and V, except for the transoral method, which is limited to levels III and IV [50, 69]. Preoperative ultrasound-guided charcoal tattooing has proven valuable for identifying metastatic lymph nodes during robotic lateral neck dissection [70].

A meta-analysis has demonstrated that critical outcomes, including the number of excised lateral lymph nodes, the extent of dissection, rates of transient RLN palsy and hypoparathyroidism, serum-stimulated thyroglobulin levels, and recurrence rates, do not differ significantly between remote-access approaches—such as robotic BABA, robotic gasless transaxillary, and endoscopic breast–chest methods—and conventional procedures [69]. However, the absence of long-term follow-up studies on remote-access lateral neck dissection precludes definitive conclusions regarding its oncologic safety. Future studies with extended follow-up periods are necessary to evaluate the long-term outcomes and efficacy of this approach.

Limitations and Barriers to Remote-Access Thyroidectomy

Remote-access thyroidectomy presents several notable limitations and challenges. Unlike minimally invasive surgeries, remote-access approaches require the creation of flaps to establish the surgical field [1]. This necessitates a wider dissection area to create adequate working space. Nevertheless, the thyroidectomy procedure itself remains as meticulous and precise as the conventional approach.

Key limitations and barriers to the broader adoption of remote-access thyroidectomy include the technical complexity of the procedure, a relatively high complication rate during the learning curve, and significant costs [1, 38]. These factors raise concerns regarding patient safety, particularly during the early stages of surgeon training. Additional barriers include high body mass index, cultural differences in perceptions of neck scarring, longer operative times, and medicolegal challenges, which are particularly pronounced in Western countries [1, 38].

Conclusions

Remote-access thyroidectomy represents a viable and safe alternative for many patients requiring thyroid surgery, provided it is performed by experienced surgeons. Surgical outcomes and major complication rates are comparable to those of conventional transcervical thyroidectomy, and oncologic outcomes are not inferior in carefully selected patients. However, unique complications associated with this approach must be weighed against patient preferences and goals. Surgeons must fully understand the advantages and limitations of various remote-access techniques. To ensure optimal outcomes, thorough training and preparation are imperative. Among its benefits, the most significant is the superior cosmetic outcome. Cosmesis and scar-related quality-of-life metrics consistently surpass those of the conventional approach over time.

Conflicts of Interest No potential conflicts of interest relevant to this article are reported.

References

1. Tae K, Ji YB, Song CM, Ryu J. Robotic and endoscopic thyroid surgery: evolution and advances. Clin Exp Otorhinolaryngol. 2019;12(1):1–11.
2. Huscher CS, Chiodini S, Napolitano C, Recher A. Endoscopic right thyroid lobectomy. Surg Endosc. 1997;11:877.
3. Miccoli P, Berti P, Conte M, Bendinelli C, Marcocci C. Minimally invasive surgery for thyroid small nodules: preliminary report. J Endocrinol Investig. 1999;22:849–51.
4. Miccoli P, Minuto MN, Ugolini C, Pisano R, Fosso A, Berti P. Minimally invasive video-assisted thyroidectomy for benign thyroid disease: an evidence-based review. World J Surg. 2008;32(7):1333–40.
5. Ikeda Y, Takami H, Tajima G, et al. Total endoscopic thyroidectomy: axillary or anterior chest approach. Biomed Pharmacother. 2002;56(Suppl 1):72s–8s.
6. Kataoka H, Kitano H, Takeuchi E, Fujimura M. Total video endoscopic thyroidectomy via the anterior chest approach using the cervical region-lifting method. Biomed Pharmacother. 2002;56(Suppl 1):68s–71s.
7. Shimizu K, Kitagawa W, Akasu H, Hatori N, Hirai K, Tanaka S. Video-assisted endoscopic thyroid and parathyroid surgery using a gasless method of anterior neck skin lifting: a review of 130 cases. Surg Today. 2002;32(10):862–8.
8. Ikeda Y, Takami H, Sasaki Y, Kan S, Niimi M. Endoscopic neck surgery by the axillary approach. J Am Coll Surg. 2000;191:336–40.
9. Yoon JH, Park CH, Chung WY. Gasless endoscopic thyroidectomy via an axillary approach: experience of 30 cases. Surg Laparosc Endosc Percutan Tech. 2006;16:226–31.
10. Kang SW, Jeong JJ, Yun JS, et al. Robot-assisted endoscopic surgery for thyroid cancer: experience with the first 100 patients. Surg Endosc. 2009;23:2399–406.
11. Ryu HR, Kang SW, Lee SH, et al. Feasibility and safety of a new robotic thyroidectomy through a gasless, transaxillary single-incision approach. J Am Coll Surg. 2010;211(3):e13–9.
12. Tae K, Kim SY, Lee YS, Lee HS. Gasless endoscopic thyroidectomy by an axillary approach: preliminary report. Korean J Otolaryngol. 2007;50:252–6.
13. Tae K, Ji YB, Cho SH, Kim KR, Kim DW, Kim DS. Initial experience with a gasless unilateral axillo-breast or axillary approach endoscopic thyroidectomy for papillary thyroid microcarcinoma: comparison with conventional open thyroidectomy. Surg Laparosc Endosc Percutan Tech. 2011;21:162–9.

14. Tae K, Ji YB, Jeong JH, Lee SH, Jeong MA, Park CW. Robotic thyroidectomy by a gasless unilateral axillo-breast or axillary approach: our early experiences. Surg Endosc. 2011;25:221–8.
15. Tae K, Ji YB, Cho SH, Lee SH, Kim DS, Kim TW. Early surgical outcomes of robotic thyroidectomy by a gasless unilateral axillo-breast or axillary approach for papillary thyroid carcinoma: 2 years' experience. Head Neck. 2012;34:617–25.
16. Ohgami M, Ishii S, Arisawa Y, et al. Scarless endoscopic thyroidectomy: breast approach for better cosmesis. Surg Laparosc Endosc Percutan Tech. 2000;10:1–4.
17. Shimazu K, Shiba E, Tamaki Y, et al. Endoscopic thyroid surgery through the axillo-bilateral-breast approach. Surg Laparosc Endosc Percutan Tech. 2003;13:196–201.
18. Choe JH, Kim SW, Chung KW, et al. Endoscopic thyroidectomy using a new bilateral axillo-breast approach. World J Surg. 2007;31:601–6.
19. Lee MC, Mo JA, Choi IJ, Lee BC, Lee GH. New endoscopic thyroidectomy via a unilateral axillo-breast approach with gas insufflation: preliminary report. Head Neck. 2013;35(4):471–6.
20. Singer MC, Seybt MW, Terris DJ. Robotic facelift thyroidectomy: I. Preclinical simulation and morphometric assessment. Laryngoscope. 2011;121:1631–5.
21. Terris DJ, Singer MC, Seybt MW. Robotic facelift thyroidectomy: II. Clinical feasibility and safety. Laryngoscope. 2011;121:1636–41.
22. Byeon HK, Kim da H, Chang JW, et al. Comprehensive application of robotic retroauricular thyroidectomy: the evolution of robotic thyroidectomy. Laryngoscope. 2016;126(8):1952–7.
23. Sung ES, Ji YB, Song CM, Yun BR, Chung WS, Tae K. Robotic thyroidectomy: comparison of a Postauricular facelift approach with a gasless unilateral axillary approach. Otolaryngol Head Neck Surg. 2016;154:997–1004.
24. Witzel K, von Rahden BH, Kaminski C, Stein HJ. Transoral access for endoscopic thyroid resection. Surg Endosc. 2008;22:1871–5.
25. Karakas E, Steinfeldt T, Gockel A, Westermann R, Kiefer A, Bartsch DK. Transoral thyroid and parathyroid surgery. Surg Endosc. 2010;24(6):1261–7.
26. Wilhelm T, Metzig A. Endoscopic minimally invasive thyroidectomy (eMIT): a prospective proof-of-concept study in humans. World J Surg. 2011;35(3):543–51.
27. Richmon JD, Holsinger FC, Kandil E, Moore MW, Garcia JA, Tufano RP. Transoral robotic-assisted thyroidectomy with central neck dissection: preclinical cadaver feasibility study and proposed surgical technique. J Robot Surg. 2011;5:279–82.
28. Nakajo A, Arima H, Hirata M, et al. Trans-oral video-assisted neck surgery (TOVANS). A new transoral technique of endoscopic thyroidectomy with gasless premandible approach. Surg Endosc. 2013;27:1105–10.
29. Wang C, Zhai H, Liu W, et al. Thyroidectomy: a novel endoscopic oral vestibular approach. Surgery. 2014;155:33–8.
30. Anuwong A. Transoral endoscopic thyroidectomy vestibular approach: a series of the first 60 human cases. World J Surg. 2016;40(3):491–7.
31. Kim HY, Chai YJ, Dionigi G, Anuwong A, Richmon JD. Transoral robotic thyroidectomy: lessons learned from an initial consecutive series of 24 patients. Surg Endosc. 2018;32(2):688–94.
32. Tae K, Lee DW, Song CM, et al. Early experience of transoral thyroidectomy: comparison of robotic and endoscopic procedures. Head Neck. 2019;41(3):730–8.
33. Tae K, Ji YB, Song CM, Park JS, Park JH, Kim DS. Safety and efficacy of transoral robotic and endoscopic thyroidectomy: the first 100 cases. Head Neck. 2020;42(2):321–9.
34. Park JO, Park YJ, Kim MR, Sun DI, Kim MS, Koh YW. Gasless transoral endoscopic thyroidectomy vestibular approach (gasless TOETVA). Surg Endosc. 2019;33(9):3034–9.
35. Park YM, Kim DH, Moon YM, et al. Gasless transoral robotic thyroidectomy using the Da Vinci SP system: feasibility, safety, and operative technique. Oral Oncol. 2019;95:136–42.
36. Chen Y, Chomsky-Higgins K, Nwaogu I, et al. Hidden in plain sight: transoral and submental thyroidectomy as a compelling alternative to "Scarless" thyroidectomy. J Laparoendosc Adv Surg Tech A. 2018;28(11):1374–7.
37. Nguyen VC, Song CM, Ji YB, Oh S, Jeong JH, Tae K. Comparison of surgical outcomes of transoral robotic and endoscopic thyroidectomy: a systematic review and network meta-analysis. Head Neck. 2024;46(3):688–701.

38. Tae K. Robotic thyroid surgery. Auris Nasus Larynx. 2021;48(3):331–8.
39. Kim KN, Lee DW, Kim JY, Han KH, Tae K. Carbon dioxide embolism during transoral robotic thyroidectomy: a case report. Head Neck. 2018;40(3):E25–8.
40. Grogan RH, Suh I, Chomsky-Higgins K, et al. Patient eligibility for transoral endocrine surgery procedures in the United States. JAMA Netw Open. 2019;2(5):e194829.
41. Kang SW, Lee SH, Ryu HR, et al. Initial experience with robot-assisted modified radical neck dissection for the management of thyroid carcinoma with lateral neck node metastasis. Surgery. 2010;148:1214–21.
42. Song CM, Ji YB, Sung ES, Kim DS, Koo HR, Tae K. Comparison of robotic versus conventional selective neck dissection and Total thyroidectomy for papillary thyroid carcinoma. Otolaryngol Head Neck Surg. 2016;154:1005–13.
43. Nguyen VC, Lee DW, Song CM, Ji YB, Park JS, Tae K. Oncologic outcomes and surgical completeness of remote-access thyroidectomy: a systematic review and network meta-analysis. Langenbeck's Arch Surg. 2024;409(1):117.
44. Kim JK, Choi SH, Choi SM, et al. Single-port transaxillary robotic thyroidectomy (START): 200-cases with two-step retraction method. Surg Endosc. 2022;36(4):2688–96.
45. Lee KE, Rao J, Youn YK. Endoscopic thyroidectomy with the da Vinci robot system using the bilateral axillary breast approach (BABA) technique; our initial experience. Surg Laparosc Endosc Percuta Tech. 2009;19(3):e71–5.
46. Kim BS, Kang KH, Park SJ. Robotic modified radical neck dissection by bilateral axillary breast approach for papillary thyroid carcinoma with lateral neck metastasis. Head Neck. 2015;37:37–45.
47. Lee DW, Bang HS, Jeong JH, et al. Cosmetic outcomes after transoral robotic thyroidectomy: comparison with transaxillary, postauricular, and conventional approaches. Oral Oncol. 2021;114:105139.
48. Lee DW, Ko SH, Song CM, Ji YB, Kim JK, Tae K. Comparison of postoperative cosmesis in transaxillary, postauricular facelift, and conventional transcervical thyroidectomy. Surg Endosc. 2020;34(8):3388–97.
49. Tae K, Kim K. Transoral robotic selective neck dissection for papillary thyroid carcinoma: dissection of levels III and IV. Head Neck. 2020;42(10):3084–8.
50. Tae K, Choi HW, Ji YB, Song CM, Park JH, Kim DS. Feasibility of transoral robotic selective neck dissection with or without a postauricular incision for papillary thyroid carcinoma: a pilot study. Front Surg. 2022;9:985097.
51. Tae K. Complications of transoral thyroidectomy: overview and update. Clin Exp Otorhinolaryngol. 2021;14(2):169–78.
52. Xing Z, Qiu Y, Abuduwaili M, et al. Surgical outcomes of different approaches in robotic assisted thyroidectomy for thyroid cancer: a systematic review and Bayesian network meta-analysis. Int J Surg. 2021;89:105941.
53. Kang YJ, Stybayeva G, Hwang SH. Surgical completeness and safety of minimally invasive thyroidectomy in patients with thyroid cancer: a network meta-analysis. Surgery. 2023;173(6):1381–90.
54. Sialakis C, Frantzana A, Iliadis C, Ouzounakis P, Antoniou Sialaki P, Kourkouta L. Comparison of robotic versus conventional open thyroidectomy for recurrent laryngeal nerve safety: a systematic review and meta-analysis. Cureus. 2024;16(2):e53860.
55. Martino B, Nitro L, De Pasquale L, et al. Conversion rates in robotic thyroid surgery: a systematic review and meta-analysis. Int J Med Robot. 2022;18(5):e2427.
56. Ji YB, Ko SH, Song CM, et al. Feasibility and efficacy of intraoperative neural monitoring in remote access robotic and endoscopic thyroidectomy. Oral Oncol. 2020;103:104617.
57. Silver Karcioglu AL, Triponez F, Solórzano CC, et al. Emerging imaging technologies for parathyroid gland identification and vascular assessment in thyroid surgery: a review from the American head and neck society endocrine surgery section. JAMA Otolaryngol Head Neck Surg. 2023;149(3):253–60.

58. Tae K, Lee DW, Bang HS, Ahn YH, Park JH, Kim DS. Sensory change in the chin and neck after transoral thyroidectomy: prospective study of mental nerve injury. Head Neck. 2020;42(11):3111–7.
59. Kim KH, Ji YB, Song CM, Kim E, Kim KN, Tae K. Learning curve of transoral robotic thyroidectomy. Surg Endosc. 2023;37(1):535–43.
60. Fassari A, Gurrado A, Iossa A, et al. Definition of learning curve for thyroidectomy: systematic review on the different approaches. Gland Surg. 2023;12(7):989–1006.
61. Nguyen VC, Song CM, Ji YB, Lee DW, Jeong JH, Tae K. Evaluation of the validity and reliability of a self-assessment questionnaire for cosmetic outcomes after thyroidectomy: a cross-sectional validation study. Eur Arch Otorrinolaringol. 2024;281(3):1505–13.
62. Ji YB, Song CM, Bang HS, Lee SH, Park YS, Tae K. Long-term cosmetic outcomes after robotic/endoscopic thyroidectomy by a gasless unilateral axillo-breast or axillary approach. J Laparoendosc Adv Surg Tech A. 2014;24:248–53.
63. Kim BH, Ryu SR, Lee JW, et al. Longitudinal changes in quality of life before and after thyroidectomy in patients with differentiated thyroid cancer. J Clin Endocrinol Metab. 2024;109(6):1505–16.
64. Song CM, Kim MS, Lee DW, et al. Comparison of postoperative voice outcomes after postauricular facelift robotic hemithyroidectomy and conventional transcervical hemithyroidectomy. Head Neck. 2019;41(9):2921–8.
65. Tae K, Kim KY, Yun BR, et al. Functional voice and swallowing outcomes after robotic thyroidectomy by a gasless unilateral axillo-breast approach: comparison with open thyroidectomy. Surg Endosc. 2012;26(7):1871–7.
66. Song CM, Park JS, Park HJ, Tae K. Voice outcomes of transoral robotic thyroidectomy: comparison with conventional trans-cervical thyroidectomy. Oral Oncol. 2020;107:104748.
67. Lee SY, Ryu SR, Yun BR, Ji YB, Song CM, Tae K. Patient-reported swallowing outcomes after transoral robotic thyroidectomy: comparison with conventional transcervical thyroidectomy. Head Neck. 2024;46(1):64–73.
68. Lee J, Nah KY, Kim RM, Ahn YH, Soh EY, Chung WY. Differences in postoperative outcomes, function, and cosmesis: open versus robotic thyroidectomy. Surg Endosc. 2010;24(12):3186–94.
69. Nguyen VC, Song CM, Ji YB, Myung JK, Park JS, Tae K. Feasibility of remote-access and minimally invasive video-assisted approaches in lateral neck dissection for papillary thyroid carcinoma: a systematic review and network meta-analysis. Eur J Surg Oncol. 2024;50(9):108469.
70. Song CM, Park JS, Park W, Ji YB, Cho SH, Tae K. Feasibility of charcoal tattooing for localization of metastatic lymph nodes in robotic selective neck dissection for papillary thyroid carcinoma. Ann Surg Oncol. 2015;22(Suppl 3):S669–75.

Complications of Thyroid Surgery

11

Vidula Mestry, Karthik N. Rao, and Prathamesh S. Pai

Editorial

Complications following thyroid surgery have reduced dramatically from what they once were. We have now entered the era of finesse and refinement. In spite of significant advances in our understanding of thyroid surgery and the availability of vastly improved imaging modalities, intraoperative nerve monitoring and magnification in the form of loupes complications can still occur.

Complications like bilateral recurrent laryngeal nerve paralysis can be devastating. Injuries to the aerodigestive tract can prove to be life-threatening. The best way to avoid complications is to have a thorough and careful approach, deep respect, and a good understanding of the thyroid and surrounding tissues accompanied by a patient and careful surgical dissection. A careful and meticulous dissection goes a long way to avoiding complications. The best way to treat a complication is to quickly identify it and treat correctly and comprehensively. Counselling the patient and their families in an honest and lucid manner prior to surgery and answering questions in a truthful and patient manner will help them deal better with the complication should it occur.

Christopher de Souza

V. Mestry
Department of Head and Neck Surgery, Apple Hospital, Kolhapur, India

K. N. Rao (✉)
Department of Head and Neck Oncology, Sri Shankara Cancer Hospital and Research Center, Bangalore, India

P. S. Pai
Department of Surgical Oncology, P D Hinduja Hospital & Medical Research Centre, Khar, Mumbai, India

P. S. Pai et al. (eds.), *Controversies in Cancer of the Thyroid and Parathyroid Glands*, https://doi.org/10.1007/978-3-032-13130-0_11

Introduction and Historical Perspective

In the eighteenth and early nineteenth centuries, thyroid surgeries were nearly abandoned due to their high mortality (~40%) and morbidity [1]. Haemorrhage and infections were the leading causes of complications. Several renowned physicians of that era, including Robert Liston, a British surgeon slated to be the fastest surgeon of his time, wrote against doing thyroid surgeries in 1846 [2]. Samuel Gross, considered one of the founders of American Surgery, called it 'Horrid Butchery' [3]. The French Academy of Medicine condemned any type of surgery on thyroid during this period.

Refinements in surgical techniques, anaesthesia drugs, invention of haemostatic instruments, and inception of sterilization gradually reduced the mortality associated with thyroid surgeries. We remember with pride Dr. Theodor Kocher, a Swiss surgeon whose ground-breaking contributions forever changed the thyroid surgery. Awarded the Nobel Prize in Physiology or Medicine in 1909—the only surgeon to ever receive this honour for refining a surgical technique—Dr. Kocher's refinements in thyroid surgery reduced mortality rates below 1%. His work not only revolutionized endocrine surgery but also set the foundation for the safe, routine procedures we rely on today. He described hypothyroidism and suggested partial removal of thyroid. In 1907, Thomas Peel Dunhill used pericapsular dissection technique for total lobectomy, which is a standard dissection technique even now [2]. In 1938, Frank Lahey advised lateral ligation of inferior thyroid artery and recorded only 0.3% nerve palsy rate [2]. Gley correlated hypocalcaemia with either excision or devascularization of parathyroid glands and suggested prevention by preserving the main trunk of the inferior thyroid artery [4]. By the advent of the First World War, thyroid surgery became an international discipline through the contributions of legendary surgeons of that era, viz., George Crile, William Mayo, Harvey Cushing, Anton Von Eisenberg, Theodore Kocher, James Berry, Thomas Peel Dunhill, Cecil Joll, and Walter E. Sistrunk [2].

We have come a long way. What was once considered a surgical nightmare is now a common procedure performed globally with excellent outcomes. Despite significant advancements in thyroid surgery over the past century, complications such as hypoparathyroidism, recurrent laryngeal nerve palsy, postoperative bleeding, chyle leak, and aerodigestive tract injuries continue to challenge surgeons. In this chapter, we describe pertinent complications, detailing their incidence, associated risk factors, and evidence-based strategies for mitigation and management. Our aim is to provide practical insights that can enhance patient outcomes and surgical safety.

Difficult Intubation

Approximately 6.8–9.6% patients undergoing thyroid surgery are difficult to intubate [5]. A meta-analysis by De Cassai et al. identified increased neck circumference, restricted neck movements, and presence of tracheal deviation as potential

Table 11.1 Difficulty in intubation

Presentation	Risk factors	Prevention	Management
Inability to ventilate Inability to visualize larynx Inability to intubate	Thick neck Large goitre Restricted neck movements due to involvement of sternocleidomastoid or prevertebral muscles	Preoperative assessment and anticipation of difficult airway Different sizes of endotracheal tubes should be available Tracheostomy support to be standby with a tracheoflex tube with adjustable flanges	Awake fibreoptic intubation Use of video laryngoscope Intubation without neuromuscular relaxant

risk factors for difficult intubation in thyroid surgery [5]. Large-volume goitres may cause tracheal deviation which not only shifts the glottic plane laterally, making laryngeal visualization difficult but also increases the lifting force needed for laryngoscopy [6].

Mere laryngotracheal deviation also does not indicate luminal narrowing. In most cases, the lumen remains patent, allowing uneventful endotracheal intubation despite the shift [7]. However, with intraluminal narrowing (shin type 3,4), laryngotracheal invasion, and impending stridor, there is a significant risk of difficult or failed intubation [8]. In these high-risk cases, 'Can't oxygenate, can't intubate' situation may occur and an emergency tracheostomy may be the only resort [9]. In extreme emergencies, a needle cricothyrotomy may be employed temporarily to maintain oxygenation while preparing for definitive airway control.

Preoperative imaging and clinical assessment, including the use of ultrasound intraoperatively, can provide valuable insights into the tracheal course and its deviation, aiding in planning emergency airway access (Table 11.1). Additionally, transillumination using a fibreoptic scope or a lighted stylet may create a visible silhouette through the skin, guiding precise incision placement during planned tracheostomy in difficult thyroid cases [10].

The cornerstone of managing difficult airways in thyroid surgery is anticipation, reinforced by a continuous and proactive dialogue between the senior anaesthetist and the operating surgeon [11, 12].

Thyroid Storm

Thyroid storm is an acute, life-threatening, decompensated state of thyrotoxic crisis caused by an excessive release of thyroid hormones into the circulation in a hyperthyroid patient posing mortality of 8–25% [13]. Surgical stress and intraoperative handling of the thyroid gland predispose a thyroid storm and the American Thyroid Association (ATA) guidelines recommend rendering the patient euthyroid with antithyroid medications with or without potassium iodide to prevent it during surgery [13].

Table 11.2 Thyroid storm

Presentation	Risk factors	Prevention	Management
Hyperthermia Hypertension (shock and hypotension in later stage) Tachycardia Wide pulse pressure Myocardial infarction/ heart failure Vomiting/diarrhoea Agitation/ confusion/ unconsciousness Extreme cases—cardiovascular collapse, hepatic failure, and death	Preoperative hyperthyroid state, which is incompletely treated Unrecognized hyperthyroid state	To render euthyroid with antithyroid medication prior to surgery Anticipation of thyroid storm in hyperthyroid patients undergoing surgery, to identify early symptoms Continuation of beta-blockers in perioperative period	Management in the ICU Steroids (hydrocortisone 100–300 mg) Beta-blockers (propranolol 4–10 mg/kg), antithyroid drugs (IV. Propylthiouracil 600 mg) Thioamides and iodides Temperature control Intravenous fluids External cooling

If thyroid storm is suspected, gland manipulation should cease immediately and the surgery should be quickly terminated. ATA guidelines recommend surgery for Graves' disease by a high-volume surgeon who performs more than 25 surgeries annually [13]. Low-volume surgeons have a higher complication rate [14].

Despite widespread clinical practices, current literature lacks high-quality evidence comparing outcomes between preoperatively treated and untreated patients. Euthyroid status does not guarantee safety from a thyroid storm, and all hyperthyroid patients undergoing elective surgery should be optimized with thionamides, iodine, β-blockers, and corticosteroids as indicated to minimize potential complications [15, 16]. Continuous intraoperative monitoring, readiness for intensive care support, and a high index of suspicion during recovery are essential, especially in patients with subclinical symptoms or poor preoperative control (Table 11.2).

Tracheomalacia

Tracheomalacia is the softening of the cartilaginous framework of the trachea due to compression by a long-standing goitre. Large long-standing multinodular goitres often raise a concern of tracheomalacia, but they are rare, with an incidence of 1.4% in the meta-analysis [17].

Tracheomalacia may be anticipated in a 'scabbard' trachea seen as a slit on axial cuts of CT cross-sectional imaging [18]. Intraoperative evidence of soft, collapsible tracheal walls [19] raising a concern and immediate extubation may precipitate respiratory distress. In any suspect case, the cuff should be deflated and checked for indrawing of the cartilages and, if collapsible, then extubation should be delayed for 24–48 h and performed under fibreoptic guidance [20]. An awake fibreoptic bronchoscopy not only confirms the diagnosis but also assists in planning definitive

Table 11.3 Tracheomalacia

Presentation	Risk factors	Prevention	Management
Inspiratory stridor after thyroidectomy, post extubation	Long-standing goitre	Intraoperative anticipation of tracheomalacia Flexible bronchoscopic extubation	Intraoperative Tracheopexy Prolonged intubation Positive pressure ventilation Tracheostomy

airway management. In patients with coexisting recurrent laryngeal nerve palsy or airway compromise, a planned tracheostomy may be necessary to prevent repeated extubation–intubation cycles and potential hypoxic events (Table 11.3).

Haematoma

Postoperative haematoma is a known complication of thyroid surgery and occurs in 0.45–4.2% [21]. Deep neck haematoma endangers airway and life mostly by laryngeal oedema which sets in due to venous obstruction and rarely by tracheal compression. Early recognition and prompt treatment are of utmost importance, and the British Association of Endocrine and Thyroid Surgeons (BAETS), British Association of Otorhinolaryngology, Head and neck surgery (BAOHNS), and Difficult Airway Society (DAS) have devised guidelines for its management [21].

The majority of bleeding events (85%) occur within 8–24 h post-surgery [22]. Common sites of bleed are from small vessels at the entry of the RLN, Berry's ligament vessels, and the anterior jugular veins caused by slippage of clips or ligatures. Major arterial bleed is rare and may arise from branches of the superior and inferior thyroid arteries or from the cricothyroid artery. Deep-seated haematomas beneath the strap muscles are more dangerous than the superficial bleeds which may present with ecchymosis but less respiratory distress.

Predictive risk factors for postoperative haematoma include patient-related factors such as male sex, older age, coagulopathies, chronic kidney or liver disease, and alcohol use [23]. Surgical factors include total or near-total thyroidectomy, malignancy, long operative duration, intraoperative hypertension, redo surgeries, and inadequate hemostasis [24].

The violent extubation or postoperative vomiting and cough can disrupt previously secured vessels. Clinical signs suggestive of bleeding include cervical pressure or tightness, dysphagia, pain, neck swelling, restlessness, blood-stained dressings, stridor, tachycardia, hypotension, and decreased oxygen saturation (Fig. 11.1).

Haematologic or imaging assessments are rarely helpful in acute scenarios and should not delay intervention. Immediate management involves releasing the wound sutures to decompress the airway followed by surgical evacuation and haemostasis. Definitive care requires securing the bleeder, usually under general anaesthesia.

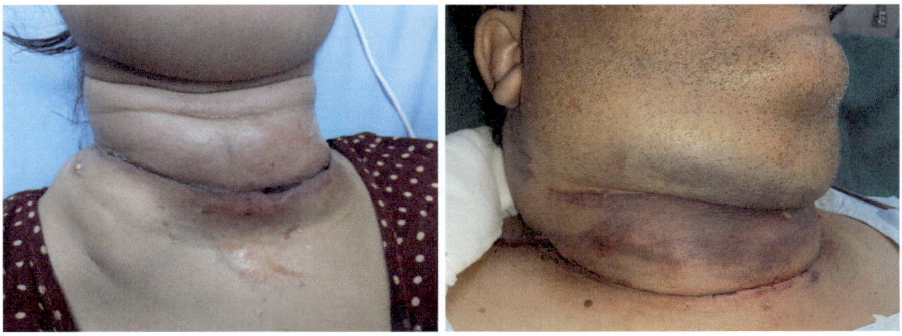

Fig. 11.1 Postoperative haematoma following thyroidectomy. Ecchymosis of the skin can be visualized

Table 11.4 Haematoma

Presentation	Risk factors	Prevention	Management
Ecchymosis of skin Increasing neck circumference Frank blood in neck drain Breathing difficulty	Reactionary hypertension Thick short neck Excessive vascularity Large size of thyroid Excessive coughing Stormy extubation	Optimum intraoperative haemostasis Stabilization of blood pressure in the postoperative period Keeping gap between strap muscles anterior to trachea to prevent peritracheal haematoma formation To avoid coughing, retching, and vomiting in the postoperative period Close watch on neck girth Drain placement for high-risk patients	Close observation for change in neck girth Emergency neck exploration in case of rapidly increasing neck girth or breathing difficulty suggestive of ongoing bleeding and enlarging haematoma

Preventive strategies include meticulous haemostasis, use of the Valsalva manoeuvre to detect occult bleeds before closure, controlled extubation, blood pressure management, and judicious use of drains. High-risk patients may benefit from extended observation and delayed discharge (Table 11.4).

Ultimately, awareness of early signs and structured postoperative monitoring protocols is crucial for timely diagnosis and intervention, potentially reducing the morbidity and mortality associated with this rare but life-threatening complication.

Seroma

Post-thyroidectomy seroma is relatively underreported but can cause delayed wound healing and has cosmetic concerns. The overall incidence of seroma formation varies by surgical technique, ranging from 5% in conventional thyroidectomy to 2.2%

with ultrasonic vessel sealing devices [25], and even lower (1.7–2.9%) in certain robotic and endoscopic approaches [26].

Intraoperative predictors include size of the surgical field, amount of flap elevation, thyroid gland volume, and tissue handling. Risk factors such as obesity, advanced age, early drain removal, and subclinical hypocalcaemia contribute significantly [27].

Seroma typically presents as a soft, fluctuant neck swelling, rarely associated with discomfort or respiratory symptoms. Immediate management includes serial percutaneous aspiration, often resolving after 1–2 sittings (Fig. 11.2). Preventive strategies include meticulous haemostasis, avoiding unnecessary dissection, optimal drain removal (output below 30 ml/day), and use of energy-based devices like ultrasonic shears, which reduce seroma incidence, although the supporting evidence is of low quality (Table 11.5).

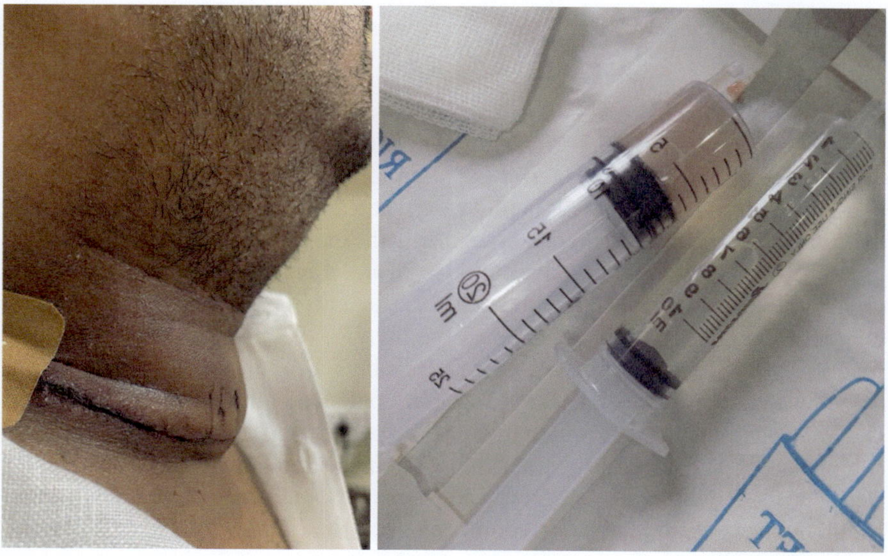

Fig. 11.2 Postoperative seroma following thyroidectomy

Table 11.5 Seroma

Presentation	Risk factors	Prevention	Management
Neck swelling with fluctuation	Large goitre Substernal goitre	Reduce dead space Optimal dissection Meticulous haemostasis Placement of drain when dead space is large Use of pressure dressing	Needle aspiration to confirm nature of collected fluid Repeated needle aspiration under aseptic precautions Pressure dressing

Hypocalcaemia

Postoperative hypocalcaemia remains one of the most common and feared complications, with temporary hypocalcaemia occurring in 1.2–40% and permanent in 1–4% of cases [28]. It is caused by either inadvertent injury, devascularization, or accidental removal of the parathyroid glands during surgery [29].

Biochemical hypocalcaemia is defined as serum calcium levels <8 mg/dl. Clinical hypocalcaemia manifests with tingling numbness in hands and feet, perioral numbness, tetany, muscle tremors, or convulsions. Hypocalcaemia which recovers within 6 months is termed as temporary, and if it continues beyond then it is termed as permanent. The most important factor determining this is the surgical expertise in preserving vascularized parathyroid glands.

Normal parathyroid glands are ~6 mm, flat, yellowish brown (caramel) coloured and lie between true and false fascia of thyroid gland. Small blood vessels can be seen on the surface of glands with a branching pattern. Parathyroid glands can be mistaken for fat, lymph nodes, or thyroid tissue. Fat globules are yellow coloured, spherical or globular, and lack branching pattern of blood vessels. Lymph nodes are pink coloured, rounded, and firm to hard if metastatic [15]. It is essential to preserve blood supply, especially the venous drainage, to ensure proper functioning. The thymic blood supply to the inferior parathyroids should be preserved, and initial ligation of any inferiorly based thyroid veins should be meticulous and towards the thyroid gland. The inferior thyroid artery being the major arterial supply to the parathyroids, ligation of its main trunk should be avoided and its terminal branches supplying the thyroid gland should be identified and ligated individually during thyroidectomy. At the superior pole of the thyroid, the terminal branches of the superior thyroid artery should be ligated individually, preserving the posterior branch which may supply the superior parathyroid gland [15].

Early identification and preservation of the parathyroid glands remain a critical component of a successful thyroidectomy. Optimal techniques include meticulous capsular dissection, judicious use of energy devices, proactive identification of all parathyroid glands, immediately addressing accidental removal or vascular injury, and incorporation of adjuncts such as surgical loupes and autofluorescence.

In contemporary thyroid surgery, the use of surgical loupes has emerged as a pivotal adjunct, with magnification typically ranging from 2.5X to 3.5X, enabling better visualization of the delicate vascular architecture of the parathyroid glands and reducing the risk of vascular compromise due to mechanical and thermal injury [29]. While endoscopic and exoscopic approaches may offer further enhancements in visualization, their role in routine practice is still evolving [30, 31].

Near-infrared autofluorescence (NIRAF) is a non-invasive imaging tool that utilizes the natural autofluorescent properties of the parathyroid glands when exposed to near-infrared light. It allows real-time, stage-independent identification of both in situ and inadvertently excised glands, enabling timely auto-transplantation and significantly reducing the risk of parathyroid insufficiency. The combination of NIRAF with indocyanine green (ICG) angiography further refines intraoperative decision-making by enabling assessment of parathyroid perfusion in addition to identification [32].

In case of accidental removal or devascularization, auto-transplantation of parathyroid glands reduces chances of permanent hypoparathyroidism more predictably than keeping devascularized gland in situ.

In addition to imaging, technological advances such as artificial intelligence (AI) models are now being developed to stratify patients at high risk for hypocalcaemia based on perioperative parameters [28, 33]. Among these, postoperative intact parathyroid hormone (iPTH) levels serve as a strong predictive marker. A iPTH value less than 15 pg/mL on the first postoperative day has a high positive predictive value for the development of hypocalcaemia, thereby guiding early calcium and vitamin D supplementation [34].

According to a recent meta-analysis, total thyroidectomy, hypomagnesemia, preoperative vitamin D deficiency, female gender, thyroid malignancy, thyroiditis, substernal multinodular goitre, parathyroidectomy, central compartment dissection, and modified radical neck dissection are significant factors associated with postoperative hypocalcaemia [35].

Clinical hypocalcaemia typically manifests as perioral numbness, paraesthesia, carpopedal spasms, or, in severe cases, tetany and arrhythmias (Table 11.6). Management strategies depend on severity and include oral calcium and calcitriol supplementation for mild cases and intravenous calcium for symptomatic or severe hypocalcaemia. Prevention, however, remains the cornerstone.

Table 11.6 Hypocalcaemia

Presentation	Risk factors	Prevention	Management
Perioral tingling Tingling numbness in hands and feet Chvostek sign Trousseau sign Muscle cramps Laryngeal spasm and stridor Tremors Tetany Seizures Cardiac arrhythmia with prolonged QT interval	Female gender Preoperative hypocalcaemia Preoperative vitamin D3 deficiency Central compartment neck dissection Redo surgery Substernal goitre Surgery for thyroid cancer Graves' disease	Meticulous bloodless surgical technique for the identification and preservation of parathyroid glands with intact blood supply Extracapsular dissection of thyroid gland Terminal ligation of inferior thyroid artery branches after it gives off the ascending and descending branches to parathyroid glands Removal, mincing, and implantation of devascularized parathyroid gland Optical magnification Use of adjuncts to identify parathyroid glands and their vascularity Early oral calcium supplementation when hypoparathyroidism is anticipated iPTh testing postop	Oral calcium supplementation (2–10 gm/day in divided doses) Addition of calcitriol 0.25–0.5 mg per day if oral calcium supplementation alone is not maintaining serum calcium Intravenous calcium gluconate in case of severe symptoms (10 ml of 10% calcium gluconate slowly over 10 min bolus dose), followed by slow infusion of up to 5 gm (5 ampules of 10%, 10 ml) calcium gluconate in 500 ml saline over 5 h

Superior and Recurrent Laryngeal Nerve Palsy

Injury to the recurrent laryngeal nerve (RLN) and the external branch of the superior laryngeal nerve (EBSLN) are among the most feared complications during thyroidectomy, significantly impacting phonation, airway protection, and overall quality of life. The incidence of temporary RLN injury ranges from 1% to 5%, while permanent RLN palsy occurs in 0.5–2% of cases. Superior laryngeal nerve injury, often underdiagnosed, is seen in up to 58% of patients postoperatively when assessed objectively, though symptomatic cases range between 0.3% and 2% [36].

Recurrent Laryngeal Nerve

Anatomical asymmetry plays a role in the oblique course of the right RLN which loops around the right subclavian artery and has a variable entry point into the larynx. In contrast, the left RLN loops around the aortic arch and has a more predictable and medial trajectory. The right RLN may be more vulnerable due to its shorter and less protected course [15, 37, 38].

The RLN is most vulnerable during the medial mobilization of the thyroid lobe and dissection at the ligament of Berry. Intraoperative predictors of RLN injury include

- Difficult or distorted anatomy (large goitres, malignancies, retrosternal extension)
- Presence of Zuckerkandl's tubercle, which may obscure visualization of the nerve
- Redo thyroid surgeries, where fibrosis and altered planes increase the risk
- Traction injuries and excessive use of electrocautery near the nerve
- Injury to the inferior thyroid artery, whose branches often intersect with the RLN
- The RLN is typically accompanied by a small vessel at its point of entry into the larynx

Unilateral RLN injury typically presents with hoarseness, breathy voice, aspiration, and reduced phonatory efficiency. Initial evaluation includes indirect laryngoscopy or flexible nasolaryngoscopy. Conservative management (voice therapy, steroids, anti-reflux measures) is the mainstay for temporary palsy (Table 11.7). In persistent cases beyond 6–12 months, injection laryngoplasty, medialization thyroplasty, or reinnervation procedures are considered.

Bilateral RLN injury, although rare, is a surgical emergency due to airway compromise. Immediate recognition is crucial. If stridor develops, urgent tracheostomy is often required. In select cases, delayed extubation with close monitoring may be attempted in the ICU setting.

Table 11.7 Unilateral RLN palsy

Presentation	Risk factors	Prevention	Management
Breathy voice (Unilateral palsy) Stridor (bilateral palsy) Cough while swallowing	Thyroid malignancies—Primary or recurrent Large goitres Presence of thyrotoxicosis Redo surgeries RLN variations (non-recurrent laryngeal nerve, branching before laryngeal entry)	Visual identification of nerve in all cases Refrain use of monopolar cautery for dissection once strap muscles are elevated off thyroid Refrain use of electrocautery near nerve	Unilateral palsy: Nasogastric tube insertion for aspiration Voice rest Deep breathing Bilateral palsy Tracheostomy Kashima's surgery—vocal cordotomy

External Branch of the Superior Laryngeal Nerve

EBSLN innervates the cricothyroid muscle, essential for pitch modulation. EBSLN is known as 'Singer's nerve' or 'Galli Curci nerve' due to its effect on the quality of voice. EBSLN injury causes vocal fatigue and inability to raise pitch and amplitude of voice [39] important in the professional voice user. EBSLN typically runs adjacent to or within the 'Joll's triangle'—bounded by the upper pole of the thyroid, the cricothyroid muscle, and the superior thyroid artery [40]. Intraoperative risks to EBSLN arise due to the variable course of EBSLN (Cernea classification) and the size of the superior pole which may endanger the nerve if the superior thyroid vessels are ligated away from the gland.

Meticulous dissection and understanding of anatomical landmarks are key. The use of surgical loupes greatly enhances the ability to identify the RLN and SLN by providing detailed visualization of small vascular and neural structures, even in the presence of Zuckerkandl's tubercle or fibrosis. Adjuncts like intraoperative neuromonitoring (IONM), both intermittent and continuous, aid in nerve identification and real-time functional assessment, especially during redo cases or large malignancies [41]. Exoscopic systems, offering high-definition magnification and shared team visualization, are being explored as promising tools for precise neural identification and documentation [42].

EBSLN injury is difficult to recognize postoperatively unless the patient is a singer or a professional voice user and specifically complains about the change in the quality of voice and thus the reported injury rate is highly variable. It can be assessed either by stroboscopy, electromyography, or expert acoustic analysis. Treatment is largely conservative, with voice therapy, though surgical options like cricothyroid approximation can be considered for professional voice users (Table 11.8).

Table 11.8 EBSLN palsy

Presentation	Risk factors	Prevention	Management
Voice change Inability to raise pitch of voice	Nerve crossing superior pole of thyroid gland Cranially extending superior pole of thyroid gland	Individual ligation of each branch of superior laryngeal artery Routine identification of EBSLN Careful dissection over cricothyroid muscle to avoid muscle injury and subsequent scarring	Nerve grafting Voice therapy

Strategies to Prevent Nerve Injury

- Routine identification of the RLN along its entire course, especially near the Berry ligament, is essential. Watch out and preserve all the branches above the level of the inferior thyroid artery. They are all motor nerves.
- Extracapsular dissection avoiding deep planes helps. No fat to be left on thyroid gland.
- Judicious and precise use of energy devices, keeping adequate distance from the nerve (ideally >2 mm).
- Terminal end artery ligation of superior thyroid vessels close to the thyroid capsule will avoid SLN injury.
- Using IONM and visual magnification (loupes or exoscopes) in complex or revision cases.
- Avoiding aggressive traction and ensuring a bloodless field for optimal visualization.

Preventing RLN and SLN injury is central to the success of thyroid surgery. The integration of surgical adjuncts like loupes, IONM, and advanced imaging systems, combined with a deep understanding of neural anatomy and careful surgical technique, greatly minimizes complication rates and ensures optimal patient outcomes.

Wound Infection

Wound infection following thyroidectomy is relatively uncommon, with reported incidence rates ranging between 0.3% and 2.9% [43]. Despite thyroidectomy being a clean surgery, several intraoperative and patient-related factors can predispose to infection. Key intraoperative predictors include prolonged operative time, excessive handling or devascularization of tissues, haematoma formation, breach of aseptic technique, and inadvertent contamination from the adjacent upper aerodigestive tract [44]. The use of surgical drains, particularly if left in situ beyond 48 h, has also been implicated as a potential risk factor, although this remains controversial.

Prevention of wound infection relies heavily on meticulous surgical technique and stringent adherence to sterile protocols. Preoperative measures include optimization of comorbid conditions such as diabetes mellitus and careful skin preparation using antiseptic solutions. Prophylactic antibiotics are generally not recommended

Table 11.9 Wound infection

Presentation	Risk factors	Prevention	Management
Redness Oedema Pain Fever Neck swelling Purulent discharge from wound or in drain	Undiagnosed laryngotracheal or oesophageal injury Undiagnosed chyle leak	Maintaining sterile technique throughout the surgery Drain care under aseptic precautions	Antibiotics Drainage of abscess and wound care

for low-risk, clean thyroid surgeries, but may be considered in selected high-risk cases such as immunocompromised patients, extensive lymph node dissection, or when upper aerodigestive tracts are injured. Intraoperatively, minimal tissue trauma, proper haemostasis, and avoidance of unnecessary dead space are essential.

When wound infection does occur, it usually presents within 5–7 days postoperatively as localized erythema, warmth, tenderness, and sometimes purulent discharge from the incision site. Management depends on severity (Table 11.9). Mild cases can often be managed conservatively, with empirical oral antibiotics targeting skin flora, primarily *Staphylococcus aureus* and *Streptococcus* species [45]. In more advanced or purulent infections, incision and drainage may be required, and culture-guided antibiotic therapy is warranted. Ultrasound may help assess underlying collections in ambiguous cases. Rarely, wound infections can progress to deep neck space infections, especially in immunocompromised individuals, warranting aggressive intervention. Importantly, postoperative wound infections can also increase the risk of hypertrophic scarring or poor cosmetic outcomes, which should be addressed during patient counselling.

With the advent of enhanced surgical visualization and meticulous surgical planning, along with evolving perioperative protocols, wound infection after thyroidectomy can largely be avoided. Nonetheless, prompt recognition and management remain key to preventing complications and ensuring optimal healing.

Chyle Leak

Chyle leak is a rare but potentially significant complication following thyroidectomy, particularly when the procedure involves central or lateral neck dissection. The reported incidence of chyle leak after thyroid surgery ranges from 0.5% to 2%, with a higher frequency observed in left-sided and extensive central neck dissections due to the anatomical course of the thoracic duct, which ascends on the right and crosses to the left behind the oesophagus and behind the carotid sheath through the left supraclavicular region before emptying into the venous system [46, 47].

Intraoperative predictors include extensive dissection above the prevertebral fascia in the left trachea-oesophageal groove, the left level IV, and the thoracic duct region, especially near the internal jugular-subclavian venous junction. High-risk scenarios also include redo, surgeries for large or invasive tumours, and presence of inflammatory or fibrotic tissues obscuring normal planes.

To prevent chyle leak, meticulous surgical technique is essential—particularly during dissection in the lower left neck. Blunt dissection should be avoided in high-risk zones, and any visible lymphatic channels should be ligated or clipped with titanium clips. The Valsalva manoeuvre helps identify chyle leak before closure. Prompt ligation of the duct with non-absorbable sutures or fibrin glue is essential to prevent postoperative morbidity.

Management of postoperative chyle leak depends on the output volume. Low-output leaks (<300 mL/day) can usually be managed conservatively with pressure dressings, a fat-free diet supplemented with medium-chain triglycerides, or even temporary nil per oral status in more persistent cases [48]. Use of octreotide, a somatostatin analogue, has been found to reduce chyle flow by reducing splanchnic blood flow and decreasing intestinal fat absorption. High-output leaks (>500 mL/day) persisting beyond 5–7 days despite conservative measures may require re-exploration and surgical repair, particularly if nutritional, immunological, or electrolyte imbalances become significant [49].

Early recognition and tailored management are crucial to minimizing morbidity, length of hospitalization, and long-term sequelae (Table 11.10).

Aerodigestive Tract (Laryngotracheal and Oesophageal) Injuries

Aerodigestive tract injuries are usually anticipated in surgeries for advanced invasive thyroid cancers with a proper reconstruction plan [8]. These injuries to the oesophagus, larynx, and trachea—during thyroidectomy, although rare—represent one of the most severe complications, with potential for significant morbidity and mortality. The reported incidence of tracheal injury ranges from 0.06% to 0.6%, followed by oesophageal injury with a prevalence of 0.02–0.15% [50]. Laryngeal cartilage injury, though seldom discussed, may occur in extensive dissections or reoperative settings, particularly in patients with distorted anatomy.

Table 11.10 Chyle leak

Presentation	Risk factors	Prevention	Management
Neck swelling Milky fluid in neck drain Neck infection	Central compartment nodes requiring extensive dissection Level IV nodes/ nodal masses Short fat neck	Intraoperative identification of chyle leak and effective control prior to closure	Fat-free diet Drain quantification Nil per oral Fluid and electrolyte replacement Antibiotics Surgical exploration

Several risk factors predispose patients to these injuries. These include large or retrosternal goitres, thyroid malignancies with extra thyroidal extension, prior radiation therapy, redo thyroid surgery, and extensive central compartment or tracheoesophageal groove dissection [51]. Intraoperative factors such as dense fibrosis from chronic thyroiditis, inadvertent excessive use of energy devices near the tracheal wall, or failure to delineate tissue planes between the thyroid capsule and tracheoesophageal fascia can increase the risk. Tumour invasion into the tracheal or oesophageal wall also poses a significant challenge, often necessitating partial resection or reconstruction.

Intraoperative predictors of impending aerodigestive injury include difficult dissection with loss of avascular planes, firm adherence of the gland to the trachea or oesophagus, and signs of mucosal breach such as air bubbling or serosanguinous fluid leakage. In suspected cases, a Valsalva manoeuvre may help detect a tracheal rent, while methylene blue dye injection via a nasogastric tube can highlight occult oesophageal injuries.

Avoidance strategies are rooted in sound surgical principles, that is, maintaining a meticulous capsular dissection technique, staying within correct anatomical planes, avoiding undue traction on the gland, and minimizing thermal spread by judicious use of energy devices. For cases with suspected invasion, a preoperative CT scan and endoscopy help in surgical planning, and en bloc resection with appropriate tracheal or oesophageal repair may be warranted.

Management depends on the extent and timing of recognition. Minor tracheal rents recognized intraoperatively can often be closed primarily with absorbable sutures, reinforced with a strap muscle or sternomastoid muscle flap. Larger defects may require patch repair or segmental tracheal resection with end-to-end anastomosis. Oesophageal injuries, especially when full-thickness, necessitate layered closure and NGT in select cases to allow healing (Table 11.11). Any mucosal exposure requires to be buttressed with a muscle patch to prevent postoperative rupture. Unrecognized intraoperative injuries may present postoperatively with subcutaneous emphysema, neck swelling, air leak from drains, dysphagia, or respiratory distress. In such cases, prompt imaging with contrast-enhanced CT or gastrografin swallow and early surgical exploration are essential to prevent mediastinitis or sepsis [8].

Table 11.11 Aerodigestive tract (laryngotracheal and oesophageal) injuries

Presentation	Risk factor	Prevention	Management
Neck (surgical) emphysema Neck pain Neck cellulitis Neck infection	Aerodigestive tract involvement by thyroid cancers Sharp dissection over trachea Displaced oesophagus due to large goitre	Nasogastric tube insertion for intraoperative identification of oesophagus Intraoperative air leak test Buttress all exposed mucosa—Larynx, tracheal, or oesophageal	Remove suction drain Pressure dressing Re-exploration in case of persistent leak, neck infection

Horner's Syndrome

Horner's syndrome is symptom complex of ptosis, miosis, enophthalmos, facial anhidrosis, and flushing. It is a rare complication of thyroid surgery with an incidence of 0.2% [52].

It occurs due to injury to cervical sympathetic chain. Individual cases have been reported in literature. Thyroid malignancies have propensity to involve retrocarotid lymph nodes, thus nodal dissection in thyroid malignancies is the most important cause of Horner's syndrome. Large goitre-displacing carotids, presence of thyroiditis, Graves' disease, postoperative haematoma formation, intraoperative injury from division, or retraction put cervical sympathetic chain at risk [53]. Topical application of alpha agonist apraclonidine confirms diagnosis of Horner's syndrome. With intact integrity of cervical sympathetic plexus, Horner's syndrome usually resolves completely at 3 months follow-up. Remote access thyroid surgery, which is done with the intent of cosmesis, is associated with a higher incidence of Horner's syndrome [54].

Hypothyroidism

Post-thyroidectomy hypothyroidism is an anticipated outcome following total or near-total thyroidectomy, given the removal of functional thyroid tissue. Transient hypothyroidism may occur in 30–60% of patients undergoing subtotal or hemithyroidectomy, depending on the residual gland function and preoperative thyroid status [15].

Several risk factors predispose to hypothyroidism post hemi or subtotal thyroidectomy, including pre-existing Hashimoto's thyroiditis or subclinical hypothyroidism, Graves' disease, radiation-induced thyroid disease, and extensive surgical resection.

Intraoperative predictors of postoperative hypothyroidism primarily depend on the volume of remnant thyroid tissue and the viability of the preserved lobe in hemithyroidectomy cases [55]. Inadvertent devascularization of the remnant lobe or unnoticed residual thyroiditis can impair the functional reserve of the thyroid remnant. Disruption of the superior and inferior thyroid arteries bilaterally, without sufficient preservation of blood supply to one lobe in hemithyroidectomy, may result in remnant gland dysfunction and subsequent hypothyroidism.

In patients with borderline thyroid function or pre-existing thyroiditis, the threshold for performing total thyroidectomy should be lower, given the high likelihood of eventual hypothyroidism. When hemithyroidectomy is performed, preserving the vascularity of the contralateral lobe, particularly through capsular dissection and avoidance of extensive manipulation, is crucial.

Management of post-thyroidectomy hypothyroidism is straightforward and revolves around levothyroxine supplementation. For patients undergoing total thyroidectomy not requiring radioiodine therapy, thyroid hormone replacement is initiated immediately postoperatively, with titration guided by TSH levels measured after 6–8 weeks. In hemithyroidectomy cases, thyroid function is monitored periodically for the first 6 months, as up to one-third may develop delayed hypothyroidism requiring replacement therapy.

Importantly, close follow-up and early recognition of hypothyroidism allow for timely intervention, preventing associated morbidities such as fatigue, weight gain, depression, and metabolic disturbances.

Poor Scar

While thyroidectomy is generally associated with excellent cosmetic outcomes, poor scar formation remains a concern, particularly among young, female, and cosmetically conscious patients. The incidence of hypertrophic or keloid scars post-thyroidectomy ranges between 2% and 8%, with additional complaints of scar hyperpigmentation, widening, and textural irregularities [56]. Several risk factors have been implicated, including younger age, female gender, darker skin types, a personal or family history of keloids, and underlying dermatoses. Intraoperative factors such as excessive tissue handling, thermal injury, haematoma formation, and infection can further compromise scar quality.

One of the most critical predictors of cosmetic outcome is incision planning and execution. A poorly planned incision can lead to an unappealing neck scar. The incision should be marked with the patient in the sitting position, ideally along a prominent transverse neck crease, which aligns with Langer's lines and ensures minimal distortion upon healing. In contrast, incisions marked in the supine position—especially in patients with a pendulous breast or large goitres—may result in poorly oriented scars that stretch or distort postoperatively. A very low-lying incision extending over the sternum carries a higher risk for hypertrophic or keloidal scars, particularly in predisposed individuals. The length of the incision must allow for adequate exposure; excessive retraction through a small incision not only hinders surgical efficiency but also damages incision edges, increasing the risk of scar complications.

During surgery, care must be taken to protect incision edges from electrocautery burns and mechanical trauma from retractors. Furthermore, precise realignment of dermal edges during closure is essential to ensure optimal healing and minimize scar tension. Subcuticular suturing using absorbable monofilament enhances edge approximation and preserves vascularity, further improving outcomes [57, 58].

Avoidance strategies include meticulous technique, appropriate incision placement, minimal thermal spread, and tension-free closure. Postoperatively, silicone gel sheeting, topical scar therapy, and pressure dressings may prevent hypertrophic scar formation. If poor scars develop despite preventive measures, treatment options include intralesional corticosteroids, fractional laser therapy, botulinum toxin, or surgical scar revision in chronic cases. Importantly, patient counselling should emphasize that scars mature over 12–18 months, and early concerns often improve with time.

A thoughtful, patient-specific approach to incision planning, handling of soft tissue, and closure is vital to achieving a satisfactory and lasting result.

References

1. Lukinović J, Bilić M. Overview of thyroid surgery complications. Acta Clin Croat. 2020;59(Supplement 1):81–6.
2. Giddings AE. The history of thyroidectomy. J R Soc Med. 1998;91(Suppl 33):3–6.
3. Minuto MN, Bertoglio S, Varaldo E. Thyroid surgery before the technologic revolution: from Samuel Gross' "torrents of blood" to Paolo Miccoli's video-assisted thyroidectomy: A history of Thyroid surgery before the 2.0-Era. Med Hist. 2019;3(3):188–95.
4. Kalra S, Baruah MP, Sahay R, Sawhney K. The history of parathyroid endocrinology. Indian J Endocrinol Metab. 2013;17(2):320–2.
5. De Cassai A, Boscolo A, Rose K, Carron M, Navalesi P. Predictive parameters of difficult intubation in thyroid surgery: a meta-analysis. Minerva Anestesiol. 2020;86(3):317–26.
6. Zhou CM, Wang Y, Xue Q, Yang JJ, Zhu Y. Predicting difficult airway intubation in thyroid surgery using multiple machine learning and deep learning algorithms. Front Public Health. 2022;10:937471.
7. Higgs A, McGrath BA, Goddard C, Rangasami J, Suntharalingam G, Gale R, et al. Guidelines for the management of tracheal intubation in critically ill adults. Br J Anaesth. 2018;120(2):323–52.
8. Rao K, Deshmukh A, Pai P, Pantvaidya G. Advanced thyroid cancer controversy and consensus. Indian J Med Paediatr Oncol. 2021;41:476–80.
9. Arora P, Arora R, Karim HMR, Neema PK, Panda CK. Transillumination and point-of-care ultrasonography to delineate tracheal deviation for challenging tracheostomy: A case report. Cureus. 2023;15(4):e37164.
10. Crewdson K, Lockey DJ. Needle, knife, or device – which choice in an airway crisis? Scand J Trauma Resusc Emerg Med. 2013;21:49.
11. Arora RD, Rao KN, Satpute S, Mehta R, Dange P, Nagarkar NM, et al. Emergency tracheostomy in locally advanced anaplastic thyroid cancer. Indian J Surg Oncol. 2023;14(3):714–22.
12. Marchis IF, Negrut MF, Blebea CM, Crihan M, Alexa AL, Breazu CM. Trends in preoperative airway assessment. Diagnostics. 2024;14(6):610.
13. Ross DS, Burch HB, Cooper DS, Greenlee MC, Laurberg P, Maia AL, et al. 2016 American Thyroid Association Guidelines for diagnosis and Management of Hyperthyroidism and Other Causes of thyrotoxicosis. Thyroid. 2016;26(10):1343–421.
14. Meltzer C, Hull M, Sundang A, Adams JL. Association between annual surgeon total thyroidectomy volume and transient and permanent complications. JAMA Otolaryngol Neck Surg. 2019;145(9):830–7.
15. Nagarkar NM, Mehta R, Rao KN. Thyroid gland. In: Nagarkar NM, Mehta R, Singh A, Rao KN, Dange PS, editors. Atlas of head neck and skull-base surgery. Singapore: Springer Nature; 2023. p. 65–91. https://doi.org/10.1007/978-981-99-6132-0_5.
16. Uludag M, Cetinoglu I, Taner Unlu M, Caliskan O, Aygun N. Preoperative preparation in hyperthyroidism and surgery in the hyperthyroid state. Med Bull Sisli Etfal Hosp. 2024;58(3):263–75.
17. Ghaloo SK, Afzal SS, Abbas SA, Ansari S, De M, Iftikhar H. Tracheomalacia in patients undergoing thyroid surgery—what is the true estimate: a systematic review and meta-analysis. World J Otorhinolaryngol-Head Neck Surg. 2024;11(1):125–37.
18. Shepard JAO, Flores EJ, Abbott GF. Imaging of the trachea. Ann Cardiothorac Surg. 2018;7(2):197–209.
19. Sulaiman A, Lutfi A, Ikram M, Fatimi S, Bin Pervez M, Shamim F, et al. Tracheomalacia after thyroidectomy for retrosternal goitres requiring sternotomy– a myth or reality? Ann R Coll Surg Engl. 2021;103(7):504–7.

20. Cooper RM, Khan S. Extubation and reintubation of the difficult airway. In: Benumof Hagbergs Airw Manag; 2013. p. 1018–1046.e7.
21. Iliff HA, El-Boghdadly K, Ahmad I, Davis J, Harris A, Khan S, et al. Management of haematoma after thyroid surgery: systematic review and multidisciplinary consensus guidelines from the Difficult Airway Society, the British Association of Endocrine and Thyroid Surgeons and the British Association of Otorhinolaryngology, Head and Neck Surgery. Anaesthesia. 2022;77(1):82–95.
22. Pontin A, Pino A, Caruso E, Pinto G, Melita G, Maria DP, et al. Postoperative bleeding after thyroid surgery: care instructions. Şişli Etfal Hastan Tıp Bül. 2019;53(4):329–36.
23. Fan C, Zhou X, Su G, Zhou Y, Su J, Luo M, et al. Risk factors for neck hematoma requiring surgical re-intervention after thyroidectomy: a systematic review and meta-analysis. BMC Surg. 2019;19:98.
24. Rao KN, Satpute S, Nagarkar NM, Singh A. Revision thyroid surgery. Indian J Surg Oncol. 2022;13(1):199–207.
25. Arora RD, Prajwal SD, Rao KN, Singh A, Nagarkar NM, Abishek AP. A comparison of harmonic scalpel and conventional techniques for thyroidectomy. Indian J Otolaryngol Head Neck Surg. 2023;75(4):3410–4.
26. Rao KN, Gangiti KK. Transoral robotic surgery. Indian J Surg Oncol. 2021;12(4):847–53.
27. Ramouz A, Rasihashemi SZ, Daghigh F, Faraji E, Rouhani S. Predisposing factors for seroma formation in patients undergoing thyroidectomy: cross-sectional study. Ann Med Surg. 2017;23:8–12.
28. Rao KN, Arora R, Rajguru R, Nagarkar NM. Artificial neural network to predict post-operative hypocalcemia following total thyroidectomy. Indian J Otolaryngol Head Neck Surg. 2024;76(4):3094–102.
29. Rao KN, Zafereo M, Rao AN, Nixon I, Robbins KT, Sreeram MP, et al. Implication of surgical loupes on complications following thyroidectomy: a meta-analysis. Eur Arch Otorrinolaringol. 2025;282(3):1159–69.
30. Sephton BM. Extracervical approaches to thyroid surgery: evolution and review. Minim Invasive Surg. 2019;2019:5961690.
31. Bernes S, Lilja-Fischer J, Petersen NK, Udholm N, Reinholdt KB, Londero S, et al. Initial experience with ultra-high-definition 3d exoscope in thyroid and parathyroid surgery. Surg Innov. 2024;31(5):513–9.
32. Rao KN, Rajguru R, Dange P, Vetter D, Triponez F, Nixon IJ, et al. Lower rates of hypocalcemia following near-infrared autofluorescence use in thyroidectomy: a meta-analysis of RCTs. Diagnostics. 2024;14(5):505.
33. Rao KN, Randolph GW, Lopez F, Zafereo M, Coca-Pelaz A, Piazza C, et al. Assessment of the risk of malignancy in Bethesda III thyroid nodules: a comprehensive review. Endocrine. 2024;85(2):473–92.
34. Riordan F, Brophy C, Murphy MS, Sheahan P. Predictive value of postoperative day 1 parathyroid hormone levels for early and late hypocalcaemia after thyroidectomy. Langenbeck's Arch Surg. 2022;407(4):1653–8.
35. Chen Z, Zhao Q, Du J, Wang Y, Han R, Xu C, et al. Risk factors for postoperative hypocalcaemia after thyroidectomy: a systematic review and meta-analysis. J Int Med Res. 2021;49(3):0300060521996911.
36. Tolley NS, Chaidas K, Bergenfelz A. Rates of RLN and SLN injury: data from national quality registries and the literature. In: Randolph GW, editor. The recurrent and superior laryngeal nerves. Cham: Springer International Publishing; 2016. p. 3–16. https://doi.org/10.1007/978-3-319-27727-1_1.
37. Gurleyik E, Gurleyik G. Incidence and surgical importance of zuckerkandl's tubercle of the thyroid and its relations with recurrent laryngeal nerve. Int Sch Res Not. 2012;2012(1):450589.
38. Kang KH, Song RY, Suh YJ, Park SJ. Safety of medial dissection of the thyroid gland along the trachea based on anatomic constancy of the laryngeal entry point of the recurrent laryngeal nerve. Ann Surg Treat Res. 2018;95(1):16–21.

39. Marchese-Ragona R, Restivo DA, Mylonakis I, Ottaviano G, Martini A, Sataloff RT, et al. The superior laryngeal nerve injury of a famous soprano, Amelita Galli-Curci. Acta Otorhinolaryngol Ital. 2013;33(1):67–71.
40. EL-Gaabary IM, EL-Sherief MM, Hablus MA, Mohamed HA. Assessment of nerve stimulation during thyroidectomy for identification of the external branch of superior laryngeal nerve. Egypt J Surg. 2020;39(4) https://doi.org/10.4103/ejs.ejs_128_20.
41. Pace-Asciak P, Russell JO, Dhillon VK. Intraoperative neuromonitoring: evaluating the role of continuous ionm and ionm techniques for emerging surgical and percutaneous procedures. Front Endocrinol. 2022;13:823117.
42. Mercante G, Costantino A, De Virgilio A, Ferreli F, Spriano G. High-definition 3d exoscope in thyroid surgery. Surg Innov. 2023;30(2):205–9.
43. Elfenbein DM, Schneider DF, Chen H, Sippel RS. Surgical site infection after thyroidectomy: a rare but significant complication. J Surg Res. 2014;190(1):170–6.
44. Huang X, Huang K, Zhang Y, Zhou L, Wu F, Qian S, et al. Risk factors for surgical site infection following thyroid surgery: a systematic review and meta-analysis. Gland Surg. 2024;13(11):2010–22.
45. Tong SYC, Davis JS, Eichenberger E, Holland TL, Fowler VG. Staphylococcus aureus infections: epidemiology, pathophysiology, clinical manifestations, and management. Clin Microbiol Rev. 2015;28(3):603–61.
46. Nagarkar NM, Rao KN, Singh A. Oral cavity and neck dissection. In: Nagarkar NM, Mehta R, Singh A, Rao KN, Dange PS, editors. Atlas of head neck and skull-base surgery. Singapore: Springer Nature; 2023. p. 105–58. https://doi.org/10.1007/978-981-99-6132-0_7.
47. Delaney SW, Shi H, Shokrani A, Sinha UK. Management of chyle leak after head and neck surgery: review of current treatment strategies. Int J Otolaryngol. 2017;2017:8362874.
48. Leović D, Pastorčić Grgić M, Gugić Radojković I, Blivajs I, Matoc L, Gršić K. Management of chyle leak following head and neck surgery: review of current treatment strategies and algorithmic approach to the treatment. Acta Clin Croat. 2022;61(Suppl 4):88–95.
49. Gupta V, Dwivedi G, Chugh R, Sahu PK, Gupta DK, Basu A, et al. Role of octreotide in conservative management of chyle leak post neck dissection in cases of head neck cancer: a retrospective analysis. Indian J Otolaryngol Head Neck Surg. 2022;74(Suppl 3):6078–86.
50. Pantvaidya G, D'Cruz A, Rao KN. Surgery in locally advanced thyroid cancer. In: IAES textbook of endocrine surgery. 1st ed. Jaypee; 2023; Available from: https://www.jaypeedigital.com/book/9789390595051/chapter/ch19.
51. Prete FP, De Luca GM, Sgaramella LI, Pasculli A, Di Meo G, Testini C, et al. Prevalence and clinical risk factors of thyroid cancer in retrosternal goiter: a retrospective comparative study with cervical multinodular goiter. J Clin Med. 2025;14(2):489.
52. Arishi AA, Abualhana F, Sferra J. Horner's syndrome following thyroid surgery. Cureus. 2023;15(9):e45825.
53. Carsote M, Nistor CE, Popa FL, Stanciu M. Horner's syndrome and lymphocele following thyroid surgery. J Clin Med. 2023;12(2):474.
54. Deng Y, Ding G. Diagnosis and treatment of HS after endoscopic thyroid surgery: case report and brief literature review. Front Surg. 2023;10:1267701. https://doi.org/10.3389/fsurg.2023.1267701. PMID: 37841812; PMCID: PMC10568127.
55. Tsai SH, Chien SC, Nguyen PA, Chien PH, Ma HP, Asdary RN, et al. Incidences of hypothyroidism associated with surgical procedures for thyroid disorders: a Nationwide population-based study. Front Pharmacol. 2019;10:1378.
56. Choi Y, Lee JH, Kim YH, Lee YS, Chang HS, Park CS, et al. Impact of postthyroidectomy scar on the quality of life of thyroid cancer patients. Ann Dermatol. 2014;26(6):693–9.
57. Ogawa R. Ideal wound closure methods for minimizing scarring after surgery. In: Téot L, Mustoe TA, Middelkoop E, Gauglitz GG, editors. Textbook on scar management: state of the art Management and emerging technologies. Cham: Springer; 2020. Available from: http://www.ncbi.nlm.nih.gov/books/NBK586099/.
58. Lee K, Ward N, Oremule B, Mani N. Optimal wound closure techniques for thyroid and parathyroid surgery: a systematic review of cosmetic outcomes. Clin Otolaryngol. 2019;44(6):905–13.

Nerve Monitoring in Thyroid Surgery

12

Amr H. Abdelhamid Ahmed and Gregory W. Randolph

Editorial

Intraoperative neural monitoring (IONM) is a tool to enhance the identification and preservation of the recurrent laryngeal nerve (RLN) and superior laryngeal nerve (SLN). It is now a mainstream tool used by a majority of surgeons when performing thyroid surgery. Thyroid surgery carries a well-recognized risk of injury to the recurrent laryngeal nerve (RLN) and also the external branch of the superior laryngeal nerves. Over the past decade, IONM has transitioned from an optional innovation to a frequently employed safety measure in thyroid surgery. Its use has increased steadily worldwide. The International Neural Monitoring Study Group (INMSG), formed in 2006, published guideline statements in 2011–2013 defining standard IONM procedures and troubleshooting, and updated consensus guidelines in 2018. IONM is increasingly recommended in high-risk cases and is considered a complementary technique to the standard visual identification of the RLN. IONM has not been shown to increase operative time significantly, and the setup is relatively straightforward, involving placement of nerve monitor electrodes and a stimulator probe. The safety profile is excellent, with essentially no risk to the patient from the monitoring itself. Thus, many endocrine surgeons now routinely employ IONM with the aim of enhancing nerve safety and improving patient outcomes.

If during a total thyroidectomy the first side's RLN loses signal and cannot be confirmed to be intact, the surgeon can halt and defer the second side (staged thyroidectomy) to avoid risking both nerves in one session. This strategy, recommended by the INMSG, can virtually eliminate the occurrence of immediate bilateral vocal

A. H. Abdelhamid Ahmed · G. W. Randolph (✉)
Division of Thyroid and Parathyroid Endocrine Surgery, Department of Otolaryngology-Head and Neck Surgery, Massachusetts Eye and Ear, Harvard Medical School, Boston, MA, USA
e-mail: amr_ahmed@meei.harvard.edu; Gregory_Randolph@meei.harvard.edu

P. S. Pai et al. (eds.), *Controversies in Cancer of the Thyroid and Parathyroid Glands*, https://doi.org/10.1007/978-3-032-13130-0_12

cord paralysis, a "zero incidence" outcome that no series without monitoring can claim.

False-positive and false-negative responses are a matter that can cause confusion intraoperatively. The authors expertly demonstrate how to discern false from true.

Overall, the cost–benefit debate continues without a one-size-fits-all answer. In a high-volume center performing complex thyroid surgeries (e.g., large goiters, recurrent disease, cancer with node dissection), the consensus leans toward IONM being justified as an investment in safety. In contrast, for a low-volume surgeon doing primarily small benign thyroidectomies, the added expense may not clearly translate into better outcomes.

The INMSG 2013 guideline recommends attempting EBSLN identification and stimulation in all cases and classifying the outcome. Monitoring the superior laryngeal nerve is feasible and has proven benefits in identifying and preserving this nerve.

Medicolegal implications form a subtle but important controversy in the use of IONM. Surgical complications like RLN injury frequently led to malpractice litigation in endocrine surgery.

The medicolegal perspective largely aligns with the clinical one: use the tool judiciously to maximize patient safety and document nerve integrity, which in turn minimizes liability.

With prudent use of technology grounded in anatomical mastery, the ultimate goal remains the same as in Kocher's era: to cure thyroid disease while preserving the patient's voice and airway—a goal now more achievable than ever.

Christopher de Souza

Introduction to Thyroid Surgery and Nerve Monitoring

Thyroid surgery carries a well-recognized risk of injury to the recurrent laryngeal nerve (RLN), which innervates the vocal folds. Unilateral RLN injury causes vocal cord paresis/paralysis with hoarseness and aspiration risk, while bilateral RLN injury can lead to acute airway obstruction that may need tracheostomy. The external branch of the superior laryngeal nerve (EBSLN), supplying the cricothyroid muscle, is also at risk during superior pole dissection—injury to this nerve can impair high-frequency voice production, a subtle but significant deficit for professional voice users. Surgeons have long sought to minimize these complications. In the late nineteenth and early twentieth centuries, pioneers like Theodor Kocher emphasized meticulous dissection to avoid nerve damage, and routine visual identification of the RLN was popularized by Frank Lahey in 1938. Historically, however, identification of the EBSLN lagged behind—indeed, Kocher's texts did not explicitly mention the SLN [1]. A famous 1935 case involved soprano Amelita Galli-Curci, who allegedly lost her upper vocal range after thyroid surgery, drawing attention to EBSLN injury (often dubbed "the nerve of Galli-Curci"). Historically, the gold standard for nerve preservation has been careful visual identification of the RLN during thyroidectomy. However, visual confirmation alone does not provide real-time information about nerve function and cannot predict or prevent functional injury if the nerve is stretched, heated, or partially damaged despite remaining anatomically intact. Indeed, studies have shown that many RLN injuries occur even when the nerve's anatomy appears intact under direct vision [2].

Modern intraoperative nerve monitoring (IONM) was first introduced in the 1960s. In 1966, Shedd and Durham described a technique using electrical stimulation of the RLN with detection of laryngeal movement via an endotracheal balloon, demonstrating the feasibility of electrophysiological RLN identification [1]. Early methods were cumbersome and not widely adopted. Over the last three decades, however, technological advances—including endotracheal tubes with embedded electrodes to record vocalis muscle electromyography—have made IONM more practical. By the 2000s, IONM became a common adjunct in thyroid surgery, with international guidelines established to standardize its use. The International Neural Monitoring Study Group (INMSG), formed in 2006, published guideline statements in 2011–2013 defining standard IONM procedures and troubleshooting, and updated consensus guidelines in 2018 [3]. Today, IONM is used in a significant proportion of thyroid surgeries worldwide, though practice patterns vary by region and surgeon training.

Controversies Surrounding IONM

Over the past decade, IONM has transitioned from an optional innovation to a frequently employed safety measure in thyroid surgery. Its use has increased steadily worldwide. For instance, an analysis of over 44,000 thyroidectomy cases in the United States found that the prevalence of IONM utilization rose from about 62% in 2016 to nearly 76% by 2022 [4]. This trend reflects a growing confidence among surgeons that nerve monitoring offers tangible benefits. Professional guidelines and expert consensus statements now acknowledge the value of IONM, especially in specific scenarios such as reoperative thyroid surgeries, surgeries for invasive thyroid cancer, and when performing a total thyroidectomy in a patient with preexisting contralateral vocal cord paralysis. While not universally mandated as the standard of care, IONM is increasingly recommended in high-risk cases and is considered a complementary technique to the standard visual identification of the RLN. Importantly, the introduction of IONM has not been shown to increase operative time significantly, and the setup is relatively straightforward, involving placement of nerve monitor electrodes and a stimulator probe. The safety profile is excellent, with essentially no risk to the patient from the monitoring itself. Given the severe consequences of nerve injury, even a modest reduction in RLN palsy incidence can have a meaningful impact. Thus, many endocrine surgeons now routinely employ IONM with the aim of enhancing nerve safety and improving patient outcomes [3].

In the following sections, we explore the major areas of debate regarding IONM in thyroid surgery. We begin with an examination of clinical efficacy data, then discuss the nuances of signal interpretation (false-positives/-negatives), economic and training considerations, impact on surgical decision-making, technological limitations and advances (including continuous monitoring), the special case of SLN monitoring, and finally medicolegal implications. Through this comprehensive review, the reader will gain an in-depth understanding of the controversies and current consensus on the role of RLN and SLN monitoring during thyroidectomy.

Clinical Efficacy of Nerve Monitoring: Does IONM Improve Outcomes?

Growing evidence from clinical studies indicates that intraoperative nerve monitoring improves key outcomes in thyroid surgery, particularly with respect to RLN injury prevention. Early studies and meta-analyses in the 2000s had mixed results, in part due to the low overall incidence of RLN palsy and heterogeneity among studies [5–9]. However, more recent high-quality studies—including large randomized controlled trials, extensive observational series, and focused meta-analyses—have provided data demonstrating that IONM has measurable benefits.

The most important outcome is the reduction of RLN palsy, and recent evidence supports that IONM use is associated with lower nerve injury rates. A landmark randomized trial by Barczyński et al. compared thyroidectomies performed with vs. without nerve monitoring (2000 nerves at risk in each arm) and found that IONM significantly decreased the incidence of transient RLN paresis. The reduction was most pronounced in high-risk patients (those with large goiters, malignancies requiring lymph node dissection, or reoperations), where the transient RLN palsy rate was about 3% lower with IONM than without [6]. Large-scale real-world data echo these findings: an analysis of 17,610 thyroidectomy cases from a national database found RLN injury rates of 5.7% with IONM vs. 6.8% without IONM, and after adjusting for other factors, IONM use was associated with a 31% lower odds of RLN injury (OR 0.69, 95% CI 0.59–0.82, $p < 0.001$) [10].

One important consideration is case complexity. In straightforward, low-risk thyroidectomies, the absolute difference made by IONM may be very small given an already low baseline injury rate. However, in high-risk situations—for example, reoperative thyroid surgery, large retrosternal goiters, or invasive thyroid cancer—monitoring might have a greater impact. A meta-analysis by Wong et al. focusing on high-risk thyroidectomies (e.g., malignancies, substernal goiters, Graves' disease, and reoperations) demonstrated that IONM had a significantly lower overall and transient RLN palsy rates [11]. These findings suggest that while IONM may not drastically alter outcomes in every routine case, it provides a safety net that is particularly valuable in challenging surgeries.

Another way IONM improves outcomes is indirect—by enabling staged procedures to avoid bilateral RLN paralysis. This benefit is difficult to capture in randomized trials (since deliberately continuing a thyroidectomy to cause bilateral injury would be unethical) but has been highlighted in guidelines [3]. If during a total thyroidectomy the first side's RLN loses signal and cannot be confirmed intact, the surgeon can halt and defer the second side (staged thyroidectomy) to avoid risking both nerves in one session [3]. This strategy, recommended by the INMSG, can virtually eliminate the occurrence of immediate bilateral vocal cord paralysis, a "zero incidence" outcome that no series without monitoring can claim. While such an event is rare, its prevention is a major patient safety victory attributable to IONM.

In light of these advantages, the consensus in the endocrine surgical community is increasingly leaning toward routine or at least selective use of IONM. Multiple meta-analyses have concluded that IONM significantly improves RLN preservation outcomes, and they specifically recommend routine nerve monitoring in bilateral thyroidectomies and thyroid cancer surgeries where the risk of nerve injury is highest.

False-Positives and False-Negatives: Interpreting EMG Signals

Interpreting the electromyographic (EMG) signals may present with false-positive loss of signal and false-negative readings. A false-positive in this context means the monitor indicates a loss of nerve function (loss of EMG signal) even though the nerve is anatomically intact and the patient has normal vocal cord movement postoperatively. This can lead the surgical team to incorrectly assume a nerve injury has occurred. A false-negative is when the monitoring shows intact responses throughout surgery, but the patient is found to have an RLN paralysis afterward—meaning the monitor failed to warn of an injury that did occur. Both situations can erode confidence in IONM and potentially compromise decision-making if not understood.

False-positive loss of signal (LOS) is not uncommon and can arise from technical issues. The most frequent cause is endotracheal tube malposition or displacement [12]. If the electrode-bearing tube shifts so that the recording surface is no longer in optimal contact with the vocal cord, the EMG amplitude may drop even though the nerve is uninjured. Blood or thick tissue between the stimulator probe and the nerve can also prevent a response, mimicking loss of signal [12]. Other causes include inadvertent use of muscle relaxants that dampen EMG responses [12]. Vagus stimulation yielding an EMG signal (typically proximal to the surgical field) indicates the monitor and neuromuscular pathway are intact, implying a true RLN issue if direct RLN stimulation still fails. If both vagal and RLN stimulation are silent, the problem is likely global or technical rather than nerve injury [12]. This diagnostic process helps distinguish a genuine nerve injury (true loss of function) from a false alarm. Nevertheless, a false-positive LOS can lead to an unnecessary staged procedure or additional dissection searching for a supposed injury, so minimizing these errors is important. Studies have shown that continuous monitoring may modestly reduce false-positive rates compared to intermittent stimulation by providing more consistent feedback on tube position and nerve status [12].

False-negative monitoring results are perhaps even more concerning, as they represent a missed injury. Several mechanisms can explain how a nerve injury might escape detection by IONM. One common scenario is segmental injury: if the RLN is stimulated distal (downstream) to an injury site, one may still obtain an EMG response from the intact distal segment even though the proximal portion was compromised. For example, if the RLN is stretched or partially injured near the ligament of Berry, a stimulation of the nerve just above the cricothyroid joint (distal to the injury) could evoke a response in the laryngeal muscles, misleading the surgeon [12]. For this reason, protocols advise a final vagus nerve stimulation at the end of thyroidectomy—a negative response on proximal (vagal) stimulation is a more reliable indicator of true RLN dysfunction than distal stimulation alone [12]. Another cause of false-negatives is a delayed neuropraxia. The nerve may conduct normally during the operation but subsequently develop edema or ischemia that leads to palsy hours later [12]. Such delayed injuries, often related to traction, would not be evident on intraoperative testing. Additionally, RLN branching and anatomical variability can play a role. The RLN often divides into anterior and posterior branches; if the anterior branch (motor to vocalis) remains intact and is stimulated, the monitor will show a response, yet if the posterior branch (to the posterior cricoarytenoid, the abductor) was injured, the patient could have an abductor palsy with a seemingly "good" intraoperative signal [12]. This subtle form of RLN injury (selective branch injury) results in impaired vocal cord abduction (e.g., unilateral fixity in midline) that might not be immediately obvious to the surgeon but would present postoperatively as dyspnea or voice issues.

To mitigate false-negatives, surgeons are taught never to rely on IONM alone to declare a field safe for transection. A fundamental principle is that a negative stimulation (no response) should not be trusted until a positive stimulation of the actual nerve has been obtained [12]. Understanding the potential for false signals and adhering to standardized troubleshooting algorithms are essential for harnessing the benefits of IONM without being misled. This interplay between technology and judgment is a recurring theme in the controversies around nerve monitoring.

Cost–Benefit Analysis of Routine IONM

Another debated aspect is the cost-effectiveness of intraoperative nerve monitoring. Several economic analyses have tackled this question with conflicting conclusions. A 2016 cost-utility analysis by Rocke et al. modeled three strategies—no monitoring, selective monitoring in high-risk cases, and universal monitoring—for total thyroidectomy [13]. Their decision-tree analysis, incorporating typical injury rates and quality-of-life impact, found that visual identification without IONM was the most cost-effective approach in general. In Rocke's model, the no-IONM strategy saved an average of $179 per patient over selective IONM and $683 over universal IONM, with negligible differences in quality-adjusted life-years (QALYs) between strategies [13]. They calculated that only if IONM could reduce RLN injury rates by over 50% (an efficacy not supported by most data) then selective use in high-risk cases becomes cost-effective [13]. This analysis, therefore, argued that routine IONM is not economically justified given the low baseline rate of permanent injury (~1–2% in experienced hands) and the substantial cost of disposables.

On the other hand, cost–benefit arguments shift when considering the avoidance of bilateral RLN paralysis. Bilateral palsy leading to tracheostomy is a catastrophic outcome with profound cost—both monetary (additional surgeries, hospitalization, rehabilitative care) and in terms of patient quality of life. IONM's ability to prompt staged thyroidectomy and thereby prevent bilateral paralysis can avert these worst-case costs. A Markov model analysis by Al-Qurayshi et al. specifically looked at the value of IONM in planned bilateral thyroid surgeries [14]. They concluded that IONM is cost-effective in the setting of planned bilateral total thyroidectomy because the cost of the monitor is outweighed by even a small reduction in the incidence of bilateral RLN injury [14]. In essence, avoiding a single permanent bilateral palsy (with its lifelong implications or need for tracheostomy) could financially justify many instances of IONM use where no injury would have happened anyway. This argument aligns with the risk-aversion perspective in endocrine surgery: while the absolute risk of bilateral RLN injury is low, the consequences are so dire that most surgeons will employ any available safeguard, cost aside.

Another factor is medicolegal cost—the potential costs of malpractice litigation from nerve injuries. Though harder to quantify, some health economists note that employing IONM might reduce lawsuits or payouts (a point discussed in the medicolegal section). If true, that could tilt cost–benefit analyses more in favor of using the technology routinely.

It is also worth noting that the cost per case of IONM can decrease with higher surgical volumes. Institutions that use the monitor frequently will amortize the capital cost of the machine and may negotiate better pricing on disposables, making the incremental cost per surgery smaller [13].

Overall, the cost–benefit debate continues without a one-size-fits-all answer. In a high-volume center performing complex thyroid surgeries (e.g., large goiters, recurrent disease, cancer with node dissection), the consensus leans toward IONM being justified as an investment in safety. In contrast, for a low-volume surgeon doing primarily small benign thyroidectomies, the added expense may not clearly translate into better outcomes [13].

Impact on Surgical Strategy and Outcomes

Beyond binary outcomes of nerve injury or not, IONM can influence surgical strategy and process in subtler ways. Examining how nerve monitoring affects intraoperative decision-making and overall surgical outcomes is an important part of the controversy.

One clear impact of IONM is on the management of bilateral thyroidectomies, as mentioned earlier. The adoption of staged thyroidectomy in the event of loss of RLN signal on the first side is now a widely accepted strategy enabled by monitoring [3]. In practical terms, this means if a surgeon is performing a total thyroidectomy and the EMG signal from the first RLN disappears (and cannot be restored with troubleshooting), the surgeon will typically stop and defer removal of the second lobe to another day, after confirming the function (or recovery) of the affected nerve. This approach has dramatically reduced the incidence of bilateral vocal cord paralysis in monitored cases [3]. While bilateral RLN palsy was already rare in the era of visual identification, IONM provides an additional safety checkpoint. Some high-volume centers have essentially eliminated bilateral paralysis by adhering to this policy. The downside is the patient may need a second surgery to complete the thyroidectomy, but this is generally considered a minor inconvenience compared to a permanent tracheostomy risk. This shift in surgical strategy—willingly staging an operation based on neural feedback—represents a paradigm change brought about by IONM [3].

In terms of operative technique, continuous feedback from IONM can guide the surgeon's maneuvers during dissection. With intermittent monitoring, the surgeon typically stimulates the nerve at specific checkpoints (after initial identification, after lobectomy, etc.). However, if using continuous IONM (C-IONM) via a vagal nerve electrode, the surgeon receives real-time EMG signals during the entire course of dissection. This can alert the surgeon to impending nerve stretch or traction. For example, if during ligation of the inferior thyroid artery the EMG amplitude begins to drop or latency increases significantly, the surgeon knows to ease off traction or reposition the thyroid lobe to relieve tension on the RLN, potentially preventing a stretch-induced neuropraxia [16]. In this way, IONM can actively shape intraoperative technique—the surgeon dynamically adjusts based on the nerve's response.

Another impact of IONM is the documentation and prognostication of nerve function at case conclusion. When a surgery is completed with intact final EMG signals (i.e., the RLN stimulated and gives a robust response), the surgical team can be fairly confident that the patient will wake up without vocal cord paralysis. This immediate confirmation can influence postoperative management: surgeons may be less inclined to perform a routine laryngoscopy on every patient postoperatively if the signal was intact (some still do to be certain, while others rely on the high negative predictive value of IONM) [3]. Conversely, if there was a loss of signal that could not be recovered, the surgeon can preemptively counsel the patient (or ICU team) that a temporary vocal cord paralysis is likely, arrange early laryngoscopy, and take precautions such as leaving the patient intubated longer or monitoring breathing closely. From a patient-centered viewpoint, knowing the nerve status immediately can alleviate anxiety—for example, telling a professional voice user that the nerve signals were perfect can provide reassurance even before they test their voice.

It is worth noting that some surgeons feel IONM adds a degree of comfort, especially in difficult cases, which might indirectly affect outcomes. When dissecting a scarred field in a reoperative neck or around a large malignant node, having the monitor might encourage more thorough dissection knowing that the nerve's function can be tested intermittently. In contrast, without a monitor, a surgeon might choose to do a slightly less aggressive dissection or leave some tissue to avoid probing too far near the nerve. This can have oncologic implications in cancer surgery—though data are sparse, one could theorize that nerve monitoring might allow more complete tumor clearance with a lower threshold for nerve preservation maneuvers (like shaving tumor off the nerve) since the function can be checked. Indeed, the INMSG 2018 Part II guidelines address management of nerves invaded by cancer and advocate using IONM to guide the decision of whether a nerve can be preserved or should be sacrificed for cure [3]. If a nerve is invaded but still conducting signal, some surgeons will leave it in place (accepting some paralysis risk) to avoid certain bilateral palsy if that is the only functioning nerve; if it is not conducting, they might resect it and plan a prompt vocal cord medialization. These nuanced decisions are facilitated by having monitoring data [3].

In terms of operative time, properly implemented IONM has minimal impact on case length. Initial adoption might add a few minutes for setup and mapping, but experienced teams integrate it smoothly. Studies have shown either no significant difference or only a slight increase in operative duration with IONM use, which is usually deemed a worthwhile trade-off for the added information [8, 13].

In summary, IONM's impact on surgical strategy is mostly positive, enabling staged operations to prevent bilateral injuries and providing real-time feedback that can improve intraoperative decisions. It allows surgeons to be proactive if nerve stress is detected and to tailor postoperative plans based on nerve integrity at closure. These benefits, while harder to quantify than raw injury rates, contribute to the argument in favor of nerve monitoring as a tool that promotes safer and smarter surgery.

Technological Limitations and Advances in IONM

Traditional IONM in thyroid surgery is intermittent—the surgeon stimulates the nerve manually at intervals and observes the EMG response. This intermittent approach can miss dynamic changes that occur between stimulations. Additionally, the standard method relies on endotracheal tube (ETT) surface electrodes to pick up laryngeal muscle signals. If the tube is even slightly mispositioned, one vocal cord might have poor contact, leading to low amplitudes or no signal from that side. The anesthesiologist must position the tube precisely and secure it well, and even then, movement from neck repositioning or surgical manipulation can shift the tube. Efforts to mitigate this include taping the tube at the lips, using nerve monitors that display baseline impedance (to infer contact quality), and employing video-assisted intubation to visually place electrodes at the cords [12].

Electrical interference is another technological issue. The electrocautery device used in surgery generates electrical noise that can saturate the EMG amplifier. Most nerve monitors have a built-in cautery filter that essentially mutes the system when cautery is active—this prevents false readings but also means the nerve cannot be monitored during those moments. Surgeons must pause cautery to test the nerve. If continuous monitoring is used, the system has to rapidly sample and differentiate true neural signals from noise. Modern systems have improved filtering and artifact rejection, but no system is completely immune to interference.

The stimulation probe itself has limitations. Most surgeons use a handheld monopolar stimulating probe; if it contacts tissue with too much pressure or surface area, current can shunt through surrounding tissue (especially if wet with saline or blood) and stimulate the nerve indirectly (or even the vagus), causing a response even when not exactly on the nerve. This "current spread" can give false-positive identifications (making one think a nerve is under the probe when it might be nearby). Bipolar stimulating probes offer more focused stimulation which can reduce shunting, but they require very close contact with the nerve and precise technique [12]. Additionally, stimulating at too high a current can cause adjacent muscle activation or contralateral responses; stimulating too low might miss the nerve. The standard range is 1–2 mA for reliable RLN stimulation. There is also a refractory period after a stimulus during which the nerve will not respond to another—most monitors have a visual or audible indicator to avoid re-stimulating too quickly. All these technical nuances mean the surgeon must understand the device's functioning well.

Continuous IONM (C-IONM) via a vagal electrode is a significant technological advance addressing some limitations of intermittent monitoring. By placing a lead on the vagus nerve (typically a small electrode clip encircling the nerve in the carotid sheath), one can continuously record RLN activity or stimulate the vagus at regular intervals automatically. Continuous stimulation can detect gradual changes in RLN function that a surgeon might not otherwise notice until a LOS occurs. For example, if during retraction the RLN starts to stretch, the EMG waveform may show a progressive drop in amplitude or an increase in latency; the system can issue a warning before complete signal loss occurs [16]. The surgeon can then relieve traction and often the EMG signal will recover, averting a permanent injury. This real-time feedback is a major improvement over only checking at the end, when it might be too late to reverse damage. Studies comparing continuous vs intermittent IONM have reported fewer transient neuropraxias and a lower rate of irreversible LOS with continuous monitoring, although outcomes in terms of permanent injuries are similar (since both methods ultimately aimed to avoid those) [16]. The trade-off is that continuous vagal monitoring requires additional steps—dissecting enough vagus nerve in the neck to apply the electrode, and the electrode itself can cause vagal irritation (some patients exhibit bradycardia or blood pressure changes during stimulation, which usually resolve by adjusting stimulus parameters or giving anticholinergic medication). The electrode must also be removed carefully at the end. These factors add complexity and a small risk of vagal nerve manipulation (which theoretically could cause its own nerve issue, though rare with proper technique).

In summary, while current IONM technology has certain limitations (ETT electrode issues, intermittent nature, artifact susceptibility), continuous improvements are addressing these. Continuous vagal monitoring has been a game-changer in how some surgeons prevent traction injuries [16]. However, continuous monitoring does introduce new complexity and cost, illustrating how advancing technology can simultaneously solve some controversies while raising new considerations.

Interpretation of EMG Signals and Standardized Protocols

For IONM to be effective, surgeons must correctly interpret the EMG data and follow standardized protocols. Misinterpretation can render the monitoring useless or even dangerous. Over the past decade, substantial effort has gone into developing consistent terminology and management algorithms for nerve monitoring results. Nevertheless, debates exist on what degree of EMG change is significant and how surgeons should respond to various signal alterations.

The International Neural Monitoring Study Group (INMSG) published a standardized checklist and protocol for IONM, sometimes called the "four-step procedure," which is now widely taught [12]. The steps are [1] **V1**—initial vagus stimulation at the start of the case to ensure the monitoring system is functioning (this yields a baseline EMG amplitude and latency); [2] **R1**—first RLN stimulation after the nerve is identified, to confirm identity and baseline response; [3] **R2**—second RLN stimulation after thyroid lobe removal or at end of dissection, to check post-manipulation nerve function; and [4] **V2**—final vagus stimulation at the end of the operation to verify the entire circuit is still intact. If V2 is lost but R2 was present, a global issue or proximal issue is suspected (like the ETT moved or a vagal stretch). If R2 is lost (and V2 lost), an RLN injury is indicated. This structured approach helps pinpoint at what stage a loss occurred and localize the problem. Adherence to this protocol has been shown to improve clarity in communication and outcomes—surgeons systematically document these steps and can compare across institutions.

A contentious point is defining what constitutes "loss of signal" (LOS) and what threshold should trigger intervention. Early guidelines defined LOS as a final EMG amplitude <100 μV (microvolts) when it was initially higher [11]. However, some nerve injury patterns present as a large drop in amplitude but not a total absence. Recent studies suggest using a relative decline—for example, >50–70% drop in amplitude combined with a significant increase in latency (e.g., 10% or 1 msec increase)—as criteria for impending dysfunction [16]. The 2018 INMSG update refined the definition of LOS to an amplitude reduction >90% from baseline (or below 100 μV) coupled with a latency prolongation, to improve specificity [11]. They also defined a "partial LOS" if amplitude drops by 50–90% [11]. The reason for these nuanced definitions is to balance sensitivity and specificity: calling LOS too early (minor fluctuations) would lead to many unnecessary staged thyroidectomies (false-positives), whereas calling it too late might miss an opportunity to prevent injury. Even with definitions, judgment is required—for instance, if a 60% amplitude drop occurs, some surgeons will pause and observe or gently explore to see if it recovers (perhaps indicating temporary stretch) [16]. If it recovers to near baseline after a positional change, they continue; if it continues to drop, they may declare LOS and stop. Thus, interpretation is dynamic.

The interpretation of subtle EMG changes is an evolving area. Surgeons have noticed patterns: a gradual latency increase (slowing of conduction) often precedes amplitude drop in stretch injuries. Latency may increase by tens of milliseconds as the nerve gets stressed, akin to a warning. Some continuous monitoring systems now provide trend graphs of latency and amplitude.

In conclusion, proper interpretation of IONM is as important as the monitoring itself. Through international guidelines and growing experience, the surgical community has made strides in demystifying EMG changes and establishing when they are meaningful. Nonetheless, minor variations and unique situations keep this an area of discussion. Surgeons must remain analytical—corroborating EMG findings with surgical findings—and avoid over-reliance on any single parameter. The controversies here will likely diminish as continuous data and large registries yield more refined criteria, but at present, decisions in the gray zones (partial LOS, subtle changes) still rely on surgeon judgment. Thus, interpretation is both art and science, and why training and experience [15] are indispensable for harnessing IONM's benefits.

Superior Laryngeal Nerve Monitoring: Feasibility and Utility

Monitoring the superior laryngeal nerve, specifically the external branch of the superior laryngeal nerve (EBSLN), presents its own set of controversies. The EBSLN is at risk during ligation of the superior thyroid vessels; unlike the RLN, EBSLN injury does not cause overt vocal cord paralysis, so its postoperative deficits are harder to detect—often manifesting as subtle voice changes (loss of high pitch, vocal fatigue). Historically, many surgeons did not routinely identify the EBSLN, partly due to its small size and variability in course. In 1992, Cernea et al. classified the EBSLN's anatomical relationship to the superior pole into three types (Cernea Type 1, 2a, 2b) based on how high or low it runs, with type 2b being the lowest and most at-risk configuration [17]. They found about 20% of nerves were type 2b (running close to the thyroid upper pole) in normal necks, but this percentage increased in large goiters due to stretching of anatomy. This underscored that certain patients (big goiters, short necks) have a higher likelihood of EBSLN injury if not identified. The question is: can and should we monitor the EBSLN to protect it?

Visually identifying the EBSLN can be challenging; it often lies under the fascia of the inferior constrictor muscle. Some surgeons rely on visual landmarks (staying far inferior with ligatures on the superior thyroid artery, or looking for the cricothyroid muscle and nerve crossing it). Others have advocated routine EBSLN stimulation to confirm its presence. When using IONM, the simplest indicator of EBSLN stimulation is observing the cricothyroid muscle twitch (since it is the only muscle the EBSLN innervates). Additionally, a high-pitched audible sound and small EMG deflection may be seen on the monitor due to activation of the intrinsic laryngeal musculature via the anastomosis between SLN and RLN. However, standard ET tube electrodes are primarily designed for the vocalis muscle, so the EBSLN EMG response is typically much smaller amplitude (as low as tens of μV). In the past, this made reliable EMG confirmation of EBSLN difficult—one study noted that using conventional monitors, only ~35% of EBSLNs were identified, versus 80% identified when using stimulation and observing the CT twitch directly. Thus, a controversy was whether it is worthwhile to attempt monitoring a nerve if the equipment cannot consistently pick it up [20].

The utility of EBSLN monitoring was dramatically demonstrated in a landmark randomized trial by Barczyński et al. in 2012 [18]. In this RCT of 210 patients (420 nerves at risk) undergoing total thyroidectomy, one group had visual identification of EBSLN only, and the other had visual + IONM for EBSLN (using CT twitch and EMG confirmation). The results were striking: the identification rate of the EBSLN soared from 34% with visual alone to 84% with IONM [18]. In other words, surgeons were able to locate and confirm the nerve in the vast majority of cases with the aid of stimulation, versus only one-third when relying on the naked eye.

The INMSG 2013 guideline recommends attempting EBSLN identification and stimulation in all cases and classifying the outcome. Thus, there is movement toward making EBSLN monitoring more commonplace. The controversies that remain include: the learning curve to consistently find the nerve (monitoring helps, but the surgeon must still expose the area where the nerve runs), and the cost–benefit specifically for SLN (one could debate if the added time is warranted in a patient with no professional voice demands). Many surgeons take a risk-based approach: if the patient is a singer, teacher, or otherwise reliant on fine voice, they will be especially vigilant about the EBSLN and often document its stimulation. In such cases, monitoring provides peace of mind that the nerve was preserved if the twitch is seen and the patient's pitch range remains intact postoperatively.

In summary, monitoring of the superior laryngeal nerve is feasible and has proven benefits in identifying and preserving this nerve, yet it is less universally adopted than RLN monitoring. The controversies here revolve around necessity and practicality. For surgeons who have seen the difference, it is convincing that IONM reduces EBSLN injuries and improves early voice outcomes [18]. Others may still rely on classical anatomic technique without stimulation. As technology improves the ease of SLN monitoring, we can expect it to become a standard part of thyroid surgery, especially given the increasing expectations of patients for perfect voice outcomes.

Medicolegal Considerations

Medicolegal implications form a subtle but important controversy in the use of IONM. Surgical complications like RLN injury frequently led to malpractice litigation in endocrine surgery. For instance, recurrent laryngeal nerve injury has been identified as the most common cause of malpractice claims related to thyroidectomy, with bilateral RLN injuries featuring prominently in lawsuits that favor plaintiffs [19]. The question arises: does using IONM protect the surgeon medicolegally, or conversely, could not using it be seen as substandard care?

From a defensive medicine perspective, many surgeons adopted IONM in part to bolster their documentation and possibly their legal defense if a nerve injury occurs. IONM provides a record (often one can save or print the EMG traces) that the nerve was functional at the end of the case (if so). This can be crucial in a courtroom to demonstrate that the surgeon took every precaution and that any injury may have been transient or unavoidable. In cases where an RLN paralysis occurred, if the intraoperative monitoring was intact throughout, a surgeon can argue that the injury was a delayed phenomenon outside their immediate control (especially if the injury was transient). In contrast, not using available technology might be painted by plaintiff attorneys as a lack of thoroughness—the absence of IONM has been questioned when bad outcomes occurred.

Conversely, if a surgeon uses IONM and still causes a nerve injury, that too can be scrutinized. However, legal case reviews have shown that juries are often sympathetic to surgeons if they demonstrate adherence to accepted protocols and careful monitoring. A 2020 analysis of malpractice trends (Swonke et al.) found that most thyroidectomy RLN injury lawsuits were decided in favor of the defense (surgeon) as long as proper precautions and documentation were evident [19]. It is often in cases of bilateral injury or clear negligence (like not identifying the nerve at all) that plaintiffs succeed. IONM use could potentially tip the balance by showing the surgeon did attempt to monitor and prevent injury.

Another medicolegal aspect is informed consent. As IONM has become prevalent, patients sometimes specifically ask if a nerve monitor will be used. In certain practice settings, not using one could conceivably require an explanation in the consent process. Currently, however, guidelines (such as from the American Thyroid Association) stop short of declaring IONM mandatory. They endorse it as a useful adjunct, particularly in high-risk cases, but state that visual identification by an experienced surgeon is the gold standard. Therefore, legally, a surgeon is not negligent per se for omitting IONM if they perform a careful thyroidectomy consistent with standard practice. That said, standard practice is evolving—in some countries like Germany, national guidelines recommend IONM in all thyroid surgeries, potentially shifting the expectation. In the United States and elsewhere, its use is about 50–70% of cases, indicating it is common but not universal. Should that percentage climb to a point where nearly everyone uses it, then not using it could be considered a deviation from the norm, influencing legal judgments.

In summary, while the decision to use IONM should be grounded in patient safety and efficacy, the medicolegal landscape undoubtedly pressures surgeons toward using it as an extra layer of documentation and assurance. Currently, most would agree that using IONM in appropriate cases represents diligence, and its proper use can strengthen a legal defense if needed. There is no legal requirement to use it in every case, but failure to use it in a high-risk situation that results in injury might be harder to defend. As IONM becomes more standard, it may eventually be seen as a required aspect of the standard of care for certain thyroidectomies. Until then, surgeons must weigh the medicolegal pros and cons themselves. Many simply feel more comfortable knowing they did everything possible—including monitoring—to protect the patient, which ethically and legally is a sound position. The medicolegal perspective largely aligns with the clinical one: use the tool judiciously to maximize patient safety and document nerve integrity, which in turn minimizes liability.

Conclusion

Intraoperative nerve monitoring in thyroid surgery resides at the intersection of surgical tradition and technological innovation. The current stance among endocrine surgeons is that IONM is a useful adjunct to optimize RLN and SLN preservation, but it does not replace the fundamental requirement for meticulous surgical technique and thorough knowledge of anatomy. The controversies that persist—regarding its impact on nerve injury rates, cost-effectiveness, and necessity in every case—are gradually being clarified as more high-quality data and experience accumulate. Evidence now suggests that IONM, when used properly, can modestly reduce transient RLN palsies, especially in challenging operations, and it provides undeniable benefits in preventing bilateral RLN paralysis through staged procedures.

In addressing the superior laryngeal nerve, what was once an afterthought in thyroid surgery is now appreciated as an important element of laryngeal function, and monitoring techniques have shown clear improvements in identifying and preserving the EBSLN. The trend is toward more routine EBSLN monitoring in thyroidectomies, particularly as technology makes it easier.

In terms of guidelines, we may see international consensus moving toward recommending IONM in most thyroid surgeries, given its low risk and the potential benefits demonstrated. The American Thyroid Association and other bodies may update their recommendations as new evidence emerges. If continuous monitoring proves to significantly reduce transient injury rates, it might prompt a broader endorsement of that technique as well.

Finally, the medicolegal climate will continue to evolve with the standard of care. Surgeons who have a good grasp of both the technical advances and the best practices guidelines will be well-positioned to provide safe care and defend their decision-making whether or not they use IONM in a given case. The emphasis will always be on outcomes—maintaining the exceedingly low rates of permanent nerve injury that expert thyroid surgeons achieve.

In conclusion, intraoperative nerve monitoring has transitioned from an experimental concept to a widely utilized tool in thyroid surgery. The controversies that accompanied this transition are being resolved through ongoing research and collective surgical experience. Most endocrine surgeons today agree that IONM adds a valuable margin of safety, particularly in difficult cases and for safeguarding voice quality, though it is not infallible. The future will likely bring even better monitoring modalities and more definitive data, further solidifying the role of nerve monitoring. For advanced surgical trainees and practicing surgeons, understanding both the capabilities and limitations of IONM—as thoroughly discussed in this chapter—is now an essential component of thyroid surgery proficiency. With prudent use of technology grounded in anatomical mastery, the ultimate goal remains the same as in Kocher's era: to cure thyroid disease while preserving the patient's voice and airway—a goal now more achievable than ever.

References

1. Shedd DP, Durham C. Electrical identification of the recurrent laryngeal nerve. I. Response of the canine larynx to electrical stimulation of the recurrent laryngeal nerve. Ann Surg. 1966;163(1):47–50.
2. Henry BM, Graves MJ, Vikse J, Sanna B, Pękala PA, Walocha JA, Barczyński M, Tomaszewski KA. The current state of intermittent intraoperative neural monitoring for prevention of recurrent laryngeal nerve injury during thyroidectomy: a PRISMA-compliant systematic review

of overlapping meta-analyses. Langenbeck's Arch Surg. 2017;402(4):663–73. https://doi.org/10.1007/s00423-017-1580-y. Epub 2017 Apr 4. PMID: 28378238; PMCID: PMC5437188
3. Schneider R, Randolph GW, Dionigi G, et al. International neural monitoring study group guideline 2018 Part I: staging bilateral thyroid surgery with monitoring loss of signal. Laryngoscope. 2018;128(Suppl 3):S1–S17.
4. Hearn M, You B, Mady LJ, Frazier KM, Morris-Wiseman L, Mathur A. Progress and outcomes of intraoperative nerve monitoring during thyroidectomy. JAMA Otolaryngol Head Neck Surg. 2025;151(3):236–42. https://doi.org/10.1001/jamaoto.2024.4452. PMID: 39820661; PMCID: PMC11907308.
5. Wojtczak B, Sutkowska-Stępień K, Głód M, Kaliszewski K, Sutkowski K, Barczyński M. Current knowledge on the use of Neuromonitoring in thyroid surgery. Biomedicine. 2024;12(3):675. https://doi.org/10.3390/biomedicines12030675. PMID: 38540288; PMCID: PMC10968482.
6. Barczyński M, Konturek A, Cichoń S. Randomized clinical trial of visualization versus neuromonitoring of recurrent laryngeal nerves during thyroidectomy. Br J Surg. 2009;96(3):240–6.
7. Pisanu A, Porceddu G, Podda M, Cois A, Uccheddu A. Systematic review with meta-analysis of studies comparing intraoperative neuromonitoring of recurrent laryngeal nerves versus visualization alone during thyroidectomy. J Surg Res. 2014;188(1):152–61.
8. Zheng S, Xu Z, Wei Y, et al. Effect of intraoperative neuromonitoring on recurrent laryngeal nerve palsy rates after thyroid surgery—a meta-analysis. J Formos Med Assoc. 2013;112(8):463–72.
9. Vasileiadis I, Karatzas T, Charitoudis G, et al. Association of intraoperative neuromonitoring with reduced recurrent laryngeal nerve injury in patients undergoing total thyroidectomy. JAMA Otolaryngol Head Neck Surg. 2016;142(10):994–1001.
10. Kim J, Graves CE, Jin C, Duh QY, Gosnell JE, Shen WT, Suh I, Sosa JA, Roman SA. Intraoperative nerve monitoring is associated with a lower risk of recurrent laryngeal nerve injury: a national analysis of 17,610 patients. Am J Surg. 2021;221(2):472–7. https://doi.org/10.1016/j.amjsurg.2020.10.013. Epub 2020 Oct 16
11. Wong KP, Mak KL, Wong CK, et al. Systematic review and meta-analysis on intraoperative neuro-monitoring in high-risk thyroidectomy. Int J Surg. 2017;38:21–30.
12. Randolph GW, Dralle H, Abdullah H, et al. Electrophysiologic recurrent laryngeal nerve monitoring during thyroid and parathyroid surgery: international standards guideline statement. Laryngoscope. 2011;121(Suppl 1):S1–S16.
13. Rocke DJ, Goldstein DP, de Almeida JR. A cost-utility analysis of recurrent laryngeal nerve monitoring in the setting of total thyroidectomy. JAMA Otolaryngol Head Neck Surg. 2016;142(12):1199–205.
14. Al-Qurayshi Z, Kandil E, Randolph GW. Cost-effectiveness of intraoperative nerve monitoring in avoidance of bilateral recurrent laryngeal nerve injury in patients undergoing total thyroidectomy. Br J Surg. 2017;104(11):1523–31.
15. Klotzka A, Iwańczyk S, Barczyński M, et al. Training in intraoperative neuromonitoring of recurrent laryngeal nerves reduces the risk of their injury during thyroid surgery. Arch Med Sci. 2021;17(5):1294–302.
16. Schneider R, Machens A, Lorenz K, Dralle H. Intraoperative nerve monitoring in thyroid surgery—shifting current paradigms. Gland Surg. 2020;9(Suppl 2):S120–8.
17. Cernea CR, Ferraz AR, Furlani J, et al. Identification of the external branch of the superior laryngeal nerve during thyroidectomy. Am J Surg. 1992;164(6):634–9.
18. Barczyński M, Konturek A, Stopa M, Honowska A, Nowak W. Randomized controlled trial of visualization versus neuromonitoring of the external branch of the superior laryngeal nerve during thyroidectomy. World J Surg. 2012;36(6):1340–7.
19. Swonke ML, Shakibai N, Chaaban MR. Medical malpractice trends in thyroidectomies among general surgeons and otolaryngologists. OTO Open. 2020;4(3):2473974X20921141.
20. Iwata AJ, Liddy W, Barczyński M, Wu CW, Huang TY, Van Slycke S, Schneider R, Dionigi G, Dralle H, Cernea CR, Kamani D, Ahmed AH, Okose OC, Wang B, Randolph GW. Superior laryngeal nerve signal attenuation influences voice outcomes in thyroid surgery. Laryngoscope. 2021;131(6):1436–42. https://doi.org/10.1002/lary.29413. Epub 2021 Jan 31. PMID: 33521945.

Dynamic Risk Stratification in Differentiated Cancer

13

Josef Madrigal, Maie St John, and Preethi Srikanthan

Editorial

Dynamic risk stratification (DRS) was introduced in 2010 as a measure that could be continually modified and be based on new data obtained at each follow-up visit. It was initially conceived for adults who underwent total thyroidectomy with adjuvant radioactive iodine ablation (RAI). The principles of DRS have also been validated in patients who have undergone either total thyroidectomy or thyroid lobectomy with or without RAI. It can also be utilized in the pediatric population. More recent work assessing the efficacy of DRS has attempted to incorporate molecular marker data in designing such risk models.

The ATA Initial Risk Stratification System was first utilized with various clinical and histopathological variables gathered both pre- and postoperatively to allow for individualized post-treatment care plans. Recognizing that risk assessment is a dynamic and ongoing process, the 2015 ATA Clinical Practice Guidelines recommended that initial risk of recurrence be continually modified throughout follow-up with DRS.

Clinicians are cautioned to consider various factors, prior to de-escalating surveillance protocols in intermediate-risk patients who are able to achieve an excellent response after follow-up. Factors that have been demonstrated to increase risk of recurrence include age $\geq$ 55 years, extrathyroidal extension, nodal burden $\geq$5,

J. Madrigal · M. S. John
Department of Surgery, Division of Head and Neck surgery, University of California, Los Angeles, Los Angeles, CA, USA
e-mail: JosefMadrigal@mednet.ucla.edu; MStJohn@mednet.ucla.edu

P. Srikanthan (✉)
Department of Medicine, Division of Endocrinology, University of California, Los Angeles, Los Angeles, CA, USA
e-mail: psrikanthan@mednet.ucla.edu

P. S. Pai et al. (eds.), *Controversies in Cancer of the Thyroid and Parathyroid Glands*, https://doi.org/10.1007/978-3-032-13130-0_13

pathologic nodes in the lateral neck, extranodal extension, and stimulated pre-ablation Tg levels >5 ng/mL.

Integration of molecular markers into dynamic risk stratification protocols has now been included. In recent years, there has been increasing interest in utilizing molecular markers to refine DRS. The impact of *BRAF* V600E and *TERT* promoter mutations on dynamic risk assessment is currently being studied. Incorporation of molecular markers may prove to refine dynamic risk assessment, but further work needs to be done in order to validate such methodology as well as to assess implications on management and treatment paradigms.

Some controversy exists as to how DRS may lead to inappropriate de-escalation of follow-up in patients initially categorized as intermediate- or high-risk but who achieve an excellent response to initial treatment. DRS, as described by the authors, has been of major importance in the treatment of thyroid cancer.

Christopher de Souza

Introduction

Over the past four decades, the estimated incidence of thyroid cancer has tripled [1]. Today, thyroid cancer remains the most common endocrine malignancy, with current estimates projecting 1.1% of individuals in the United States receiving this diagnosis during their lifetime [2]. Fortunately, the vast majority of these patients (90%) develop differentiated thyroid cancer (DTC). With its papillary, follicular, and oncocytic variants, DTC often carries an excellent prognosis, with an overall estimated 5-year survival rate of 98.5% [3]. In nearly all cases, thyroid surgery with or without adjuvant radioactive iodine ablation (RAI) has curative intent [4].

Given DTC's increasing incidence and excellent prognosis, significant efforts over the past two decades have been focused on developing management strategies that derive individualized treatment and follow-up protocols from patient-specific risk assessments. Thus, multiple staging systems have been validated to estimate the risk of mortality and recurrence in patients with DTC. In its 2015 Clinical Practice Guidelines, the American Thyroid Association (ATA) recommended the American Joint Cancer Commission/Union Internationale Contre le Cancer (AJCC/UIC) TNM staging system as a tool to predict disease-specific mortality [5]. Since the TNM staging system was not designed to predict the risk of recurrence in patients with DTC, the ATA Guidelines also recommended the utilization of a three-tiered stratification system that categorized individuals as having low, intermediate, or high risk of recurrent disease. First introduced in 2009, this ATA Initial Risk Stratification System utilized various clinical and histopathological variables gathered both pre- and postoperatively to allow for individualized post-treatment care plans [6]. While such a stratification system allows clinicians to determine the initial follow-up plan for their patients within 1–2 years of treatment, the ATA Initial Risk Stratification System remains a static representation that cannot be modified based on the clinical course of the individual patient's disease or their response to treatment. Recognizing this, Tuttle and colleagues first proposed dynamic risk stratification (DRS) in patients who underwent total thyroidectomy followed by radioactive iodine ablation for DTC [7]. By considering clinical, biochemical, and structural variables gathered throughout a patient's post-treatment course, DRS provides clinicians the opportunity to assess risk of recurrence at each follow-up visit.

Recognizing that risk assessment is a dynamic and ongoing process, the 2015 ATA Clinical Practice Guidelines recommended that initial risk of recurrence be continually modified throughout follow-up with DRS [5]. Although DRS was initially developed and validated in patient cohorts that underwent total thyroidectomy with adjuvant RAI, more recent work has demonstrated its applicability in individuals who underwent thyroid lobectomy and who did not undergo radioactive iodine ablation [8–10]. Ultimately, adoption of DRS into clinical practice has allowed for the identification of not only individuals who are at increased risk for persistent or recurrent disease that require further evaluation and treatment but also (and equally as important) those who have undergone remission that may have de-escalated follow-up.

Utilization of Initial Risk Assessments in Differentiated Thyroid Cancer

Unlike the vast majority of other malignancies, the risk of recurrence in differentiated thyroid cancer does not parallel the risk of mortality [11]. In most instances, the risk of recurrence far exceeds the risk of disease-specific mortality in DTC. Because of this, staging systems that are designed to predict mortality, such as the AJCC/UIC TNM system, are unable to accurately predict recurrence.

In order to address the paucity in measures that assess risk of recurrence, the 2009 ATA Clinical Practice Guidelines first endorsed a three-tiered system that classified patients as having low, intermediate, or high risk of developing recurrent disease (Table 13.1) [6]. Risk was calculated by a clinician after completion of initial treatment (thyroid lobectomy or total thyroidectomy with or without RAI) utilizing both histopathologic findings and unstimulated serum thyroglobulin levels. In summary, low-risk patients were those individuals found to have intrathyroidal DTC without any evidence of extrathyroidal extension, vascular or lymphatic invasion, or metastasis, whereas high-risk patients were defined as those found to have aggressive histopathologic variants, gross extrathyroidal extension, incomplete tumor resection, or distant metastasis found on imaging studies or suggested by inappropriately elevated serum thyroglobulin levels. The intermediate-risk group comprised individuals with microscopic extrathyroidal extension, vascular or lymphatic invasion, cervical nodal disease, or aggressive tumor histology. The validity of such an initial risk stratification system has been demonstrated in various international cohorts with patients categorized as intermediate- or high-risk experiencing significantly higher rates of persistent or recurrent structural disease [7, 12, 13].

In their 2015 guidelines, the ATA further modified its recommendation on initial risk assessment with the addition of other clinical and histopathologic variables: number and size of metastatic lymph nodes, number of foci of vascular invasion, as

Table 13.1 American Thyroid Association 2009 Initial Risk Stratification System

Initial risk assessment	Clinical and pathologic features
ATA low-risk	Papillary thyroid cancer with all the following features: No local or distant metastasis All macroscopic tumor has been resected No tumor invasion of locoregional tissues or structures No aggressive histology (tall cell, hobnail variant, columnar cell carcinoma, etc.) If ^{131}I is given, there is no uptake outside the thyroid bed on the first post-treatment whole-body RAI scan
ATA intermediate-risk	Microscopic invasion of tumor into the perithyroidal soft tissue Papillary thyroid cancer with vascular invasion Cervical lymph node metastasis Aggressive histology (tall cell, hobnail variant, columnar cell carcinoma, etc.) ^{131}I uptake outside of the thyroid bed on the first post-treatment whole-body RAI scan
ATA high-risk	Macroscopic invasion of tumor into the perithyroidal soft tissue Incomplete tumor resection Distant metastases Postoperative serum thyroglobulin suggestive of distant metastasis

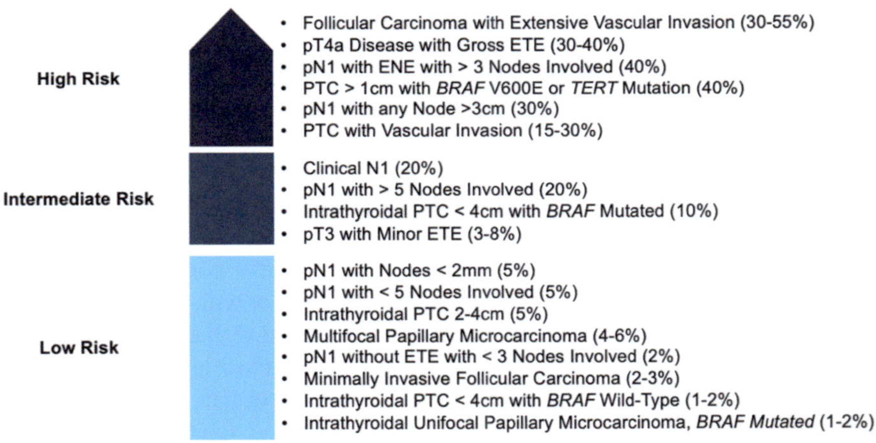

Fig. 13.1 American Thyroid Association 2015 Initial Risk Stratification System

well as *BRAF* and *TERT* mutational status. Furthermore, it encouraged clinicians to view the initial risk stratification system as a continuum, with patients ranging from very low risk to very high risk of persistent or recurrent structural disease (Fig. 13.1) [5, 14]. Under the revised initial risk stratification system, entities that include intrathyroidal papillary thyroid cancer with low number (≤5 nodes) or low-volume

(<0.2 cm) metastatic cervical nodes as well as papillary microcarcinoma regardless of *BRAF* mutational status were included in the low-risk category. Similarly, the high-risk category was expanded to include papillary thyroid cancer with a *TERT* mutation, follicular thyroid cancer with extensive vascular invasion, as well as the presence of any lymph node >3 cm. Like its precursor, the validity of this modified initial risk stratification system has been supported in multiple studies [8, 9, 15–17].

By estimating the risk of recurrence following treatment of DTC, clinicians may utilize the ATA Initial Risk Stratification System to develop follow-up plans for their patients within the first 1–2 years after treatment [18]:

1. *Low risk* (intrathyroidal DTC, ≤5 lymph nodes with micrometastasis): Follow-up occurs within 6–12 months after initial risk assessment with a neck ultrasound planned 12 months post-treatment.
2. *Intermediate risk* (aggressive histology, minor extrathyroidal extension, vascular invasion, >5 lymph nodes involved): Follow-ups occur at 6-month intervals with neck ultrasound performed 6 months post-treatment. Additional imaging [subsequent ultrasounds or computed tomography (CT) scan of the neck] is dependent on the burden of cervical nodal disease and thyroglobulin levels.
3. *High risk* (gross extrathyroidal extension, incomplete tumor resection, distant metastasis, lymph nodes >3 cm): Follow-up is individualized as a majority of these patients will have known or suspected persistent disease. These patients will often undergo follow-up imaging of the neck and chest 2–3 months after initial risk stratification with subsequent treatment plans developed on a case-by-case basis.

While the initial risk of recurrence stratification system is important in determining follow-up for patients in the first 1–2 years after treatment of DTC, it is a static measure that does not account for the clinical course of an individual patient's disease or their response to treatments received. Data acquired during the course of a patient's follow-up, such as thyroglobulin and anti-thyroglobulin levels, as well as evidence of structural recurrence on imaging results, may alter the estimated risk of recurrence. For example, a patient who was initially classified as having a low risk of recurrence who is then found to have rising serum thyroglobulin levels or is noted to have suspicious lymphadenopathy on follow-up ultrasound may have higher risk than that initially predicted. On the other hand, a patient who was initially classified as having high risk but remains without any evidence of structural or biochemical recurrence decades after initial treatment may have decreased risk compared to initial estimates. Such examples demonstrate that estimating risk of recurrence is an ongoing and dynamic process that must be continually modified with newly acquired data at each follow-up visit.

Utilization of Dynamic Risk Stratification in Patients with Differentiated Thyroid Cancer

Validation of Dynamic Risk Stratification in Patients Who Underwent Total Thyroidectomy with Radioactive Iodine Ablation

Recognizing the limitations of the ATA Initial Risk Stratification Systems, Tuttle and colleagues first proposed dynamic risk stratification in 2010 [7]. In their landmark study, 588 adult patients who underwent treatment of differentiated thyroid cancer with total thyroidectomy followed by radioactive iodine ablation at the Memorial Sloan-Kettering Cancer Center were identified. The median follow-up time was 7 years. These patients were first categorized as low, intermediate, or high risk of recurrence utilizing the 2009 ATA Initial Risk Stratification System. Response to initial treatment was categorized as excellent, acceptable, or incomplete based on data gathered at subsequent follow-up visits, including serum thyroglobulin (Tg) levels and imaging results. Patients were re-stratified according to their best response calculated within 2 years of treatment. In assessing patient outcomes, Tuttle and colleagues noted that persistent or recurrent disease occurred at an incidence of 3%, 21%, and 68% in the low-, intermediate-, and high-risk groups, respectively. However, after re-stratification, they found that the incidence of persistent or recurrent disease decreased significantly in patients reclassified as having excellent response to therapy (2% in low-risk, 2% in intermediate-risk, 14% in high-risk). Conversely, individuals who were re-stratified as having incomplete response to initial therapy had increased incidence compared to initial estimates (13% in low-risk, 41% in intermediate-risk, 79% in high-risk). Tuttle and colleagues further calculated the proportion of variance explained (PVE), which is a statistic that estimates the proportion of outcome variation that can be attributed to each stratification system. They found that the ATA Initial Risk Stratification System was only able to account for 34% of the variance in developing persistent or recurrent disease in their patient cohort while their proposed dynamic risk assessment accounted for 84%.

Such findings supporting utilization of DRS were subsequently validated in international cohorts [12, 19–22]. These studies noted that patients who achieved an excellent response after initial treatment with total thyroidectomy followed by RAI had a 1–4% estimated incidence of developing recurrent disease during long-term follow-up while 50–85% of patients who had an incomplete response were likely to remain with persistent disease despite additional treatment [22].

Overall, the results of these studies demonstrate the superiority of dynamic risk assessment in identifying individuals who are at increased risk of developing recurrent disease and require closer follow-up as well as those patients who have decreased risk and thus may be de-escalated. Thus, in their 2015 guidelines, the ATA recommended that initial risk of recurrence be continuously modified as more data is acquired during the follow-up period. The ATA defined four response-to-therapy categories based on biochemical testing (stimulated/nonstimulated Tg, anti-Tg antibody) and imaging results (Table 13.2) [5]:

Table 13.2 American Thyroid Association 2015 dynamic risk stratification response groups in patients who underwent total thyroidectomy with radioactive iodine ablation

Response group	Definition
Excellent response	Negative imaging *and either* Nonstimulated Tg < 0.2 ng/mL *or* TSH-stimulated Tg < 1.0 ng/mL
Biochemical incomplete response	Negative imaging *and* Nonstimulated Tg > 1.0 ng/mL *or* TSH-stimulated Tg > 10.0 ng/mL *or* Rising anti-Tg antibody levels
Structural incomplete response	Structural or functional evidence of disease
Indeterminate response	Nonspecific findings on imaging studies *or* Nonstimulated Tg detectable but <1.0 ng/mL *or* Stimulated Tg detectable but <10.0 ng/mL *or* Anti-Tg antibodies stable or declining in the absence of structural or functional disease

1. *Excellent responders*: no clinical, biochemical, or structural evidence of disease.
2. *Biochemical incomplete responders:* abnormal Tg or rising anti-Tg antibody levels without imaging correlates.
3. *Structural incomplete responders*: persistent or recurrent disease found on imaging.
4. *Intermediate responders*: nonspecific biochemical or structural findings that cannot be classified as either benign or malignant.

Implications of Dynamic Risk Stratification on Follow-Up

In their review of dynamic risk stratification in patients with differentiated thyroid cancer, Pitoia and Jerkovich provided management and follow-up recommendations for each response-to-therapy category defined by the ATA [22].

Excellent Responders

Given that individuals who achieve an excellent response to initial treatment have been found to have decreased incidence of structural recurrence at final follow-up (1–4%), the majority of patients in this response-to-therapy category may be considered for de-escalation in frequency of follow-up and degree of thyroid-stimulating hormone (TSH) suppression. Although this has minimal therapeutic implications for individuals initially classified as having a low risk of recurrence, it may have a significant impact on the estimated 57–63% of intermediate-risk and 14–16% of high-risk patients that achieve this response. Based on initial retrospective studies, the re-stratification of a patient initially calculated to have an intermediate risk of recurrence to the excellent response to treatment group implies a significant reduction in incidence of recurrent or persistent disease from 36–43% to 1–2% at final follow-up [7, 12, 13, 23]. Pitoia and Jerkovich thus recommended that low- and intermediate-risk patients who sustain an excellent response may be followed with clinical assessments and serum Tg levels every 1–2 years without the need for routine neck ultrasounds [20]. Although this may have little significance to those who were initially stratified as low risk who follow-up annually, such de-escalation would reduce the frequency of follow-up for those in the intermediate-risk group who follow-up every 6 months. Significant controversy, however, exists regarding de-escalating surveillance and TSH suppression in certain populations, which will be discussed further below.

Biochemical Incomplete Responders

Management of patients with biochemical incomplete response (elevated Tg or anti-Tg antibody levels without imaging correlates) is largely based on trends in Tg and anti-Tg antibody levels over time [20]. Fortunately, prognosis in patients re-stratified as having an incomplete biochemical response remains favorable, with 56–68% achieving an excellent response at final follow-up with or without additional therapy and with only 8–17% eventually developing structural [7, 12, 13, 23–25]. In their review, Pitoia and Jerkovich recommended that cross-sectional imaging with CT or 18-FDG-PET/CT be reserved only for patients with increasing Tg or anti-Tg antibody levels. Conversely, those with declining levels may continue observation with neck ultrasound performed every 2–3 years.

Structural Incomplete Responders

Unfortunately, a patient who sustains a structural incomplete response after initial treatment exhibits a 50–85% risk of persistent disease at final follow-up despite additional treatments [14, 22]. Management of these patients is highly personalized, accounting for various clinical and histopathologic variables, including size and location of disease, rate of progression, as well as avidity to radioactive iodine and 18-FDG. These individuals often require multidisciplinary care with experts from endocrinology, medical oncology, radiation oncology, and head and neck surgery. Management of these patients may involve revision surgery, external beam radiation therapy, systemic chemotherapy/tyrosine kinase inhibitors, or active surveillance [22].

Indeterminate Responders

Management of patients with nonspecific structural or biochemical findings that cannot be reliably classified as benign or malignant (indeterminate response) relies on serial imaging and serum Tg or anti-Tg levels, with the goal of re-stratifying individuals as excellent or incomplete responders [14]. Similar to those who sustain a biochemical incomplete response after initial therapy, patients who have an indeterminate response develop structural recurrence at a rate of approximately 13–20%.

Controversies in Dynamic Risk Stratification

In a study of 217 intermediate-risk individuals who were re-stratified as excellent responders after total thyroidectomy and RAI, Llamas-Olier and colleagues noted a surprisingly elevated early recurrence rate of 7.4% within a median follow-up time of 42 months [26]. Detection of recurrent structural or biochemical disease was significantly associated with several factors, including lateral neck lymph node metastasis, lateral neck RAI uptake in post-therapy whole-body scans, and pre-ablation Tg levels >10 ng/mL. This study postulated that these early recurrences may in fact be due to subclinical residual or micrometastatic disease that fails to reach the threshold for detection upon re-stratification. Therefore, clinicians are cautioned to consider various factors, described below, prior to de-escalating surveillance protocols in intermediate-risk patients who are able to achieve an excellent response after follow-up. Such factors that have been demonstrated to increase risk of recurrence in this population include age ≥55 years, extrathyroidal extension, nodal burden ≥5, pathologic nodes in the lateral neck, extranodal extension, and stimulated pre-ablation Tg levels >5 ng/mL [27–30].

Similarly, a recent study of 236 patients with high-risk DTC treated with total thyroidectomy and RAI noted that individuals re-stratified as having excellent response to initial therapy still suffered from a recurrence rate of 14%, which is in stark contrast to the 1–4% risk for all excellent responders. Indeed, such discrepancy can be explained by the fact that high-risk individuals comprise a minority of excellent responders, with low- and intermediate-risk patients accounting for much of the estimated risk of recurrence in this response group. These findings serve as cautionary reminders to clinicians, underscoring the need to interpret DRS in the context of a patient's initial risk assessment. As noted, certain intermediate-risk patients who are at higher risk of harboring subclinical residual or micrometastatic disease may benefit from further follow-up prior to de-escalation. In addition, all high-risk patients should undergo closer follow-up with additional imaging to rule out persistent or recurrent disease prior to de-escalation.

Extension of Dynamic Risk Stratification to Special Populations

Total Thyroidectomy or Thyroid Lobectomy Without Radioactive Iodine

In their 2015 Clinical Practice Guidelines, the ATA recommended less aggressive treatment for select individuals with differentiated thyroid cancer [5]. Per their recommendations, patients with very low-risk tumors, defined as papillary microcarcinomas (tumors less than 1 cm) without evidence of aggressive histology, local invasion, or nodal/distant metastasis, may elect for active surveillance and defer immediate surgery. Similarly, patients with tumors less than 4 cm without such aggressive features may be offered thyroid lobectomy as initial treatment. The 2015 ATA Guidelines also narrowed candidacy for RAI, not recommending routine administration for low-risk patients and only recommending it for certain populations within the intermediate-risk group. Given that dynamic risk stratification was validated in patients who underwent total thyroidectomy followed by RAI, the 2015 ATA Guidelines made no recommendations regarding utilization of DRS in patients who underwent total thyroidectomy or thyroid lobectomy without RAI.

Fortunately, more recent studies have demonstrated that the principles of dynamic risk assessment can also be applied to these patients. In their multi-institutional study of 507 patients who underwent total thyroidectomy or thyroid lobectomy without RAI, Momesso and colleagues used similar principles to define four response-to-therapy groups (Table 13.3). After re-stratification, the incidence of persistent or recurrent disease was noted to be 0%, 1.3%, 31.6%, and 100% in the excellent, indeterminate, biochemical incomplete, and structural incomplete response groups, respectively [8]. Such findings were further validated in two separate studies from South Korea, demonstrating that response to initial therapy in non-radioactive iodine-ablated patients was associated with disease-free survival. In both studies, the PVE of dynamic risk stratification was superior to the ATA Initial Risk Stratification System [9, 10]. Although specific follow-up recommendations in patients who underwent thyroid lobectomy or total thyroidectomy without RAI have yet to be published, the above studies demonstrate that DRS remains effective in guiding clinicians in tailoring individualized management plans for their patients.

Table 13.3 Dynamic risk stratification response groups in patients who underwent total thyroidectomy without radioactive iodine ablation or thyroid lobectomy

Response group	Total thyroidectomy w/o RAI	Thyroid lobectomy
Excellent response	Negative imaging Nonstimulated Tg < 0.2 ng/mL Undetectable anti-Tg	Negative imaging Stable nonstimulated Tg <30.0 ng/mL Undetectable anti-Tg
Biochemical incomplete response	Negative imaging Nonstimulated Tg levels >5.0 ng/mL Increasing anti-Tg levels	Negative imaging Nonstimulated Tg levels >30.0 ng/mL Increasing Tg or anti-Tg levels
Structural incomplete response	Structural or functional evidence of disease	Structural or functional evidence of disease
Indeterminate response	Nonspecific findings on imaging studies Nonstimulated Tg levels 0.2–5.0 ng/mL Stable or declining TgAb levels	Nonspecific findings on imaging studies Stable or declining TgAb levels

Children and Adolescents

Pediatric thyroid cancer has been rapidly increasing in the United States, with a recent study published from the Surveillance, Epidemiology, and End Results (SEER) database estimating a nearly 10% annual increase in incidence over the past two decades [31]. Compared to younger children, adolescents have a nearly ten-fold increase in risk of developing pediatric thyroid cancer. While a female preponderance is observed in adolescents, no such association exists in younger children [32]. Compared to adults, children and adolescents are more likely to present with regional metastasis to the neck or distant metastasis to the lungs [33]. Traditionally, total thyroidectomy has been recommended as initial treatment given prior studies that have demonstrated lower risk of recurrent disease (6% in total thyroidectomy vs 35% in thyroid lobectomy) [34]. More recent work, however, has demonstrated that thyroid lobectomy may be offered to select populations, such as patients with unifocal T1a papillary thyroid cancer without evidence of nodal disease [35]. Regardless, differentiated thyroid cancer maintains an excellent prognosis in children and adolescents with estimated 10-year survival rates of 97–99% [36].

Prior to the ATA 2015 Management Guidelines for Children with Thyroid Nodules and Differentiated Thyroid Cancer, there were no published recommendations regarding pediatric DTC [32]. In their 2015 guidelines, the ATA acknowledged the low utility of extrapolating the AJCC/UIC TNM staging system to predict prognosis in pediatric populations given extremely low disease-specific mortality as well as the lack of granularity in classifying these patients as stage I (no distant metastasis) or stage II (distant metastasis). Instead, they recommended the utilization of a similar three-tiered stratification system that categorized children and adolescents as having low, intermediate, or high risk of persistent cervical disease. While low-risk patients were defined as those whose disease was confined to the thyroid or only had microscopic metastasis to a small number of central neck nodes, high-risk individuals were defined as those with locally invasive tumors, extensive lateral neck involvement, or distant metastasis. Patients who did not belong in either group, those with extensive central neck involvement or minimal lateral neck involvement, were classified as intermediate risk. As demonstrated in Table 13.4, the ATA recommended post-treatment guidelines for each of these risk groups [32]:

Table 13.4 American Thyroid Association 2015 Initial Risk Stratification System for pediatric patients

Initial risk assessment	Clinical and pathologic features
Pediatric low-risk	Disease grossly confined to thyroid with N0/Nx disease *or* Incidentally found N1a disease (microscopic metastasis to small number of central neck nodes)
Pediatric intermediate-risk	Extensive N1a disease *or* Minimal N1b disease
Pediatric high-risk	Regionally extensive disease (extensive N1b) *or* Locally invasive disease (T4 tumors) with or without distant metastases

1. *Pediatric low risk:* Initial postoperative staging is performed with a TSH-suppressed Tg. If there is no evidence of disease, surveillance is performed with an ultrasound at 6 months postoperatively, then annually as well as Tg every 3–6 months for 2 years then annually.
2. *Pediatric intermediate and high risk:* Initial postoperative staging is performed with TSH-stimulated Tg and diagnostic ^{123}I scan. If no evidence of disease, ultrasound is performed every 6 months for 5 years, then annually as well as Tg every 3–6 months for 3 years then annually. A repeat TSH-stimulated Tg and diagnostic ^{123}I scan is recommended in high-risk patients in 1–2 years. This can also be considered in intermediate-risk patients.

In 2017, Sung and colleagues published the first study assessing the utility of dynamic risk stratification in pediatric patients with DTC [37]. In summary, 77 pediatric patients who underwent total thyroidectomy with RAI or thyroid lobectomy alone for treatment of DTC were identified. The median follow-up was 5.3 years. These patients were first categorized as low-, intermediate-, or high-risk based on the ATA's Management Guidelines for Children [32]. They were then subsequently re-stratified as having excellent, indeterminate, biochemical incomplete, or structural incomplete response to initial therapy based on previous definitions utilized in the adult population [5, 8]. In assessing outcomes, Sung and colleagues noted similar incidence of recurrent disease in the ATA low- and intermediate-risk groups but significantly higher rates in the high-risk group (65%). More importantly, this study noted that only 1 of 38 patients who were re-stratified as having an excellent response to initial treatment developed recurrent disease. Such an observation has a significant impact on follow-up plans given only 22% of patients were initially classified as ATA low risk while 49% of individuals achieved excellent response during follow-up.

Further studies have validated the efficacy of DRS in predicting recurrent or persistent disease in pediatric populations [38–41]. As such, clinicians may utilize dynamic risk assessment to tailor individualized management and follow-up plans for children and adolescents with DTC who underwent thyroid lobectomy or total thyroidectomy with or without RAI, similar to adults.

Integration of Molecular Markers to Dynamic Risk Stratification

In recent years, there has been increasing interest in utilizing molecular markers to refine DRS. The impact of *BRAF* V600E and *TERT* promoter mutations on dynamic risk assessment is currently being studied.

BRAF V600E is an oncogenic mutation that remains highly prevalent in papillary thyroid carcinoma (PTC), with approximately 45% of tumors harboring this mutation. Such a mutation in *BRAF* renders the mitogen-activated protein kinase signaling pathway constitutively activated. Prior studies have demonstrated that *BRAF* V600E is associated with aggressive features in PTC, including extrathyroidal extension, lymph node metastasis, distant metastasis, and recurrence [42, 43]. Similarly, *TERT* promoter mutations are also oncogenic, with its presence leading to unchecked activity of telomerase, which functions in adding telomeres to promote chromosomal integrity and genomic stability [44]. In one study of *TERT* promoter mutations in DTC, Melo and colleagues found that 7.5% of papillary thyroid carcinomas and 17.1% of follicular thyroid carcinomas harbored such mutations, portending more aggressive tumor behavior, as well as heightened risk of recurrence/persistence and mortality [45]. The combination of these two mutations has also been demonstrated to exhibit synergistic effects [43].

In 2017, Kim and colleagues conducted the first study assessing the ability of molecular markers to augment dynamic risk assessment [46]. They identified 357 patients with DTC but without evidence of distant metastasis on initial evaluation. These patients were then stratified by their response-to-therapy groups as well as by the presence of *TERT* promoter mutations. Using adjusted hazard ratios (AHRs), they were able to define four prognostic groups that were found to be associated with recurrence as well as cancer-related death: AHR 1 (excellent response and wild-type [WT] *TERT*), AHR 2 (intermediate response and WT *TERT*), AHR 3 (biochemical/structural incomplete response and WT *TERT* or excellent/intermediate response and mutant *TERT*), and AHR 4 (biochemical/structural incomplete response with mutant *TERT*). This study found that recurrence-free survival decreased with each AHR group: 94.9% in AHR 1, 82.7% in AHR 2, 50.2% in AHR 3, and 23.1% in AHR 4.

Similarly, in 2023, Pérez-Fernández and colleagues assessed the utility of incorporating *BRAF* V600E mutational status in DRS [47]. In a retrospective study of 685 patients who underwent total thyroidectomy with or without RAI, 53.4% were found to harbor a *BRAF* V600E mutation. Although the presence of this oncogene was inversely associated with achievement of an excellent response to initial treatment, incorporation of *BRAF* V600E did not add additional benefit in DRS.

Incorporation of molecular markers may prove to refine dynamic risk assessment, but further work needs to be done in order to validate such methodology as well as assess implications on management and treatment paradigms.

Summary

Given its increasing incidence and favorable prognosis, clinicians caring for patients with DTC require tools that effectively identify patients who are at heightened risk of recurrence and require further evaluation and treatment as well as patients who have entered remission and may benefit from less intensive follow-up. Although the ATA Initial Risk Stratification System was found to correlate with risk of recurrence, such measures were unable to account for the clinical course of an individual patient's disease and their response to treatment. Dynamic risk stratification was thus introduced in 2010 as a means of continually modifying risk of recurrence calculations based on new data gathered at each follow-up visit. While DRS has been demonstrated to predict outcomes more reliably than ATA Risk Groups, some controversy exists as to how DRS may lead to inappropriate de-escalation of follow-up in patients initially categorized as intermediate- or high-risk but who achieve an excellent response to initial treatment. Caution must be exercised prior to de-escalating certain intermediate-risk patients and all high-risk individuals. Although initial recommendations cautioned against utilization of DRS in patients who did not receive RAI, more recent work has demonstrated its validity in non-radioactive iodine-ablated individuals. Furthermore, DRS has also been validated in children and adolescents. More work is required to allow incorporation of molecular markers to our risk calculations, which may further refine DRS and allow clinicians to better tailor individualized treatment plans for their patients.

References

1. Lim H, Devesa SS, Sosa JA, Check D, Kitahara CM. Trends in thyroid cancer incidence and mortality in the United States, 1974-2013. JAMA. 2017;317(13):1338–48. https://doi.org/10.1001/JAMA.2017.2719.
2. Thyroid Cancer — Cancer Stat Facts. https://seer.cancer.gov/statfacts/html/thyro.html. Accessed March 16, 2025.
3. Siegel RL, Miller KD, Wagle NS, Jemal A. Cancer statistics, 2023. CA Cancer J Clin. 2023;73(1):17–48. https://doi.org/10.3322/CAAC.21763.
4. Boucai L, Zafereo M, Cabanillas ME. Thyroid cancer: a review. JAMA. 2024;331(5):425–35. https://doi.org/10.1001/JAMA.2023.26348.
5. Haugen BR, Alexander EK, Bible KC, et al. 2015 American Thyroid Association management guidelines for adult patients with thyroid nodules and differentiated thyroid cancer: the American Thyroid Association guidelines task force on thyroid nodules and differentiated thyroid cancer. Thyroid. 2016;26(1):1–133. https://doi.org/10.1089/thy.2015.0020.
6. Cooper DS, Doherty GM, Haugen BR, et al. Revised American thyroid association management guidelines for patients with thyroid nodules and differentiated thyroid cancer. Thyroid. 2009;19(11):1167–214. https://doi.org/10.1089/thy.2009.0110.
7. Tuttle RM, Tala H, Shah J, et al. Estimating risk of recurrence in differentiated thyroid cancer after total thyroidectomy and radioactive iodine remnant ablation: using response to therapy variables to modify the initial risk estimates predicted by the new American Thyroid Association staging system. Thyroid. 2010;20(12):1341–9. https://doi.org/10.1089/THY.2010.0178.
8. Momesso DP, Vaisman F, Yang SP, et al. Dynamic risk stratification in patients with differentiated thyroid cancer treated without radioactive iodine. J Clin Endocrinol Metab. 2016;101(7):2692–700. https://doi.org/10.1210/JC.2015-4290.
9. Park S, Kim WG, Song E, et al. Dynamic risk stratification for predicting recurrence in patients with differentiated thyroid cancer treated without radioactive iodine remnant ablation therapy. Thyroid. 2017;27(4):524–30. https://doi.org/10.1089/THY.2016.0477.
10. Cho JW, Lee YM, Lee YH, Hong SJ, Yoon JH. Dynamic risk stratification system in post-lobectomy low-risk and intermediate-risk papillary thyroid carcinoma patients. Clin Endocrinol. 2018;89(1):100–9. https://doi.org/10.1111/CEN.13721.
11. Mazzaferri EL, Kloos RT. Clinical review 128: current approaches to primary therapy for papillary and follicular thyroid cancer. J Clin Endocrinol Metab. 2001;86(4):1447–63. https://doi.org/10.1210/JCEM.86.4.7407.
12. Castagna MG, Maino F, Cipri C, et al. Delayed risk stratification, to include the response to initial treatment (surgery and radioiodine ablation), has better outcome predictivity in differentiated thyroid cancer patients. Eur J Endocrinol. 2011;165(3):441–6. https://doi.org/10.1530/EJE-11-0466.

13. Pitoia F, Bueno F, Urciuoli C, Abelleira E, Cross G, Tuttle RM. Outcomes of patients with differentiated thyroid cancer risk-stratified according to the American Thyroid Association and Latin American Thyroid Society risk of recurrence classification systems. Thyroid. 2013;23(11):1401–7. https://doi.org/10.1089/THY.2013.0011. https://home.liebertpub.com/thy
14. Tuttle RM, Alzahrani AS. Risk stratification in differentiated thyroid cancer: from detection to final follow-up. J Clin Endocrinol Metab. 2019;104(9):4087–100. https://doi.org/10.1210/JC.2019-00177.
15. Pitoia F, Jerkovich F, Urciuoli C, Falcón F, de Lima AP. Impact of historic histopathologic sample review on the risk of recurrence in patients with differentiated thyroid cancer. Arch Endocrinol Metab. 2018;62(2):157–63. https://doi.org/10.20945/2359-3997000000020.
16. Van Velsen EFS, Stegenga MT, Van Kemenade FJ, et al. Evaluating the 2015 American Thyroid Association risk stratification system in high-risk papillary and follicular thyroid cancer patients. Thyroid. 2019;29(8):1073–9. https://doi.org/10.1089/THY.2019.0053.
17. Wu J, Hu XY, Ghaznavi S, et al. The prospective implementation of the 2015 ATA guidelines and modified ATA recurrence risk stratification system for treatment of differentiated thyroid cancer in a Canadian tertiary care referral setting. Thyroid. 2022;32(12):1509–18. https://doi.org/10.1089/THY.2022.0055.
18. Tarasova VD, Tuttle RM. A risk-adapted approach to follow-up in differentiated thyroid cancer. Rambam Maimonides Med J. 2016;7(1):e0004. https://doi.org/10.5041/RMMJ.10231.
19. Hong CM, Lee WK, Jeong SY, Lee SW, Ahn BC, Lee J. Superiority of delayed risk stratification in differentiated thyroid cancer after total thyroidectomy and radioactive iodine ablation. Nucl Med Commun. 2014;35(11):1119–26. https://doi.org/10.1097/MNM.0000000000000183.
20. Pitoia F, Jerkovich F, Urciuoli C, et al. Implementing the modified 2009 American Thyroid Association risk stratification system in thyroid cancer patients with low and intermediate risk of recurrence. Thyroid. 2015;25(11):1235–42. https://doi.org/10.1089/THY.2015.0121.
21. Kowalska A, Walczyk A, Pałyga I, et al. The delayed risk stratification system in the risk of differentiated thyroid cancer recurrence. PLoS One. 2016;11(4):e0153242. https://doi.org/10.1371/JOURNAL.PONE.0153242.
22. Pitoia F, Jerkovich F. Dynamic risk assessment in patients with differentiated thyroid cancer. Endocr Relat Cancer. 2019;26(10):R553–66. https://doi.org/10.1530/ERC-19-0213.
23. Vaisman F, Momesso D, Bulzico DA, et al. Spontaneous remission in thyroid cancer patients after biochemical incomplete response to initial therapy. Clin Endocrinol. 2012;77(1):132–8. https://doi.org/10.1111/J.1365-2265.2012.04342.X.
24. Vaisman F, Tala H, Grewal R, Tuttle RM. In differentiated thyroid cancer, an incomplete structural response to therapy is associated with significantly worse clinical outcomes than only an incomplete thyroglobulin response. Thyroid. 2011;21(12):1317–22. https://doi.org/10.1089/THY.2011.0232.
25. Pitoia F, Abelleira E, Tala H, Bueno F, Urciuoli C, Cross G. Biochemical persistence in thyroid cancer: is there anything to worry about? Endocrine. 2014;46(3):532–7. https://doi.org/10.1007/S12020-013-0097-6.
26. Llamas-Olier AE, Cuéllar DI, Buitrago G. Intermediate-risk papillary thyroid cancer: risk factors for early recurrence in patients with excellent response to initial therapy. Thyroid. 2018;28(10):1311–7. https://doi.org/10.1089/THY.2017.0578.
27. Lee SH, Roh JL, Gong G, et al. Risk factors for recurrence after treatment of N1b papillary thyroid carcinoma. Ann Surg. 2019;269(5):966–71. https://doi.org/10.1097/SLA.0000000000002710.
28. Kim Y, Roh JL, Song DE, et al. Risk factors for posttreatment recurrence in patients with intermediate-risk papillary thyroid carcinoma. Am J Surg. 2020;220(3):642–7. https://doi.org/10.1016/j.amjsurg.2020.01.049.
29. Chen Q, Zou X, Liu F, et al. Impact of different categories of intermediate risk factors on the recurrence of papillary thyroid carcinoma: a retrospective cohort study. Int J Surg. 2024; https://doi.org/10.1097/JS9.0000000000001945.

30. Maino F, Botte M, Dalmiglio C, et al. Prognostic factors improving ATA risk system and dynamic risk stratification in low- and intermediate-risk DTC patients. J Clin Endocrinol Metab. 2024;109(3):722–9. https://doi.org/10.1210/CLINEM/DGAD591.
31. Qian ZJ, Jin MC, Meister KD, Megwalu UC. Pediatric thyroid cancer incidence and mortality trends in the United States, 1973-2013. JAMA Otolaryngol Head Neck Surg. 2019;145(7):617–23. https://doi.org/10.1001/JAMAOTO.2019.0898.
32. Francis GL, Waguespack SG, Bauer AJ, et al. Management guidelines for children with thyroid nodules and differentiated thyroid cancer. Thyroid. 2015;25(7):716–59. https://doi.org/10.1089/THY.2014.0460.
33. Verburg FA, Van Santen HM, Luster M. Pediatric papillary thyroid cancer: current management challenges. Onco Targets Ther. 2016;10:165–75. https://doi.org/10.2147/OTT.S100512.
34. Hay ID, Gonzalez-Losada T, Reinalda MS, Honetschlager JA, Richards ML, Thompson GB. Long-term outcome in 215 children and adolescents with papillary thyroid cancer treated during 1940 through 2008. World J Surg. 2010;34(6):1192–202. https://doi.org/10.1007/S00268-009-0364-0.
35. Sudoko CK, Jenks CM, Bauer AJ, et al. Thyroid lobectomy for T1 papillary thyroid carcinoma in pediatric patients. JAMA Otolaryngol Head Neck Surg. 2021;147(11):943–50. https://doi.org/10.1001/JAMAOTO.2021.2359.
36. Zhang B, Wu W, Shang X, Huang D, Liu M, Zong L. Incidence and prognosis of thyroid cancer in children: based on the SEER database. Pediatr Surg Int. 2022;38(3):445. https://doi.org/10.1007/S00383-022-05069-3.
37. Sung TY, Jeon MJ, Lee YH, et al. Initial and dynamic risk stratification of pediatric patients with differentiated thyroid cancer. J Clin Endocrinol Metab. 2017;102(3):793–800. https://doi.org/10.1210/JC.2016-2666.
38. Sohn SY, Kim YN, Kim HI, Kim TH, Kim SW, Chung JH. Validation of dynamic risk stratification in pediatric differentiated thyroid cancer. Endocrine. 2017;58(1):167–75. https://doi.org/10.1007/S12020-017-1381-7.
39. Zanella AB, Scheffel RS, Nava CF, et al. Dynamic risk stratification in the follow-up of children and adolescents with differentiated thyroid cancer. Thyroid. 2018;28(10):1285–92. https://doi.org/10.1089/THY.2018.0075.
40. Kim K, Kim WW, Choi JB, et al. Usefulness of dynamic risk stratification in pediatric patients with differentiated thyroid carcinoma. Ann Surg Treat Res. 2018;95(4):222–9. https://doi.org/10.4174/ASTR.2018.95.4.222.
41. Majeed AK, Satapathy S, Ballal S, Bal C. Dynamic risk stratification for predicting long-term outcomes in pediatric differentiated thyroid cancers. J Clin Endocrinol Metab. 2023;108(6):e208–15. https://doi.org/10.1210/CLINEM/DGAC731.
42. Tufano RP, Teixeira GV, Bishop J, Carson KA, Xing M. BRAF mutation in papillary thyroid cancer and its value in tailoring initial treatment: a systematic review and meta-analysis. Medicine (Baltimore). 2012;91(5):274–86. https://doi.org/10.1097/MD.0B013E31826A9C71.
43. Xing MM, Alzahrani AS, Carson KA, et al. Association between BRAF V600E mutation and mortality in patients with papillary thyroid cancer. JAMA. 2013;309(14):1493–501. https://doi.org/10.1001/JAMA.2013.3190.
44. Liu R, Xing M. TERT promoter mutations in thyroid cancer. Endocr Relat Cancer. 2016;23(3):R143. https://doi.org/10.1530/ERC-15-0533.
45. Melo M, Da Rocha AG, Vinagre J, et al. TERT promoter mutations are a major indicator of poor outcome in differentiated thyroid carcinomas. J Clin Endocrinol Metab. 2014;99(5):E754–65. https://doi.org/10.1210/JC.2013-3734.
46. Kim TH, Ki CS, Kim HS, et al. Refining dynamic risk stratification and prognostic groups for differentiated thyroid cancer with TERT promoter mutations. J Clin Endocrinol Metab. 2017;102(5):1757–64. https://doi.org/10.1210/JC.2016-3434.
47. Pérez-Fernández L, Sastre J, Zafón C, et al. Validation of dynamic risk stratification and impact of BRAF in risk assessment of thyroid cancer, a nation-wide multicenter study. Front Endocrinol (Lausanne). 2023;13:1071775. https://doi.org/10.3389/FENDO.2022.1071775.

Radioiodine Therapy in the Management of Differentiated Thyroid Cancer

14

Kunal Ramesh Chandekar, Shubha Gadde Ravindra, Swayamjeet Satapathy, and Chandrasekhar Bal

Editorial

Dr. Bal and his colleagues from the All India Institute of Medical Sciences in New Delhi have addressed current controversies in the management of differentiated thyroid cancer, with a particular focus on risk stratification in major decision-making. They clearly support the use of radioactive iodine (RAI) therapy in high-risk patients while acknowledging that its role remains controversial in the intermediate-risk group. For low-risk patients, they affirm that RAI is not indicated. The authors also discuss the issues of a remnant ablation and emphasize the importance of precision and individualized treatment decisions. Additionally, they highlight potential complications of RAI therapy, including sialadenitis and the risk of second primary malignancies.

There have been significant advances in the postoperative application of radioactive iodine (RAI) therapy. The updated 2025 American Thyroid Association (ATA) guidelines recommend a more selective use of RAI, generally reserving it for patients with high-risk pathological features. The previous practice of administering multiple doses is now largely obsolete. One of the most notable developments is the use of recombinant TSH (Thyrogen), eliminating the need to induce hypothyroidism prior to the treatment. This is particularly beneficial for younger patients, many of whom struggle with the effects of being hypothyroid for 4–6 weeks. The shift to Thyrogen represents a major advancement in patient-centered care. Overall, this document reflects the extensive experience of the authors at the All India Institute of Medical Sciences in New Delhi and provides a thoughtful, evidence-based approach to modern RAI therapy.

Ashok R. Shaha

We confirm that the images/tables included are original and have not been published earlier.

K. R. Chandekar · S. G. Ravindra · S. Satapathy · C. Bal (✉)
Department of Nuclear Medicine, All India Institute of Medical Sciences, New Delhi, India

P. S. Pai et al. (eds.), *Controversies in Cancer of the Thyroid and Parathyroid Glands*, https://doi.org/10.1007/978-3-032-13130-0_14

Introduction

Thyroid cancer is the most common endocrine malignancy with approximately 821,173 new cases and 47,485 deaths each year as per recent global estimates [1]. The increasing incidence of thyroid cancer is mainly due to effective screening and widespread use of imaging, leading to enhanced detectability of these cancers [2]. Differentiated thyroid cancers (DTCs) arise from the thyroid follicular cells and account for more than 90% of all thyroid cancers. DTC has an excellent long-term prognosis and a 10-year overall survival (OS) rate of >90% following standard treatment with surgery ± postoperative radioiodine (RAI) therapy [3].

Since its introduction eight decades ago, RAI therapy has remained an important cornerstone in postoperative management of DTC, serving three main purposes: (i) ablation of thyroid remnant tissue, (ii) adjuvant therapy for suspected but unconfirmed microscopic residual disease, and (iii) treatment of persistent or recurrent structural disease [4, 5]. The current American Thyroid Association (ATA) guidelines (2015) introduced an updated initial risk stratification system for DTC, categorizing post-thyroidectomy patients into three distinct risk groups: low, intermediate, and high—based on the probability of disease recurrence or persistence [5]. While RAI therapy is routinely recommended for high-risk or metastatic DTC patients, its utility in low- and intermediate-risk patients is increasingly debated, given evidence suggesting no significant impact on long-term recurrence rates and survival outcomes in these groups [5–10]. Several important factors must be considered to determine whether postoperative RAI therapy is justified and likely to benefit these patients (Fig. 14.1).

In recent years, a "less-is-more" strategy for RAI therapy has emerged, reflecting a broader shift in thyroid cancer management from a one-size-fits-all approach to a more risk-adapted treatment paradigm [5, 11]. This approach acknowledges the indolent nature of the disease in most patients. Recognition of a separate entity of low-risk tumors such as noninvasive follicular thyroid neoplasm with papillary-like nuclear features (NIFTP), adoption of active surveillance and/or limited surgery (lobectomy) as a viable option for small primary tumors, relaxing needs for thyroid-stimulating hormone (TSH) suppression, and less rigorous follow-up in carefully selected patients are all extensions of the same [5, 12, 13].

Existing literature on RAI therapy is primarily based on retrospective, observational data. Heterogeneity in terms of histological variants, RAI avidity, and completeness of resection are potential confounding factors that are difficult to account for. Further, the intent of therapy is often poorly defined with limited data strictly pertaining to adjuvant treatment. The lack of prospective randomized controlled trials (RCTs) makes it difficult to answer several pertinent questions regarding the optimal use of RAI therapy in DTC [6, 7]. Conducting such prospective RCTs requires large-scale multidisciplinary collaboration, supported by adequate financial and technical resources. The inherently low risk of cancer recurrence and mortality in DTC necessitates the recruitment of a very large number of patients and long-term follow-up, making feasibility a real challenge.

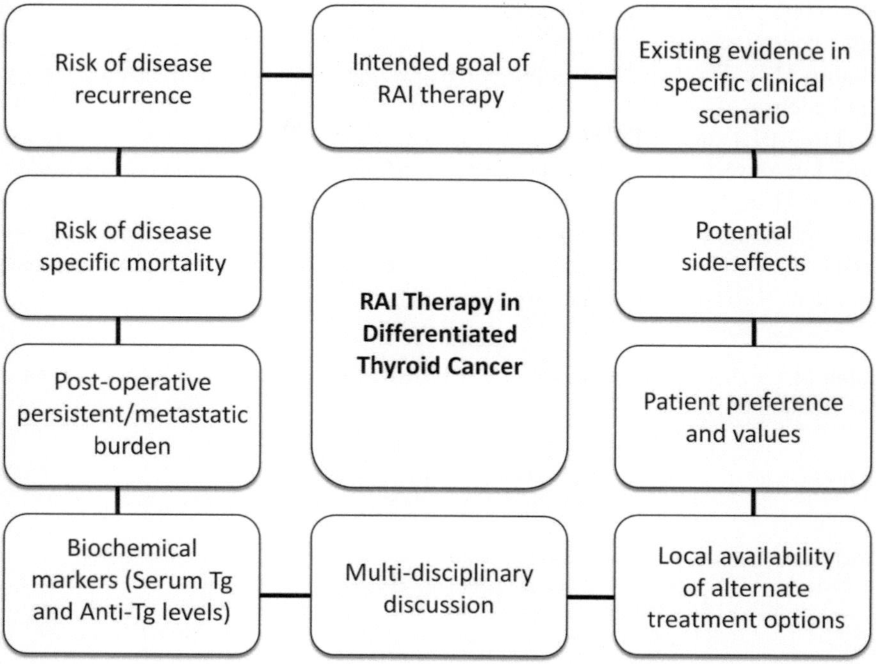

Fig. 14.1 Key factors in radioiodine (RAI) therapy decision-making

In this review, we aim to examine the important controversies surrounding utility of postoperative RAI in DTC management in light of the latest evidence.

How Much RAI Activity Is Needed for Thyroid Remnant Ablation?

The goal of remnant ablation is to destroy residual thyroid tissue following surgical total thyroidectomy so as to facilitate detection of nodal and distant metastases on iodine-131(^{131}I) whole-body scintigraphy (WBS) and improve the sensitivity of serum thyroglobulin (Tg) measurements in initial staging and follow-up studies [14].

The amount of radioactivity that would result in successful remnant ablation was a matter of debate until a few years in the past due to lack of large, prospective RCTs. An initial pilot study by Bal et al. demonstrated that activities above 50 mCi do not confer any additional benefit with regard to the rate of successful ablation (ablation rates, 30 mCi, 63%; 50 mCi, 77.8%; 90 mCi, 73.7%; 155 mCi, 76.7%) [15]. A subsequent RCT by the same group showed that a minimum activity of 25 mCi would be required for effective ablation (ablation rates in patients receiving less than 25 mCi vs those receiving at least 25 mCi, 61.8% vs 81.6%,

$P = 0.006$) [16]. Furthermore, the rates of short-term adverse events were higher after administration of 100 mCi when compared to 30 mCi as reported in some studies [17]. The two most important RCTs that established the non-inferiority/equivalence of 30 mCi as against 100 mCi ^{131}I for remnant ablation were the ESTIMABL1 and HiLo trials [18–20]. The recurrence rates in patients treated with low-dose RAI were not significantly different from those treated with high-dose RAI on long-term follow-up results of these trials. The salient features of these trials are presented in Table 14.1. Thus, in light of evidence from various trials, the current ATA guidelines recommend against the use of activities over 30 mCi ^{131}I for remnant ablation in DTC [5].

Table 14.1 Salient features of major trials on thyroid remnant ablation with 30 mCi (1.11 GBq) radioiodine therapy

	ESTIMABL1	HiLo
Type of trial	Randomized phase 3 equivalence trial conducted across 24 centres in France ($n = 752$)	Randomized phase 3 non-inferiority trial conducted across 29 centres in the UK ($n = 438$)
Inclusion criteria	M0 DTC patients (excluding aggressive histologic subtypes) with the following T and N stages: pT1 (tumor diameter ≤1 cm) and N1 or Nx or pT1 (tumor diameter 1–2 cm) and any N or pT2N0	M0 DTC patients (excluding aggressive histologic subtypes) with the following T and N stages: T1– T3 with N0/N1/Nx disease
Definition of successful ablation	Normal neck ultrasound and Tg/rhTSH ≤1 ng/mL at 6–10 months	Negative ^{131}I WBS (uptake <0.1%) and/or Tg < 2.0 ng/mL at 6–9 months
Ablation rate	Equivalent between the ^{131}I doses [1.1 GBq (30 mCi) vs 3.7 GBq (100 mCi)]—91.5% vs 93.5%, equivalence margin = 10% and stimulation methods (thyroid hormone withdrawal vs rhTSH)	Non-inferior across the ^{131}I doses [1.1 GBq (30 mCi) vs 3.7 GBq (100 mCi)]—85.0% vs 88.9%, non-inferiority margin = 10% and stimulation methods (thyroid hormone withdrawal vs rhTSH)
Long-term follow-up results with disease recurrence rates	726 patients had a median follow-up of 5.4 years since randomization No. of patients with recurrent disease: 1.1 GBq vs 3.7 GBq: Six patients vs five patients	434 patients had a median follow-up of 6.5 years since randomization No. of patients with recurrent disease: 1.1 GBq vs 3.7 GBq: 11 patients vs 10 patients

Role of RAI Therapy for Remnant Ablation and/or Adjuvant Treatment in Low-Risk DTC

The 2015 ATA low-risk group includes patients having intrathyroidal DTC (T1-T3a tumors) with or without lymph node micrometastases (N0/N1, ≤5 lymph nodes and size ≤0.2 cm) [5]. Existing guidelines strongly recommend against RAI use in patients with unifocal papillary microcarcinoma, in the absence of other adverse features [5, 21]. However, the recommendations for no-iodine (no-RAI) follow-up in patients with other low-risk DTCs are still weak and need to be personalized.

Schvartz et al. performed a retrospective study to analyze the survival benefit of RAI in low-risk patients. A total of 1298 DTC patients (pT1-T2 and pN0/Nx) with a median follow-up of 10.3 years were included in the study, with 911 patients in the RAI group and 387 patients in the no-RAI group. The study failed to demonstrate any survival benefit of RAI in terms of OS and disease-free survival (DFS) in these patients (Cox univariate *P*-values of 0.35 and 0.48, respectively) [22]. Subsequent data from a prospective multi-institutional registry of the National Thyroid Cancer Treatment Cooperative Study Group (NTCTCSG) failed to prove any OS benefit in low-risk DTC patients receiving RAI. This study included a total of 4941 patients with a median follow-up of 6 years, with 43% of patients in the "low-risk category." [23]

ESTIMABL2, a prospective RCT, assessed the non-inferiority of follow-up alone as opposed to 30 mCi RAI in patients with low-risk DTC. A total of 776 patients with localized pT1a/T1b (including multifocal tumors) and pN0/Nx tumors with nonaggressive histology and normal postoperative neck ultrasonography (USG) underwent randomization. A composite of abnormal RAI scan (in patients randomized to RAI group), abnormal neck USG, and elevated levels of Tg or anti-Tg antibodies were used as predictors of recurrent disease. A total of 95.6% and 95.9% of the patients had no events at 3 years in the follow-up group and ablation group, respectively, thus demonstrating the non-inferiority of follow-up alone strategy (difference 0.3%, non-inferiority margin = 5%). The selective inclusion of T1, N0/Nx patients, and short follow-up of 3 years, however, limits the generalizability of this trial to all low-risk patients [8].

Satapathy et al., from AIIMS, New Delhi, assessed the recurrence rate and recurrence-free survival (RFS) in 2074 patients encompassing all low-risk categories as defined by ATA 2015 guidelines receiving RAI vis-à-vis no-RAI validated by propensity score-matched analysis. The patients had a median follow-up of 8 years. They concluded that there was no added benefit of RAI in low-risk DTC in terms of recurrence rate (1.3% vs 3.3%, RAI vs no-RAI in propensity score-matched cohort, $P = 0.095$) and 10-year RFS (96.3% vs 96.2%, RAI vs no-RAI in propensity score-matched cohort, $P = 0.788$). However, on subgroup regression analysis, they observed that RAI could be advantageous in certain select subgroups such as those with age < 55 years ($P = 0.044$), male sex ($P = 0.015$), pT3a tumors ($P = 0.049$), and baseline stimulated Tg ≥ 5 ng/mL ($P = 0.002$) [9]. Thus, future prospective randomized studies should aim to evaluate the role of RAI versus no-RAI follow-up in low-risk patients with pT3a tumors and those with high postoperative Tg levels.

Role of RAI Therapy for Remnant Ablation and/or Adjuvant Treatment in Intermediate-Risk DTC

ATA intermediate-risk category encompasses DTC patients with microscopic extrathyroidal extension (ETE), or lymph nodal metastases (>0.2 cm but <3 cm size of tumor deposit), or more specifically papillary thyroid cancer (PTC) with vascular invasion and aggressive histological subtypes (such as tall-cell, columnar-cell, or hobnail variants) [5]. Despite a favorable 10-year disease-specific survival (DSS) rate of >95%, ATA-defined intermediate-risk DTC represents a heterogeneous group carrying a variable risk (range ~ 5–30%) of disease recurrence [5, 24]. This makes it difficult to provide uniform recommendations for the entire category. The 2015 ATA guidelines specify that RAI adjuvant therapy (in the absence of persistent structural disease) "should be considered" after TT in intermediate-risk DTC patients [5]. However, this is a weak recommendation based on low-quality retrospective studies, which have often yielded conflicting findings.

In a large, retrospective study from Korea, Kim et al. evaluated the impact of RAI therapy on locoregional recurrence (LRR) in 8297 intermediate-risk PTC patients. The RFS rates were 95.7% versus 94.9% (229/252) at 5 years and 89.0% versus 91.6% at 10 years, in the no-RAI and RAI groups, respectively. There was no significant difference according to RAI ablation ($P = 0.627$, by log-rank test). After accounting for clinic-pathological factors, RAI ablation did not significantly reduce the risk of LRR (adjusted hazard ratio (HR) = 0.852; $P = 0.413$). Furthermore, on subgroup analysis, RAI ablation did not significantly lower the LRR risk even in intermediate-risk PTC patients with aggressive features such as BRAF positivity (adjusted HR = 0.729; $P = 0.137$), multifocality (adjusted HR = 1.032; $P = 0.926$), ETE (adjusted HR = 0.870; $P = 0.541$), and regional lymph node metastasis (adjusted HR = 0.804; $P = 0.349$) [10].More recently, however, Tian et al. published a retrospective propensity score-matched analysis examining the impact of RAI therapy in intermediate-risk PTC patients with low Tg levels (unstimulated Tg levels ≤1 ng/mL or stimulated Tg levels ≤10 ng/mL). Of the included patients, 690 were successfully matched (552 in the RAI group and 138 in the non-RAI group) with a median follow-up of 51 months. Recurrence rates were significantly lower in the RAI group compared to the non-RAI groups, being 0.9% versus 3.6% for structural recurrence ($P = 0.007$) and 0.7% vesus 4.3% for biochemical recurrence ($P = 0.005$), respectively. The authors concluded that postoperative RAI therapy significantly reduces the risk of structural and biochemical recurrence in intermediate-risk PTC patients, despite low Tg levels [25].

Given such conflicting results, a recent meta-analysis tried to consolidate evidence (from 11 articles with 56,266 patients) on the utility of RAI therapy in intermediate-risk PTC over no-RAI follow-up. RAI therapy showed no significant reduction in structural disease recurrence rates compared to no-RAI follow-up (pooled univariate odds ratio (OR), 0.73; 95% CI, 0.29–1.87; $I^2 = 75\%$). However, the authors proposed that possible explanation for this could be difference in baseline characteristics between RAI and no-RAI groups. In several of these studies, the patients who were kept on no-RAI follow-up had significantly lower proportion of higher-risk or adverse features compared to the RAI groups. Moreover, the included studies demonstrated substantial variation in treatment approaches. These specific clinic-pathological features and treatment decisions are significant risk modifiers that affect structural recurrence and may have influenced the results of the meta-analysis [26]. Ballal et al., from AIIMS, New Delhi, have suggested a "middle path," i.e., only "surgically ablated" intermediate-risk DTC patients (patients with a negative initial diagnostic WBS, 24-h neck RAI uptake value of ≤0.2%, and a stimulated Tg level of ≤10 ng/ml), should be kept on no-RAI follow-up [27]. This strategy appears clinically reasonable and helps us provide more personalized treatment.

The abovementioned meta-analysis also reported that RAI therapy was associated with improved OS compared to no-RAI follow-up (pooled multivariate HR, 0.63; 95% CI, 0.48–0.82; $I^2 = 79\%$) in intermediate-risk PTC patients [26]. Another study by Zhao et al., based on the Surveillance, Epidemiology, and End Results (SEER) database (2004–2018), used propensity score matching to account for differences in clinic-pathological characteristics between the RAI and no-RAI groups. They also reported that TT was associated with poorer OS compared with TT + RAI treatment with an HR of 1.52 (95% CI, 1.11–2.07) in intermediate-risk PTC patients [28].

Despite the paucity of risk group-specific data, RAI therapy appears to be beneficial for intermediate-risk DTC in patients belonging to certain age groups (e.g., ≥65 years), in those with lateral compartment nodal metastasis, and in patients with larger primary tumours, multifocal primary, and ETE [24, 29, 30]. Further, there is also a lack of clarity on the optimal amount of RAI activity to be used for adjuvant treatment in intermediate-risk DTC. The 2015 ATA guidelines recommend using activities >30 mCi and up to 150 mCi for adjuvant treatment. Higher administered activities in this setting are unlikely to improve therapeutic outcomes and entail greater risk of side effects [5]. Future research should aim to specifically identify subgroups within the intermediate-risk category where the advantages of RAI therapy clearly outweigh any drawbacks, thereby justifying its application.

Role of RAI Therapy in High-Risk or Metastatic DTC

What Is the Risk of Second Primary Malignancy (SPM) Post-RAI Therapy?

SPMs are largely a problem of long-term survivors of thyroid cancer. Children, young adults, and adolescents may be at a higher risk, owing to tissue susceptibility and longer life expectancy. The relationship between RAI usage and occurrence of SPM is however debatable. According to the ATA 2015 guidelines, the absolute increase in risk of developing a SPM attributable to RAI is small when compared to the general population and does not warrant any additional screening measures [5].

Early reports from a combined European (Swedish, Italian, and French) cohort of 6841 DTC patients suggested that RAI therapy was associated with increased relative risk (RR) for SPM of bone and soft tissue (RR = 4.0), female genital organs

(RR = 2.2), central nervous system (RR = 2.2), and leukemia (RR = 2.5). Further, an increased risk of both solid tumors and leukemia as was seen with increasing cumulative activity of RAI with an excess absolute risk of 14.4 solid cancers and of 0.8 leukemias per GBq of ^{131}I and10 [5] person-years of follow-up [31]. In a systematic review and meta-analysis by Yu et al., the pooled risk ratio for any subsequent malignant neoplasm in RAI-treated thyroid cancer patients (n = 10 studies, 65,539 patients) was 0.98 (95% CI, 0.76–1.27, $P < 0.001$). However, when adjusted for confounders (n = 6 studies, 11,241 patients), the pooled risk ratio was 1.16 (95% CI = 0.97–1.39; $P = 0.054$). In secondary analyses examining specific malignancies, the risk of leukemia was increased, but the risk of multiple myeloma was reduced in RAI-treated thyroid cancer patients. Further, there was no significant increased RR of breast cancer, salivary cancer, and combined hematologic malignancies associated with RAI treatment status [32]. In another critical review by Reinecke et al., the relative effect of RAI versus no RAI for SPM ranged between 1.14 and 1.84 in various studies, with most being statistically insignificant. The relative effect for secondary hematologic malignancy (SHM) ranged between 1.30 and 2.50, with two-thirds of the studies showing statistically significant difference. The risk increased with increasing cumulative activity of RAI [33]. Thus, patients receiving RAI for treatment of thyroid cancers seem to have an increased risk for SHMs with inconsistent results for other solid SPMs.

A recent study by Pasqual et al. examined the RR of developing solid and hematologic malignancies in patients diagnosed with thyroid cancer at ages less than 45 years and treated with RAI using the US SEER cancer database. The median duration of follow-up in the study was 15 years. The RR of developing solid malignancies was 1.23 (95% CI, 1.11–1.37) in 27,050 ≥5-year survivors of thyroid cancer. The RR of developing hematologic malignancies was 1.51 (95% CI, 1.08–2.01) in 32,171 ≥2-year survivors of thyroid cancer [34].

Given the heterogeneity in existing literature, more studies are needed to evaluate the relationship between RAI and risk of developing subsequent neoplasms (solid and hematological) and generate high-quality evidence regarding the same. Till then, RAI needs to be used judiciously, ascertaining the risk-benefit ratio on a case-to-case basis.

What Is the Optimal Cumulative RAI Activity that Can Be Safely Administered in Metastatic DTC?

In a pivotal study, Durante et al. reported long-term outcomes of RAI therapy in 444 patients with metastatic DTC. They found that post-treatment, 48% of negative imaging (diagnostic WBS and conventional radiographs) studies were observed after the administration of a cumulative activity of less than 7.4 GBq (200 mCi), 36% with 7.4–14.8 GBq (201–400 mCi), 12% with 14.8–22.2 GBq (401–600 mCi), and only 4% with a cumulative activity higher than 22.2 GBq (600 mCi) [35]. Given that the risk of SPMs (particularly hematologic malignancies), bone marrow suppression, and lacrimal and salivary toxicity increases with the cumulative activity,

ATA guidelines usually recommend that the use of RAI therapy beyond 600 mCi should be personalized on a case-to-case basis [5, 36, 37]. This arbitrary threshold (cumulative activity of 600 mCi or 22.2 GBq) is well recognized, as it has also been used by prospective clinical trials evaluating the role of multi-targeted kinase inhibitors in metastatic DTC to define "RAI-refractory" disease [38, 39].

More recently, Bharadwaj et al., from AIIMS, New Delhi. reported the largest retrospective cohort of metastatic DTC patients ($n = 671$) treated with RAI therapy with a median follow-up duration of ~10 years. Patients were classified into three groups based on the cumulative RAI activity received, group A (≤600 mCi), group B (>600–1000 mCi), and group C (>1000 mCi). Further, they found that ~32.5% of the patients in group B (600–1000 mCi) achieved complete/excellent response, which was markedly higher than the results reported by Durante et al., where only ~4% of patients achieved excellent response beyond 600 mCi. Importantly, the incidence of SPMs did not rise with greater RAI activity, indicating that the risk of SPM may not be linked to higher cumulative doses. However, cumulative RAI activity greater than 1000 mCi was associated with significant increase in bone marrow suppression, decreased pulmonary function, and xerostomia ($P < 0.001$). The authors suggested that a maximum up to 1000 mCi (37 GBq) strikes a favorable balance between potential benefits and toxicity profile in DTC patients with RAI-concentrating extensive metastases [40].

The ATA recognizes that a cutoff of 600 mCi RAI should not be interpreted and implemented as absolute criterion for RAI-refractory disease [6]. In such patients, the decision on further treatment with RAI should be guided by a multidisciplinary approach and personalized based on several parameters such as presence of significant RAI uptake, response to previous treatment courses, low ^{18}F-FDG avidity at disease sites, side effect profile from the RAI therapy, available alternate treatment options, availability of clinical trials, and most importantly, patient preference [41].

Role of Empirical RAI Therapy in Patients with TENIS

After initial therapy, follow-up in DTC is usually performed by serum Tg, neck USG, and diagnostic WBS. Approximately 20–25% of DTC patients develop Tg elevation and negative iodine scintigraphy (TENIS) syndrome during follow-up [42, 43]. This condition highlights a diagnostic and therapeutic dilemma, as functional imaging often fails to localize residual disease despite biochemical evidence. Empiric RAI therapy has been tried in patients with TENIS with the dual goal of potential disease localization on post-therapy WBS and consequent therapeutic benefit. The 2015 ATA guidelines suggest considering empiric RAI therapy (typically 100–200 mCi) in TENIS patients without evidence of structural disease that is not amenable to locoregional or directed therapy (surgery, external beam radiotherapy (EBRT), thermal ablation, alcohol ablation, and others) [5]. However, this is a weak recommendation based on low-quality evidence.

There is no universally accepted cutoff value of serum Tg above which empiric RAI therapy should be considered in a TENIS patient. Most studies suggest Tg levels (after levothyroxine withdrawal) of 10 ng/mL or higher as a "clinically actionable" finding [44, 45]. The appropriate first step in such patients with TENIS is to look for evidence of structural disease. ^{18}F-FDG PET/CT, as a hybrid imaging tool, has excellent utility in this setting. In addition to assessing structural disease burden, it also has treatment and prognostic implications. As DTC cells undergo dedifferentiation, they lose their ability to concentrate RAI due to decreased expression of the sodium-iodide symporter (NIS) protein. Simultaneously, these cells exhibit increased glucose uptake driven by upregulation of glucose transporter 1 (GLUT1) receptors. This inverse pattern of RAI uptake and glucose metabolism, often termed the "flip-flop phenomenon," is indicative of increased tumor proliferation and aggressiveness [46]. Hence, TENIS patients with positive ^{18}F-FDG PET are unlikely to respond to empiric RAI therapy.

Early retrospective studies on utility of empiric RAI therapy reported localization of persistent disease on post-therapy WBS in up to 50% of TENIS patients. Despite reports of reduction in serum Tg levels post-empiric RAI therapy, no significant benefit in OS was observed [47–50]. However, more recently, a study from Italy assessed the impact of empiric RAI therapy in a propensity score-matched cohort of 238 DTC patients with Tg elevation and without evidence of structural disease. They found a significantly higher event rate (disease progression, relapse, need for additional therapy or death) in patients who did not receive empiric RAI therapy (no-ET group) compared to those who did (ET group), with rates of 30% and 18%, respectively ($P < 0.001$). Multivariate Cox regression analysis identified age ($P < 0.01$), pre-therapy Tg levels ($P < 0.05$), and the use of empiric RAI therapy ($P < 0.01$) as independent predictors of outcomes. Additionally, the Kaplan-Meier survival analysis revealed that progression-free survival (PFS) was notably shorter in the no-ET group compared to the ET group ($P < 0.01$) [51]. A recent meta-analysis of 14 studies involving 690 patients treated with high-dose empiric RAI therapy for TENIS syndrome revealed that those with micrometastases often demonstrated new lesions on post-treatment WBS that were not visible on diagnostic WBS (proportion = 0.64; 95% CI, 0.51–0.77). Additionally, these patients experienced a significant reduction in serum Tg levels (proportion = 0.69; 95% CI, 0.52–0.84) after treatment. In contrast, patients with macrometastases did not show similar beneficial findings following empiric RAI therapy [52]. Overall, the most compelling evidence for benefit from empiric RAI therapy is for pulmonary metastases, which are not amenable to directed therapies [53, 54]. Hence, for TENIS patients, particularly those with a large tumor burden, alternative systemic treatment options such as tyrosine kinase inhibitors (TKIs) should be explored, and empiric RAI therapy should not be routinely encouraged. However, it is important to acknowledge no prospective study has been conducted on empiric RAI therapy, which makes it difficult to provide definitive recommendations.

Definition of RAI-Refractory Thyroid Cancer

RAI-refractory DTC (RR-DTC), though uncommon, is a challenging clinical entity with poor long-term outcomes. The mean life expectancy of RR-DTC is 3–5 years and the OS is less than 10% at 10 years [55].The prevalence of RR-DTC is estimated to be approximately 15% of all DTC patients [56]. Multiple studies have suggested several clinicopathological characteristics such as older age at diagnosis (≥55 years); pT3/T4 stage; extensive vascular invasion; ETE; aggressive histological subtypes; synchronous cervical, pulmonary, and bone metastases at initial work-up; high ^{18}F-FDG avidity; and the presence of *TERT* promoter mutations, as risk factors associated with RAI refractoriness [56–58]. The primary mechanisms contributing to development of RR-DTC involve the activation of extracellular signal-regulated kinase (ERK) or mammalian target of rapamycin (mTOR) pathways, characterized by reduced expression of the NIS and increased expression of GLUT1 [56].

Various groups have suggested different definitions, classifications, and criteria for identifying patients with RAI-refractory thyroid cancer [6, 59, 60]. The 2015 ATA guidelines classify RR-DTC into four broad categories, which include (i) tumor that never concentrated RAI (no uptake outside thyroid bed at the first RAI therapy) or de novo refractory disease, (ii) tumor that has lost the ability to concentrate RAI after previous evidence of RAI avidity, (iii) tumor heterogeneity where only some lesions show RAI concentration while others do not, and (iv) tumors that progress despite significant RAI concentration [5]. The 2019 "Martinique principles," a multidisciplinary consensus statement, identified the progression of DTC metastases despite receiving a cumulative ^{131}I dose exceeding 22.2 GBq (600 mCi) as an additional clinical scenario indicating RAI refractoriness, alongside these four broad categories [6]. Ensuring appropriate preparation with avoidance of iodine excess and TSH stimulation is a must prior to labeling any patient as RR-DTC. Further, it is important that protocols for RAI scintigraphy are optimized and standardized across institutions. At present, it is unclear whether low-dose diagnostic WBS can be used to define RAI refractoriness as several parameters such as administered RAI activity, acquisition time, γ-camera model, and reconstruction algorithm scan influence its accuracy [56]. Corroborative SPECT/CT, wherever available, should be used so as to ensure that no patient is inappropriately classified as having RR-DTC. Additional imaging modalities such as CT, MRI, and/or ^{18}F-FDG PET/CT may be utilized for accurate assessment of structural disease burden in these patients.

The ATA recognizes that no current definition, classification, or clinical scenario is sacrosanct, i.e., it cannot be an absolute indicator that a patient has RR-DTC. The goal is to stratify patients based on the likelihood that their tumor will respond to RAI therapy so as to ensure its judicious use [6]. Our understanding of RR-DTC will continue to evolve as future research addresses the limitations and technical issues confounding existing literature. Further, improvements in radioiodine imaging and associated technology with increasing clinical adoption of redifferentiation therapies and molecular genomics will enhance the practice of RAI theranostics [61–63].

Miscellaneous

Should We Be Worried About "Thyroid Stunning"?

"Stunning" refers to the phenomenon of reduced RAI uptake by thyroid remnant tissue (or less commonly by functioning DTC metastases) on post-therapy scans due to a preceding dose of RAI administered for diagnostic WBS. Multiple studies have examined this phenomenon and reported conflicting results. Debated issues include whether stunning is a real phenomenon, whether it arises from differences in nuclear imaging techniques, its exact mechanism, and its potential impact on clinical outcomes. Proponents of stunning suggest that radiation from the diagnostic dose may lead to (i) cell death, reducing the number of viable cells available to trap iodine; (ii) impaired gene expression and membrane translocation of the NIS protein; and (iii) increased serum iodide levels secondary to thyroid follicle damage, ultimately reducing RAI uptake from the subsequent therapeutic dose [64].

Jeevanram et al. analyzed the radiation delivered to thyroid remnants following five different diagnostic activities in 52 patients. When the diagnostic dose delivered 35 Gy or more, subsequent treatment uptake decreased by 75%, whereas a diagnostic dose delivering 17.5 Gy resulted in a 25% reduction in uptake [65]. Park et al. observed a noticeable decrease in iodine-avid tissue activity on post-treatment scans (100–200 mCi ^{131}I) compared to diagnostic scans (3–10 mCi) performed a few days earlier. Therapeutic uptake was reduced in 40% (2/5) of patients who received 3 mCi, 67% (2/3) of patients who received 5 mCi, and 89% (16/18) of patients who received 10 mCi [66]. However, not all groups have reported similar results. Cholewinski et al. found no indication of stunning in a study of 122 patients, even though they were administered a diagnostic dose of 5 mCi (185 MBq), and scans were performed 72 h later [67]. McDougall et al. observed stunning in only 1.4% (2/147) of patients with a 2 mCi diagnostic dose [68].

Interestingly, Nordén et al. documented the effect of ^{131}I on NIS gene expression in porcine thyroid cells. Cells stimulated with TSH or insulin-like growth factor-1 (IGF-1) were exposed to ^{131}I (7.5 Gy) for 48 h, resulting in a 60–90% reduction in NIS transcription at all time points [69]. While this study provides important in vitro evidence for stunning, it does not answer the more critical question of whether stunning affects RAI treatment efficacy. Morris et al. retrospectively compared ablation success rates between 37 patients who underwent diagnostic scans with 3–5 mCi (111–185 MBq) of ^{131}I and 63 patients treated directly. Ablation rates were similar at 65% and 67%, respectively, indicating stunning was not a concern [70]. Dam et al. also reported comparable rates of successful remnant ablation (91% vs 89%, respectively) in patients with and without stunning on post-therapy WBS [71]. These results suggest that stunning may not necessarily impact treatment outcomes. Ultimately, nuclear medicine physicians must remember that thyroid stunning can be avoided by using the alternate isotope ^{123}I or lower doses (1–3 mCi) of ^{131}I for diagnostic WBS and by minimizing the time interval between diagnostic WBS and the therapeutic administration of RAI [64].

What Is the Role of Personalized Dosimetry for RAI Therapy in DTC?

The efficacy of RAI therapy is related to the radiosensitivity of the tumor/remnant tissue and the mean radiation dose delivered to it. In routine clinical practice, therapeutic ^{131}I is administered based on empiric fixed amounts taking into account the patient's risk profile and biochemical/imaging evidence of disease burden. Personalized dosimetry is often reserved for challenging scenarios such as diffuse pulmonary metastases, extensive skeletal/marrow involvement, extremes of age, and in the presence of medical comorbidities (e.g., chronic kidney disease and coexisting lung conditions) [72–75]. Dosimetric approaches include blood and whole-body dosimetry and quantitative tumor lesion dosimetry [76, 77]. Iodine-124 (^{124}I) PET-based dosimetry may be superior to conventional dosimetry using ^{131}I or iodine-123 (^{123}I) planar scintigraphy and SPECT-CT. However, ^{124}I is expensive and not universally available [78].

Dosimetric estimates of RAI activity to be administered should ensure ≤ 2 Gy radiation absorbed dose to blood and ≤ 80 mCi whole-body retention at 48 h [5, 79]. The whole-body threshold becomes important in cases of diffuse pulmonary metastases where the critical organ might be lungs and not the red bone marrow. These prescribed thresholds are often breached in a sizeable proportion of patients receiving fixed empiric doses, particularly older (>70 years) patients [80, 81].

Personalized dosimetry is time consuming, expensive, and technically demanding requiring specialized equipment and trained personnel. Moreover, the biological variability of iodine kinetics and tumor heterogeneity in DTC further complicates the standardization of personalized dosimetry. In contrast, empiric fixed dosing is simpler, cost-effective, and considered sufficient for most DTC patients, particularly those in the low- or intermediate-risk groups, where the likelihood of clinical remission is high. Literature comparing the two strategies is mostly retrospective with no large-scale, prospective data [82]. Unless we generate robust clinical evidence to demonstrate superiority of the dosimetric approach, guidelines are unlikely to mandate or recommend their adoption for routine clinical use.

Conclusion

RAI therapy in DTC must be tailored based on individual patient and tumor characteristics (Fig. 14.2). The controversies surrounding its use underscore the complexity of balancing treatment efficacy with potential risks and side effects. Advances in hybrid imaging, pathological and molecular profiling, and targeted therapy have transformed the management paradigm. While RAI remains a cornerstone for high-risk DTC, its utility in low- and intermediate-risk patients continues to be debated, necessitating further robust evidence to refine clinical guidelines. Prospective, well-structured, and focused RCTs, guided by multidisciplinary collaboration among endocrinologists, oncologists, and nuclear medicine physicians, will be pivotal in advancing the standard of care and ensuring improved outcomes and quality of life for patients with differentiated thyroid cancer.

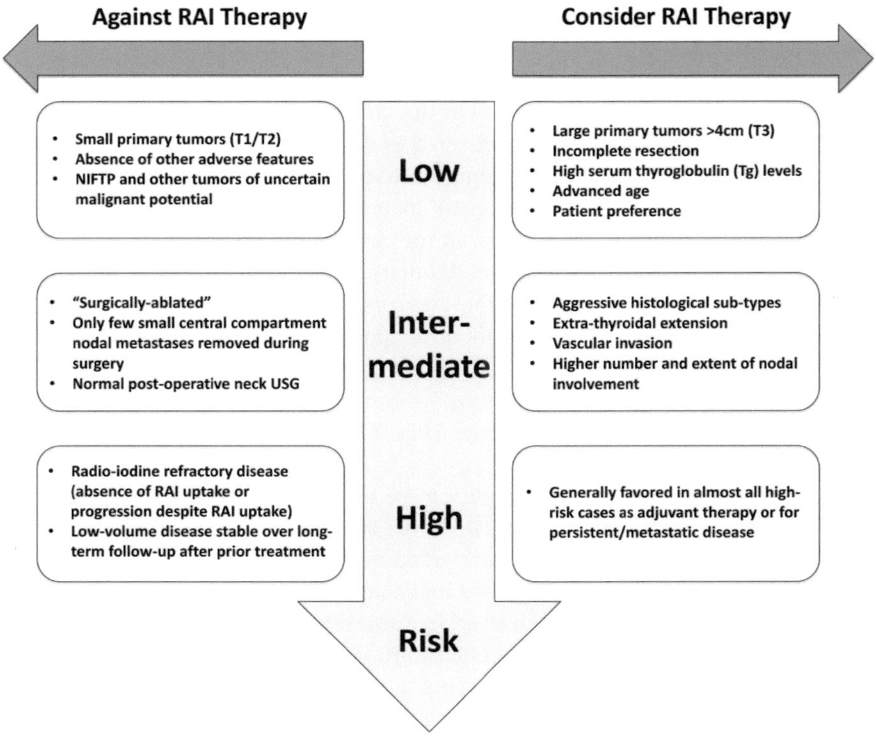

Fig. 14.2 Individual patient and tumor characteristics that guide use of radioiodine (RAI) therapy in different risk categories of thyroid cancer

References

1. Bray F, Laversanne M, Sung H, et al. Global cancer statistics 2022: GLOBOCAN estimates of incidence and mortality worldwide for 36 cancers in 185 countries. CA Cancer J Clin. 2024;74(3):229–63.
2. Sajisevi M, Caulley L, Eskander A, et al. Evaluating the rising incidence of thyroid cancer and thyroid nodule detection modes: a multinational, multi-institutional analysis. JAMA Otolaryngol Head Neck Surg. 2022;148(9):811–8.
3. Davies L, Welch HG. Thyroid cancer survival in the United States: observational data from 1973 to 2005. Arch Otolaryngol Head Neck Surg. 2010;136(5):440–4.
4. Greenspan BS, Hofman MS, Buscombe J. The accomplishments and legacy of Saul Hertz, MD. J Nucl Med. 2024;65(4):659–63.
5. Haugen BR, Alexander EK, Bible KC, et al. 2015 American Thyroid Association management guidelines for adult patients with thyroid nodules and differentiated thyroid cancer: the American Thyroid Association guidelines task force on thyroid nodules and differentiated thyroid cancer. Thyroid. 2016;26(1):1–133.
6. Tuttle RM, Ahuja S, Avram AM, et al. Controversies, consensus, and collaboration in the use of ^{131}I therapy in differentiated thyroid cancer: a joint statement from the American Thyroid Association, the European Association of Nuclear Medicine, the Society of Nuclear Medicine and Molecular Imaging, and the European Thyroid Association. Thyroid. 2019;29(4):461–70.

7. Buscombe J. Controversies in the radioiodine treatment of patients with differentiated thyroid cancer. Semin Nucl Med. 2023;53(4):475–80.
8. Leboulleux S, Bournaud C, Chougnet CN, et al. Thyroidectomy without radioiodine in patients with low-risk thyroid cancer. N Engl J Med. 2022;386(10):923–32.
9. Satapathy S, Tupalli A, Chandekar KR, Ballal S, Bal C. Radioiodine versus no radioiodine outcomes in low-risk differentiated thyroid cancers: a propensity-score matched analysis. Clin Endocrinol (Oxf). 2023;99(5):483–91.
10. Kim SK, Woo JW, Lee JH, et al. Radioactive iodine ablation may not decrease the risk of recurrence in intermediate-risk papillary thyroid carcinoma. Endocrine-Related Cancer. 2016;23(5):367–76.
11. Tuttle RM. Controversial issues in thyroid cancer management. J Nucl Med. 2018;59(8):1187–94.
12. Baloch ZW, Asa SL, Barletta JA, et al. Overview of the 2022 WHO classification of thyroid neoplasms. Endocr Pathol. 2022;33(1):27–63.
13. Kim MJ, Moon JH, Lee EK, et al. Active surveillance for low-risk thyroid cancers: a review of current practice guidelines. Endocrinol Metab (Seoul). 2024;39(1):47–60.
14. Indrasena BS. Use of thyroglobulin as a tumour marker. World J Biol Chem. 2017;8(1):81–5.
15. Bal C, Padhy AK, Jana S, Pant GS, Basu AK. Prospective randomized clinical trial to evaluate the optimal dose of 131 I for remnant ablation in patients with differentiated thyroid carcinoma. Cancer. 1996;77(12):2574–80.
16. Bal CS, Kumar A, Pant GS. Radioiodine dose for remnant ablation in differentiated thyroid carcinoma: a randomized clinical trial in 509 patients. J Clin Endocrinol Metab. 2004;89(4):1666–73.
17. Mallick U, Harmer C, Yap B, et al. Ablation with low-dose radioiodine and thyrotropin alfa in thyroid cancer. N Engl J Med. 2012;366(18):1674–85.
18. Schlumberger M, Catargi B, Borget I, et al. Strategies of radioiodine ablation in patients with low-risk thyroid cancer. N Engl J Med. 2012;366(18):1663–73.
19. Schlumberger M, Leboulleux S, Catargi B, et al. Outcome after ablation in patients with low-risk thyroid cancer (ESTIMABL1): 5-year follow-up results of a randomised, phase 3, equivalence trial. Lancet Diabetes Endocrinol. 2018;6(8):618–26.
20. Dehbi HM, Mallick U, Wadsley J, Newbold K, Harmer C, Hackshaw A. Recurrence after low-dose radioiodine ablation and recombinant human thyroid-stimulating hormone for differentiated thyroid cancer (HiLo): long-term results of an open-label, non-inferiority randomised controlled trial. Lancet Diabetes Endocrinol. 2019;7(1):44–51.
21. Pacini F, Fuhrer D, Elisei R, et al. 2022 ETA consensus statement: what are the indications for post-surgical radioiodine therapy in differentiated thyroid cancer? Eur Thyroid J. 2022;11(1):e210046.
22. Schvartz C, Bonnetain F, Dabakuyo S, et al. Impact on overall survival of radioactive iodine in low-risk differentiated thyroid cancer patients. J Clin Endocrinol Metab. 2012;97(5):1526–35.
23. Carhill AA, Litofsky DR, Ross DS, et al. Long-term outcomes following therapy in differentiated thyroid carcinoma: NTCTCS registry analysis 1987-2012. J Clin Endocrinol Metab. 2015;100(9):3270–9.
24. Wang X, Zhu J, Li Z, Wei T. The benefits of radioactive iodine ablation for patients with intermediate-risk papillary thyroid cancer. PLoS One. 2020;15(6):e0234843.
25. Tian T, Qi Z, Huang S, Wang H, Huang R. Radioactive iodine therapy decreases the recurrence of intermediate-risk PTC with low thyroglobulin levels. J Clin Endocrinol Metab. 2023;108(8):2033–41.
26. Chandekar KR, Satapathy S, Bal C. Impact of radioiodine therapy on recurrence and survival outcomes in intermediate-risk papillary thyroid carcinoma -a systematic review and meta-analysis. Clin Endocrinol (Oxf). 2024;100(2):181–91.
27. Ballal S, Soundararajan R, Garg A, Chopra S, Bal C. Intermediate-risk differentiated thyroid carcinoma patients who were surgically ablated do not need adjuvant radioiodine therapy: long-term outcome study. Clin Endocrinol (Oxf). 2016;84(3):408–16.

28. Zhao H, Gong Y. Radioactive iodine in low- to intermediate-risk papillary thyroid cancer. Front Endocrinol (Lausanne). 2022;13:960682.
29. Ruel E, Thomas S, Dinan M, Perkins JM, Roman SA, Sosa JA. Adjuvant radioactive iodine therapy is associated with improved survival for patients with intermediate-risk papillary thyroid cancer. J Clin Endocrinol Metab. 2015;100(4):1529–36.
30. Tang J, Kong D, Cui Q, et al. The role of radioactive iodine therapy in papillary thyroid cancer: an observational study based on SEER. Onco Targets Ther. 2018;11:3551–60.
31. Rubino C, de Vathaire F, Dottorini ME, et al. Second primary malignancies in thyroid cancer patients. Br J Cancer. 2003;89(9):1638–44.
32. Yu CY, Saeed O, Goldberg AS, et al. A systematic review and meta-analysis of subsequent malignant neoplasm risk after radioactive iodine treatment of thyroid cancer. Thyroid. 2018;28(12):1662–73.
33. Reinecke MJ, Ahlers G, Burchert A, et al. Second primary malignancies induced by radioactive iodine treatment of differentiated thyroid carcinoma - a critical review and evaluation of the existing evidence. Eur J Nucl Med Mol Imaging. 2022;49(9):3247–56.
34. Pasqual E, Schonfeld S, Morton LM, et al. Association between radioactive iodine treatment for pediatric and young adulthood differentiated thyroid cancer and risk of second primary malignancies [published correction appears in J ClinOncol. 2022 Jul 10;40(20):2283. 10.1200/JCO.22.01222]. J ClinOncol. 2022;40(13):1439–49.
35. Durante C, Haddy N, Baudin E, et al. Long-term outcome of 444 patients with distant metastases from papillary and follicular thyroid carcinoma: benefits and limits of radioiodine therapy. J Clin Endocrinol Metab. 2006;91(8):2892–9.
36. Alexander C, Bader JB, Schaefer A, Finke C, Kirsch CM. Intermediate and long-term side effects of high-dose radioiodine therapy for thyroid carcinoma. J Nucl Med. 1998;39(9):1551–4.
37. Prinsen HT, Klein Hesselink EN, Brouwers AH, et al. Bone marrow function after (131) I therapy in patients with differentiated thyroid carcinoma. J Clin Endocrinol Metab. 2015;100(10):3911–7.
38. Brose MS, Nutting CM, Jarzab B, et al. Sorafenib in radioactive iodine-refractory, locally advanced or metastatic differentiated thyroid cancer: a randomised, double-blind, phase 3 trial. Lancet. 2014;384(9940):319–28.
39. Schlumberger M, Tahara M, Wirth LJ, et al. Lenvatinib versus placebo in radioiodine-refractory thyroid cancer. N Engl J Med. 2015;372(7):621–30.
40. Bharadwaj MS, Ballal S, Bal C. Optimal cumulative I-131 activity in metastatic differentiated thyroid cancer: balancing efficacy and adverse events. J Clin Endocrinol Metab. 2024;109(11):e2120–30.
41. Mayson SE, Chan CM, Haugen BR. Tailoring the approach to radioactive iodine treatment in thyroid cancer. Endocr Relat Cancer. 2021;28(10):T125–40.
42. Shinohara S, Kikuchi M, Suehiro A, et al. Characteristics and prognosis of patients with thyroglobulin-positive and radioactive iodine whole-body scan-negative differentiated thyroid carcinoma. Jpn J Clin Oncol. 2015;45(5):427–32.
43. Vijayan R, Palaniswamy SS, Vadayath UM, Nair V, Kumar H. Clinicopathological features and outcome of thyroglobulin elevation and negative iodine scintigraphy (TENIS) patients with negative neck ultrasound: experience from a thyroid carcinoma clinic in India. World J Nucl Med. 2021;20(4):361–8.
44. Donohoe KJ, Aloff J, Avram AM, et al. Appropriate use criteria for nuclear medicine in the evaluation and treatment of differentiated thyroid cancer. J Nucl Med. 2020;61(3):375–96.
45. de Keizer B, Koppeschaar HP, Zelissen PM, et al. Efficacy of high therapeutic doses of iodine-131 in patients with differentiated thyroid cancer and detectable serum thyroglobulin. Eur J Nucl Med. 2001;28(2):198–202.
46. Chandekar KR, Satapathy S, Bal C. Positron emission tomography/computed tomography in thyroid cancer: an updated review. PET Clin. 2024;19(2):131–45.
47. Fatourechi V, Hay ID, Javedan H, Wiseman GA, Mullan BP, Gorman CA. Lack of impact of radioiodine therapy in tg-positive, diagnostic whole-body scan-negative patients with follicular cell-derived thyroid cancer. J Clin Endocrinol Metab. 2002;87(4):1521–6.

48. Koh JM, Kim ES, Ryu JS, Hong SJ, Kim WB, Shong YK. Effects of therapeutic doses of 131I in thyroid papillary carcinoma patients with elevated thyroglobulin level and negative 131I whole-body scan: comparative study. Clin Endocrinol (Oxf). 2003;58(4):421–7.
49. Sabra MM, Grewal RK, Tala H, Larson SM, Tuttle RM. Clinical outcomes following empiric radioiodine therapy in patients with structurally identifiable metastatic follicular cell-derived thyroid carcinoma with negative diagnostic but positive post-therapy 131I whole-body scans. Thyroid. 2012;22(9):877–83.
50. Tramontin MY, Nobre GM, Lopes M, et al. High thyroglobulin and negative whole-body scan: no long-term benefit of empiric radioiodine therapy. Endocrine. 2021;73(2):398–406.
51. Piscopo L, Zampella E, Volpe F, et al. Efficacy of empirical radioiodine therapy in patients with differentiated thyroid cancer and elevated serum thyroglobulin without evidence of structural disease: a propensity score analysis. Cancers (Basel). 2023;15(16):4196.
52. Kim K, Hong CM, Ha M, et al. Efficacy of empirical 131 I radioiodine therapy in well-differentiated thyroid carcinoma patients with thyroglobulin-elevated negative iodine scintigraphy syndrome : a systematic review and meta-analysis. Clin Nucl Med. 2024;49(8):741–7.
53. Schlumberger M, Arcangioli O, Piekarski JD, Tubiana M, Parmentier C. Detection and treatment of lung metastases of differentiated thyroid carcinoma in patients with normal chest X-rays. J Nucl Med. 1988;29(11):1790–4.
54. Pacini F, Agate L, Elisei R, et al. Outcome of differentiated thyroid cancer with detectable serum Tg and negative diagnostic (131)I whole body scan: comparison of patients treated with high (131)I activities versus untreated patients. J Clin Endocrinol Metab. 2001;86(9):4092–7.
55. Schmidt A, Iglesias L, Klain M, Pitoia F, Schlumberger MJ. Radioactive iodine-refractory differentiated thyroid cancer: an uncommon but challenging situation. Arch Endocrinol Metab. 2017;61(1):81–9.
56. Volpe F, Nappi C, Zampella E, et al. Current advances in radioactive iodine-refractory differentiated thyroid cancer. Curr Oncol. 2024;31(7):3870–84.
57. Liu J, Liu R, Shen X, Zhu G, Li B, Xing M. The genetic duet of *BRAF* V600E and *TERT* promoter mutations robustly predicts loss of radioiodine avidity in recurrent papillary thyroid cancer. J Nucl Med. 2020;61(2):177–82.
58. Stegenga MT, van Velsen EFS, Oudijk L, et al. Clinical and histopathological risk factors for radioactive iodine-refractory follicular and oncocytic thyroid carcinoma. J Clin Endocrinol Metab. 2024;109(12):e2334–41.
59. Schlumberger M, Brose M, Elisei R, et al. Definition and management of radioactive iodine-refractory differentiated thyroid cancer. Lancet Diabetes Endocrinol. 2014;2(5):356–8.
60. Kiyota N, Robinson B, Shah M, et al. Defining radioiodine-refractory differentiated thyroid cancer: efficacy and safety of Lenvatinib by radioiodine-refractory criteria in the SELECT trial. Thyroid. 2017;27(9):1135–41.
61. Karapanou O, Simeakis G, Vlassopoulou B, Alevizaki M, Saltiki K. Advanced RAI-refractory thyroid cancer: an update on treatment perspectives. Endocr Relat Cancer. 2022;29(5):R57–66.
62. Aashiq M, Silverman DA, Na'ara S, Takahashi H, Amit M. Radioiodine-refractory thyroid cancer: molecular basis of redifferentiation therapies, management, and novel therapies. Cancers (Basel). 2019;11(9):1382.
63. Laschinsky C, Theurer S, Herold T, et al. Molecular markers are associated with onset of radioiodine refractoriness in patients with papillary thyroid carcinoma. J Nucl Med. 2023;64(12):1865–8.
64. McDougall IR, Iagaru A. Thyroid stunning: fact or fiction? Semin Nucl Med. 2011;41(2):105–12.
65. Jeevanram RK, Shah DH, Sharma SM, Ganatra RD. Influence of initial large dose on subsequent uptake of therapeutic radioiodine in thyroid cancer patients. Int J Rad Appl Instrum B. 1986;13(3):277–9.
66. Park HM, Perkins OW, Edmondson JW, Schnute RB, Manatunga A. Influence of diagnostic radioiodines on the uptake of ablative dose of iodine-131. Thyroid. 1994;4(1):49–54.
67. Cholewinski SP, Yoo KS, Klieger PS, O'Mara RE. Absence of thyroid stunning after diagnostic whole-body scanning with 185 MBq 131I. J Nucl Med. 2000;41(7):1198–202.

68. McDougall IR. 74 MBq radioiodine 131I does not prevent uptake of therapeutic doses of 131I (i.e. it does not cause stunning) in differentiated thyroid cancer. Nucl Med Commun. 1997;18(6):505–12.
69. Nordén MM, Larsson F, Tedelind S, et al. Down-regulation of the sodium/iodide symporter explains 131I-induced thyroid stunning. Cancer Res. 2007;67(15):7512–7.
70. Morris LF, Waxman AD, Braunstein GD. The nonimpact of thyroid stunning: remnant ablation rates in 131I-scanned and nonscanned individuals. J Clin Endocrinol Metab. 2001;86(8):3507–11.
71. Dam HQ, Kim SM, Lin HC, Intenzo CM. 131I therapeutic efficacy is not influenced by stunning after diagnostic whole-body scanning. Radiology. 2004;232(2):527–33.
72. Van Nostrand D, Atkins F, Yeganeh F, Acio E, Bursaw R, Wartofsky L. Dosimetrically determined doses of radioiodine for the treatment of metastatic thyroid carcinoma. Thyroid. 2002;12(2):121–34.
73. Kumar P, Damle NA, Bal C. Radioiodine therapy in pediatric differentiated thyroid cancer: dosimetry, clinical care, and future challenges. Clin Nucl Med. 2023;48(2):158–67.
74. Song H, He B, Prideaux A, et al. Lung dosimetry for radioiodine treatment planning in the case of diffuse lung metastases. J Nucl Med. 2006;47(12):1985–94.
75. Holst JP, Burman KD, Atkins F, Umans JG, Jonklaas J. Radioiodine therapy for thyroid cancer and hyperthyroidism in patients with end-stage renal disease on hemodialysis. Thyroid. 2005;15(12):1321–31.
76. Van Nostrand D, Atkins F, Moreau S, et al. Utility of the radioiodine whole-body retention at 48 hours for modifying empiric activity of 131-iodine for the treatment of metastatic well-differentiated thyroid carcinoma. Thyroid. 2009;19(10):1093–8.
77. Maxon HR, Thomas SR, Hertzberg VS, et al. Relation between effective radiation dose and outcome of radioiodine therapy for thyroid cancer. N Engl J Med. 1983;309(16):937–41.
78. Jentzen W, Freudenberg L, Eising EG, Sonnenschein W, Knust J, Bockisch A. Optimized 124I PET dosimetry protocol for radioiodine therapy of differentiated thyroid cancer. J Nucl Med. 2008;49(6):1017–23.
79. Benua RS, Cicale NR, Sonenberg M, Rawson RW. The relation of radioiodine dosimetry to results and complications in the treatment of metastatic thyroid cancer. Am J Roentgenol Radium Ther Nucl Med. 1962;87:171–82.
80. Kulkarni K, Van Nostrand D, Atkins F, Aiken M, Burman K, Wartofsky L. The relative frequency in which empiric dosages of radioiodine would potentially overtreat or undertreat patients who have metastatic well-differentiated thyroid cancer. Thyroid. 2006;16(10):1019–23.
81. Tuttle RM, Leboeuf R, Robbins RJ, et al. Empiric radioactive iodine dosing regimens frequently exceed maximum tolerated activity levels in elderly patients with thyroid cancer [published correction appears in J Nucl Med. 2007 Jan;48(1):7]. J Nucl Med. 2006;47(10):1587–91.
82. Klubo-Gwiezdzinska J, Van Nostrand D, Atkins F, et al. Efficacy of dosimetric versus empiric prescribed activity of 131I for therapy of differentiated thyroid cancer. J Clin Endocrinol Metab. 2011;96(10):3217–25.

External Beam Radiation Therapy in Thyroid Cancer

15

Sarbani Ghosh Laskar, Anuj Kumar, Shwetabh Sinha, and Samarpita Mohanty

Editorial

Thyroid cancers are a surgical disease. Most resectable cancers in the younger population have a good prognosis and have a 99% 20-year survival. The other extreme where the tumours are of a higher grade, those that do not respond to radioiodine and those that are not amenable to complete surgery might benefit from external beam radiation therapy. These cases are few, but merit discussion on the utility of radiation in thyroid cancers as they are a different entity both in terms of pathology and effectiveness.

The authors have highlighted several guidelines that formulated indications for the same. In light of the new developments, EBRT might take a further back seat. The indications for radiation today might evolve to molecular pathology and targeted therapy, redifferentiation and surgical resection following therapy. Radiation therapy is more beneficial in skeletal metastasis prior to surgery, preventing symptoms due to oedema developing during the period of thyroxin withdrawal.

Radiotherapy in the adjuvant therapy should be considered with caution and with a multidisciplinary decision since subsequent surgery in the neck might become difficult. Outcomes in ongoing trials will emerge and only time will tell how the indications evolve.

Prathamesh S. Pai.

S. G. Laskar (✉)
Department of Radiation Oncology & Head & Neck Disease Management Group, Tata Memorial Hospital & Homi Bhabha National Institute, Tata Memorial Centre, Mumbai, Maharashtra, India

A. Kumar · S. Sinha · S. Mohanty
Department of Radiation Oncology & Head & Neck Disease Management Group, Advanced Centre for Treatment, Research and Education in Cancer (ACTREC) & Homi Bhabha National Institute, Tata Memorial Centre, Mumbai, Maharashtra, India

P. S. Pai et al. (eds.), *Controversies in Cancer of the Thyroid and Parathyroid Glands*, https://doi.org/10.1007/978-3-032-13130-0_15

Introduction

Thyroid cancer, comprising various histological subtypes, is primarily managed through surgical resection and radioactive iodine (RAI) therapy [1]. However, in cases with unresectable disease, RAI-refractory tumours, aggressive biological behaviour and/or anaplastic cancers, external beam radiation therapy (EBRT) becomes an essential adjunct to enhance locoregional control [2]. This chapter explores the role of EBRT in thyroid cancer, covering its indications, advanced radiation techniques and guideline-based application. Given the scarcity of randomised trial data, most recommendations are derived from retrospective studies, underscoring the complexities in applying EBRT across thyroid cancer subtypes [3–5]. Recent advancements, including intensity-modulated radiation therapy (IMRT) and proton therapy, have improved targeting accuracy, thereby minimising radiation exposure to surrounding healthy structures [6–8]. This chapter aims to provide an evidence-based perspective on the optimal application of EBRT to maximise patient outcomes while minimising risks.

Anatomical Considerations and Patterns of Spread

The thyroid gland is located at the C5-T1 level, close to several critical structures, including the trachea, oesophagus and carotid arteries. Careful planning in EBRT is essential to minimise radiation exposure to adjacent structures and prevent adverse effects. The thyroid gland's lymphatic drainage primarily begins in the central compartment (Level VI) and can extend to lateral cervical nodes (Levels II–V) in advanced cases, necessitating meticulous EBRT planning to address potential nodal involvement [9, 10]. Understanding patterns of distant metastasis is essential, as lung and bone metastases are common in advanced thyroid cancers, while brain and liver involvement is rare. Such knowledge guides treatment planning, particularly for high-risk or metastatic disease where systemic therapies may be used alongside EBRT to control locoregional disease [11].

Staging and Classification of Thyroid Cancer

The American Joint Committee on Cancer (AJCC) TNM staging system, based on tumour size (T), nodal involvement (N) and metastasis (M), provides a standardised framework for assessing thyroid cancer [12]. Specific histological subtypes influence the role of EBRT:

Differentiated thyroid carcinoma (DTC): Comprising papillary and follicular cancers, DTC generally responds well to RAI therapy. EBRT is reserved for high-risk cases, including those with extensive extrathyroidal extension, recurrent disease or RAI-refractory tumours, as it offers additional locoregional control.

The role of age is also an important consideration while considering adjuvant EBRT.

Medullary thyroid carcinoma (MTC): Originating from parafollicular C cells, MTC does not take up RAI, making EBRT critical in unresectable disease, or for residual disease after surgery, particularly in cases with a high risk of locoregional recurrence or extensive nodal involvement.

Anaplastic thyroid carcinoma (ATC): As the most aggressive thyroid cancer subtype, ATC has a poor prognosis with rapid local and distant progression. EBRT is primarily used for palliation in ATC to relieve symptoms such as airway obstruction, dysphagia and painful metastases, especially when other treatment options are limited. In cases that have undergone complete resection, adjuvant EBRT with concurrent chemotherapy is usually recommended.

Poorly differentiated thyroid carcinoma (PDTC): Intermediate in aggressiveness between DTC and ATC, PDTC often requires a multimodal approach, integrating EBRT with surgery and RAI/systemic therapy for locoregional control.

Indications for External Beam Radiotherapy in Thyroid Cancer [13]

EBRT is indicated in specific clinical scenarios as follows:

1. **Radical treatment**

   Unresectable tumours without RAI uptake: EBRT serves as a primary treatment for unresectable thyroid cancers that lack RAI uptake, particularly in aggressive cases like ATC. The goal is local control, given that other treatment options may be inadequate.

   Unresectable bulky tumours with RAI uptake: In bulky, unresectable tumours, EBRT can be combined with RAI to achieve locoregional control, aiming to reduce tumour size and limit disease progression.

2. **Adjuvant treatment**

   Gross tumour invasion detected during surgery: For extensive local invasion identified intraoperatively, EBRT is recommended to target residual microscopic or macroscopic disease, particularly for tumours unresponsive to RAI.

   Extensive pT4 disease in older patients: For patients over 60 with extensive pT4 disease (extrathyroidal extension), EBRT is indicated to reduce recurrence risk and improve locoregional control.

   Recurrent disease uncontrolled by surgery and RAI: High-dose EBRT is considered for recurrent disease when surgery or RAI is ineffective, especially in cases of persistent or recurrent neck involvement.

   RAI-refractory tumours with adverse pathological features: For RAI-non-avid differentiated thyroid cancers with high-risk features (e.g. extensive nodal involvement or extrathyroidal extension), adjuvant EBRT offers locoregional control, reducing the risk of recurrence.

3. **Palliative treatment**

   Symptomatic bone metastases: For symptomatic bone metastases not controlled by RAI, EBRT provides pain relief and helps prevent fractures.

   Spinal cord compression: EBRT is indicated with surgical stabilisation to alleviate spinal compression and prevent neurological complications.

   Cerebral metastases: For brain metastases, EBRT (often stereotactic radiosurgery or whole-brain radiotherapy) helps control intracranial disease and alleviates symptoms.

   Locoregional symptoms due to tumour growth: EBRT can relieve specific symptoms such as airway obstruction (stridor), swallowing difficulty (dysphagia), superior vena cava obstruction and bleeding in tumours prone to haemorrhage.

Guideline Overview for EBRT in Thyroid Cancer

American Thyroid Association (ATA) Guidelines for DTC [14]

Adjuvant RT: The use of adjuvant EBRT in DTC patients is controversial, with no strong support for routine use post-thyroidectomy. However, in patients over 60 years with extrathyroidal extension and no gross residual disease, EBRT may improve relapse-free and cause-specific survival [15–17]. Selective EBRT may also be considered for those undergoing frequent neck re-explorations for palliation of recurrent disease, weighing the risks of surgery against EBRT. Generally, EBRT is not recommended after complete tumour resection but may be considered for high-risk patients with aggressive histologic subtypes [4].

Invasive aerodigestive tract tumours: For tumours invading the aerodigestive tract, surgery combined with RAI and/or EBRT is advised. EBRT provides palliation in cases with airway compromise [3].

Distant metastases: Symptomatic distant metastases are managed with stereotactic radiation or thermal ablation (e.g. SBRT or RFA), especially if surgery is contraindicated. For CNS metastases, SRS may be considered, with RAI administered if there is uptake.

ATA Guidelines for ATC [18]

Adjuvant EBRT: After R0 or R1 resection, patients with good performance status, no metastatic disease and a preference for an aggressive approach should be offered standard fractionation IMRT alongside concurrent systemic therapy. Age over 60 years is linked to poorer outcomes, while younger age is considered a favourable prognostic factor in survival [19, 20].

Unresectable or residual disease: IMRT with systemic therapy is recommended for unresectable or residual ATC. BRAF/MEK inhibitors are considered for BRAFV600E mutation cases.

Timing of RT: Radiation should be started within 6 weeks post-surgery for maximising locoregional control.

Palliative RT for bone metastases: Palliative RT is recommended for symptomatic bone metastases. If structural integrity is compromised, orthopaedic fixation is advised before RT. Bisphosphonates or RANK ligand inhibitors are also recommended to support bone health.

British Thyroid Association (BTA) Guidelines [21]

High-risk cases: EBRT is generally avoided post-surgery unless there is significant residual or unresectable disease. It is recommended for high-risk differentiated thyroid cancer patients with gross residual or recurrent disease unmanageable by surgery or RAI, with IMRT used to enhance precision and locoregional control. Unlike ATA, BTA does not specify age as a factor in patient selection

Timing of EBRT: The timing of EBRT relative to RAI is unclear. Typically, EBRT is given post-RAI to prevent potential thyroid cell stunning effect. However, if residual disease threatens critical structures like the airway, EBRT may be prioritised before RAI to minimise RAI-induced complications.

MTC and ATC: EBRT is selectively used in MTC for locoregional control, while it is recommended in ATC, particularly in extensive or unresectable cases. However, unlike ATA, BTA does not use age-specific criteria for ATC or specify precise timing details for initiating EBRT.

AHNS (American Head and Neck Society) 2016 Guidelines [22]

Gross residual disease: Both AHNS and ATA recommend EBRT for patients with gross residual or unresectable disease. AHNS, however, provides specific dosing guidance, suggesting IMRT doses over 60 Gy for long-term control, while ATA does not set a specific dose.

Adjuvant EBRT for high-risk patients: In patients over 45 with a high likelihood of residual disease and poor RAI response, adjuvant EBRT may be indicated, particularly with extrathyroidal extension. This is similar to ATA's approach, although ATA applies an older threshold (age over 60) for high-risk DTC patients and sets an age-based prognostic criterion (age $\leq$ 65) specifically for ATC.

Cervical lymph node involvement: AHNS, like ATA, does not typically recommend EBRT solely for cervical lymph node involvement, unless additional high-risk features are present.

National Comprehensive Cancer Network (NCCN) Guidelines [23]

DTC-papillary and follicular carcinoma: NCCN aligns with ATA for considering EBRT in patients with gross unresectable disease or rapid progression threatening vital structures. RAI-refractory cases also benefit from EBRT for local control.

MTC: NCCN, like ATA, advises EBRT for residual or recurrent disease post-surgery, especially in high-risk cases prone to recurrence.

ATC: Given ATC's aggressive nature, EBRT is essential for palliative treatment and symptom relief in unresectable cases, often integrated with systemic therapy. While similar to ATA's approach, NCCN does not include age-related prognostic considerations or specific timing recommendations for EBRT initiation, as recommended by ATA.

Scoring Systems for EBRT in Differentiated Thyroid Carcinoma (DTC)

Billan et al. proposed a scoring system for EBRT in DTC to provide a systematic framework for evaluating patients who may benefit from EBRT [24]. This scoring system incorporates multiple clinical and pathological factors, including patient age, tumour resectability, presence of extrathyroidal disease, extent of nodal involvement and histological subtype, among others. Each factor is assigned a point value based on its association with higher recurrence risk or adverse prognosis in DTC. The cumulative score helps guide clinicians on whether EBRT should be considered or is strongly recommended, offering a more tailored approach for high-risk DTC cases where traditional treatments, like surgery and radioiodine, may not be fully effective. A total score greater than 4 suggests that EBRT should be considered as a potential treatment option and discussed with the patient. A score exceeding 6 indicates a strong recommendation for EBRT, as it reflects a higher risk profile where additional therapy may be beneficial. Table 15.1 demonstrates the criteria and corresponding point values from the scoring system.

Table 15.1 Scoring criteria for EBRT in DTC [Billian et al.]

Criteria	0 points	1 point	2 points	4 points
Age	<45 years	45–60 years	>60 years	
Gender	Female	Male		
Resectability	Resectable			Unresectable
Extensive extra-capsular nodal spread	No		Yes	
Extra-thyroidal disease	T3		T4	
Surgical margins (R0, R1, R2)	R0		R1	R2
Histological variants	Common variants		Aggressive variants (e.g. tall cell and Hürthle cell)	
Recurrent disease	No		Yes	
Tumours with radioiodine fixation	Yes		No	

Table 15.2 Scoring criteria for EBRT in DTC [Sun et al.]

Criteria	0 points	1 point	2 points	4 points
Age	<45	45–60	>60	–
Gender	Female	Male	–	–
Resectability	Resectable	Unresectable	–	–
Extensive extracapsular nodal spread	No	Yes	–	–
Extrathyroidal disease	T3	T4	–	–
R0–R1–R2	R0	R1	R2	–
Histological variants (e.g. tall cell, Hürthle cell, columnar, diffuse sclerosing and solid variant)	No	Yes	–	–
Recurrent disease (risk of recurrent nerve damage, etc.)	No	Yes	–	–
Tumours with radioiodine fixation	Yes	No	–	–

In another scoring system developed by Sun et al., EBRT is recommended selectively for DTC patients with specific high-risk characteristics [25]. This system assigns scores based on factors such as patient age, gender, extent of disease, presence of extracapsular nodal spread, extrathyroidal extension, residual disease post-surgery, histologic subtype, recurrence status and radioiodine uptake. Higher scores indicate a greater likelihood that EBRT will provide locoregional control, especially for patients less responsive to other treatments like surgery and radioiodine therapy. This structured scoring method enables clinicians to make data-informed decisions about EBRT use based on individual risk profiles. Table 15.2 outlines the scoring criteria.

For patients with a score of 4–6, EBRT may be considered as part of the treatment plan, particularly in cases where other treatments may not provide adequate locoregional control. For patients scoring ≥6, EBRT is strongly recommended, as these individuals present with multiple high-risk factors indicating a greater likelihood that EBRT will significantly contribute to improved outcomes by minimising recurrence risks and enhancing locoregional disease management.

Planning for EBRT

In EBRT planning for thyroid cancers, precise patient positioning is critical for accurate radiation delivery and sparing of healthy tissues. Patients are positioned head first supine, with a neutral neck rest and arms by the side. A custom thermoplastic mask is used to immobilise the head and neck region, ensuring reproducibility and optimising tumour targeting while minimising exposure to non-target areas. Figure 15.1 illustrates a patient immobilised in a head-first supine position with a custom thermoplastic mask, ensuring precise and reproducible positioning for accurate radiation delivery in thyroid cancer treatment.

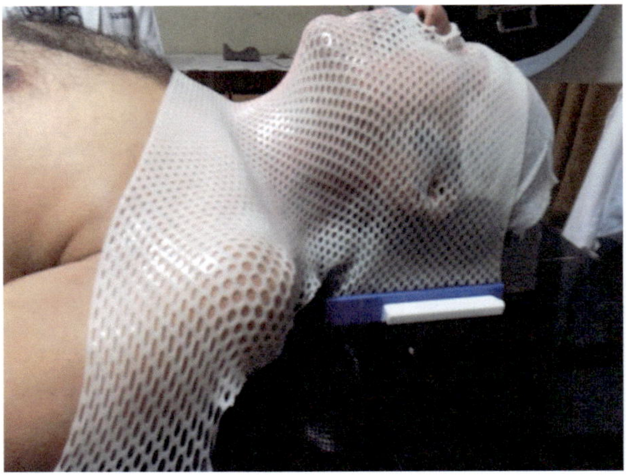

Fig. 15.1 Patient immobilisation with thermoplastic mask for EBRT planning

Table 15.3 Target volume definition for EBRT in thyroid cancer

Target area	Description
Thyroid bed	Primary volume extending from the hyoid bone to the sternal notch, covering the carotid sheaths and tracheoesophageal groove
Regional lymph nodes	Includes perithyroidal, paratracheal, pretracheal, superior mediastinum and cervical lymph nodes in the presence of nodal involvement

Target Volumes

In EBRT for thyroid cancer, defining target volumes is essential for effective locoregional control while sparing nearby structures. The primary focus is the thyroid bed, extending from the hyoid bone to the sternal notch, including the carotid sheath and tracheoesophageal groove. When there is suspected or confirmed nodal involvement, regional lymph nodes such as the perithyroidal, paratracheal, pretracheal, superior mediastinum and cervical nodes may also be included based on the patient's risk profile and disease extent. Table 15.3 demonstrates target volumes for EBRT planning.

Radiation Technique

Previously, conventional radiotherapy techniques were commonly used to treat thyroid cancer. However, these techniques had limitations, including less precision in targeting the tumour, resulting in greater exposure of surrounding healthy tissues to radiation. This lack of specificity could lead to higher risks of side effects, especially to critical structures such as the spinal cord and parotid glands.

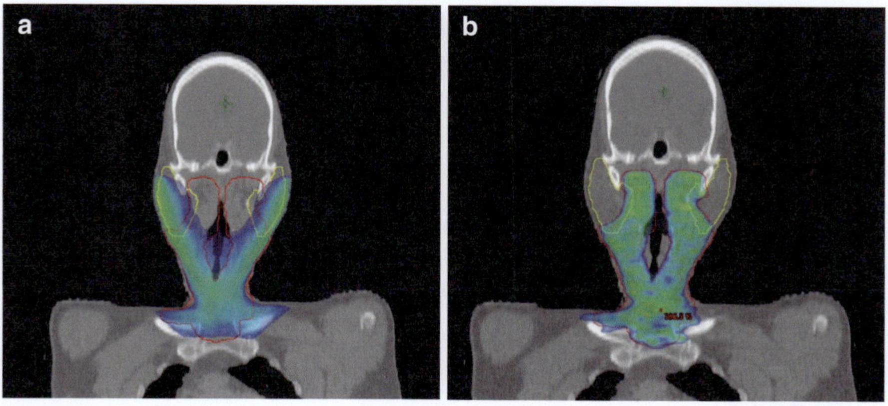

Fig. 15.2 Comparison of target dose coverage in (**a**) conventional radiotherapy and (**b**) IMRT planning

Intensity-modulated radiation therapy (IMRT) addresses these drawbacks by enabling highly precise radiation delivery to concave and irregularly shaped structures. IMRT enhances target volume coverage, allowing for focused radiation on the tumour site while significantly reducing exposure to nearby healthy tissues. The accompanying figure provides a comparison between conventional radiotherapy and IMRT, highlighting IMRT's advantage in concentrating radiation on the tumour and sparing surrounding tissues more effectively. Figure 15.2a and b illustrates the differences in target dose coverage between conventional radiotherapy and IMRT planning, highlighting the improved precision and tissue sparing achieved with IMRT.

Target Doses for EBRT

In EBRT for thyroid cancer, target doses are tailored to disease extent and risk of residual microscopic disease. A dose of 70 Gy is recommended for controlling visible tumour in areas with gross disease, while 66 Gy is designated for areas with positive margins or residual disease. For high-risk areas of microscopic disease, such as the thyroid bed, tracheoesophageal groove and Level VI nodes, 60 Gy is advised. Low-risk regions, including uninvolved lymph nodes in Levels II–V and VII, are recommended to receive 54 Gy to minimise exposure to healthy tissues. This dose distribution maximises treatment efficacy while reducing toxicity. Table 15.4 shows the target doses for EBRT planning.

Table 15.4 Target doses for EBRT in thyroid cancer

Target dose	Description
70 Gy	Gross disease
66 Gy	Areas with positive surgical margins
60 Gy	Areas with high risk of microscopic disease, including the thyroid bed, tracheoesophageal groove and Level VI cervical nodes
54 Gy	Areas with low risk of microscopic disease, including uninvolved Levels II–V and VII nodes

Toxicities with EBRT

Acute Toxicities

Skin: Erythema, dry desquamation, and in severe cases, moist desquamation

Mucositis and pharyngitis: Pain and discomfort due to inflammation in the oesophageal and laryngeal regions

Dysphagia: Swallowing difficulties resulting from radiation-induced mucosal irritation

Late Toxicities

Skin: Telangiectasias, pigmentation changes, and fibrosis

Xerostomia: Salivary gland damage resulting in chronic dry mouth

Oesophageal stricture: Long-term narrowing of the oesophagus, leading to chronic swallowing difficulties

Conclusion

EBRT is a selective yet valuable treatment modality for high-risk thyroid cancers. Factors such as age, resectability, RAI avidity and histological variants aid in patient selection. Structured scoring systems and evolving guidelines support decision-making, maximising benefits of EBRT while managing risks. Given the complexity of these cases, a multidisciplinary approach is essential for optimising patient selection and ensuring that potential benefits of EBRT are carefully weighed against the anticipated adverse effects. Randomised controlled trials are necessary to build a stronger evidence base, allowing for more precise recommendations and better integration of EBRT in the treatment paradigm for high-risk thyroid cancer patients.

References

1. Nguyen QT, Lee EJ, Huang MG, et al. Diagnosis and treatment of patients with thyroid cancer. Am Health Drug Benefits. 2015;8(1):30–40. PMID: 25964831; PMCID: PMC4415174
2. Powell C, Newbold K, Harrington KJ, Bhide SA, Nutting CM. External beam radiotherapy for differentiated thyroid cancer. Clin Oncol (R Coll Radiol). 2010;22(6):456–63. https://doi.org/10.1016/j.clon.2010.03.012.
3. Keum KC, Suh YG, Koom WS, et al. The role of postoperative external beam radiotherapy in the management of patients with papillary thyroid cancer invading the trachea. Int J Radiat Oncol Biol Phys. 2006;65(2):474–80. https://doi.org/10.1016/j.ijrobp.2005.12.010.
4. Brierley J, Tsang R, Panzarella T, Bana N. Prognostic factors and the effect of treatment with radioactive iodine and external beam radiation on patients with differentiated thyroid cancer seen at a single institution over 40 years. Clin Endocrinol. 2005;63(4):418–27.
5. Chow SM, Yau S, Kwan CK, Poon PC, Law SC. Local and regional control in patients with papillary thyroid carcinoma: specific indications of external radiotherapy and radioactive iodine according to T and N categories in AJCC 6th edition. Endocr Relat Cancer. 2006;13(4):1159–72.
6. Nutting CM, Convery DJ, Cosgrove VP, et al. Improvements in target coverage and reduced spinal cord irradiation using intensity-modulated radiotherapy (IMRT) in patients with carcinoma of the thyroid gland. Radiother Oncol. 2001;60(2):173–80.
7. Urbano TG, Clark CH, Hansen VN, et al. Intensity modulated radiotherapy (IMRT) in locally advanced thyroid cancer: acute toxicity results of a phase I study. Radiother Oncol. 2007;85(1):58–63.
8. Youssef I, Yoon J, Mohamed N, et al. Outcomes and toxicities of nonmedullary thyroid tumors treated with proton beam radiation therapy. Int J Part Ther. 2022;9(2):20–30. https://doi.org/10.14338/IJPT-22-00005.1.
9. Muulte KM. Central cervical lymph node metastases in papillary thyroid cancer: a systematic review of imaging-guided and prophylactic removal of the central compartment. Clin Endocrinol. 2012;76(1):131–6.
10. Lang BH, Wo KY, Lo CY. Impact of routine unilateral central neck dissection on preablative and postablative stimulated thyroglobulin levels after total thyroidectomy in papillary thyroid carcinoma. Ann Surg Oncol. 2012;19:60–7.
11. Duaddy N, Baudin E, Leboulleux S, et al. Long-term outcome of 444 patients with distant metastases from papillary and follicular thyroid carcinoma: benefits and limits of radioiodine therapy. J Clin Endocrinol Metab. 2006;91:2892–9.
12. Amin MB, Edge S, Greene F, et al. AJCC cancer staging manual. 8th ed. New York, NY: Springer; 2017.
13. Perros P. Report of the thyroid cancer guidelines update group. In: Guidelines for the management of thyroid cancer. 2nd ed. London: Royal College of Physicians; 2007.
14. Haugen BR, Alexander EK, Bible KC, et al. 2015 American Thyroid Association management guidelines for adult patients with thyroid nodules and differentiated thyroid cancer: the American Thyroid Association guidelines task force on thyroid nodules and differentiated thyroid cancer. Thyroid. 2016;26(1):1–133. https://doi.org/10.1089/thy.2015.0020.
15. Ford D, Giridharan S, McConkey C, et al. External beam radiotherapy in the management of differentiated thyroid cancer. Clin Oncol (R Coll Radiol). 2003;15(6):337–41.
16. Terezakis SA, Lee KS, Ghossein RA, et al. Role of external beam radiotherapy in patients with advanced or recurrent nonanaplastic thyroid cancer: Memorial Sloan-Kettering Cancer Center experience. Int J Radiat Oncol Biol Phys. 2009;73(3):795–801.
17. Chow SM, Law SC, Mendenhall WM, et al. Papillary thyroid carcinoma: prognostic factors and the role of radioiodine and external radiotherapy. Int J Radiat Oncol Biol Phys. 2002;52(3):784–95. https://doi.org/10.1016/s0360-3016(01)02686-4.

18. Bible KC, Kebebew E, Brierley J, et al. 2021 American Thyroid Association guidelines for management of patients with anaplastic thyroid cancer. Thyroid. 2021;31(3):337–86. https://doi.org/10.1089/thy.2020.0944.
19. Glaser SM, Mandish SF, Gill BS, et al. Anaplastic thyroid cancer: prognostic factors, patterns of care, and overall survival. Head Neck. 2016;38(Suppl 1):E2083.
20. Kim TY, Kim KW, Jung TS, et al. Prognostic factors for Korean patients with anaplastic thyroid carcinoma. Head Neck. 2007;29:765–72.
21. Perros P, Boelaert K, Colley S, et al. Guidelines for the management of thyroid cancer. Clin Endocrinol. 2014;81(Suppl 1):1–122. https://doi.org/10.1111/cen.12515.
22. Kiess AP, Agrawal N, Brierley JD, et al. External-beam radiotherapy for differentiated thyroid cancer locoregional control: a statement of the American Head and Neck Society. Head Neck. 2021;43(3):659–71. https://doi.org/10.1002/hed.24357.
23. National Comprehensive Cancer Network (NCCN). NCCN clinical practice guidelines in oncology: thyroid carcinoma. Version 1.2024. Published 2024. Accessed November 15, 2024. Available at: NCCN Guidelines.
24. Billan S, Charas T. External beam radiation in differentiated thyroid carcinoma. Rambam Maimonides Med J. 2016;7(1) https://doi.org/10.5041/RMMJ.10235.
25. Sun XS, Sun SR, Guevara N, et al. Indications of external beam radiation therapy in non-anaplastic thyroid cancer and impact of innovative radiation techniques. Crit Rev Oncol Hematol. 2013;86(1):52–68. https://doi.org/10.1016/j.critrevonc.2012.09.007.

Neoadjuvant Treatment of Thyroid Cancer

16

Amr H. Abdelhamid Ahmed, Marika D. Russell, and Gregory W. Randolph

Editorial

Thyroid cancers are a surgical disease!! This has been thus far the often-quoted comment that all trainees are ingrained with. A lot has transpired in the past decade with better understanding of the disease process of thyroid cancers. Pathology has undergone reclassification and at a molecular level, the thyroid cancer is better understood. High-grade cancers of the thyroid still have poor outcomes and surgery no longer may be enough and effective.

Chemotherapy and immunotherapy have taken major strides and are part of the discussions in multidisciplinary joint clinics and are part of the treatment guidelines in squamous cell head neck cancers. Likewise in thyroid cancers, there seems to be a role for these therapeutics.

Thyroid cancer is a spectrum of mutations. Literature is replete with further understating of the type mutation, be it BRAF or RET versus nonmutated pathology. Indolent differentiated cancers have excellent prognosis. On the other hand, poorly differentiated and anaplastic cancers have extremely poor outcomes especially in those that are not resectable. This chapter outlines the neoadjuvant approaches including targeted therapy and immunotherapy in improving survival outcomes, their combinations, duration of therapy, and potential benefits and risks. Neoadjuvant therapy has potential and it is for us to understand it and offer it to our patients.

Prathamesh S. Pai.

A. H. Abdelhamid Ahmed · M. D. Russell · G. W. Randolph (✉)
Division of Thyroid and Parathyroid Endocrine Surgery, Department of Otolaryngology-Head and Neck Surgery, Massachusetts Eye and Ear, Harvard Medical School, Boston, MA, USA
e-mail: amr_ahmed@meei.harvard.edu; mrussell20@meei.harvard.edu; Gregory_Randolph@meei.harvard.edu

P. S. Pai et al. (eds.), *Controversies in Cancer of the Thyroid and Parathyroid Glands*, https://doi.org/10.1007/978-3-032-13130-0_16

Molecular Mechanisms of Oncogenesis in Thyroid Cancer

Thyroid epithelial follicular cells give rise to several different subtypes of differentiated thyroid cancer (DTC), of which papillary thyroid carcinoma (PTC) is the most common. PTC may harbor driver mutations in *BRAF* (most frequently *BRAF V600E*) and *RAS* genes, or gene fusions involving *RET*, *NTRK*, *ALK*, or *ROS1*. Follicular thyroid carcinomas are frequently driven by fusions in *RAS*, *PPAR* gamma genes, or *PTEN* mutations. Oncocytic thyroid carcinoma (previously referred to as Hürthle cell carcinoma) demonstrates extensive mitochondrial DNA mutations and can also be associated with *RAS* mutations and *PPAR* gamma fusions [1, 2]. Dedifferentiation of these cancers can occur through accumulation of additional mutations as seen with poorly differentiated thyroid carcinoma (PDTC), which is characterized by additional mutations in *TP53*, *TERT* promoter, *NF1*, *PI3K/AKT/mTOR* pathway genes, and SWI/SNF chromatin remodeling genes (e.g., *SMARCA4* and *ARID1A*). The most aggressive dedifferentiated thyroid cancer is anaplastic thyroid carcinoma (ATC), which carries a poor prognosis, and the most common genetic alterations associated with ATC are mutations in *TP53*, *TERT* promoter, *BRAF*, *RAS*, and *PI3K-AKT* pathway genes among numerous other genetic alterations. Medullary thyroid carcinoma (MTC) does not originate from follicular cells but instead from parafollicular c-cells and can harbor *RET* or *RAS* mutations, or rarely *RAS* fusions [3].

Candidacy: Who Should Receive Neoadjuvant Treatment?

Determining patient candidacy for neoadjuvant therapy hinges on multiple factors, including tumor histology, molecular biomarkers, and disease extent. Neoadjuvant treatment for aggressive cancers such as *BRAF*-altered ATC can result in significant tumor shrinkage, which can lower the morbidity associated with surgical treatment and is associated with improved survival [4]. On the other hand, the impact of neoadjuvant therapy on surgical outcomes for advanced differentiated thyroid cancer is less clear. Currently, there is no accepted role for treatment of early-stage or small thyroid cancers. Presently, there is a critical need for clinical trials to establish treatment parameters and develop guidelines for use of neoadjuvant therapy in advanced thyroid cancer management.

Which Treatment to Give?

Advances in molecular testing have shown it to be of benefit for diagnostic and prognostic purposes and in guiding treatment strategies [5–7]. We will focus in this chapter on the following three general categories of systemic treatment: antiangiogenic therapies, oncogenic pathway inhibitors, and immunotherapy.

- Antiangiogenic therapies (multikinase inhibitors)
- Tumor growth in thyroid cancer often depends on angiogenesis. Multikinase inhibitors such as lenvatinib target tumor vasculature by inhibiting key pro-angiogenic signaling pathways, notably vascular endothelial growth factor (VEGF), FGF, and PDGF receptors. By blocking these pathways, new blood vessel formation is suppressed, effectively starving the tumor of nutrients. Additionally, some of these agents also inhibit oncogenic kinases (e.g., RET) in the tumor, directly curbing pro-growth signaling in cancer cells. This dual action—anti-vascular and direct tumor inhibition—underlies their therapeutic role in advanced, radioiodine-refractory thyroid carcinomas [8].
- Oncogenic pathway inhibitors (BRAF, RET, NTRK, RAS)
- *BRAF*, *RET*, *NTRK*, and *RAS* are major oncogenic drivers in thyroid tumorigenesis. Mutations or fusions in these genes constitutively activate growth signaling cascades (especially the MAPK pathway), leading to unchecked cell proliferation [9]. For example, the common *BRAF V600E* mutation in papillary thyroid carcinoma causes continuous MEK–ERK signaling; inhibitors like vemurafenib competitively block the mutant BRAF's ATP-binding site, thereby shutting down aberrant MAPK signaling [10]. Similarly, selective RET and TRK inhibitors inactivate oncogenic RET mutants or NTRK fusions, and RAS-driven tumors can be treated with downstream MEK pathway inhibitors. By disrupting these driver oncoproteins, targeted therapies halt their downstream signaling, suppress tumor growth, and induce tumor regression or redifferentiation.
- Immunotherapy strategies
- Immunotherapy aims to overcome tumor immune evasion in thyroid cancer. Immune checkpoint inhibitors—antibodies against PD-1/PD-L1 or CTLA—work by disrupting inhibitory signals that normally dampen T-cell responses. Blocking these checkpoints reinvigorates T lymphocytes to recognize and destroy tumor cells. This approach is being applied especially in aggressive or refractory thyroid cancers that express immune checkpoint ligands. Other immune-modulating strategies (e.g., tumor vaccines or T-cell therapies) are under exploration, but immune checkpoint blockade currently represents the primary immunotherapeutic avenue, leveraging the patient's immune system to attack the cancer [11].

BRAF-Mutated Anaplastic Thyroid Cancer

Anaplastic thyroid cancer (ATC) is an aggressive form of thyroid malignancy characterized by rapid progression and poor prognosis with limited treatment options [12]. Approximately 20–50% of ATC cases harbor the *BRAF V600E* mutation, which has become a critical target for therapy [13].

Treatment with combined BRAF and MEK inhibitors (dabrafenib and trametinib) has shown remarkable efficacy in this molecular subset, yielding high response rates and improved outcomes. In a phase II trial (NCT02034110), dabrafenib plus trametinib achieved an objective response rate of ~56% and a median overall survival of ~14.5 months in *BRAF V600E*-mutant ATC, far exceeding historical outcomes, and leading to FDA approval of this regimen for unresectable ATC [13, 14].

Accordingly, routine *BRAF V600E* testing in ATC and the use of dabrafenib and trametinib in *BRAF*-mutant cases—including as neoadjuvant therapy—can downstage locally advanced (stage IVA/IVB) disease and maintain disease control [13]. A large cohort study observed that patients who underwent surgery after BRAF-directed neoadjuvant therapy had a 94% 1-year survival, significantly higher than in those treated with other modalities [12].

Importantly, neoadjuvant BRAF/MEK inhibition can render initially inoperable tumors resectable. Wang et al. reported that preoperative dabrafenib plus trametinib enabled complete (R0) surgical resection in 100% of six patients with initially unresectable, *BRAF V600E*-positive ATC without requiring tracheostomy or other radical procedures for locoregional control. Pathologic examination of the resected specimens showed a dramatic response, with markedly decreased viable anaplastic carcinoma cells and only residual differentiated thyroid carcinoma components, reflecting intratumor heterogeneity. This neoadjuvant approach translated to prolonged survival: 6-month and 1-year survival rates were 100% and 83%, respectively, in the above series [4].

Despite these advances, emerging mechanisms of resistance to BRAF-targeted therapy in ATC—such as acquired secondary *RAS* mutations or upregulation of compensatory pathways—have been reported. This has prompted investigations of combination regimens to improve the durability of response [15].

Recent studies have explored the addition of immune checkpoint inhibitors, such as pembrolizumab (anti-PD-1 antibody), to the standard dabrafenib and trametinib regimen. The rationale is that targeted therapies may increase tumor antigen presentation and T-cell infiltration, potentially enhancing the efficacy of immunotherapy. A retrospective, single-center study suggested improved overall survival with the addition of pembrolizumab to combined dabrafenib and trametinib [16]. Ongoing clinical trials are further evaluating the efficacy and safety of combining BRAF/MEK inhibitors with immune checkpoint inhibitors in *BRAF*-mutated ATC. These studies aim to determine whether this combination can improve response rates and overall survival compared to targeted therapy alone. The emerging data support the potential role of immunotherapy in combination with targeted agents as a promising strategy for managing *BRAF*-mutated ATC.

BRAF-Wild-Type Anaplastic Thyroid Cancer

For patients with *BRAF*-wild-type (non-mutated) ATC, treatment options are more limited, and the prognosis remains poor, as *BRAF*-wild-type tumors lack FDA-approved targeted options [12, 17]. Recent studies have explored the use of targeted and immunotherapy to improve surgical outcomes and survival. The role of neoadjuvant therapy in this setting remains an active area of research.

Cabanillas et al. (NCT03181100) reported on the addition of anti-PD-L1 immunotherapy (atezolizumab) to tailored targeted therapy (vemurafenib/cobimetinib for cohort 1 of *BRAF V600E*-mutated ATC; cobimetinib for cohort 2 of *RAS* or *NF*-mutated ATC; or bevacizumab for cohort 3 of wild-type *BRAF/RAS/NF* ATC). The trial achieved a median overall survival of 19 months across the three cohorts, vastly exceeding historical outcomes [17]. Notably, the 19 patients enrolled in cohort 1 (*BRAF*-mutant ATC) had a median overall survival of 43 months (95% CI, 16 months—not estimable), while in the 21 patients enrolled in cohort 2 (*BRAF*-wild-type but had mutations in *RAS*, *NF1*, or *NF2*), it was 8.7 months (95% CI, 5.1–37.0). The three patients enrolled in the third cohort with *BRAF* wild type and no other identifiable mutations of significance had a median OS of just 6.2 months.

In NRG/RTOG 0912 trial, pazopanib plus cytotoxic chemotherapy (e.g., weekly paclitaxel) plus intensity-modulated radiation therapy (IMRT) showed no difference in overall survival compared to placebo plus chemoradiation [18].

The ATLEP trial tested a combination of lenvatinib/pembrolizumab and reported that the best overall response for patients with *BRAF*-wild-type ATC within two treatment years was partial response in 51.9% of patients (14/27) and stationary disease in 44.4% of patients (12/27) [19].

Few studies have examined the potential use of targeted and/or immunotherapy in *BRAF*-wild-type ATC in the neoadjuvant setting. A 2023 study reported on 4 weeks of neoadjuvant therapy with combined lenvatinib and pembrolizumab (an immune checkpoint inhibitor) for two patients with *BRAF*-wild-type ATC. Surgical resection was reconsidered only if re-staging showed a decrease in tumor size of more than 50%. Neoadjuvant therapy in these two patients induced a response sufficient to achieve local resectability in initially non-resectable ATC. Postoperative histopathological findings confirmed significant tumor necrosis or regressive fibrotic tissue, highlighting the potential of combining targeted therapy with immunotherapy to enhance treatment efficacy in *BRAF*-wild-type ATC [20].

Similarly, a retrospective series of six patients with metastatic *BRAF*-wild-type ATC who received a combined lenvatinib and pembrolizumab reported a complete response in four patients and a stable disease in one patient, with a median progression-free survival of 16.5 months [21]. All patients with long-term (>2 years) or complete responses had either increased TMB or a PD-L1 TPS of >50%, suggesting an immune-driven tumor clearance in some *BRAF*-wild-type ATCs.

Another case report reporting use of anti-PD-1 (camrelizumab) plus multikinase inhibitor (famitinib) regimen enabled complete resection of a locally advanced *BRAF*-wild-type ATC [22].

Beyond immunochemotherapy, neoadjuvant targeted therapies are being explored in *BRAF*-wild-type ATC harboring other oncogenic alterations: for example, ALK inhibitor crizotinib produced dramatic responses in ALK-rearranged ATC [23]. Additionally, RET inhibitors (selpercatinib and pralsetinib) showed efficacy in *RET*-fusion-positive cases. Collectively, these emerging neoadjuvant strategies—spanning conventional chemoradiation, immunotherapy, and targeted precision drugs—are facilitating tumor downstaging, enabling margin-negative resections, and enhancing locoregional disease control. Moreover, in early clinical trials, these therapies are markedly extending survival for patients with *BRAF*-wild-type ATC compared to historical outcomes. Continued research, including prospective trials, is needed to clarify optimal combinations and sequencing of neoadjuvant therapies in *BRAF*-wild-type ATC and to overcome resistance mechanisms.

BRAF-Mutated Differentiated Thyroid Cancer

Differentiated thyroid cancer (DTC) is generally associated with a favorable prognosis; however, a subset of patients presents with a locally advanced disease that is challenging to surgically manage. In cases where DTC harbors the *BRAF V600E* mutation, neoadjuvant therapy has been explored as a strategy to downstage tumors, thereby facilitating surgical resection and potentially improving outcomes.

A case report detailed the use of neoadjuvant targeted therapy with dabrafenib and trametinib in a patient with unresectable *BRAF V600E*-mutated locally invasive PTC (the most common subtype of DTC). The combination therapy led to significant tumor shrinkage, allowing for subsequent surgical resection. This approach underscores the potential of neoadjuvant targeted therapy to convert unresectable tumors into resectable ones, thereby enhancing the prospects for curative surgery [24]. Likewise, a recent report described a patient with recurrent, radioactive iodine-resistant PTC invading the larynx who was spared a total laryngectomy after neoadjuvant dabrafenib–trametinib dramatically reduced the tumor, permitting a less extensive partial laryngectomy and preservation of vocal function [25].

In addition to downstaging, neoadjuvant therapy with targeted BRAF and MEK inhibitors has emerged as a strategy to restore radioactive iodine (RAI) avidity in advanced differentiated thyroid cancers (DTC). *BRAF V600E*-mutated PTC may be associated with resistance to RAI therapy due to constitutive MAPK pathway activation that represses thyroid differentiation gene expression [26]. Thus, inhibiting the aberrant BRAF–MEK–ERK signaling (e.g., with the BRAF inhibitors vemurafenib or dabrafenib and the MEK inhibitor trametinib) can re-induce expression of the sodium–iodide symporter (NIS), thyroglobulin, and other iodine-handling proteins, thereby increasing iodine uptake. Clinically, multiple trials since 2015 demonstrate substantial efficacy of these agents in *BRAF V600E*-positive PTC. In a phase II study of metastatic RAI-refractory (RAI-R) PTC, vemurafenib yielded a 38.5% partial response rate and significant tumor regression, establishing its activity in this setting [27]. Similarly, dabrafenib monotherapy has shown objective responses in progressive PTC, with one randomized trial reporting response rates of ~42% with dabrafenib versus ~48% with combined dabrafenib–trametinib (no significant difference) [28]. Beyond tumor shrinkage, these neoadjuvant approaches can re-sensitize tumors to RAI.

In one study, a short course of dabrafenib induced new RAI uptake on post-treatment scans in 60% of patients (six of ten), enabling therapeutic RAI administration; two patients achieved partial remission and four had stable disease after

RAI, indicative of clinical benefit from this redifferentiation strategy [29]. More recently, a phase II trial combining dabrafenib and trametinib before RAI reported restored RAI avidity in the majority of cases and tumor downstaging: abnormal RAI uptake was seen in 65% of lesions after the combo therapy (vs. 5% at baseline), and at 6 months post-RAI, 38% of patients had a partial response with disease stabilization in 52% [30]. These findings highlight that dual MAPK pathway blockade can not only directly shrink *BRAF*-mutant PTC tumors but also re-differentiate them to respond to RAI.

In addition to *BRAF*-directed therapies, a recent therapeutic approach is multikinase inhibitors like lenvatinib. Its efficacy in RAI-refractory (RAI-R) DTC was established in the SELECT trial, which demonstrated a significant improvement in progression-free survival compared to placebo (18.3 vs. 3.6 months) and a higher response rate of 65% [31]. Importantly, lenvatinib's effectiveness appears to be independent of *BRAF* mutation status.

DTC: *BRAF*-Wild-Type-Differentiated Thyroid Cancer

For patients with *BRAF*-wild-type DTC, treatment options are more limited. Lenvatinib is most effective in this patient population, alone or in combination with immunotherapy. An early case report detailed the use of lenvatinib as neoadjuvant therapy in a patient with locally advanced PTC. The patient received lenvatinib for 14 months, leading to significant tumor shrinkage and subsequent successful surgical resection [32].

In a retrospective analysis of real-world data, lenvatinib was shown to have efficacy in treatment of patients with *BRAF*-mutated radioactive iodine (RAI)-refractory DTC. Patients with *BRAF V600E* and *K601E* mutations, as well as those with *BRAF*-wild-type DTC or those with untested mutational status, exhibited favorable outcomes with lenvatinib. The progression-free survival for *BRAF*-mutant patients was approximately 56 months, with overall survival not reached, suggesting a strong therapeutic benefit. There were no significant differences in outcomes between *BRAF V600E* and *K601E* mutations, though the sample size for *K601E* was smaller [33]. Provider-reported overall response rate (complete or partial response) was 76.4% in *BRAF*-mutated DTC, 75.0% in *BRAF*-wild-type DTC, and 69.3% in untested patients treated with lenvatinib, which is significantly higher than those reported with BRAF/MEK inhibitors (~30–35%). Adverse effects differ between therapies, with lenvatinib-associated hypertension, bleeding, and fatigue, whereas BRAF/MEK inhibitors primarily cause fever and fatigue. Patient-specific comorbidities should guide treatment selection. Neoadjuvant treatment may be particularly advantageous for patients with bulky or rapidly progressing disease, where early disease control is critical [34]. Emerging clinical trial results will be useful in guiding management [35].

Length of Treatment

The optimal duration of neoadjuvant therapy in thyroid cancer is not well defined and varies based on individual patient factors, tumor characteristics, and the specific agents used. Clinical experience and case reports provide some guidance on treatment length.

A systematic review analyzing neoadjuvant targeted therapy in locally advanced thyroid carcinoma found that treatment duration typically ranged from 4 to 6 months. The review emphasized that prolonged neoadjuvant therapy might increase the risk of drug-related adverse events, suggesting a need to balance treatment efficacy with potential toxicity [36]. In a study evaluating the efficacy and safety of lenvatinib as neoadjuvant therapy in locally advanced differentiated thyroid cancer, patients received lenvatinib for a median duration of 8 weeks (range, 4–32 weeks). The study concluded that lenvatinib could be an effective neoadjuvant treatment, but the optimal duration requires further investigation [37].

Multiple groups have developed metrics to evaluate tumor burden improvement by performing serial imaging every two cycles and assessing changes from baseline. These metrics classify patient response into specific categories (such as the Thyroid Surgical Morbidity Score) [38] or use point-based systems, which assigns higher points based on the extent of tumor invasion into surrounding structures and track patient improvement throughout the treatment journey (MMM score) [39].

These findings suggest that duration of neoadjuvant treatment can range from a few weeks to several months, depending on the therapeutic response and tolerability. Individualized treatment plans should consider tumor response, patient tolerance, and potential adverse effects in determining the appropriate length of therapy.

Potential Complications

Neoadjuvant therapy in thyroid cancer aims to reduce tumor size and improve surgical outcomes. However, it may be associated with complications that must be carefully identified and managed promptly.

Fistula formation is a recognized complication of neoadjuvant therapy, particularly with treatments that affect tissue integrity and healing. The risk of fistula development may be influenced by factors such as tumor location, the extent of invasion into adjacent structures, and the specific agents used in therapy. For instance, antiangiogenic agents like lenvatinib can impair wound healing through inhibition of vascular endothelial growth factor (VEGF) pathways, potentially increasing the risk of fistula formation [40, 41]. This is especially relevant in tumors with tracheal or vascular invasion, which can result in the development of airway or large vessel fistula formation as tumor regresses with treatment.

Tissue changes following neoadjuvant treatment can also be challenging at surgery. This is especially the case following treatment with tyrosine kinase inhibitors, which can induce desmoplastic reaction characterized by fibrous tissue formation. These tissue changes can complicate surgical resection by obscuring tissue planes and increasing the difficulty of complete tumor removal. While it may be difficult to anticipate these surgical challenges, close monitoring of tumor response through imaging and clinical assessment can aid in determining the optimal timing for surgery to minimize these complications [9].

Recovery of Invaded Recurrent Laryngeal Nerve (RLN) Function

Invasion of the recurrent laryngeal nerve (RLN) by locally advanced thyroid leads to vocal fold paralysis, which can negatively impact quality of life and complicates surgical management. However, recent work suggests there may be benefit with neoadjuvant therapy leading to reversal of RLN dysfunction. Our group reported on a series of seven patients with initially unresectable thyroid cancers invading the RLN who experienced recovery of vocal fold motion after neoadjuvant treatment. Six of these subjects had *BRAF V600E*-positive ATC treated with neoadjuvant dabrafenib and trametinib; by 13.5 months, all patients (100%) had regained normal vocal fold mobility (mean time to recovery ~5 months). The median number of therapy cycles to achieve initial motion return was 3 (range 1–13.5). In this series, the RLN was able to be surgically preserved in five subjects [42].

A follow-up study characterizing the six nerves, which were surgically managed, found that tumor involvement was limited to the nerve's epineurium in all cases. Intraoperative electrophysiology showed normal proximal nerve stimulation in two-thirds of patients. Of the five patients (83.3%) who received nerve-sparing surgical treatment, four had full preservation of neural function postoperatively.

While the rate of this occurrence is not known, recovery of RLN function has major implications for planned bilateral surgery, as it reduces risk of bilateral vocal fold paralysis and associated airway compromise. As such, reduction of tumor burden through neoadjuvant treatment can have significant implications for both oncologic and functional outcomes [43].

References

1. Nikiforov YE. RET/PTC rearrangement in thyroid tumors. Endocr Pathol. 2002;13(1):3–16. https://doi.org/10.1385/ep:13:1:03.
2. Vuong HG, AMA A, Abdelhamid AH, et al. The changing characteristics and molecular profiles of papillary thyroid carcinoma over time: a systematic review. Oncotarget. 2016;8(6):10637–49. https://doi.org/10.18632/oncotarget.12885.
3. Accardo G, Conzo G, Esposito D, et al. Genetics of medullary thyroid cancer: an overview. Int J Surg Lond Engl. 2017;41(Suppl 1):S2–6. https://doi.org/10.1016/j.ijsu.2017.02.064.
4. Wang JR, Zafereo ME, Dadu R, et al. Complete surgical resection following Neoadjuvant Dabrafenib plus Trametinib in BRAFV600E-mutated anaplastic thyroid carcinoma. Thyroid Off J Am Thyroid Assoc. 2019;29(8):1036–43. https://doi.org/10.1089/thy.2019.0133.
5. Alzumaili B, Sadow PM. Update on Molecular Diagnostics in Thyroid Pathology: A Review. Genes (Basel). 2023;14(7):1314 https://doi.org/10.3390/genes14071314. PMID: 37510219; PMCID: PMC10379610.

6. Randolph GW, Sosa JA, Hao Y, et al. Preoperative identification of medullary thyroid carcinoma (MTC): clinical validation of the Afirma MTC RNA-sequencing classifier. Thyroid. 2022;32(9):1069–76. https://doi.org/10.1089/thy.2022.0189.
7. Sajisevi M, Caulley L, Eskander A, et al. Evaluating the rising incidence of thyroid cancer and thyroid nodule detection modes. JAMA Otolaryngol Head Neck Surg. 2022;148(9):811–8. https://doi.org/10.1001/jamaoto.2022.1743.
8. Zhu C, Ma X, Hu Y, et al. Safety and efficacy profile of lenvatinib in cancer therapy: a systematic review and meta-analysis. Oncotarget. 2016;7(28):44545–57. https://doi.org/10.18632/oncotarget.10019.
9. Navas Moreno V, Sebastián Valles F, Lahera Vargas M, et al. Neoadjuvant treatment in locally advanced thyroid carcinoma. J Clin Med. 2024;13(19):5769. https://doi.org/10.3390/jcm13195769.
10. Crispo F, Notarangelo T, Pietrafesa M, et al. BRAF inhibitors in thyroid cancer: clinical impact, mechanisms of resistance and future perspectives. Cancer. 2019;11(9):1388. https://doi.org/10.3390/cancers11091388.
11. Neto AP, Lucchesi HL, Valsecchi VA d S, et al. Immunotherapy for patients with thyroid cancer: a comprehensive appraisal. Chin Clin Oncol. 2024;13(3):36. https://doi.org/10.21037/cco-23-133.
12. Maniakas A, Dadu R, Busaidy NL, et al. Evaluation of overall survival in patients with anaplastic thyroid carcinoma, 2000-2019. JAMA Oncol. 2020;6(9):1397–404. https://doi.org/10.1001/jamaoncol.2020.3362.
13. Subbiah V, Kreitman RJ, Wainberg ZA, et al. Dabrafenib plus trametinib in patients with BRAF V600E-mutant anaplastic thyroid cancer: updated analysis from the phase II ROAR basket study. Ann Oncol Off J Eur Soc Med Oncol. 2022;33(4):406–15. https://doi.org/10.1016/j.annonc.2021.12.014.
14. Research Center for Drug Evaluation and. FDA approves Dabrafenib plus Trametinib for anaplastic thyroid vancer with BRAF V600E mutation. FDA; 2019. Available from: https://www.fda.gov/drugs/resources-information-approved-drugs/fda-approves-dabrafenib-plus-trametinib-anaplastic-thyroid-cancer-braf-v600e-mutation. Last accessed: March 23, 2025
15. Cabanillas ME, Dadu R, Iyer P, et al. Acquired secondary RAS mutation in BRAFV600E-mutated thyroid cancer patients treated with BRAF inhibitors. Thyroid Off J Am Thyroid Assoc. 2020;30(9):1288–96. https://doi.org/10.1089/thy.2019.0514.
16. Hamidi S, Iyer PC, Dadu R, et al. Checkpoint inhibition in addition to Dabrafenib/Trametinib for BRAFV600E-mutated anaplastic thyroid carcinoma. Thyroid®. 2024;34(3):336–46. https://doi.org/10.1089/thy.2023.0573.
17. Cabanillas ME, Dadu R, Ferrarotto R, et al. Anti–programmed death ligand 1 plus targeted therapy in anaplastic thyroid carcinoma. JAMA Oncol. 2024;10(12):1672–80. https://doi.org/10.1001/jamaoncol.2024.4729.
18. Sherman EJ, Harris J, Bible KC, et al. Randomized phase II study of radiotherapy and paclitaxel with Pazopanib or placebo in anaplastic thyroid cancer: NRG/RTOG 0912. Lancet Oncol. 2023;24(2):175–86. https://doi.org/10.1016/S1470-2045(22)00763-X.
19. Dierks C, Ruf J, Seufert J, et al. 1646MO phase II ATLEP trial: final results for lenvatinib/pembrolizumab in metastasized anaplastic and poorly differentiated thyroid carcinoma. Ann Oncol. 2022;33:S1295. https://doi.org/10.1016/j.annonc.2022.07.1726.
20. Maurer E, Eilsberger F, Wächter S, et al. Mutation-based, short-term "neoadjuvant" treatment allows resectability in stage IVB and C anaplastic thyroid cancer. European Archives of Oto-Rhino-Laryngology. 2023;280(3):1509–18. https://doi.org/10.1007/s00405-023-07827-y.
21. Dierks C, Seufert J, Aumann K, et al. Combination of Lenvatinib and Pembrolizumab is an effective treatment option for anaplastic and poorly differentiated thyroid carcinoma. Thyroid. 2021;31(7):1076–85. https://doi.org/10.1089/thy.2020.0322.
22. Yang S, Ji D, Xue F, et al. Neoadjuvant famitinib and camrelizumab, a new combined therapy allowing surgical resection of the primary site for anaplastic thyroid carcinoma. Cancer Rep. 2022;6(1):e1770. https://doi.org/10.1002/cnr2.1770.

23. de Salins V, Loganadane G, Joly C, et al. Complete response in anaplastic lymphoma kinase–rearranged oncocytic thyroid cancer: a case report and review of literature. World J Clin Oncol. 2020;11(7):495–503. https://doi.org/10.5306/wjco.v11.i7.495.
24. Bapat N, Ferraro T, Esper L, et al. Treatment of unresectable BRAF V600E, TERT-mutated differentiated papillary thyroid cancer with Dabrafenib and Trametinib. JCEM Case Rep. 2024;2(8):luae112. https://doi.org/10.1210/jcemcr/luae112.
25. Farlow JL, McCrary HC, Sipos JA, et al. Neoadjuvant dabrafenib and trametinib for functional organ preservation in recurrent BRAF V600E-mutated papillary thyroid cancer. Oral Oncol. 2023;147:106625. https://doi.org/10.1016/j.oraloncology.2023.106625.
26. Dunn LA, Sherman EJ, Baxi SS, et al. Vemurafenib redifferentiation of BRAF mutant, RAI-refractory thyroid cancers. J Clin Endocrinol Metab. 2018;104(5):1417–28. https://doi.org/10.1210/jc.2018-01478.
27. Brose MS, Cabanillas ME, Cohen EEW, et al. Vemurafenib in patients with BRAFV600E-positive metastatic or unresectable papillary thyroid cancer refractory to radioactive iodine: a non-randomised, multicentre, open-label, phase 2 trial. Lancet Oncol. 2016;17(9):1272–82. https://doi.org/10.1016/S1470-2045(16)30166-8.
28. Busaidy NL, Konda B, Wei L, et al. Dabrafenib versus Dabrafenib + Trametinib in BRAF-mutated radioactive iodine refractory differentiated thyroid cancer: results of a randomized, phase 2, open-label multicenter trial. Thyroid Off J Am Thyroid Assoc. 2022;32(10):1184–92. https://doi.org/10.1089/thy.2022.0115.
29. Rothenberg SM, McFadden DG, Palmer EL, et al. Redifferentiation of iodine-refractory BRAF V600E-mutant metastatic papillary thyroid cancer with dabrafenib. Clin Cancer Res Off J Am Assoc Cancer Res. 2015;21(5):1028–35. https://doi.org/10.1158/1078-0432.CCR-14-2915.
30. Leboulleux S, Do Cao C, Zerdoud S, et al. A phase II Redifferentiation trial with Dabrafenib-Trametinib and 131I in metastatic radioactive iodine refractory BRAF p.V600E-mutated differentiated thyroid cancer. Clin Cancer Res Off J Am Assoc Cancer Res. 2023;29(13):2401–9. https://doi.org/10.1158/1078-0432.CCR-23-0046.
31. Schlumberger M, Tahara M, Wirth LJ, et al. Lenvatinib versus placebo in radioiodine-refractory thyroid cancer. N Engl J Med. 2015;372(7):621–30. https://doi.org/10.1056/NEJMoa1406470.
32. Katoh H, Kajita, Sabine, Yokota, Mitsuo, et al. Neoadjuvant use of Lenvatinib in locally advanced papillary thyroid carcinoma involving critical vessels. Int J Endocr Oncologia. 2020;7(3):IJE33. https://doi.org/10.2217/ije-2020-0014.
33. Sava J. Real-world study confirms Lenvatinib's benefit in RAI-refractory DTC; 2024. Available from https://www.targetedonc.com/view/real-world-study-confirms-lenvatinib-s-benefit-in-rai-refractory-dtc. Last accessed: March 24, 2025.
34. Worden FP, Wirth LJ, Reynolds N, et al. Patients with radioiodine-refractory differentiated thyroid cancer (RAI-R DTC) with BRAF V600E and/or K601E mutation status: a real-world view of effectiveness of lenvatinib monotherapy. J Clin Oncol. 2024;42(16_suppl):6098. https://doi.org/10.1200/JCO.2024.42.16_suppl.6098.
35. Randolph G. A phase 2 study of Neoadjuvant Lenvatinib in locally advanced invasive thyroid cancer. Clinical trial registration clinicaltrialsgov; 2023.
36. Huang N, Wang Y, Wei W, et al. A systematic review of neoadjuvant targeted therapy in locally advanced thyroid cancer. Holist Integr Oncol. 2022;1(1):16. https://doi.org/10.1007/s44178-022-00016-7.
37. Yu J, Wu Y. 2227P The efficacy and safety of lenvatinib in neoadjuvant therapy in patients with locally advanced thyroid cancer: a single-arm phase II clinical trial. Ann Oncol. 2023;34:S1147. https://doi.org/10.1016/j.annonc.2023.09.1006.
38. Zhao X, Wang JR, Dadu R, et al. Surgery after BRAF-directed therapy is associated with improved survival in BRAFV600E mutant anaplastic thyroid cancer: a single-center retrospective cohort study. Thyroid Off J Am Thyroid Assoc. 2023;33(4):484–91. https://doi.org/10.1089/thy.2022.0504.
39. Russell M, Gild ML, Wirth LJ, et al. Neoadjuvant therapy to improve resectability of advanced thyroid cancer: a real-world experience. Head Neck. 2024;46(10):2496–507. https://doi.org/10.1002/hed.27735.

40. Dang RP, McFarland D, Le VH, et al. Neoadjuvant therapy in differentiated thyroid cancer. Int J Surg Oncol. 2016;2016:3743420. https://doi.org/10.1155/2016/3743420.
41. Shonka DC, Ho A, Chintakuntlawar AV, et al. American Head and Neck Society Endocrine Surgery Section and International Thyroid Oncology Group consensus statement on mutational testing in thyroid cancer: defining advanced thyroid cancer and its targeted treatment. Head Neck. 2022;44(6):1277–300. https://doi.org/10.1002/hed.27025.
42. Silver Karcioglu A, Abdelhamid Ahmed AH, Feng Z, et al. Return of vocal fold motion and surgical preservation of invaded recurrent laryngeal nerves after the use of Neoadjuvant therapy in patients presenting with advanced thyroid cancer and vocal fold paralysis: the Lazarus effect. Thyroid®. 2023;33(10):1259–63. https://doi.org/10.1089/thy.2023.0136.
43. Russell MD, Abdelhamid Ahmed AH, Feng Z, et al. Recovery of recurrent laryngeal nerve function with Neoadjuvant treatment: neural characterization. Laryngoscope. 2024;134(7):3415–9. https://doi.org/10.1002/lary.31304.

Management of Metastatic Thyroid Cancer

17

Armando Patrizio, Lina Pedraza-Sanchez,
and Samantha Kass Newman

Editorial

Although thyroid carcinoma generally has an excellent cause-specific survival or overall survival, the incidence of metastasis/recurrence is not low. Clinicians often enface recurred thyroid carcinoma and struggle with management for metastasis/recurrence. This chapter widely states the management of recurred lesions of thyroid carcinoma. Authors described about prophylactic lymph node dissection at an initial surgery, and completion total thyroidectomy after lobectomy as an initial surgery, of which indications are still controversial. Next, they stated the controversy about RAI administration and EBRT in the adjuvant setting and for controlling distant metastasis/recurrence. Lastly, they made a brief comment on molecular testing, preparing for molecular targeted medicines. This chapter involves a wide range of important clinical issues, but writing is well established and very understandable for readers.

Ashok R. Shaha.

Background

The concept of "metastatic disease" is interpreted by many to mean aggressive cancer that is spreading, life limiting, and requiring prompt intervention. The development of sensitive biomarkers across the field of oncology, such as thyroglobulin for thyroid cancer, as well as PSA, CEA, CA-125, and circulating tumor DNA for other tumor types, which demonstrate metastatic involvement during the course of a cancer's trajectory, has called this concept into question. These markers have suggested

A. Patrizio · L. Pedraza-Sanchez · S. K. Newman (✉)
Memorial Sloan Kettering Cancer Center, New York, NY, USA
e-mail: patriza1@mskcc.org; pedrazl@mskcc.org; kasss@mskcc.org

P. S. Pai et al. (eds.), *Controversies in Cancer of the Thyroid and Parathyroid Glands*, https://doi.org/10.1007/978-3-032-13130-0_17

that cells of multiple tumor types have the ability to circulate and survive in a state of relative dormancy, where they enter the G0 phase of the cell cycle but maintain the potential for growth depending on dynamic microenvironment factors such as blood and oxygen supply [1, 2]. Follicular-derived differentiated thyroid cancers have long demonstrated this ability to remain indolent, and as a result, are often prognostically favorable, even with both local and regional metastatic disease involvement. In this chapter, we discuss the natural history of metastatic thyroid cancer and the most controversial aspects of its management.

Papillary thyroid carcinoma is understood to begin with a triggering oncogenic event that allows a follicular thyroid cell to escape regulatory mechanisms, permitting tumor growth and early subclinical metastatic spread. At time of diagnosis and initial surgery, microscopic cervical lymph node metastases are identifiable in more than 50% of individuals [3], though some studies quote as high as 80%, even for primary tumors under 1 cm in size [4]. Despite lymph node involvement observed on pathological examination, most patients with papillary thyroid carcinoma enter a quiescent phase after an initial period of early tumor growth, which is characterized by either long-term stable disease or very slow growth over time in all disease sites [5]. What is often described as disease recurrence at either local or distant sites is more likely to represent growth of preexisting metastases that were biologically inactive or growing at such a slow pace that they were previously below a threshold of detection by conventional methods [2].

Standard initial management for newly diagnosed thyroid cancer, without evidence of clinical or radiographic lymph node metastatic disease, is surgery with either lobectomy or total thyroidectomy without prophylactic lymph node dissection. However, given the above, these patients risk having residual disease left behind in this initial treatment approach. Most commonly, this residual disease takes the form of microscopic invasion by cancer cells in small central compartment lymph nodes in the neck, but more rarely appears elsewhere in the body. Less than 5% of patients present with distant metastases at the time of diagnosis [6]; however, as full body staging is not routinely recommended in those with a newly diagnosed thyroid cancer, this is likely a significant underestimate. The fact that residual cancer cells are likely to be left behind after surgical intervention, and that they may not require intervention, can be a challenging concept for patients to accept.

The American Thyroid Association (ATA) recognizes the likely indolent nature of these micrometastases in the neck and, accordingly, stratifies intrathyroidal papillary cancers with less than five involved lymph nodes into the low-risk category. This is based on a substantial body of data, which suggests that recurrence rates and mortality remain exceedingly low for those with presumed or biopsy-proven residual neck disease. Accordingly, the role of upfront prophylactic neck dissection, with the goal of targeting this presumed disease, or other more aggressive upfront therapies at the time of diagnosis, in those without clear radiographic or clinical lymph node involvement, is only one of many controversial topics in this area. As such, from MSKCC and others suggests that prophylactic central neck dissection provides no advantage in recurrence risk or overall survival in the absence of clinically apparent nodal disease preoperatively [4, 7]. This suggests a bigger picture concept—that detectable metastatic disease may behave in an idle manner and does not necessarily require intervention.

The decision variables involved in the intervention of metastatic follicular-derived thyroid cancer are therefore complex and controversial, and we seek to describe this below.

Locoregional Metastatic Disease

Prevalence and Natural History

Nodal metastasis in differentiated thyroid cancer (DTC) is common and often arises early in the disease. The metastatic pattern typically begins in the central neck compartments (levels 6 and 7) and then extends to the lateral compartments (levels 2–5) [8]. The size and number of the metastatic lymph nodes are directly related to recurrence risk, with micrometastases (<0.2 cm) and fewer than five total involved nodes posing the lowest risk, and larger metastatic nodes >1.5 cm or more than ten involved nodes posing the highest risk [9, 10]. The pattern of spread in PTC follows a predictable sequence, though skip metastasis—where cancer bypasses the central nodes and spreads directly to lateral nodes—is seen in around 20% of cases [10]. Additional factors such as extranodal extension and histologic subtype also contribute to initial assessment of risk of neck lymphadenopathy.

Notably, lymph node involvement does not appear to significantly impact overall survival rates [11], which highlights the need for careful patient selection for interventions.

Prophylactic Neck Dissection

The role of prophylactic neck dissection in the central compartment is primarily to enhance staging and risk stratification. However, its routine use in clinically node-negative patients is not supported by evidence for survival benefits [12] and may carry unnecessary risks including hypoparathyroidism and injury to the recurrent laryngeal nerve. Current recommendations suggest central compartment dissection mainly for patients with locally advanced tumors (T3 or T4) or clinically involved lateral nodes (cN1b), only when it may help guide further treatment. In cases of recurrent or persistent disease, treatment decisions are complex and should involve weighing the risks and benefits of both surgical intervention and conservative approaches, particularly given that small volume disease often stays stable over time. This approach emphasizes the important of personalization in these decisions to avoid overtreatment [13, 14].

Prophylactic central neck dissection (pCND) is generally not recommended for small, solitary papillary thyroid carcinomas (T1, T2) unless high-risk factors, such as extrathyroid extension or BRAF mutation, are present. However, pCND may be considered for clinically node-negative (cN0) cases with advanced tumors (T3 or

T4) or lateral neck disease (cN1b) to aid in staging and treatment planning. This approach aims to minimize overtreatment while providing targeted management for higher-risk patients [15].

Harries et al. demonstrated that in PTC patients with clinically involved lateral neck lymph nodes (cN1b) but no central compartment involvement, those who did not undergo pCND had a low rate of central neck recurrence, with outcomes comparable to those who did undergo the procedure. These findings suggest that pCND offers limited benefit in this group, especially considering the risks of injury to the parathyroid glands and recurrent laryngeal nerves. Therefore, pCND may not be necessary for certain cN1b patients, in line with guidelines recommending pCND only for high-risk cases [12].

Viola et al. evaluated the benefits and risks of adding pCND to total thyroidectomy (TTx) in PTC patients with no clinically detectable lymph node metastases (cN0). They found no significant differences in disease recurrence or persistence between those who underwent TTx alone and those who received TTx with pCCND. Although the TTx-only group required more radioactive iodine (RAI) treatments to achieve remission, the pCCND group experienced a higher rate of permanent hypoparathyroidism, highlighting the additional surgical risks of this procedure [11]. While pCCND led to a minor upstaging in a few patients over age 45, it did not generally affect therapeutic decisions or outcomes, given the trend toward conservative RAI use in low-risk cases. The authors concluded that routine pCCND may not be justified in all cN0 PTC patients due to the lack of substantial clinical benefits and increased surgical morbidity [11].

Completion Thyroidectomy

As discussed in prior chapters, management for differentiated thyroid cancer (DTC) typically involves either total thyroidectomy (TT) or lobectomy. The choice between lobectomy and TT is guided by tumor size, histopathological features, and patient risk factors. Lobectomy is preferred for unilateral, intrathyroidal tumors ≤1 cm without contralateral disease or high-risk features, such as a history of radiation exposure or familial thyroid cancer. However, in the recent iteration of the American Thyroid Association guidelines on DTC released in 2025, lobectomy is the preferred approach in cases of intrathyroidal tumors less than or equal to 2 cm, and may be adopted for low risks cancers between 2 and 4 cm. TT is generally indicated for tumors >4 cm or those with aggressive histologic features, extrathyroidal extension, or metastases [16, 17].

Recent studies suggest that for low-risk tumors, lobectomy provides similar survival outcomes to TT while minimizing complications such as hypoparathyroidism and RLN injury. A meta-analysis by Bi and Zhang demonstrated comparable recurrence rates between TT (1.87%) and lobectomy (2.20%) for papillary thyroid microcarcinoma (PTMC), with TT offering slightly better recurrence-free survival. However, TT was associated with higher rates of complications, highlighting lobectomy's advantages in reducing surgical risks for appropriately selected case [18, 19].

Completion thyroidectomy (CT) involves the surgical removal of the remaining thyroid tissue after an initial lobectomy. It is most often required in the setting of a staged operation due to high preoperative risk or when pathology from initial surgery is worse than expected. Indications for CT include gross extrathyroidal extension, residual disease involving critical structures (e.g., the esophagus, RLN, or tracheal wall), major vascular or capsular invasion, and aggressive subtypes such as poorly differentiated or high-grade carcinomas [20].

However, a study by Alameer [21] highlights that in well-selected patients with incidental N1a metastases, observation and close follow-up may suffice, avoiding the risks of additional surgery. In their cohort, only one regional recurrence occurred over a median follow-up of 48 months, resulting in a 97.4% recurrence-free survival rate. This aligns with the trend toward conservative management in low- to intermediate-risk thyroid cancer, as supported by the American Thyroid Association (ATA) guidelines [13].

Dedhia [18] demonstrated that CT achieves comparable thyroid resection completeness to TT, as evidenced by similar unstimulated thyroglobulin (uTg) levels 6 months postoperatively. Furthermore, CT was associated with significantly lower rates of transient hypoparathyroidism and symptomatic hypocalcemia compared to TT, with no differences in permanent complications or RLN injury. The timing of CT, ideally no sooner than 6 weeks post-lobectomy, allows for parathyroid revascularization and reduces transient hypoparathyroidism [18].

High-volume surgical expertise is critical for optimizing outcomes in both TT and CT. Overall, the decision to pursue CT or TT should be individualized, considering patient risk factors, tumor characteristics, and the potential benefits of avoiding overtreatment in low-risk cases [20].

Recurrent Nodal Metastases

The frequent occurrence of regional lymph node metastases in differentiated thyroid cancer has been established above. For those who have structurally and biochemically incomplete response after initial treatment, local recurrence occurs in up to 30% of patients, with actual percentages varying based on the American Thyroid Association's risk stratification system [13]. While recurrences often happen early in the disease course (within 3–5 years from initial diagnosis), they can occur decades afterward.

The decision on whether to intervene for recurrent nodal metastases remains controversial as prognosis generally remains favorable even in the setting of local recurrence, with studies reporting >90% survival at 10 years [10, 22, 23]. Patients with recurrence must therefore be carefully chosen for intervention, after the confirmation of the malignant nature through a FNA biopsy with cytology and/or Tg analysis. While there is no controversy surrounding operative intervention for bulky nodal metastases [10], the benefit to operative intervention on low-volume disease is less clear. There is no high-quality data that clearly suggests that resection of small volume disease improves mortality; however, even small volume disease has the potential for growth and invasion, rendering surgery more complex and increasing morbidity and mortality [24].

The ability to detect low-volume recurrence has been enhanced by high-sensitivity thyroglobulin assays and improvements in imaging techniques. However, it is crucial to discuss with patients the difference between detectable disease and actionable disease and the fact that low-volume disease does not always require treatment. Factors that may prompt treatment are similar to factors that might make one unsuitable for active surveillance at initial diagnosis—rapid growth of the lesion, anatomical location adjacent to critical structures, tumors with more aggressive histology (i.e., BRAF positive), and personal preferences. Multiple studies suggest stability of recurrent disease with a risk of further progression approaching 20% [25–27]. Those who are appropriate for active surveillance of a local recurrence traditionally have low-volume disease, high surgical risk, or both.

For those who have undergone total thyroidectomy, TSH suppression is a straightforward strategy that should be employed in those with local recurrence, though the recommended TSH of <0.1 can be challenging to tolerate in some. For those who have undergone lobectomy and experience recurrence in the thyroid but have a remaining functional lobe, the role of TSH suppression is less clear but may still provide some benefit; data is lacking significantly in this area. It also remains unclear whether TSH suppression after lobectomy reduces recurrence risk [28].

When active treatment is deemed necessary, surgery remains the gold standard with the highest response rates. The 2015 ATA guidelines state that surgery is indicated for central neck nodes >8 mm or lateral neck nodes >10 mm in the smallest dimension [13]. Reoperation is associated with the same, but more frequently occurring surgical risks as primary operation, and a specialized high-volume thyroid cancer surgical specialist is indicated in these cases [24]. While an initial reoperation boasts relatively high rates of success, measured by reduction in thyroglobulin and detectable structural disease, further operations yield both lower success rates and higher complications [29]. In the presence of distant disease, resection of locoregional metastases can still be beneficial to prevent compromise of critical neck anatomy or to help facilitate increased iodine delivery to distant metastatic disease [24].

In addition to surgery, radioactive iodine, EBRT, radiofrequency ablation, and percutaneous ethanol injection can be used to control local disease. RAI and EBRT are discussed below.

Radioactive Iodine

Radioactive iodine (RAI) therapy has been a cornerstone in the treatment of differentiated thyroid cancer (DTC) since the 1940s, utilizing the thyroid follicular cell's unique ability to concentrate iodine through the sodium-iodide symporter [30].

Radioactive iodine serves three primary purposes in the management of thyroid carcinoma, each with a different goal. In the case of most patients with thyroid cancer after a complete surgery with, the most utilized is *remnant ablation*, targeting residual healthy thyroid tissue, which improves accuracy of follow-up diagnostics. If residual microscopic disease is suspected and the patient is at high risk of recurrence, *adjuvant therapy* can be given to reduce the risk of recurrence and enhance progression-free and overall survival. The third is *treatment of known disease*, with the goal of destroying either structural or biochemical disease that may not be amenable to a surgical intervention [24]. Identification of the goal of iodine therapy must preclude its use. By integrating risk stratification systems, molecular profiling, and advanced imaging [31], clinicians can tailor RAI use to maximize its benefits while minimizing unnecessary exposure and associated risks. This personalized approach ensures that RAI therapy is applied where it is most effective, aligning treatment decisions with patient-specific factors and preferences.

In the case of locoregional disease metastases, including small volume nodal metastases, the role of iodine therapy remains controversial. Presumed benefit is influenced by nodal characteristics such as size, location, and extranodal extension. While adjuvant RAI can lower recurrence risk, its benefits vary based on tumor characteristics and postoperative thyroglobulin (Tg) levels; for example, patients with low postoperative Tg (<1 ng/mL) may gain limited benefit. Advanced imaging modalities, including SPECT/CT and FDG PET/CT, improve the detection of iodine-avid nodal disease and help distinguish benign thyroid remnants from metastatic nodes [32, 33].

Reflecting this shift toward individualized care, the 2022 NCCN guidelines no longer recommend RAI solely for minor extrathyroidal extension [9]. Similarly controversial, a study demonstrated that low-dose RAI (1.1 GBq) is as effective as high-dose RAI (5.5 GBq) for intermediate-risk DTC patients with small tumors (≤2 cm), microscopic extrathyroidal extension, and no lymph node metastasis. Over a 7.2-year follow-up, both groups showed comparable success rates (97% vs. 90%) and no recurrences, highlighting the sufficiency of low-dose RAI in this subgroup, minimizing side effects, and reinforcing the importance of risk-based treatment strategies [34].

For high-risk DTC patients, including those with gross extrathyroidal extension, large nodal metastases, or distant metastases (discussed separately below), RAI therapy is a standard treatment, shown to improve both disease-specific and overall survival [35]. By targeting subclinical or macroscopic residual disease, RAI significantly reduces recurrence rates and enhances progression-free survival. Post-treatment imaging, such as whole-body scans, is essential for identifying iodine-avid metastases and evaluating the response to therapy. High-risk patients typically require higher cumulative RAI doses, ranging from 100 to 600 mCi, although this is also controversial, as lower-dose regimens may be effective in select cases with minimal disease burden [35].

For locoregional disease recurrence, radioactive iodine is generally not recommended as primary treatment. RAI is often ineffective in treating bulky nodal recurrence [24] and is most effective when targeting microscopic disease as an adjuvant therapy after surgery. A study by Wu [36] done in 2018 showed that in patients who were treated with RAI for lymph node metastases, only 28% of patients achieved a complete remission, and those who did had smaller sized targeted nodes (5 mm as opposed to 9 mm, on average). Further, those who achieved complete remission required three treatments of I-131 [36].

External Beam Radiation Therapy

As discussed above, indications for radioactive iodine in the postoperative setting are controversial, yet well established.

External beam radiation therapy (EBRT) in the adjuvant setting has traditionally been avoided, due to conflicting data on efficacy and survival, as well as increased risk of morbidity. Its use is not typically considered unless surgery and radioactive iodine fail to achieve local control. Even then, patients with residual neck disease maintain a decent prognosis in most scenarios, so the risk of treatment toxicity must be carefully weighed.

However, advances in molecular profiling of differentiated thyroid cancers have provided insights into the behavior of less common histologies that were not previously known. For example, we know that both oncocytic carcinoma of the thyroid and tall cell variant papillary thyroid cancers downregulate the sodium-iodide symporter on the membrane of the follicular cell as they dedifferentiate, thereby making these cell types less likely to concentrate iodine [37]. Whether or not radioactive iodine serves any purpose whatsoever in these cancer types remains controversial and is discussed at length below.

This rapidly expanding knowledge of thyroid cancer histology that may be resistant to iodine helps clinicians develop more precise treatments and avoid unnecessary toxicity. However, the loss of RAI as an adjuvant tool in those at intermediate or high risk of recurrence is significant. It is critical to examine the role of prophylactic adjuvant EBRT for these patients.

Currently, EBRT is effective in achieving local control when radioactive iodine and/or repeated surgery has failed to prevent recurrence. Bulky recurrences in the neck can be problematic if they compromise critical anatomy, such as the esophagus, trachea, or carotid artery [24]. Patients felt to benefit from EBRT tended to be older, with more extensive disease at presentation and significant extrathyroidal extension [24]. It can be inferred from clinical experience and the data currently available that EBRT is most useful to those at highest risk of recurrence.

The American Thyroid Association (ATA) and the American Head and Neck Society (AHNS) offer differing recommendations for EBRT use in differentiated thyroid cancer. The ATA's 2009 guidelines recommended EBRT for patients >45 years with gross extrathyroidal extension (ETE) and high-risk residual disease [38]. However, their 2016 update was less specific, suggesting EBRT for tumors invading critical structures [13], with clarification expected in the ATA 2025 guidelines.

The American Head and Neck Society released a statement in 2016 recommending EBRT for those with gross residual or unresectable disease, except if the patient is <45 or has disease that is RAI avid [39]. This recommendation was based on primarily retrospective studies, which showed evidence of improved regional control in this patient population [40–44]. The second recommendation states that EBRT should not be routinely used as adjuvant therapy if the resection of gross disease was felt to be complete and advises a "multidisciplinary approach" that will vary by institution [39]. However, they also state that those >45 with high likelihood of microscopic disease and low likelihood of responding to RAI, EBRT maybe considered, based on several studies suggesting those with pT4a disease had improved local progression-free survival [39]. Finally, an oft-cited study from the Princess Margaret Cancer Center showed improvement in 10-year cause-specific survival and local relapse-free rate in those >60 without evidence of gross residual disease [45]. Based on this, postoperative EBRT was incorporated into guidelines for standard of care for management of thyroid cancer.

The reality is that much of these recommendations are based on retrospective data. To our knowledge, there are no randomized controlled trials that compare efficacy of RAI versus EBRT, or EBRT versus observation alone for the above groups. And though much has been said about the use of EBRT for local control, a paucity of data suggests its impact on overall survival.

The controversy surrounding EBRT is not only related to its efficacy but also its morbidity and mortality. Those who received EBRT for thyroid cancer have actually been shown to have higher rates of death [46]. This relationship, however, is likely inseparable from the reality that EBRT has been reserved for those who are older and have more advanced disease and whose prognosis is worse at the outset. The toxicity associated with high-dose radiation to the neck is not insignificant and include mucositis, dysphagia, and voice changes, with some requiring feeding support initially if severe in the short term. Late toxicities may include fibrosis, esophageal or tracheal stenosis, and the risk of secondary malignancy in the radiated area [39].

Distant Metastatic Disease

Distant metastases occur in approximately 10–35% of follicular cell-derived thyroid cancers, with specific risk factors depending on tumor histology [6]. Less than 5% of patients present with distant metastatic disease at diagnosis, though this is likely an underestimate given that full-body staging is not standard of care. Though thyroid cancer can metastasize to any anatomical location, the most common sites are the lung and bone. A majority of those with distant disease have lung metastases only (up to 75%) with less than 25% presenting with disease in the bone and even fewer (~10%) with disease in both sites [6]. Distant metastases are more commonly found in older patients, those with aggressive histologies, and those with more extensive disease at time of initial diagnosis. While associated with lower overall survival, many patients with distant disease survive for more than a decade after diagnosis [47]. To help differentiate between those whose disease may remain indolent from those more likely to experience early progression, clinical characteristics, mutational analysis, cross-sectional imaging, and serial thyroglobulin measurements to assess doubling time are useful tools.

Staging and Imaging

Since more than 50% of differentiated thyroid cancer (DTC) demonstrate indolence, routine full-body staging at time of diagnosis is not considered standard of care. In DTC, most of the information that guides postoperative management are based on the pathology report, the postsurgical thyroglobulin (Tg) plasma level and, when available, molecular analysis [37]. Pathological characteristics such as degree of vascular invasion, the presence of disease in the surgical margins, the extent of nodal involvement, and the subtype of papillary cancer itself guide aggressiveness of monitoring.

Therefore, all current guidelines recommend limiting the pre-surgical imaging for DTC to only a high-definition neck ultrasound (US) able to characterize the tumor mass and the central and bilateral neck compartments. In a historical study from Japan, the neck US in expert hands showed satisfactory sensitivity for estimating the tumor dimension (80%) and local minimal extension (77%), but not for evaluating the eventual involvement of gross structure such as the esophagus (28.6%) and the trachea (42.9%); and only 36.7% of the metastatic lymph nodes were correctly identified pre-surgically [48]. It is well established that 30–40% of patients are noted to have "unexpected" lymph node metastases after the surgery, especially in the central compartment since its ultrasonographic exploration is often hampered by the overlying thyroid gland [49].

For this reason, in case of large, locally aggressive tumor and/or with extensive nodal involvement, a thorough imaging assessment with cross-sectional imaging of the neck (magnetic resonance imaging (MRI), computed tomography (CT) with contrast) should be considered to plan the adequate extension of the surgery and the optimal postoperative management. Many centers also perform preoperative laryngoscopy to evaluate the vocal cord mobility and to exclude their impairments that could lead to a different surgical strategy (lobectomy vs. total thyroidectomy and even, and even the sacrifice of paralyzed nerve), as vocal cord paralysis or paresis is found in up to 70% of cases with locally advanced disease [50, 51].

Elevated post-therapy Tg usually correlates with the burden of residual disease, which could be confined to the neck or already be present distantly. In such cases, a diagnostic whole-body scan (WBS) with radioactive iodine (RAI) can help assess disease extent and determine the appropriate dose of iodine-131 (I131). However, there is no consensus on this approach, especially in the light of the potential stunning of the thyroid remnants and metastasis, avoidable only with the not widely available and expensive radionuclide I123 and I124 [52]. In a study by Chen [53], 25% of 122 patients who received a pre-ablation I123 WBS eventually received a different dose than anticipated due to discovery of unsuspected regional and distant metastases. On the other hand, the post-treatment WBS performed after 2–7 days from the administration of the therapeutic dose remains of paramount importance in disease re-staging and may be sufficient to disclose the presence of high-risk disease [54]. When feasible, adding the WBS with the single-photon emission computed tomography/computed tomography (SPECT/CT) can significantly improve the staging, risk stratification, and follow-up compared to the traditional scintigraph planar images, facilitating the discernment of cervical lymph node metastases from the physiological uptakes and of distant metastatic lesions in less common sites [55].

In the case of highly aggressive disease or suspected distant metastases, a PET/CT is strongly recommended, especially with an elevated thyroglobulin but absence of iodine-avid disease. PET/CT in this context showed a sensitivity and specificity of 80 and 90%, respectively [56]. Moreover, the FDG PET/CT scan has been demonstrated to be more sensitive than WBS with more aggressive DTC histology, including tall cell variant, oncocytic thyroid carcinoma, and, especially for the poorly differentiated thyroid cancer (PTDC), where its use is considered mandatory for a correct staging [13].

For the 50% of patients with distant metastatic disease who unfortunately do not achieve remission after adequate surgical and RAI treatment, PET/CT has proved an important tool in assessing prognosis and predicting further iodine responsiveness. A retrospective study from France showed that in 80 patients with metastatic DTC, PET/CT uptake was the only prognostic factor for survival ($p = 0.02$), and the prognosis was significantly related both to standardized uptake value (SUV) max and to the number of [18F]FDG-avid lesions ($p = 0.03$ and 0.009, respectively) [57].

Finally, the I124 PET/CT is emerging as a critical tool in postoperative detection of metastatic lesions, which may be amenable to RAI [58]. Thanks to its high sensitivity, this specific type of functional imaging study is also used for the estimation of an absorbed individual dose to a single lesion, which serves to modulate the activity of I131 in the setting of distant metastatic disease [59]. This emerging technology is known as lesional dosimetry.

Radioactive Iodine Therapy in Distant Metastatic Disease

Beyond the purposes of remnant ablation and adjuvant therapy, radioactive iodine (RAI) with I131 plays a role in the treatment of gross local disease, regional lymph nodes, and distant metastatic disease. It can be delivered by three approaches in this setting: (1) empiric high dose, which usually ranges from 150 mCi in case of neck and mediastinum lymph node involvement, to 200 mCi in case of lung metastases, (2) blood dosimetry, and (3) lesional dosimetry. To date, no compelling data from randomized clinical trials are available to compare these three methods. The evidence is mainly from retrospective series and has suggested superiority of lesional dosimetry approach especially in pediatric patients, those with extensive lung disease, and those with renal failure and elderly [13]. Among those older than 70 years, the maximum tolerated dose is conventionally 150 mCi, based on a study that found an empiric dose of 200 mCi to exceed the maximum tolerated radiation-absorbed dose (MTRD) in 22–38% of patients in this age group [60].

Prior to treatment with I131, induction of a transient hypothyroid state is mandatory to allow the maximum uptake of RAI. However, while in context of remnant ablation and adjuvant therapy, the use of recombinant TSH is universally preferred, in patients with distant metastatic disease, it is debated. Indeed, a rapid increase of TSH and subsequent stimulated growth of metastatic lesions raise concern about the potential for local mass effect that could in turn cause severe symptomatic disease or compromise critical structures, especially in case of brain metastases, spinal cord metastases, or lesions in close proximity to aerodigestive structures. In those with contraindication to thyroid hormone withdrawal but still potentially vulnerable to dangerous swelling of disease sites, steroids may be utilized.

Diffuse RAI-avid pulmonary micrometastases (<2 mm) have the highest rates of remission, even after repetitive cycles of treatment [61]. Solitary lung lesions, while less common, may be amenable to a surgical approach. The effectiveness of RAI treatment for bone metastases is less evident; though has been associated with improved survival, it is rarely curative, and local approaches such as surgery, or radiotherapy, should be considered [62]. The role of I131 for the treatment of brain metastases is limited, especially because of the unpredictable and usually low uptake of radioiodine within the brain and the severe side effects due to direct toxicity or to the development of peritumoral edema [63].

Finally, it is important to consider that up to two-thirds of patients with distant metastases will eventually become RAI refractory [47]. Therefore, we must always assess iodine avidity of the tumor prior to repeated dose of RAI.

Recently, thanks to the increased use of molecularly targeted therapies such as dabrafenib and trametinib, patients with metastatic and progressive disease may benefit from redifferentiation treatments, which enable iodine-refractory cancer cells to regain the ability to concentrate iodine. This approach demands the identification of an underlying driver mutation and the use of diagnostic pre-treatment scanning to assess radiosensitivity of lesions [64].

Radiation Therapy in Distant Metastatic Disease

In the management of advanced differentiated thyroid cancer (DTC), EBRT is usually reserved for invasive aerodigestive disease resulting from an incomplete surgical resection. However, EBRT should be also considered in the case of progressive and symptomatic distant metastatic disease, refractory to radioiodine and not susceptible to surgery. Bone, soft tissue, and central nervous system (CNS) metastases are potential targets for radiotherapy [65]. EBRT also serves a palliative purpose. It may help with pain control and locally compressive symptoms in the spine. It may control asymptomatic bone lesion localized in worrisome weightbearing segments of the skeleton.

Stereotactic body radiation therapy (SBRT) is a more precise modality of delivering targeted radiation to a tumor, limiting the effect to adjacent normal tissue. It should be reserved for patients with resistant and symptomatic bone metastases resistant to a standard course of EBRT and for those who have longer life expectancy (>6 months), with a definite curative intent. SBRT is also recommended for the treatment of vertebral metastases and bone oligometastases [66]. Although SBRT is feasible for oligometastases in the lung [3], the pattern of spread of DTC to the lungs is typically as multiple bilateral micrometastases. Therefore, once these tumors lose their iodine avidity, conventional external multifractionated radiation therapy can help control symptoms of dyspnea, chest pain, and hemoptysis with few side effects. This approach should be reserved only for palliation intent, while patients with better prognosis should first attempt SBRT or systemic therapy where improvements in local control are the primary goal [67].

Metastasectomy

As described above, the most affected site of distant metastasis from DTC are the lungs and bones. While presentation of lung metastases is multiple bilateral micrometastases, bone disease may be solitary and therefore managed with a surgical approach. This is especially true when the lesions involve the weightbearing long bones or the acetabulum, causing complete or impending pathological fractures. Prophylactic fixation in this case may have a palliative role, reducing pain and maximizing skeletal functionality. In the case of a single bone metastatic focus, this approach would not only reduce local symptoms but also improve prognosis, even if the lesion is not associated with impending fracture [68].

This approach can also be extended to single and amenable metastasis involving other organs such as the lung, liver, and brain. While the available data are limited by the small samples size, several studies have shown encouraging results in favor of the neurosurgical option: Choi et al. [69] showed that a sample of 37 patients with brain metastases from DTC who had neurosurgical intervention had better overall survival than those without treatment (30.7 vs. 5 months). Furthermore, Yoo et al. [70] confirmed a statistically significant survival benefit for neurosurgery in case of less than three sites of brain metastases. One must consider, however, that surgical resection of brain lesions exposes the patient to several potential complications including seizure, worsening neurologic status, perioperative hemorrhagic and ischemic stroke, infections, and prolonged hospitalization.

Stereotactic radiosurgery (SRS) involves a focused high dose of radiation delivered to a precise target rather than a larger radiation field, as in the case of whole brain radiation therapy (WBRT). Usually, SRS is indicated in case of small (not larger than 2 cm) and surgically unresectable brain metastases and has shown a better local control than conventional WBRT. Moreover, also in patients with BM from DTC, SRS showed an excellent safety profile in terms of headache, seizure, nausea vomiting, and cognitive decline [71]. However, even if WBRT has shown uncertainty in terms of overall survival and is associated with higher toxicity, it is still preferred to achieve local disease control in patients with multiple brain lesions or lesion too large to be treated with SRS or surgery [63].

Molecular Testing

Starting from program as The Cancer Genome Atlas (TCGA), which has genetically characterized more than 30 primary tumors, groundbreaking advancements have been accomplished in identifying targetable mutations in papillary thyroid cancer

[72]. In a single-institution large-scale sequencing initiative of more than 10,000 patients affected by advanced cancer, thyroid cancer resulted to be, after GIST, the cancer type with the highest number of actionable mutations, which were present in 61% of cases [73]. More recent studies have elucidated somatic genetic alterations, such as TERT promoter, RBM10 mutations, and chromosome 1q gain, underlying the most aggressive phenotypes and RAI-resistant DTC [37, 74].

With this premise, several targeted therapies have been approved for the treatment of advanced thyroid cancer, improving the outcomes of patients with known actionable mutations. The 2024 NCCN guidelines now recommend performing somatic testing in locally recurrent, advanced, metastatic, or RAI-refractory disease, to detect these mutations and identify those who may benefit from targeted therapies [65]. A recent joint consensus of the American Head and Neck Society (AHNS) and the International Thyroid Oncology Group (ITOG) has been released to clarify the use of somatic genetic alteration detection for therapeutic intervention in advanced thyroid cancer. Based on their statements, all patients with advanced thyroid cancer, including metastatic disease, should be tested for BRAFV600E somatic mutation and, if negative, for fusion mutations of RET, NTRK1, NTRK3, and ALK. In case of positive BRAFV600E mutation, the first-line therapy is an approved antiangiogenic multikinase inhibitor (aaMKI, lenvatinib or sorafenib), but if there is a preexisting contraindication, development of severe side effects, or disease progression, a specific BRAF inhibitor, such as dabrafenib, should be considered. For those who harbors somatic fusion mutation of RET, NTRK1, and NTRK3, the targeted drug represents the first choice as systemic therapy (i.e., selpercatinib/ pralsetinib and larotrectinib/ entrectinib, respectively) [75]. This approach has also been endorsed by the recent 2025 ATA guidelines, which suggest tissue-based biomarker testing to identify actionable oncogenic drivers in those who are candidates for systemic therapy in RAIR and progressive structural disease.

Somatic mutations are usually analyzed from a sample collected from the primary tumor, preferably with a next-generation sequencing (NGS) assay, but in metastatic disease, testing tissue could also derive from a secondary lesion. In a retrospective mutational profiling analysis with NGS of 216 patients with advanced thyroid cancer, researchers from the MD Anderson included also samples deriving from 69 lymph node metastases and 16 distant metastases. In six patients (3%), the authors performed genetical analysis in two different tumor blocks for each patient, and in two cases, they found an additional mutation (PIK3CA, TP53, and AKT1) different from the one shared with the primary site (BRAFV600E) [76]. This small but significant report suggests that metastatic lesions may acquire novel mutations during their progression, which may be susceptible to different targeted therapies than the primary tumor.

A time and cost-sparing alternative to the NGS analysis is the recently introduced antibodies for the immunohistochemistry analysis of BRAF V600E (clone VE1), NRAS/HRAS/KRAS (pan-RAS Q61R), NTRK1-3 (pan-TRK), and ALK fusions (5A4) that have shown strong concordance with molecular techniques [77]. Another widely available tool for the detection of fusion and rearrangement mutations is fluorescence in situ hybridization (FISH), though this technique is not as sensitive as NGS assays [76]. As such, when an alternative methodology has negative results, an NGS assay should be utilized.

As with many other areas in oncology, precision medicine has found its way to the management of advanced thyroid cancer, and its future is promising.

References

1. van der Toom EE, Verdone JE, Pienta KJ. Disseminated tumor cells and dormancy in prostate cancer metastasis. Curr Opin Biotechnol. 2016;40:9–15.
2. Rajan N, Khanal T, Ringel MD. Progression and dormancy in metastatic thyroid cancer: concepts and clinical implications. Endocrine. 2020;70(1):24–35.
3. Falcinelli L, et al. Stereotactic radiotherapy for lung oligometastases. Rep Pract Oncol Radiother. 2022;27(1):23–31.
4. Gyorki DE, Untch B, Tuttle RM, Shaha AR. Prophylactic central neck dissection in differentiated thyroid cancer: an assessment of the evidence. Ann Surg Oncol. 2013;20(7):2285–9.
5. Newman SK, et al. Invasion of a recurrent laryngeal nerve from small well-differentiated papillary thyroid cancers: patient selection implications for active surveillance. Thyroid. 2022;32(2):164–9.
6. Shaha AR, Shah JP, Loree TR. Patterns of nodal and distant metastasis based on histologic varieties in differentiated carcinoma of the thyroid. Am J Surg. 1996;172(6):692–4.
7. Ricarte-Filho J, et al. Papillary thyroid carcinomas with cervical lymph node metastases can be stratified into clinically relevant prognostic categories using oncogenic BRAF, the number of nodal metastases, and extra-nodal extension. Thyroid. 2012;22(6):575–84.
8. Wang LY, Ganly I. Nodal metastases in thyroid cancer: prognostic implications and management. Future Oncol. 2016;12(7):981–94.
9. Haddad RI, et al. Thyroid carcinoma, NCCN clinical practice guidelines in oncology. J Natl Compr Canc Netw. 2022; https://doi.org/10.6004/jnccn.2022.0040.
10. Randolph GW, et al. The prognostic significance of nodal metastases from papillary thyroid carcinoma can be stratified based on the size and number of metastatic lymph nodes, as well as the presence of extranodal extension. Thyroid. 2012;22(11):1144–52.
11. Viola D, et al. Prophylactic central compartment lymph node dissection in papillary thyroid carcinoma: clinical implications derived from the first prospective randomized controlled single institution study. J Clin Endocrinol Metab. 2015;100(4):1316–24.
12. Harries V, et al. Is a prophylactic central compartment neck dissection required in papillary thyroid carcinoma patients with clinically involved lateral compartment lymph nodes? Ann Surg Oncol. 2021;28(1):512–8.
13. Haugen BR, et al. 2015 American Thyroid Association management guidelines for adult patients with thyroid nodules and differentiated thyroid cancer: the American Thyroid Association guidelines task force on thyroid nodules and differentiated thyroid cancer. Thyroid. 2016;26(1):1–133.
14. Mizrachi A, Shaha AR. Lymph node dissection for differentiated thyroid cancer. Mol Imaging Radionucl Ther. 2017;26(Suppl 1):10–5.
15. Pavlidis ET, Pavlidis TE. Role of prophylactic central neck lymph node dissection for papillary thyroid carcinoma in the era of de-escalation. World J Clin Oncol. 2023;14(7):247–58.
16. Adam MA, et al. Extent of surgery for papillary thyroid cancer is not associated with survival: an analysis of 61,775 patients. Ann Surg. 2014;260(4):601–5; discussion 605–7.
17. Barney BM, et al. Overall and cause-specific survival for patients undergoing lobectomy, near-total, or total thyroidectomy for differentiated thyroid cancer. Head Neck. 2011;33(5):645–9.
18. Dedhia PH, et al. Outcomes after completion thyroidectomy versus total thyroidectomy for differentiated thyroid cancer: a single-center experience. J Surg Oncol. 2020;122(4):660–4.

19. Bi J, Zhang H. A meta-analysis of total thyroidectomy and lobectomy outcomes in papillary thyroid microcarcinoma. Medicine (Baltimore). 2023;102(50):e36647.
20. Shaha AR, Michael Tuttle R. Completion thyroidectomy-indications and complications. Eur J Surg Oncol. 2019;45(7):1129–31.
21. Alameer E, et al. Partial thyroidectomy with incidental metastatic lymph nodes. JAMA Otolaryngol Head Neck Surg. 2024;150(1):49–56.
22. Chereau N, et al. Recurrence of papillary thyroid carcinoma with lateral cervical node metastases: predictive factors and operative management. Surgery. 2016;159(3):755–62.
23. Ito Y, et al. Prognosis of patients with papillary thyroid carcinoma showing postoperative recurrence to the central neck. World J Surg. 2011;35(4):767–72.
24. Roman SA, Shen WT, Sosa JA, editors. Controversies in thyroid nodules and differentiated thyroid cancer. Cham: Springer; 2023.
25. Maciel J, Donato S, Simoes H, Leite V. Clinical outcomes of a conservative approach in cervical lymph node metastases of thyroid cancer. Clin Endocrinol. 2021;94(3):460–5.
26. Robenshtok E, et al. Suspicious cervical lymph nodes detected after thyroidectomy for papillary thyroid cancer usually remain stable over years in properly selected patients. J Clin Endocrinol Metab. 2012;97(8):2706–13.
27. Tomoda C, et al. Cervical lymph node metastases after thyroidectomy for papillary thyroid carcinoma usually remain stable for years. Thyroid. 2016;26(12):1706–11.
28. Bae MR, et al. Thyroid stimulating hormone suppression and recurrence after thyroid lobectomy for papillary thyroid carcinoma. Endocrine. 2022;75(2):487–94.
29. Onuma AE, et al. Long-term efficacy of lymph node reoperation for persistent papillary thyroid cancer: 13-year follow-up. Ann Surg Oncol. 2019;26(6):1737–43.
30. Spitzweg C, et al. Clinical review 132: the sodium iodide symporter and its potential role in cancer therapy. J Clin Endocrinol Metab. 2001;86(7):3327–35.
31. Leboulleux S, et al. Thyroidectomy without radioiodine in patients with low-risk thyroid cancer. N Engl J Med. 2022;386(10):923–32.
32. Chidambaranathan N, et al. The significance of the presence of extranodal extension in the metastatic node of differentiated thyroid cancer: a proposal for modification in the American Thyroid Association (ATA) risk stratification. Eur Arch Otorrinolaringol. 2024;281(4):1923–31.
33. van Velsen EFS, Verburg FA. Adjuvant radioiodine for intermediate-risk papillary thyroid cancer-to treat or not to treat. J Clin Endocrinol Metab. 2023;108(10):e1149–50.
34. Han JM, et al. Effects of low-dose and high-dose postoperative radioiodine therapy on the clinical outcome in patients with small differentiated thyroid cancer having microscopic extrathyroidal extension. Thyroid. 2014;24(5):820–5.
35. Tuttle RM, et al. Controversies, consensus, and collaboration in the use of (131)I therapy in differentiated thyroid cancer: a joint statement from the American Thyroid Association, the European Association of Nuclear Medicine, the Society of Nuclear Medicine and Molecular Imaging, and the European Thyroid Association. Thyroid. 2019;29(4):461–70.
36. Wu X, et al. Clinical outcomes and prognostic factors of radioiodine ablation therapy for lymph node metastases from papillary thyroid carcinoma. Nucl Med Commun. 2018;39(1):22–7.
37. Boucai L, et al. Genomic and transcriptomic characteristics of metastatic thyroid cancers with exceptional responses to radioactive iodine therapy. Clin Cancer Res. 2023;29(8):1620–30.
38. American Thyroid Association Guidelines Taskforce on Thyroid, N, et al. Revised American Thyroid Association management guidelines for patients with thyroid nodules and differentiated thyroid cancer. Thyroid. 2009;19(11):1167–214.
39. Kiess AP, et al. External-beam radiotherapy for differentiated thyroid cancer locoregional control: a statement of the American head and neck society. Head Neck. 2016;38(4):493–8.
40. Servagi Vernat S, et al. 10-year Locoregional control with postoperative external beam radiotherapy in patients with locally advanced high-risk non-anaplastic thyroid carcinoma De novo or at relapse, a propensity score analysis. Cancers (Basel). 2019;11(6):849.
41. Fussey JM, et al. External beam radiotherapy in differentiated thyroid carcinoma: a systematic review. Head Neck. 2016;38(Suppl 1):E2297–305.

42. Groen AH, et al. Postoperative external beam radiotherapy for locoregional control in iodine refractory differentiated thyroid cancer. Eur Thyroid J. 2022;11(1):e210033.
43. Jacomina LE, et al. The role of postoperative external beam radiotherapy for differentiated thyroid carcinoma: a systematic review and meta-analysis. Head Neck. 2020;42(8):2181–93.
44. Chow SM, et al. Local and regional control in patients with papillary thyroid carcinoma: specific indications of external radiotherapy and radioactive iodine according to T and N categories in AJCC 6th edition. Endocr Relat Cancer. 2006;13(4):1159–72.
45. Brierley J, Tsang R, Panzarella T, Bana N. Prognostic factors and the effect of treatment with radioactive iodine and external beam radiation on patients with differentiated thyroid cancer seen at a single institution over 40 years. Clin Endocrinol. 2005;63(4):418–27.
46. Yang Z, et al. Comparison of survival outcomes following postsurgical radioactive iodine versus external beam radiation in stage IV differentiated thyroid carcinoma. Thyroid. 2017;27(7):944–52.
47. Durante C, et al. Long-term outcome of 444 patients with distant metastases from papillary and follicular thyroid carcinoma: benefits and limits of radioiodine therapy. J Clin Endocrinol Metab. 2006;91(8):2892–9.
48. Shimamoto K, et al. Preoperative staging of thyroid papillary carcinoma with ultrasonography. Eur J Radiol. 1998;29(1):4–10.
49. Abboud B, et al. Correlations of neck ultrasound and pathology in cervical lymph node of papillary thyroid carcinoma. Acta Chir Belg. 2020;120(4):238–44.
50. Randolph GW, Kamani D. The importance of preoperative laryngoscopy in patients undergoing thyroidectomy: voice, vocal cord function, and the preoperative detection of invasive thyroid malignancy. Surgery. 2006;139(3):357–62.
51. Shaha AR. Routine laryngoscopy in thyroid surgery: a valuable adjunct. Surgery. 2007;142(6):865–6.
52. Pacini F, et al. ETA consensus statement: what are the indications for post-surgical radioiodine therapy in differentiated thyroid cancer? Eur Thyroid J. 2022;11(1):e210046.
53. Chen MK, et al. The utility of I-123 pretherapy scan in I-131 radioiodine therapy for thyroid cancer. Thyroid. 2012;22(3):304–9.
54. Souza Rosario PW, et al. Post I-131 therapy scanning in patients with thyroid carcinoma metastases: an unnecessary cost or a relevant contribution? Clin Nucl Med. 2004;29(12):795–8.
55. Xue YL, Qiu ZL, Song HJ, Luo QY. Value of (1)(3)(1)I SPECT/CT for the evaluation of differentiated thyroid cancer: a systematic review of the literature. Eur J Nucl Med Mol Imaging. 2013;40(5):768–78.
56. Schutz F, Lautenschlager C, Lorenz K, Haerting J. Positron emission tomography (PET) and PET/CT in thyroid cancer: a systematic review and meta-analysis. Eur Thyroid J. 2018;7(1):13–20.
57. Deandreis D, et al. Do histological, immunohistochemical, and metabolic (radioiodine and fluorodeoxyglucose uptakes) patterns of metastatic thyroid cancer correlate with patient outcome? Endocr Relat Cancer. 2011;18(1):159–69.
58. Santhanam P, et al. Utility of I-124 PET/CT in identifying radioiodine avid lesions in differentiated thyroid cancer: a systematic review and meta-analysis. Clin Endocrinol. 2017;86(5):645–51.
59. Jentzen W, et al. 124I PET assessment of response of bone metastases to initial radioiodine treatment of differentiated thyroid cancer. J Nucl Med. 2016;57(10):1499–504.
60. Tuttle RM, et al. Empiric radioactive iodine dosing regimens frequently exceed maximum tolerated activity levels in elderly patients with thyroid cancer. J Nucl Med. 2006;47(10):1587–91.
61. Ilgan S, et al. Iodine-131 treatment and high-resolution CT: results in patients with lung metastases from differentiated thyroid carcinoma. Eur J Nucl Med Mol Imaging. 2004;31(6):825–30.
62. Proye CA, et al. Is it still worthwhile to treat bone metastases from differentiated thyroid carcinoma with radioactive iodine? World J Surg. 1992;16(4):640–5; discussion 645–6.
63. Prinzi A, et al. Brain metastases in differentiated thyroid cancer: clinical presentation, diagnosis, and management. Thyroid. 2024;34(10):1194–204.

64. Buffet C, et al. Redifferentiation of radioiodine-refractory thyroid cancers. Endocr Relat Cancer. 2020;27(5):R113–32.
65. Tuttle RM, et al. Thyroid Carcinoma, version 2.0214. J Natl Compr Canc Netw. https://doi.org/10.6004/jnccn.2014.0169.
66. Lutz S, et al. Palliative radiation therapy for bone metastases: update of an ASTRO evidence-based guideline. Pract Radiat Oncol. 2017;7(1):4–12.
67. Fleming C, et al. Palliative efficacy and local control of conventional radiotherapy for lung metastases. Ann Palliat Med. 2017;6(Suppl 1):S21–7.
68. Wood TJ, et al. Surgical management of bone metastases: quality of evidence and systematic review. Ann Surg Oncol. 2014;21(13):4081–9.
69. Choi J, Kim JW, Keum YS, Lee IJ. The largest known survival analysis of patients with brain metastasis from thyroid cancer based on prognostic groups. PLoS One. 2016;11(4):e0154739.
70. Yoo J, Kim HJ, Kim SM, Park HH. Prognostic factors to predict the efficacy of surgical interventions against brain metastasis secondary to thyroid cancer. Eur Thyroid J. 2022;11(5):e220087.
71. Kedia S, Santhoor H, Singh M. Adverse radiation effects following gamma knife radiosurgery. Neurol India. 2023;71(Supplement):S59–67.
72. Cancer Genome Atlas Research, N. Integrated genomic characterization of papillary thyroid carcinoma. Cell. 2014;159(3):676–90.
73. Zehir A, et al. Mutational landscape of metastatic cancer revealed from prospective clinical sequencing of 10,000 patients. Nat Med. 2017;23(6):703–13.
74. Ibrahimpasic T, et al. Genomic alterations in fatal forms of non-anaplastic thyroid cancer: identification of MED12 and RBM10 as novel thyroid cancer genes associated with tumor virulence. Clin Cancer Res. 2017;23(19):5970–80.
75. Shonka DC Jr, et al. American head and neck society endocrine surgery section and international thyroid oncology group consensus statement on mutational testing in thyroid cancer: defining advanced thyroid cancer and its targeted treatment. Head Neck. 2022;44(6):1277–300.
76. Chen H, et al. Molecular profile of advanced thyroid carcinomas by next-generation sequencing: characterizing tumors beyond diagnosis for targeted therapy. Mol Cancer Ther. 2018;17(7):1575–84.
77. Baloch ZW, et al. Overview of the 2022 WHO classification of thyroid neoplasms. Endocr Pathol. 2022;33(1):27–63.
78. Ringel MD, Sosa JA, Baloch Z, Bischoff L, Bloom G, Brent GA, Brock PL, Chou R, Flavell RR, Goldner W, Grubbs EG, Haymart M, Larson SM, Leung AM, Osborne J, Ridge JA, Robinson B, Steward DL, Tufano RP, Wirth LJ. 2025 American Thyroid Association Management Guidelines for Adult Patients with Differentiated Thyroid Cancer. Thyroid. 2025 Aug;35(8):841-985. https://doi.org/10.1177/10507256251363120. Erratum in: Thyroid. 2025 Nov;35(11):1350. doi: 10.1177/10507256251387671. PMID: 40844370.

Chemotherapy and Immunotherapy in Advanced and Metastatic Thyroid Cancers

18

Kevin J. Zhang, Wanxing Chai-Ho, and Deborah J. Wong

Editorial

The emergence of immunotherapies and targeted therapies involving the PI3K/Akt/mTOR and MAPK cell signaling pathways, which are most often implicated in thyroid cancer, has changed the landscape of treatment for radioactive iodine refractory and metastatic disease. The multikinase inhibitors lenvatinib, sorafenib, and cabozantinib, targeted inhibitors for BRAF, RET, and TRK, and immunotherapies in combination with tyrosine kinase inhibitors (TKIs) have demonstrated significant treatment efficacy. When recurrent locoregional or distant metastatic disease is not amenable to RAI therapy, systemic therapy can be considered. Thyroid cancer generally develops from aberrant signaling in cell growth, proliferation, and survival pathways. The PI3K/Akt/mTOR and MAPK signaling pathways are most critical to thyroid cancer development. The PI3K/Akt/mTOR pathway is triggered through the binding of signaling molecules to receptors on the cell membrane, leading to the activation of a receptor tyrosine kinase. PI3K phosphorylates PIP2 to create PIP3, which then activates AKT. mTOR acts downstream from AKT and promotes tumorigenesis. The MAPK pathway is similarly activated through the binding of an external signal to a receptor tyrosine kinase. This RTK then activates RAS, leading to downstream kinase cascade including RAF kinase and BRAF activation of MEK and ERK. This is followed by nuclear activation by ERK of genes responsible for tumorigenesis. Kinase inhibitors target the activity of the PI3K/Akt/mTOR and

K. J. Zhang
Division of Endocrinology, Department of Medicine, University of California, Los Angeles, CA, USA
e-mail: KJZhang@mednet.ucla.edu

W. Chai-Ho · D. J. Wong (✉)
Division of Hematology/Oncology, Department of Medicine, University of California, Los Angeles, CA, USA
e-mail: WChaiHo@mednet.ucla.edu; DeWong@mednet.ucla.edu

P. S. Pai et al. (eds.), *Controversies in Cancer of the Thyroid and Parathyroid Glands*, https://doi.org/10.1007/978-3-032-13130-0_18

MAPK pathways, which make them a useful tool in the treatment of metastatic thyroid cancer. Radioactive iodine resistance in thyroid cancer portends a poor prognosis with a 10-year survival rate of 10%. Resistance most commonly develops through alterations in the sodium-iodine symporter or constitutive MAPK signaling. Redifferentiation is a process involving restoration of the radioactive iodine uptake in previously RAIR DTC. MAPK inhibitors have demonstrated efficacy in redifferentiation and permitting RAI treatment. The MKI's lenvatinib and sorafenib are recommended as first-line options for systemic therapy. For second-line treatment, cabozantinib is recommended as it has demonstrated efficacy after progression with lenvatinib or sorafenib. More recently, the advent of successful targeted therapies for advanced and metastatic thyroid cancer has introduced the question of optimal sequencing for currently available therapies.

Microsatellite instability (MSI), mismatch repair deficiency (dMMR), tumor mutation burden (TMB), and PD1/PD-L1 (programmed cell death protein 1/programmed cell death ligand 1) expression may serve as biomarkers for prediction of efficacy of immunotherapy in anaplastic thyroid cancer. Current recommendations at this time state that immunotherapy can be considered for thyroid carcinoma with TMB-high (>10 mutations/MB) and in MSI-high or dMMR tumors in the absence of better alternate treatment options.

A current active area of research is the combination of TKIs and immunotherapeutic agents in the treatment of thyroid cancer. The potential of these treatment regimens has been purported through several recent studies of advanced thyroid cancer.

Chemotherapy may also play a role in improving radiosensitivity of DTC in patients with metastatic unresectable or gross residual disease where external beam radiation therapy (EBRT) is considered for preservation of the aerodigestive tracts.

Chris de Souza

Introduction

In recent years, the incidence of thyroid cancer in the United States has been increasing. There were 43,720 new thyroid carcinoma cases diagnosed in the United States in 2023. The lifetime risk of developing thyroid carcinoma is estimated at 1.2%. Women are at higher risk than men, with thyroid cancer being the fifth most common malignancy in women. The prognosis from thyroid cancer is generally very good, with low mortality and 10-year survival estimated to be 90–95% for differentiated thyroid cancers. However, specific patient factors, disease states, and cancer subtypes may significantly impact prognosis [3].

The most common subtypes of thyroid cancer include differentiated thyroid cancer, medullary thyroid cancer (MTC), and anaplastic thyroid cancer (ATC). Papillary thyroid cancer (PTC), follicular thyroid cancer, and Hurthle cell cancer account for 89, 4.5, and 1.8% of all diagnoses, respectively. MTC and ATC make up 1.6 and 0.8%, respectively.

Management of thyroid cancer follows a multimodal treatment course and may include surgical resection, postoperative radioactive iodine, thyroid-stimulating hormone (TSH) suppression with thyroid hormone replacement, and external beam radiation therapy (EBRT). Locoregionally recurrent thyroid cancer may be managed with local therapy with surgery, EBRT, or ablation through cryotherapy, ethanol, or radiofrequency therapy. Radioactive iodine may also be utilized in recurrent and metastatic iodine-avid disease. When recurrent locoregional or distant metastatic disease is not amenable to RAI therapy, systemic therapy is generally considered. Cytotoxic agents have limited efficacy for metastatic thyroid cancer. However, targeted therapies and immunotherapies have demonstrated utility in these cases and have changed the landscape of treatment for radioactive iodine refractory and metastatic disease.

Pathogenesis

Similar to other cancers, thyroid cancer generally develops from aberrant signaling in cell growth, proliferation, and survival pathways. The PI3K/Akt/mTOR and MAPK signaling pathways are most critical to TC development (Fig. 18.1).

The PI3K/Akt/mTOR pathway is triggered through the binding of signaling molecules to receptors on the cell membrane, leading to the activation of a receptor tyrosine kinase. PI3K phosphorylates PIP2 to create PIP3, which then activates AKT. mTOR acts downstream from AKT and promotes tumorigenesis.

The MAPK pathway is similarly activated through the binding of an external signal to a receptor tyrosine kinase. This RTK then activates RAS, leading to downstream kinase cascade including RAF kinase and BRAF activation of MEK and ERK. This is followed by nuclear activation by ERK of genes responsible for tumorigenesis. In thyroid cancer, 80% of mutations can be explained by genes within the MAPK pathway, including RAS, BRAF, and RET fusions. RET is a RTK that can be activated through mutations or fusions with other genes such as PTC1 or PTC3. Aberrant RET signaling causes constitutive activation of MAPK and is strongly associated with the development of PTCs, familial MTC, and sporadic MTC.

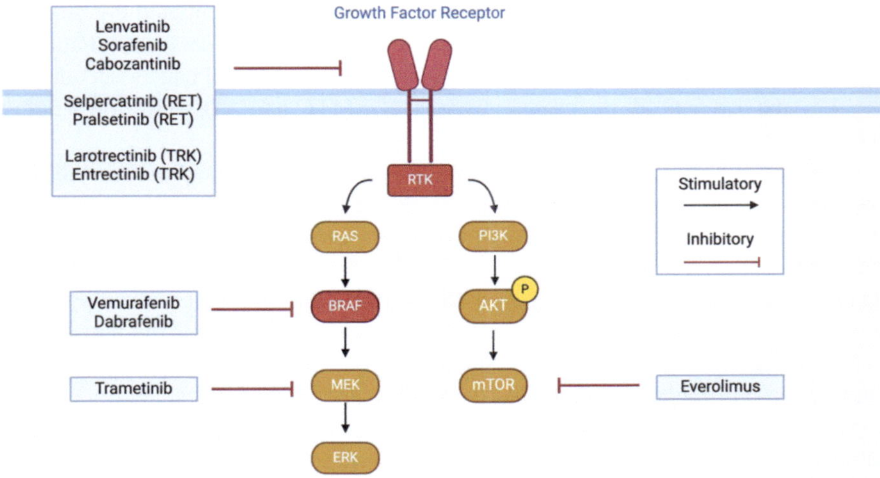

Fig. 18.1 Molecular pathogenesis of thyroid cancer. The main signaling pathways responsible for thyroid cancer pathogenesis are the RAS/RAF/MEK and PI3K/AKT/mTOR pathways. BRAF mutations lead to constitutive MAPK pathway activation, which allows for tumorigenesis and proliferation. Multikinase inhibitors (lenvatinib, sorafenib, cabozantinib), RET inhibitors (selpercatinib, pralsetinib), and TRK inhibitors (larotrectinib, entrectinib) inhibit receptor tyrosine kinases at the cell surface, preventing downstream activity. BRAF inhibitors (vemurafenib, dabrafenib) and the MEK inhibitor (trametinib) inhibit BRAF V600E mutation activity. Everolimus is a mTOR inhibitor that is utilized for RAIR TC with mutations in the PI3K/AKT/mTOR pathway

Molecular Targets and Current Agents

BRAF V600E and BRAF Inhibitors

BRAF V600E is a well-known target in the treatment of melanoma and NSCLC, and treatment with inhibitors of BRAF and MEK has demonstrated efficacy. In thyroid cancer, BRAF V600E mutation portends a poorer prognosis in early-stage disease. About 40% of PTC and 20–50% of ATC patients have a BRAF V600E mutation [10, 16, 29].

Vemurafenib is a BRAF inhibitor that is utilized in the treatment of BRAF V600E mutation-positive thyroid cancer and melanoma. In a non-randomized, multicenter, open-label, phase 2 trial, vemurafenib was given to patients with BRAF V600E-positive metastatic unresectable RAIR PTC. Among treatment-naive patients, 10 of 26 (38%) had PR [7]. Common adverse effects include squamous cell carcinoma of the skin, lymphopenia, and increased GGT.

Dabrafenib is a BRAF inhibitor that has been used in combination with trametinib, a MEK inhibitor, for FDA-approved treatment of locally advanced or metastatic BRAF V600E-mutated anaplastic thyroid cancer. In a cohort of 23 patients with BRAF V600E-mutated ATC, 57% had partial response and 4% had a complete response. In addition, 9 of 14 (64%) of these responders had ongoing response for more than 6 months. Commonly seen side effects of this combination therapy include fever, chills, rash, headache, joint pain, and cough [26].

RET and RET Inhibitors

RET signaling is important in normal physiologic neural and genitourinary system development. However, it also has a major role in the development of various cancer types, most notably DTC, NSCLC, and urothelial carcinoma. There are two major mechanisms for RET oncogene activation, which are RET fusions with genes, such as KIF5B in NSCLC and CCDC6 and NCOA4 in DTC, and gain-of-function RET point mutations in MTC.

Selpercatinib is an oral selective RET kinase inhibitor that is FDA approved for the treatment of advanced MTC with RET mutation and advanced and RAI refractory thyroid cancer with RET gene fusion. The phase III LIBRETTO-531 trial evaluated the performance of selpercatinib compared to multikinase inhibitors cabozantinib or vandetanib in RET-mutated MTC. At a median follow-up of 12 months, the primary endpoint of mPFS by BICR was not reached with selpercatinib and 16.8 months in the control group, with a hazard ratio for disease progression of 0.28 (95% CI, 0.16–0.48, $p < 0.001$). Selpercatinib had a significant overall response rate of 69.4% (95% CI, 62.4–75.8) versus 38.9% in the control group. Side effects were less impactful on treatment course than other multikinase inhibitors, with most common notable ones including hypertension, dry mouth, transaminase elevation, QT prolongation, and rash. The rate of treatment discontinuation from side effects of selpercatinib was 4.7% versus 26.8% [19].

Pralsetinib is another RET kinase inhibitor with utility in multiple cancer types including RET-fusion-positive MTC and lung cancer. In the ARROW phase I/II trial, 13 RET-fusion-positive TC patients had an ORR of 91%. A greater response rate was seen in treatment naive MTC patients (74%) compared to previously treated patients (60%). Common side effects include hypertension, edema, diarrhea, constipation, fatigue, and transaminase elevation [27].

NTRK and TRK Inhibitors

Neurotropic tyrosine receptor kinase (NTRK) signaling is important for physiologic neuronal development in the CNS. Unlike RET, mutations in NTRK genes do not appear to be oncogenic driver events. The primary mechanism for tumorigenesis is through activating NTRK fusions, leading to the production of an intracellular fusion protein with a constitutively activated or overexpressed kinase domain. NTRK fusions are relatively rare and more often associated with thyroid cancer and GIST along with salivary and secretory breast cancer.

TRK inhibitors including larotrectinib and entrectinib may be used for metastatic thyroid cancers with a TRK gene fusion. In pooled data from phase I/II larotrectinib trials, 29 patients with TRK-fusion-positive TC showed an overall response rate of

86% for PTC/FTC and 29% for ATC, including CR in two patients [28]. In a phase II trial, entrectinib also demonstrated efficacy with overall response rate of 54% in patients with TRK inhibitor naive locally advanced or metastatic NTRK-mutated thyroid cancer with an estimated mPFS of 19.9 months with mOS 19.9 months [14]. The most common adverse effects of TRK inhibitor therapy include CNS effects such as dizziness, hepatotoxicity, QT prolongation (entrectinib only), and weight gain.

Multikinase Inhibitors

Kinase inhibitors target the activity of the PI3K/Akt/mTOR and MAPK pathways, which make them a useful tool in the treatment of metastatic thyroid cancer. Multikinase inhibitors have a clinical benefit rate of 50–60%, comprised of PR and stable disease. Duration of response is noted to be around 12–24 months on average. They offer a PFS benefit but no overall survival benefit. Current FDA-approved multikinase inhibitors for use in thyroid cancer include lenvatinib, sorafenib, cabozantinib, pazopanib, axitinib, sunitinib, everolimus, and vandetanib.

Lenvatinib is an inhibitor of VEGFR 1–3, FGFR 1–4, platelet-derived growth factor alpha, RET, and KIT and is approved for radioactive iodine-resistant DTC. It is prescribed at a dose of 24 mg daily. Median PFS was 18.3 months (HR, 0.21; CI, 0.14–0.31; $p < 0.001$). PFS was longer in TKI-naive patients with PFS 18.7 months compared to 15.1 months in patients who had previously received TKI therapy. A significant overall response rate of 64.8% was observed with four documented complete responses but no overall survival benefit. Most common adverse effects included hypertension, diarrhea, fatigue, decreased appetite, weight loss, and nausea [24].

Sorafenib is an inhibitor of VEGFR 1–3, platelet-derived growth factor beta, RAF-1, RET, and BRAF and is approved for radioactive iodine-resistant DTC. Sorafenib has demonstrated an improvement in PFS of 10.8 months (HR, 0.59; CI, 0.45–0.76; $p < 0.0001$) with an objective response rate of 12.2% but no difference in overall survival [6]. Sorafenib is prescribed at a dose of 400 mg BID. There is a large side effect profile, with the most common including hand-foot skin reaction, diarrhea, alopecia, rash or desquamation, fatigue, and weight loss.

Cabozantinib, an inhibitor of VEGFR 2, AXL, MET, RET, and c-MET, was approved by the FDA for treatment of locally advanced or metastatic and radioactive iodine-resistant DTC. The COSMIC-311 study enrolled a cohort of patients who had previously received at least two multikinase inhibitors including lenvatinib or sorafenib, 76% of which had developed progression while on these MKI. In this group, cabozantinib was shown to have an overall response rate of 15% versus 0% in placebo by blinded independent radiology committee (BIRC) [8]. This included 69% stable disease and 6% progression of disease versus 42 and 55% in placebo, respectively. Common side effects of cabozantinib include palmar-plantar erythrodysesthesia, hypertension, fatigue, diarrhea, and hypocalcemia (Table 18.1).

Table 18.1 Tyrosine kinase inhibitors with activity for thyroid cancers

Drug	Indication	Target	PFS (months)	ORR	Adverse effects (most common)
Lenvatinib	DTC	VEGF1-3, FGF1-4, PDGF, KIT, RET	18.3 vs 3.6 placebo	64.80%	Hypertension, diarrhea, fatigue, decreased appetite, weight loss, nausea
Sorafenib	DTC	VEGF1-3, PDGF, FGF, KIT, RET	10.8 vs 5.8 placebo	12.20%	Hand-foot skin reaction, diarrhea, alopecia, rash or desquamation, fatigue, weight loss
Cabozantinib	MTC	c-MET, RET, VEGF2	11.2 vs 4 placebo	28%	Palmar-plantar erythrodysesthesia, hypertension, fatigue, diarrhea, hypocalcemia
Selpercatinib	MTC	RET	NR	73%	Hypertension, dry mouth, transaminase elevation, QT prolongation, rash
Pralsetinib	MTC	RET	NR	74%	Hypertension, edema, diarrhea, constipation, fatigue, transaminase elevation
Larotrectinib	DTC/ ATC	TRK	2.2 (ATC)	86% (DTC) 29% (ATC)	Dizziness, hepatotoxicity, weight gain
Entrectinib	DTC/ ATC	TRK	19.9	54%	Dizziness, hepatotoxicity, weight gain, QT prolongation
Vemurafenib	PTC	BRAF V600E	18.2	39%	Squamous cell carcinoma of the skin, lymphopenia, increased GGT
Dabrafenib/ trametinib	ATC	BRAF V600E/ MEK1&2	NR	69%	Fever, chills, rash, headache, joint pain, cough

PFS progression-free survival, *ORR* overall response rate, *DTC* differentiated thyroid carcinoma, *MTC* medullary thyroid carcinoma, *PTC* papillary thyroid carcinoma, *ATC* anaplastic thyroid carcinoma, *NR* not reached

Mechanisms of Resistance

Radioactive Iodine Resistance

Radioactive iodine resistance in thyroid cancer portends a poor prognosis with a 10-year survival rate of 10%. Resistance most commonly develops through alterations in the sodium-iodine symporter or constitutive MAPK signaling. The sodium-iodine symporter (NIS) is a plasma membrane glycoprotein on thyroid follicular cells that is responsible for the transport of iodide into the cell. Likewise, radioactive iodine is taken up into thyroid cells through NIS. NIS may be downregulated through alterations in the RTK/BRAF/MAPK/ERK and PI3K/AKT/mTOR pathways and therefore is thought to be a mechanism of radioactive iodine resistance. Constitutive MAPK activation, especially when involving a BRAF activating mutation such as V600E, is also thought to lead to increased dedifferentiation of thyroid cells through increased cell division and alterations in thyroid metabolism through inhibition of sodium-iodide symporter and thyroid peroxidase. The activity of MAPK and dedifferentiation is highest in BRAF mutations, followed by RET and NTRK fusions, and lowest in RAS mutations.

Redifferentiation is a process involving restoration of the radioactive iodine uptake in previously RAIR DTC. MAPK inhibitors have demonstrated efficacy in redifferentiation and permitting RAI treatment. One example is selumetinib, a MEK 1 and 2 inhibitor, which was shown to increase uptake after treatment for 4 weeks in 20 patients with RAIR metastatic thyroid cancer, of which nine had BRAF mutations and five had NRAS mutations. Of the 12 patients who had increased uptake after treatment, eight patients reached the dosimetry threshold and were treated, resulting in five patients with PR and three with stable disease [22]. Treatment with dabrafenib and vemurafenib has also been shown to have efficacy in re-establishing increased radioactive iodine uptake.

BRAF Resistance

Resistance to BRAF inhibitors may be primary or secondary in nature. Mechanisms of primary resistance may include concurrent inhibition of the B-cell CLL/lympha 2 (BCL2) apoptosis pathway or the PI3K/AKT/mTOR pathway. BCL2 signaling may be interfered by mechanisms such as copy number gain of myeloid cell leukemia 1 (MCL1) or loss of cyclin-dependent kinase inhibitor 2A (CDK2NA). In these cases, the use of BCL2 inhibitors in combination with BRAF inhibitors has shown enhanced sensitivity to treatment. Mutations in PI3KCA may lead to inhibition of the PI3K/AKT/mTOR pathway. Agents like everolimus, targeted inhibitors for this pathway, may be considered in these instances. Everolimus has demonstrated some clinical efficacy for the treatment of thyroid cancer in both advanced DTC and ATC. In a phase II clinical trial, 17 patients (65% of total) with advanced DTC or ATC who were treated with everolimus 10 mg daily demonstrated stable disease with durable response, with 15 of these patients maintaining SD for more than 24 weeks [21].

Known causes of acquired resistance to BRAF inhibitors include secondary mutations in the MAPK pathway, including the acquisition of NRAS Q61K or KRAS G12V, and FGFR alterations and upregulation in the setting of VEGFR inhibitor use. Further research is needed in this area to evaluate the potential use of MEK inhibitors or novel MAPK inhibitors and FGFR inhibitors, respectively.

Current Controversies and Areas of Investigation

Sequencing of Therapies

In general, the MKIs lenvatinib and sorafenib are recommended as first-line options for systemic therapy. For second-line treatment, cabozantinib is recommended as it has demonstrated efficacy after progression with lenvatinib or sorafenib. More recently, the advent of successful targeted therapies for advanced and metastatic thyroid cancer has introduced the question of optimal sequencing for currently available therapies.

The selection of initial treatment for radioactive iodine refractory BRAF-mutated DTC is an area of ongoing investigation. There is limited randomized data comparing BRAF-targeted therapy with multikinase agents. Current studies suggest that objective response rates along with progression-free survival may be higher in MKI compared to BRAF-targeted therapy, as in the RECIST trial with ORR 65% versus 30–35%, respectively, and mPFS of 18.3 months versus 10–15 months, respectively [24]. However, interpretation of this data is difficult as the patient populations in these trials were heterogeneous in relation to BRAF-mutation status and previous treatments. Side effect tolerability appears to be lower in dabrafenib/trametinib compared to lenvatinib (76% vs 48–58%) [9]. Multikinase agents such as lenvatinib remain the preferred agent for RAIR BRAF-mutated DTC.

On the other hand, it appears that targeted therapies for RET-mutated and NTRK-mutated thyroid cancers have much greater efficacy and tolerability when compared to BRAF-targeted therapy. Current clinical practice favors utilizing a targeted agent in these cases versus a multikinase inhibitor as initial therapy. However, there is also a lack of comparative randomized data. Until further comparative trial data becomes available, providers are recommended to utilize an individualized and shared decision-making approach when making the decision for frontline agent selection for their patients.

Predictive Markers for Immunotherapy

Microsatellite instability (MSI), mismatch repair deficiency (dMMR), tumor mutation burden (TMB), and PD1/PD-L1 (programmed cell death protein 1/programmed cell death ligand 1) expression may serve as biomarkers for prediction of efficacy of immunotherapy in anaplastic thyroid cancer [13, 18].

PD-L1 expression has been shown to be associated with decreased survival in DTC, PDTC, and ATC, but not in MTC. In one study, PD-L1 was reported to be found in around 53.2% of papillary thyroid cancers [4]. However unlike for other cancers, there currently are no validated expression scores for thyroid cancer specifically. In a phase II trial investigating spartalizumab, a PD-1 receptor antagonist, in patients with ATC, greater response was seen in PD-L1 positive vs PD-L1 negative (29% vs 0%) with a 1-year survival of 52.1% in PD-L1-positive population [12].

Current recommendations state that immunotherapy can be considered for thyroid carcinoma with TMB-high (>10 mutations/MB) and in MSI-high or dMMR tumors in the absence of better alternate treatment options [1].

Combination Therapy for Advanced ATC and Poorly Differentiated TC

A current active area of research is the combination of TKIs and immunotherapeutic agents in the treatment of thyroid cancer. The potential of these treatment regimens has been purported through several recent studies of advanced thyroid cancer. Particular attention on trials has been focused on ATC and poorly differentiated TC, in which treatment options are limited.

In the phase II ATLEP trial, lenvatinib (20 mg daily) and pembrolizumab (200 mg every 3 weeks) were given to patients with metastatic ATC and poorly differentiated thyroid cancer without BRAF V600E mutations. This regimen demonstrated a significant clinical benefit rate, with 34.3% overall response rate at 3 months, with the best overall response within 2 years being 96.73% for ATC and 100% for PDTC. Benefits were also seen in mPFS of 9.5 months and overall survival of 1.25 months in ATC with 25.9% survival greater than 2 years, as well as PDTC with mPFS of 20 months [17].

A retrospective analysis was conducted of patients with BRAF V600E-positive ATC who were treated with dabrafenib plus trametinib along with pembrolizumab compared to those who had not received immunotherapy. The overall response rate in the immunotherapy arm was higher, 73% compared to 65%, with increased modified PFS of 11 months versus 4 months, and a median overall survival of 17 months versus 9 months [20].

A recent nonrandomized phase II trial evaluating a combination of vemurafenib, cobimetinib, and atezolizumab in BRAF V600E-mutated ATC demonstrated the longest mOS at 43.2 months and mPFS 13.9 months. Nine of 18 patients were able to undergo surgical resection [11].

Role of Cytotoxic Chemotherapy

Cytotoxic chemotherapy for treatment of advanced thyroid cancers has limited efficacy. In general, TKI demonstrates much higher efficacy and tolerability for the management of advanced or metastatic RAIR thyroid cancer. A retrospective study comparing sorafenib with chemotherapy as initial treatment of locally advanced or metastatic RAIR thyroid cancer demonstrated significantly longer PFS of 25.5 months versus 4.7 months respectively [23].

Although data is limited, cytotoxic chemotherapy may be considered in disease that is refractory to TKI therapies. In past trials, most favorable outcomes were seen with combination chemotherapy regimens that included doxorubicin [25]. In a systematic review of 16 studies evaluating chemotherapy in advanced DTC, the

Table 18.2 Combination therapy (tyrosine kinase inhibitors and immunotherapy)

Drug combination	Indication	PFS (months)	ORR
Lenvatinib/pembrolizumab	ATC/PDTC with BRAF V600E	9.5	34.30% (at 3 months)
Dabrafenib/trametinib/pembrolizumab	ATC with BRAF V600E	11 versus 4 (no immunotherapy)	73%
Vemurafenib/cobimetinib/atezolizumab	ATC with BRAF V600E	13.9	59%

PFS progression-free survival, *ORR* overall response rate, *ATC* anaplastic thyroid carcinoma, *PDTC* poorly differentiated thyroid cancer

average ORR was 22.1% with 2.5% CR [2]. Treatment was also significantly limited by poor tolerability. A case was reported of a patient with RAIR PDTC who had progression with three different MKI (vandetanib, sorafenib, sunitinib) but achieved complete response to a doxorubicin-cisplatin combination lasting 10 months and paclitaxel-carboplatin regimen lasting 5 months (Table 18.2) [15].

Chemotherapy may also play a role in improving radiosensitivity of DTC in patients with metastatic unresectable or gross residual disease where external beam radiation therapy (EBRT) is considered for preservation of the aerodigestive tracts. In a retrospective review, 88 patients who received intensity-modulated radiation therapy were identified, 45 of which received concurrent doxorubicin, and it was found that patients who received doxorubicin had higher local progression-free survival (85.8% vs 68.8%, $p = 0.036$) as well as higher 4-year OS (68.0% vs 47.0%, $p = 0.043$) with similar rates of acute and late toxicities [5].

References

1. Agosto Salgado S, et al. NCCN guidelines version 5.2024 thyroid carcinoma. 2024. https://www.ncbi.nlm.nih.gov/.
2. Albero A, Lopéz JE, Torres A, de la Cruz L, Martín T. Effectiveness of chemotherapy in advanced differentiated thyroid cancer: a systematic review. Endocr Relat Cancer. 2016;23(2):R71–84. https://doi.org/10.1530/ERC-15-0194.
3. American Cancer Society. Cancer facts & figures 2024. Atlanta: American Cancer Society; 2024.
4. Bai Y, Niu D, Huang X, Jia L, Kang Q, Dou F, Ji X, Xue W, Liu Y, Li Z, Feng Q, Lin D, Kakudo K. PD-L1 and PD-1 expression are correlated with distinctive clinicopathological features in papillary thyroid carcinoma. Diagn Pathol. 2017;12(1):72. https://doi.org/10.1186/s13000-017-0662-z.
5. Beckham TH, Romesser PB, Groen AH, Sabol C, Shaha AR, Sabra M, Brinkman T, Spielsinger D, McBride S, Tsai CJ, Riaz N, Tuttle RM, Fagin JA, Sherman EJ, Wong RJ, Lee NY. Intensity-modulated radiation therapy with or without concurrent chemotherapy in nonanaplastic thyroid cancer with Unresectable or gross residual disease. Thyroid. 2018;28(9):1180–9. https://doi.org/10.1089/thy.2018.0214.
6. Brose MS, Nutting CM, Jarzab B, DECISION investigators, et al. Sorafenib in radioactive iodine-refractory, locally advanced or metastatic differentiated thyroid cancer: a randomised, double-blind, phase 3 trial. Lancet. 2014;384(9940):319–28.
7. Brose MS, Cabanillas ME, Cohen EE, Wirth LJ, Riehl T, Yue H, Sherman SI, Sherman EJ. Vemurafenib in patients with BRAF(V600E)-positive metastatic or unresectable papillary

thyroid cancer refractory to radioactive iodine: a non-randomised, multicentre, open-label, phase 2 trial. Lancet Oncol. 2016;17(9):1272–82. https://doi.org/10.1016/S1470-2045(16)30166-8. Epub 2016 Jul 23

8. Brose MS, Robinson B, Sherman SI, et al. Cabozantinib for radioiodine-refractory differentiated thyroid cancer (COSMIC-311): a randomised, double-blind, placebo-controlled, phase 3 trial. Lancet Oncol. 2021;22(8):1126–38.
9. Busaidy NL, Konda B, Wei L, et al. Dabrafenib versus Dabrafenib + Trametinib in BRAF-mutated radioactive iodine refractory differentiated thyroid cancer: results of a randomized, phase 2, open-label multicenter trial. Thyroid. 2022;32(10):1184–92.
10. Cabanillas ME, Ryder M, Jimenez C. Targeted therapy for advanced thyroid cancer: kinase inhibitors and beyond. Endocr Rev. 2019;40:1573–604.
11. Cabanillas ME, Dadu R, Ferrarotto R, et al. Anti–programmed death ligand 1 plus targeted therapy in anaplastic thyroid carcinoma: a nonrandomized clinical trial. JAMA Oncol. 2024;10(12):1672–80. https://doi.org/10.1001/jamaoncol.2024.4729.
12. Capdevila J, Wirth LJ, Ernst T, Ponce Aix S, Lin CC, Ramlau R, Butler MO, Delord JP, Gelderblom H, Ascierto PA, Fasolo A, Führer D, Hütter-Krönke ML, Forde PM, Wrona A, Santoro A, Sadow PM, Szpakowski S, Wu H, Bostel G, Faris J, Cameron S, Varga A, Taylor M. PD-1 blockade in anaplastic thyroid carcinoma. J Clin Oncol. 2020;38(23):2620–7. https://doi.org/10.1200/JCO.19.02727. Epub 2020 May 4
13. Carneiro HC, de Andrade Natal R, Farias EC, et al. Predictive biomarkers in thyroid cancer in the current molecular-morphology paradigm. Surg Exp Pathol. 2024;7:14. https://doi.org/10.1186/s42047-024-00157-1.
14. Cho BC, Chiu CH, Massarelli E, Buchschacher GL, Goto K, Overbeck TR, Loong HHF, Chee CE, Garrido P, Dong X, Fan Y, Lu S, Schwemmers S, Bordogna W, Zeuner H, Osborne S, John T. Updated efficacy and safety of entrectinib in NTRK fusion-positive non-small cell lung cancer. Lung Cancer. 2024;188:107442. https://doi.org/10.1016/j.lungcan.2023.107442.
15. Crouzeix G, Michels JJ, Sevin E, Aide N, Vaur D, Bardet S, French TUTHYREF Network. Unusual short-term complete response to two regimens of cytotoxic chemotherapy in a patient with poorly differentiated thyroid carcinoma. J Clin Endocrinol Metab. 2012;97(9):3046–50. https://doi.org/10.1210/jc.2012-1630. Epub 2012 Jun 21.
16. Davies H, Bignell GR, Cox C, Stephens P, Edkins S, Clegg S, Teague J, Woffendin H, Garnett MJ, Bottomley W, Davis N, Dicks E, Ewing R, Floyd Y, Gray K, Hall S, Hawes R, Hughes J, Kosmidou V, Menzies A, Mould C, Parker A, Stevens C, Watt S, Hooper S, Wilson R, Jayatilake H, Gusterson BA, Cooper C, Shipley J, Hargrave D, Pritchard-Jones K, Maitland N, Chenevix-Trench G, Riggins GJ, Bigner DD, Palmieri G, Cossu A, Flanagan A, Nicholson A, Ho JW, Leung SY, Yuen ST, Weber BL, Seigler HF, Darrow TL, Paterson H, Marais R, Marshall CJ, Wooster R, Stratton MR, Futreal PA. Mutations of the BRAF gene in human cancer. Nature. 2002;417(6892):949–54. https://doi.org/10.1038/nature00766.
17. Dierks C, Ruf J, Seufert J, Kreissl M, Klein C, Spitzweg C, Kroiss M, Thomusch O, Lorenz K, Zielke A, Miething C. Phase II ATLEP trial: Final results for lenvatinib/pembrolizumab in metastasized anaplastic and poorly differentiated thyroid carcinoma. Annals of Oncology. 33:S1295.
18. Fan S, Yuan Y, Su Y, Sang D. Advanced anaplastic thyroid carcinoma with positive expression of PD-L1 response to immune checkpoint inhibitors: a case report. SAGE Open Med Case Rep. 2025;13:2050313X241313084. https://doi.org/10.1177/2050313X241313084.
19. Hadoux J, Elisei R, Brose MS, Hoff AO, Robinson BG, Gao M, Jarzab B, Isaev P, Kopeckova K, Wadsley J, Führer D, Keam B, Bardet S, Sherman EJ, Tahara M, Hu MI, Singh R, Lin Y, Soldatenkova V, Wright J, Lin B, Maeda P, Capdevila J, Wirth LJ, LIBRETTO-531 Trial Investigators. Phase 3 trial of Selpercatinib in advanced RET-mutant medullary thyroid cancer. N Engl J Med. 2023;389(20):1851–61. https://doi.org/10.1056/NEJMoa2309719. Epub 2023 Oct 21.
20. Hamidi S, Iyer PC, Dadu R, Gule-Monroe MK, Maniakas A, Zafereo ME, Wang JR, Busaidy NL, Cabanillas ME. Checkpoint inhibition in addition to Dabrafenib/Trametinib for

BRAF^{V600E}-mutated anaplastic thyroid carcinoma. Thyroid. 2024;34(3):336–46. https://doi.org/10.1089/thy.2023.0573. Epub 2024 Feb 13

21. Harris EJ, Hanna GJ, Chau N, Rabinowits G, Haddad R, Margalit DN, Schoenfeld J, Tishler RB, Barletta JA, Nehs M, Janne P, Huang J, Groden P, Kacew A, Lorch J. Everolimus in anaplastic thyroid cancer: a case series. Front Oncol. 2019;9:106. https://doi.org/10.3389/fonc.2019.00106.
22. Ho AL, Grewal RK, Leboeuf R, Sherman EJ, Pfister DG, Deandreis D, Pentlow KS, Zanzonico PB, Haque S, Gavane S, Ghossein RA, Ricarte-Filho JC, Domínguez JM, Shen R, Tuttle RM, Larson SM, Fagin JA. Selumetinib-enhanced radioiodine uptake in advanced thyroid cancer. N Engl J Med. 2013;368(7):623–32. https://doi.org/10.1056/NEJMoa1209288.
23. Majidova N, Aghamaliyeva S, Guliyev M, Dinc G, Akyıldız A, Ozcan E, Akdağ Kahvecıoglu F, Çağrı Yıldırım H, Sever N, Guren AK, Kocaaslan E, Erel P, Agyol Y, Celebi A, Arıkan R, Isık S, Bayoglu IV, Demirci NS, Dizdar Ö, Hacıbekiroğlu I, Kostek O, Sarı M. Sorafenib vs chemotherapy in the treatment of locally advanced or metastatic, radioactive iodine-refractory differentiated thyroid cancer: real-world data from Turkey. J Chemother. 2024:1–6. https://doi.org/10.1080/1120009X.2024.2430845. Epub ahead of print.
24. Schlumberger M, Tahara M, Wirth LJ, et al. Lenvatinib versus placebo in radioiodine-refractory thyroid cancer. N Engl J Med. 2015;372(7):621–30.
25. Sherman SI. Cytotoxic chemotherapy for differentiated thyroid carcinoma. Clin Oncol (R Coll Radiol). 2010;22(6):464–8. https://doi.org/10.1016/j.clon.2010.03.014. Epub 2010 May 8
26. Subbiah V, Kreitman RJ, Wainberg ZA, Cho JY, Schellens JHM, Soria JC, Wen PY, Zielinski C, Cabanillas ME, Urbanowitz G, Mookerjee B, Wang D, Rangwala F, Keam B. Dabrafenib and Trametinib treatment in patients with locally advanced or metastatic BRAF V600-mutant anaplastic thyroid cancer. J Clin Oncol. 2018;36(1):7–13. https://doi.org/10.1200/JCO.2017.73.6785. Epub 2017 Oct 26
27. Subbiah V, Hu MI, Wirth LJ, Schuler M, Mansfield AS, Curigliano G, Brose MS, Zhu VW, Leboulleux S, Bowles DW, Baik CS, Adkins D, Keam B, Matos I, Garralda E, Gainor JF, Lopes G, Lin CC, Godbert Y, Sarker D, Miller SG, Clifford C, Zhang H, Turner CD, Taylor MH. Pralsetinib for patients with advanced or metastatic RET-altered thyroid cancer (ARROW): a multi-cohort, open-label, registrational, phase 1/2 study. Lancet Diabetes Endocrinol. 2021;9(8):491–501. https://doi.org/10.1016/S2213-8587(21)00120-0. Epub 2021 Jun 9. Erratum in: Lancet Diabetes Endocrinol. 2021 Oct;9(10):e4. 10.1016/S2213-8587(21)00247-3.
28. Waguespack SG, Drilon A, Lin JJ, Brose MS, McDermott R, Almubarak M, Bauman J, Casanova M, Krishnamurthy A, Kummar S, Leyvraz S, Oh DY, Park K, Sohal D, Sherman E, Norenberg R, Silvertown JD, Brega N, Hong DS, Cabanillas ME. Efficacy and safety of larotrectinib in patients with TRK fusion-positive thyroid carcinoma. Eur J Endocrinol. 2022;186(6):631–43. https://doi.org/10.1530/EJE-21-1259.
29. Xing M, Alzahrani AS, Carson KA, Viola D, Elisei R, Bendlova B, Yip L, Mian C, Vianello F, Tuttle RM, Robenshtok E, Fagin JA, Puxeddu E, Fugazzola L, Czarniecka A, Jarzab B, O'Neill CJ, Sywak MS, Lam AK, Riesco-Eizaguirre G, Santisteban P, Nakayama H, Tufano RP, Pai SI, Zeiger MA, Westra WH, Clark DP, Clifton-Bligh R, Sidransky D, Ladenson PW, Sykorova V. Association between BRAF V600E mutation and mortality in patients with papillary thyroid cancer. JAMA. 2013;309(14):1493–501. https://doi.org/10.1001/jama.2013.3190.

Anaplastic Thyroid Carcinoma

19

Abhishek Vaidya and Prathamesh S. Pai

Editorial

ATC is regarded as one of the most fatal of all solid tumours, with an overall disease-specific mortality approaching ~100%. This reality underscores the importance of rapid intervention and consideration of clinical trials when managing ATC. The molecular profile of ATC is characterized by accumulation of multiple mutations: an initial oncogenic driver (BRAF or RAS) followed by TERT promoter mutations and p53 inactivation, amongst others, leading to a highly undifferentiated, treatment-resistant phenotype. A key decision is to assess if curable (confined to the thyroid/neck and surgically resectable) or incurable (widely metastatic or unresectable). This stratification guides the intensity of therapy and goals of care.

Post-surgery, adjuvant external beam radiotherapy (EBRT) is advised to all patients to prevent local recurrences. Intensity-modulated radiation therapy (IMRT) is preferred, allowing delivery of high doses (60–66 Gy in conventional fractionation) to the thyroid bed and involved nodal regions while sparing critical structures as much as possible.

Aggressive combined treatment can meaningfully extend life in a select group of patients. The majority, however, still succumb very quickly, reinforcing the need for early palliative care involvement.

It is now standard of care to screen all ATC tumours for BRAF mutation at diagnosis and if positive to start dabrafenib/trametinib combination promptly. The advent of BRAF/MEK-targeted therapy has substantially improved outcomes for the subset of ATC patients with BRAF^V600E some of whom have experienced

A. Vaidya (✉)
National Cancer Institute, Nagpur, India

P. S. Pai
Department of Surgical Oncology, P D Hinduja Hospital & Medical Research Centre, Khar, Mumbai, India

P. S. Pai et al. (eds.), *Controversies in Cancer of the Thyroid and Parathyroid Glands*, https://doi.org/10.1007/978-3-032-13130-0_19

complete remissions lasting a year or longer, which was virtually unheard of previously.

The poor prognosis of ATC and its resistance to conventional therapy have prompted investigation into immunotherapy. Ongoing studies are evaluating combinations of BRAF/MEK inhibitors with immunotherapy in BRAF-mutant ATC, as well as dual checkpoint blockade (e.g. CTLA-4 plus PD-1 inhibition) in ATC irrespective of mutation status, in an effort to overcome resistance and augment antitumour immune activity. It is likely that integrating immunotherapy into upfront ATC management will become a new standard, especially for patients with no contraindications to immunotherapy.

Introduction

Anaplasia means "to form backward", which implies loss of the structural and functional differentiation. Anaplastic thyroid cancer (ATC) is a rare, highly aggressive cancer with a poor prognosis and a high mortality rate. Although thyroid cancer is typically known for being one of the more treatable cancers, the anaplastic variant defies this trend, with a median survival of less than 6 months. The rapid progression of this cancer and its propensity for metastasis make it one of the most difficult cancers to treat effectively.

Despite guidelines and research [1–4], the management of ATC remains a subject of significant controversy, particularly concerning the optimal treatment strategies, the role of surgery, radiotherapy, systemic therapy, and the use of targeted therapies as well as immunotherapy. This chapter explores the key controversies in the management of ATC, highlighting differences in expert opinion, evolving clinical evidence, and unresolved challenges.

Pathogenesis and Molecular Features

ATC is believed to often arise from preexisting multinodular goitre or a differentiated thyroid carcinoma (DTC) through a process of dedifferentiation [3]. Approximately 20–30% of ATCs are thought to develop from a prior well-differentiated thyroid cancer (most commonly papillary thyroid carcinoma), and in another subset of cases, an ATC tumour coexists alongside a differentiated or poorly differentiated component within the thyroid [3, 5]. Studies have shown identical mutations (BRAFV600E, TERT promotor, TP53 mutations) in coexisting ATC and papillary carcinoma components of the same tumour, indicating clonal evolution from the differentiated to anaplastic form [5, 6].

Genetic profiling of ATC reveals a high burden of mutations and chromosomal alterations consistent with its aggressive behaviour (see Table 19.1) [7–11]. Early "driver" mutations common in well-differentiated thyroid cancers (such as BRAF or RAS mutations) are often present in ATC, but ATC tumours typically harbour additional mutations in tumour suppressors and genome stability genes that are

Table 19.1 Genetic alterations and drivers in anaplastic thyroid cancer

(a) Well-established alterations			
Gene/alteration	Frequency	Clinical implication	Notes
BRAF V600E [8, 10, 46]	~45%	Targetable with BRAF + MEK inhibitors	Often coexists with TERT promoter mutation
TERT promoter [9]	65–75%	Marker of aggressive course	Synergistic with BRAF/RAS
TP53 [8, 10]	50–63%	Loss of tumour suppressor	Hallmark of dedifferentiation
RAS (NRAS/KRAS/HRAS) [8, 10]	22–24%	MAPK pathway activation	No approved targeted therapy
PIK3CA [7]	~18%	Activates PI3K/AKT/mTOR	Often co-mutated
PTEN [11]	~14%	Loss activates PI3K pathway	Contributes to resistance
CDKN2A/B [10]	Variable	Cell cycle dysregulation	Potential CDK4/6 inhibitor sensitivity
(b) Rarer/emerging alterations			
Gene/alteration	Frequency	Clinical implication	Notes
PD-L1 (CD274) [10]	~60–70% expression	Predicts PD-1/PD-L1 inhibitor response	9p24.1 amplification in subset
SWI/SNF (ARID1A, SMARCA4) [8]	Frequent (variable)	Epigenetic therapy potential	Often co-mutated with TP53
MSI-H / MMR deficiency	~5–8%	Predicts pembrolizumab sensitivity	Tumour-agnostic approval
NTRK fusions [10]	<1%	Targetable with TRK inhibitors	Larotrectinib/entrectinib approved tumour-agnostic
RET fusions [8]	Very rare	RET inhibitors	Selpercatinib/pralsetinib approved

infrequent in differentiated tumours [8, 11]. TP53, the tumour suppressor gene, is mutated in the majority of ATCs, contributing to loss of cell cycle control. TERT promoter mutations are found in roughly 40–60% of ATCs and frequently co-occur with BRAF or RAS mutations, synergistically promoting aggressive behaviour. [8, 9] Activating BRAF V600E mutations themselves are present in a substantial subset of ATC (estimates range from ~25% up to 50% of cases in different series), especially in those that arose from an antecedent papillary carcinoma (tall-cell variant PTC is often implicated) [10, 12]. RAS mutations (NRAS or HRAS) account for another 20–30% of ATCs, more often in tumours arising from follicular or Hürthle cell carcinoma lineage [8, 10]. Other commonly altered pathways include the PI3K/AKT/mTOR pathway (mutations in PIK3CA, PTEN, etc.), alterations in cell cycle regulators (e.g. CDKN2A/B deletions), and aberrations in genes like PTC/RET fusions or NTRK fusions in a minority of cases [6, 7, 11]. Overall, the molecular profile of ATC is characterized by accumulation of multiple mutations: an initial oncogenic driver (BRAF or RAS) followed by TERT promoter mutations and p53 inactivation, amongst others, leading to a highly undifferentiated, treatment-resistant phenotype [8, 10].

Clinical Presentation and Diagnosis

ATC typically presents in older adults (sixth–seventh decade) with a rapidly enlarging neck mass. There is often a relatively short history of symptoms, sometimes only a few weeks of noticing a growth in the anterior neck. Patients may develop compressive symptoms due to the tumour's aggressive local invasion: dysphagia (from oesophageal compression), dyspnoea or stridor (from tracheal compression/invasion), and hoarseness from recurrent laryngeal nerve involvement are common presenting features. The tumour is usually hard, immobile, and rapidly enlarging on exam, and regional lymphadenopathy is frequently present. At diagnosis, most patients have locoregionally advanced disease, and almost 50% on investigation have distant metastases often to the lungs followed by the bone and brain.

The diagnosis of ATC is usually a clinical suspicion based on symptoms of rapid growth in weeks and a hard midline mass with restricted mobility. Fine-needle aspiration (FNA) is the first-line diagnostic test for any thyroid nodule, and cytology is quite diagnostic in ATC with smears showing high cellularity and pleomorphic malignant cells (giant cells, spindle cells, and squamoid cells) along with atypical mitoses [13]. Ultrasound (US)-guided core needle biopsy is a crucial diagnostic step, since urgent diagnosis is paramount as well as it is vital to get tissue for molecular pathology [14, 15].

On histopathology, ATC has an undifferentiated appearance and may show varying histologic patterns (spindle-cell-sarcomatoid, pleomorphic giant cell, and epithelioid carcinoma), and multiple patterns may coexist. In around 20% of cases, a spectrum ranging from areas of residual differentiated thyroid carcinoma to a transitional poorly differentiated carcinoma can be found alongside an anaplastic component, supporting the dedifferentiation pathogenesis. Immunohistochemistry can aid in confirming thyroid origin of an anaplastic tumour as most ATCs will express cytokeratins (pancytokeratin positive) and often epithelial membrane antigen (EMA). They typically lose thyroid-specific markers like thyroglobulin and TTF-1, but may retain patchy positivity for PAX-8 (a transcription factor marker of thyroid lineage) in about one-third of cases, which can be a helpful clue to thyroid origin [16]. This is important because the differential diagnosis of ATC includes metastases to the thyroid (e.g. from lung, which can be keratin positive but PAX-8 negative) and primary thyroid lymphoma or sarcoma. ATC by definition should be negative for lymphoid markers (to exclude lymphoma) and negative for mesenchymal markers like desmin (to exclude a sarcoma) [17]. When needed, a broad IHC panel and molecular studies can be employed to confirm the diagnosis [16].

Staging and Prognosis

The AJCC/UICC TNM staging system classifies all anaplastic thyroid carcinomas as Stage IV disease due to their extremely poor prognosis. Under the eighth edition AJCC staging [18], tumours confined to the thyroid (regardless of size) are Stage

IVA; tumours with extrathyroidal extension (local invasion) are Stage IVB; and any case with distant metastasis is Stage IVC.

These stage groupings reflect the grave prognosis even with a small intrathyroidal ATC. Clinically, the distinction between IVA and IVB (locally resectable vs unresectable disease) and the presence of metastases (IVC) guide management decisions [18], but they all should be considered as advanced cancers.

Prognostic factors in ATC are uniformly poor, but nuances do exist [19, 20]. Patients with disease confined to the thyroid (IVA) at presentation have a slightly better prognosis than those with gross extrathyroidal extension or distant spread. Complete surgical resection of the primary tumour is associated with improved survival. Patients under 50–65 years tend to survive few months more than older patients [1, 21]. Tumour genetic profile might predict responsiveness to targeted therapy. Those with a presence of a BRAF mutation might do better than the tumours with no actionable mutations. Those with markers of high-risk behaviour (TERT and p53 mutations) or extremely high proliferative index may behave even more aggressively [22].

Without treatment, ATC is universally fatal within few months [19, 20]. Even with maximal multimodal therapy, historical survival rates show <10% of patients alive at 2 years. In a large SEER database analysis from 1983 to 2002, the median survival was only 4 months, and the 5-year survival was under 5% [23]. A more recent SEER analysis reported a median overall survival (OS) of 4 months and a 6-month OS of 35% [24]. Contemporary series from high-volume centres suggest that a small subset of patients who have locoregionally confined disease who undergo complete surgery followed by chemoradiation have lived beyond 12–24 months, and rare cases of disease-free survival at 3 or more years are reported [25]. Nevertheless, ATC is regarded as one of the most fatal of all solid tumours, with an overall disease-specific mortality approaching ~100%. This reality underscores the importance of rapid intervention and consideration of clinical trials when managing ATC.

Management

Given the complexity and urgency of ATC management, care should be delivered by a multidisciplinary team, ideally at centres experienced with this rare disease. The ATA 2021 guidelines strongly emphasize assembling an ATC care team (including endocrinology, surgery, medical and radiation oncology, palliative care, etc.) as soon as the diagnosis is suspected [1]. Initial management steps include securing the airway if compromised (some patients require prompt intubation or tracheostomy due to tracheal invasion), assessing resectability of the tumour, and evaluating for distant metastases with appropriate imaging (CT/MRI of the neck and chest, plus brain imaging since brain metastases are not uncommon) [1]. Due to the rapid progression, time is of the essence—staging and treatment decisions are often made within days, and in parallel, molecular testing of the tumour is initiated urgently (especially for BRAF status, which can now be determined within 1–2 days by immunohistochemistry or expedited PCR) [1]. A key decision is to assess if curable (confined to the thyroid/neck and surgically resectable) or incurable (widely metastatic or unresectable). This stratification guides the intensity of therapy and goals of care.

Locoregional Resectable Disease: Surgery and Radiotherapy

In ATC that is localized to the thyroid and neck, and is resectable, without distant metastasis (Stage IVA), an aggressive multimodal treatment with intent of cure is pursued. Surgery is the cornerstone of curative-intent therapy and involves a complete thyroidectomy with en bloc resection of involved surrounding tissues along with neck dissection. Unlike differentiated thyroid cancer, the goal in ATC surgery is maximal tumour clearance. Achieving an R0 or R1 resection (microscopic positive margin) significantly improves survival chances compared to having unresected or grossly residual disease [26]. A systematic review found that surgical resection (especially R0/R1) was associated with improved 1-year survival in ATC, whereas patients who did not undergo surgery did not survive beyond a year [26]. Therefore, when feasible, an experienced head-neck or endocrine surgeon should do prompt surgery, even if that requires extensive resection of adjacent structures (e.g. strap muscles and jugular vein) [1]. However, it is vitally important that aggressive surgical approach has to be balanced with the patient's performance status and preferences. Surgery that anticipates either R1 resection or resection of major structures (parts of trachea or oesophagus) to achieve R0, such that the quality of life will be severely affected, should be avoided [1].

Role of Adjuvant Therapy

Surgery alone is not sufficient therapy except in the most exceptional circumstance of a tiny intrathyroidal ATC discovered incidentally where you would still consider adjuvant therapy. Post-surgery, adjuvant external beam radiotherapy (EBRT) is advised to all patients to prevent local recurrence [1]. Intensity-modulated radiation therapy (IMRT) is preferred, allowing delivery of high doses (60–66 Gy in conventional fractionation) to the thyroid bed and involved nodal regions while sparing critical structures as much as possible [1]. The addition of radiotherapy after surgery improves locoregional control and is associated with longer survival in retrospective analyses. A population-based study found that patients who received surgery followed by radiotherapy lived longer than those who had surgery alone for ATC with extrathyroidal extension [23]. Likewise, institutional series have reported that aggressive combined modality therapy (complete surgery + adjuvant radiotherapy, often with chemotherapy) can roughly double median survival in comparison to one modality alone [27]. In a study, trimodality treatment (surgery, radiation, and systemic therapy) had markedly improved survival compared to those treated with single-modality or palliative approaches. The 1-year overall survival in the multimodal cohort was ~42%, compared to ~10% in the earlier cohort managed more conservatively [27]. These data support using all available modalities for fit patients with nonmetastatic ATC.

Concurrent Chemoradiation

When either the primary tumour is unresectable (Stage IVB) or the patient is not a surgical candidate, definitive chemoradiation is offered to control the locoregional disease. This typically involves high-dose radiation to the thyroid tumour and neck (60–66 Gy) delivered with IMRT or proton therapy, combined with concurrent chemotherapy as a radiosensitizer [1, 27]. However, outcomes with definitive chemoradiation alone are poor and rare. Nonetheless, some cases achieve temporary tumour control and palliation of local symptoms. For unresectable disease, the goal is to prevent imminent airway or oesophageal obstruction and buy time for systemic therapy to work if an actionable mutation is present.

Systemic Therapy

Chemotherapy

Chemotherapy in ATC has historically been of limited benefit when used alone, but it is frequently used in combination with radiation (concurrent or sequential) in the curative-intent setting. Doxorubicin was the first chemotherapeutic agent used for ATC and remained a mainstay for decades despite modest efficacy—response rates to doxorubicin monotherapy are only to the order of 20%, and responses are usually partial and not durable [3, 28]. In modern practice, taxane-based chemotherapy has supplanted doxorubicin for ATC. Small studies have shown that paclitaxel or docetaxel, given weekly or in high-dose short courses, can induce tumour shrinkage and radiosensitize ATC [28]. A Phase II study of concurrent docetaxel with hyperfractionated radiotherapy reported appreciable locoregional control and some pathological responses in ATC patients [25]. Weekly paclitaxel is often used during radiation due to its radiosensitizing properties and relatively tolerable toxicity profile; some centres continue it as maintenance therapy for a short period after radiation as well. Combination regimens such as paclitaxel + carboplatin have also been used and can have higher response rates than single agents, though no randomized trials exist [28]. A retrospective analysis from a tertiary centre showed that amongst patients treated with palliative intent, those who received chemotherapy (often taxane-based) lived longer than those who got best supportive care alone, suggesting some benefit to systemic therapy even in the metastatic setting [29]. However, no conventional cytotoxic regimen has demonstrated a significant improvement in overall survival in controlled studies, and the role of chemotherapy in ATC is largely adjunctive (to surgery/radiation) or palliative. Outcomes of multimodal therapy in ATC remain poor overall, but significantly better than with single-modality treatment. An illuminating real-world dataset comes from a large Indian tertiary cancer centre (Tata Memorial Hospital), which reported their 12-year experience managing 134 ATC patients [29]. In that cohort, only 39% of patients were able to receive curative-intent therapy (surgery and adjuvant therapy or definitive chemoradiation), whereas 61% received only palliative treatments or best supportive care (12). The differences in outcomes were stark: patients treated with curative intent had a median overall survival (OS) of ~134 days (~4.5 months) versus only ~50 days (~1.6 months) in those treated palliatively. Furthermore, within the curative-intent subgroup, those who underwent surgery (followed by adjuvant therapy) fared better than those who received nonsurgical definitive chemoradiation (median OS 155 days vs 76 days, respectively). Notably, patients who had surgery followed by adjuvant chemoradiation achieved the best outcomes—in that subset, median OS was 540 days (approximately 18 months), compared to only 91 days (~3 months) in patients who had surgery but no adjuvant therapy. This study suggests that aggressive combined treatment can meaningfully extend life in a select group of patients. The majority, however, still succumb very quickly, reinforcing the need for early palliative care involvement.

Neoadjuvant Systemic Therapy

Neoadjuvant therapy before surgery has been tried in ATC management [30, 31]. Traditionally, due to the rapid progression, most patients underwent upfront surgery if resectable. But with the advent of very active systemic agents for certain subsets of ATC (see below), there have been attempts to shrink tumours preoperatively to improve resectability especially in BRAF-mutated ATC [1, 30, 31]. Small [31] series have documented instances of initially unresectable ATC becoming surgically removable after short-term targeted therapy, leading to unexpectedly prolonged survival. This approach is not yet standard, but is being studied in clinical trials (such approaches are investigating neoadjuvant dabrafenib + trametinib with immunotherapy in BRAF-mutated ATC) [32, 33].

Targeted Therapy

Until recently, systemic therapy for ATC was limited to conventional chemotherapy, with minimal impact on long-term survival. However, the emergence of targeted therapies against specific mutations has dramatically changed the management of a subset of ATC patients (see Table 19.2) [34–37]. The discovery of actionable mutations in ATC has opened new therapeutic avenues. The most important of these is BRAF. Approximately 40% (range ~ 25–50%) of ATC tumours carry the BRAF^V600E mutation, the same mutation common in papillary thyroid carcinoma [12]. In 2018, results from an international basket trial (the ROAR study) patients with BRAF^V600- mutated ATC were treated with a combination of the BRAF inhibitor dabrafenib and MEK inhibitor trametinib, yielding a confirmed

Table 19.2 Current chemotherapy, targeted therapy, and immunotherapy regimens in ATC

(a) FDA/EMA-approved regimen			
Regimen	Mechanism	Setting	Key outcomes
Dabrafenib + trametinib [34]	BRAF + MEK inhibition	BRAF V600E-mutant unresectable/metastatic ATC	ORR ~56%; improved OS; FDA approval for BRAF V600E ATC
b) Other regimens (off-label or in trials)			
Regimen	Mechanism	Setting	Key outcomes
Paclitaxel ± carboplatin [47]	Taxan ± platinum chemo	First-line cytotoxic	ORR 10–20%; median OS <6 months
Lenvatinib [36]	Multi-targeted TKI (VEGFR/FGFR/PDGFR/RET)	Off-label/advanced ATC	ORR ~15%; mPFS ~3.2 months
Pembrolizumab [35]	Anti-PD-1 immunotherapy	PD-L1 high/MSI-H ATC	Modest response rates in small series; durable responses in some patients
Lenvatinib + pembrolizumab [37]	TKI + PD-1 inhibitor	Investigational	Retrospective cohorts show promising responses

response rate of about 69% [34]. The responses were rapid and dramatic, leading to relief of symptoms, and notably, the median duration of response, progression-free survival, and overall survival in that cohort was not reached at the time of reporting (median follow-up 47 weeks), with a 12-month overall survival estimated at 80% [34]. As a result of this trial, dabrafenib + trametinib became the first FDA-approved systemic therapy for BRAF-mutated ATC4. It is now standard of care to screen all ATC tumours for BRAF mutation at diagnosis and, if positive, to start dabrafenib/trametinib combination promptly [1]. The advent of BRAF/MEK-targeted therapy has substantially improved outcomes for the subset of ATC patients with BRAF^V600E, some of whom have experienced complete remissions lasting a year or longer, which was virtually unheard of previously.

In addition to BRAF, other targetable alterations such as NTRK gene fusions, while less common, are studied in ATC. These fusions drive oncogenic TRK kinase activity. The TRK inhibitors larotrectinib and entrectinib have shown extraordinary efficacy in TRK fusion-positive cancers of various types, with response rates around 75% and often prolonged remissions even in advanced disease. ATC with an NTRK fusion would be expected to respond similarly [38].

ATC rarely can harbour RET fusions or RET mutations. The selective RET inhibitor selpercatinib has demonstrated efficacy in RET-altered thyroid cancers—in a 2020 trial, patients with RET fusion-positive thyroid cancers (mostly PTC) had an objective response rate of 79%, including some responses in aggressive cases [39]. If an ATC patient were found to have a RET fusion, selpercatinib or a similar RET inhibitor (like pralsetinib) would be a rational off-label choice.

ALK fusions are exceedingly rare in ATC but have been reported. There are case reports of ATC patients with an ALK rearrangement achieving near-complete tumour regression when treated with ALK inhibitors (such as crizotinib or newer-generation ALK inhibitors) [40]. While these cases are anecdotal, they illustrate the importance of comprehensive molecular testing for targetable mutations, which might be detected and are the key to survival.

In addition to these specific mutation-directed therapies, multitargeted kinase inhibitors that have activity against the angiogenic pathways have been used in ATC. Lenvatinib, a VEGFR-targeted TKI (approved for radioiodine-refractory differentiated thyroid carcinoma), has shown some activity in ATC. A Phase II study of lenvatinib in advanced thyroid cancers reported partial responses in a subset of ATC patients (overall response ~24%) and some disease stabilization, though progression typically occurred within a few months [41]. Sorafenib, another anti-angiogenic TKI, was tested in a small Phase II trial in ATC and achieved a few partial responses but no major survival benefit [42]. These multi-kinase inhibitors can be considered for ATC patients who lack a clear driver mutation or after failure of other therapies, as they may slow tumour progression. Their benefit is mostly palliative, however, and they come with significant side effects (hypertension, fatigue, mucositis, etc.), which in a frail ATC patient can be hard to manage.

Immunotherapy and Emerging Approaches

The poor prognosis of ATC and its resistance to conventional therapy have prompted investigation into immunotherapy. ATC tumours often have abundant tumour-associated macrophages and can express immune checkpoints like PD-L1 [35], providing a rationale for trying immune checkpoint inhibitors. Early results have been mixed but somewhat encouraging. While 19% overall response rate may seem modest, it is notable in ATC, and responders in that trial had a median duration of response of about dozen months, far exceeding the typical survival of nonresponders. The median overall survival in the spartalizumab trial was about 5.7 months, which underscores the fact that a small subset may benefit [35]. Importantly, responses to PD-1 blockade were more likely in tumours with PD-L1 expression of ≥50%, suggesting a biomarker; approximately 25% of ATCs in that study had high PD-L1, and most of the responders were in that category. These findings have opened the door to using PD-1 inhibitors (like pembrolizumab or nivolumab) in ATC, particularly in patients who have no other targetable mutations or who have stable disease after initial therapy.

Checkpoint inhibitors are also being combined with other treatments in ATC in hopes of synergy. One promising approach is the combination of immunotherapy with anti-angiogenic therapy. In a German multicentre series, the combination of lenvatinib and pembrolizumab produced tumour responses in several patients with advanced thyroid carcinoma, including ATC, whereas either agent alone may not have been effective. This synergy is thought to arise because lenvatinib can remodel the tumour microenvironment, reducing immunosuppressive cell populations and enhancing T-cell infiltration, thereby increasing the efficacy of PD-1 blockade [37]. Similarly, ongoing studies are evaluating combinations of BRAF/MEK inhibitors with immunotherapy in BRAF-mutant ATC, as well as dual checkpoint blockade (e.g. CTLA-4 plus PD-1 inhibition) in ATC irrespective of mutation status, in an effort to overcome resistance and augment antitumour immune activity [43].

Adjuvant Immunotherapy

One of the most promising developments has been the use of immunotherapy in the adjuvant setting after initial aggressive therapy to prevent recurrence. Traditionally, after surgery and chemoradiation for Stage IVB ATC (locally advanced, no distant metastasis), patients would relapse quickly, often with distant metastases. Building on the efficacy of pembrolizumab in other refractory cancers, investigators at MD Anderson Cancer Centre launched a trial of adjuvant pembrolizumab following definitive surgery and radiation in ATC. Amongst 16 patients treated with pembrolizumab after chemoradiation, the 1-year relapse-free survival has vastly improved and reduced the recurrence rate from 82% to 19%. The median progression-free and overall survival were not reached compared with 5.4 months and 31 months in controls, respectively, with all patients in the pembrolizumab arm alive at 12 and 24 months versus 80 and 52% in the control group [44]. This translated into a statistically significant improvement in progression-free and overall survival for the adjuvant pembrolizumab group. These data, although from a small non-randomized study, suggest that immunotherapy given immediately after initial treatment may eradicate microscopic residual disease and dramatically delay or prevent relapse in ATC. Based on these findings, some major cancer centres have already adopted adjuvant PD-1 inhibitor therapy (often for 1 year) as part of their ATC treatment protocol for Stage IVB disease. Ongoing trials (such as ITOG's trials) will shed more light, but it is likely that integrating immunotherapy into upfront ATC management will become a new standard, especially for patients with no contraindications to immunotherapy. Table 19.3 details ongoing trials and new directions in the management of ATC.

In addition to systemic therapy, there are other emerging approaches being explored for ATC. These include targeted radiotherapy (such as iodine-125 seed implants or intensity-modulated proton therapy for unresectable disease), gene therapy and oncolytic viruses, and various experimental drugs targeting pathways like PI3K/mTOR or cell cycle checkpoints (some early-phase trials have tested agents like everolimus, CDK inhibitors, etc., with limited success so far) [1]. Given ATC's aggressive biology, experimental approaches are often justified, and clinical trial enrolment is strongly encouraged whenever available.

Table 19.3 Future directions and ongoing/planned clinical trials in ATC

Agent/approach	Phase	Study ID/key site
NTRK inhibitors (larotrectinib, entrectinib) [38, 48]	II (basket trials)	STARTRK-2 (entrectinib); NAVIGATE (larotrectinib)
RET inhibitors (selpercatinib [39], pralsetinib)	I/II (basket trials)	LIBRETTO-001 (selpercatinib)
CDK4/6 inhibitors (palbociclib) [49]	I/II	Preclinical support; trials in other cancers
FTase inhibitor (tipifarnib) [50]	I/II	Preclinical support in HRAS-mutant ATC
Oncolytic virotherapy (GLV-1 h68) [51]	I	Early-phase/preclinical only
Dual ICI (nivolumab + ipilimumab) [37]	II	NCT03246958 (UCSF); ORR ~30% in ATC cohort
TKI + ICI (lenvatinib + pembrolizumab) [5]	II/III	ATLEP trial; anecdotal + real-world reports
Pembrolizumab (MSI-H tumours) [52]	II/III (site-agnostic)	Tumour-agnostic approval; relevant to ~5–8% of ATC
Adoptive cell therapy (CAR-T, TILs) [53]	I	Experimental; no ATC-specific trials registered yet

Palliative Care and Supportive Measures

Parallel to aggressive oncologic management, early palliative care involvement is essential in ATC [1]. Patients deteriorate rapidly, and symptoms need to be managed proactively. Airway compromise is frequent in anaplastic thyroid carcinoma; tracheal invasion is reported in about 25% of patients, and published series report that roughly 20–30% may develop acute airway obstruction necessitating tracheostomy during the disease course [1 , 45]. Reported rates vary by series and setting. Elective tracheostomy is generally avoided if possible; emergency tracheostomy is performed for life-threatening obstruction after multidisciplinary discussion [1, 45]. Pain control is another priority, as ATC invading nerves or surrounding structures can cause severe pain. Nutritional support (feeding tube placement) may be needed if swallowing becomes impaired.

Given the extremely poor prognosis, goals-of-care discussions should be initiated early. The healthcare team should help patients and families understand the likely course of the disease and assist with advanced care planning for ventilation, bleeding, dysphagia, etc. Frank discussions about the intent of treatment (curative vs palliative) and involvement of palliative care specialists from the time of diagnosis is critical [1].

Even during active treatment, quality of life can be improved by palliative treatment interventions such as external beam radiation for palliating painful bone metastases and stenting of the trachea or oesophagus to alleviate obstruction [1].

Thyroid cancer, including ATC, can produce thyrotoxic symptoms if large amounts of hormone are released from destroyed thyroid tissue, so beta-blockers or even anti-thyroid medications are occasionally used to control hyperthyroid symptoms (though true thyrotoxicosis is uncommon in ATC since the tumour is largely non-functioning). Family and psychosocial support is likewise crucial, as the shock of an ATC diagnosis and its rapid progression are emotionally devastating.

Key Advances in Anaplastic Thyroid Carcinoma Management: Latest Emerging Evidence

Evidence emerging in 2025 has consolidated immuno-targeted combinations as a new therapeutic backbone in anaplastic thyroid carcinoma (ATC), particularly in BRAF-mutant disease.A landmark phase II non-randomized trial from MD Anderson demonstrated that mutation-matched targeted therapy combined with PD-L1 blockade (atezolizumab) achieved a median overall survival of 19 months across cohorts, with BRAF V600E–mutated patients achieving a median overall survival exceeding 40 months—far surpassing historical benchmarks of 4–6 months [54].

Most notably, a multicenter phase II ASCO 2025 trial evaluating *neoadjuvant pembrolizumab combined with dabrafenib and trametinib (DTP)* in BRAF V600E–mutated ATC reported unprecedented surgical conversion rates, with over 80% of patients proceeding to resection and a high proportion achieving R0/R1 margins, alongside encouraging 1- and 2-year survival outcomes [55].

Neoadjuvant Immuno-Targeted Therapy in BRAF-Mutant ATC

ASCO 2025—Zafereo et al. [55]

A multicenter phase II trial evaluated neoadjuvant pembrolizumab combined with dabrafenib and trametinib in patients with BRAF V600E–mutated anaplastic thyroid carcinoma. The regimen produced rapid and substantial tumor regression, enabling surgical resection in the majority of patients who were initially deemed borderline resectable or unresectable. High rates of R0/R1 resection were achieved, with encouraging 1- and 2-year survival outcomes compared with historical controls. These findings support neoadjuvant immuno-targeted therapy as a viable strategy to facilitate curative-intent surgery in selected BRAF-mutant ATC patients.

Mutation-Matched Targeted Therapy Plus PD-L1 Blockade

ASCO Updates/JAMA Oncology Publication—Cabanillas et al. [54]

Prospective phase II data presented and updated through ASCO meetings demonstrated that combining PD-L1 inhibition (atezolizumab) with mutation-matched targeted therapy significantly prolongs survival in ATC. The greatest benefit was observed in BRAF V600E–mutated tumors treated with BRAF/MEK inhibition plus immunotherapy, achieving median overall survival exceeding 40 months. Non-BRAF cohorts showed more modest benefit. These results represent one of the most substantial survival improvements reported in ATC to date, albeit from non-randomized data.

Dual Immune Checkpoint Blockade

ASCO 2024–2025—Dual ICI cohorts4

Phase II studies evaluating combined PD-1 and CTLA-4 inhibition (nivolumab plus ipilimumab) in aggressive thyroid cancers, including ATC, reported objective responses in a subset of patients irrespective of driver mutation status. However, responses were heterogeneous and associated with increased immune-related toxicity. These data suggest potential activity in molecularly unselected ATC but emphasize the need for careful patient selection and experienced multidisciplinary management.

Peri-operative and Adjuvant Immunotherapy

ASCO Updates/Thyroid 2025—Cabanillas et al. [58]

ASCO updates reinforced earlier institutional data demonstrating that adjuvant pembrolizumab administered after definitive surgery and chemoradiation in stage IVB ATC may significantly delay recurrence and improve survival. While derived from non-randomized cohorts, these findings complement neoadjuvant data and suggest a broader peri-operative role for immune checkpoint inhibition in ATC management.

Interpretation and Clinical Context

Collectively, ASCO 2024–2025 data indicate a paradigm shift toward *systemic disease control upfront*, particularly in BRAF-mutant ATC, using *combined targeted therapy and immunotherapy*, with surgery increasingly integrated as a downstream consolidative modality. These data strengthen the paradigm shift toward upfront systemic disease control followed by surgery, rather than immediate surgery alone, in selected patients with locally advanced ATC. Parallel phase II experiences with dual immune checkpoint blockade and TKI–immunotherapy combinations continue to suggest activity in molecularly unselected ATC, though with higher toxicity and less predictable benefit. While these advances represent a meaningful departure from historical outcomes, the evidence remains largely phase II and non-randomized, underscoring the importance of treatment at experienced centers and continued enrollment in prospective trials (Table 19.4).

Table 19.4 Major clinical trials and evidence updates in anaplastic thyroid carcinoma

Study/Year	Trial ID	Phase	Population	Regimen	Key outcomes
Cabanillas et al. 2024–2025 [54]	NCT03181100	Phase II	Advanced ATC (mutation-matched cohorts)	Atezolizumab + targeted therapy (BRAF/MEK, MEK alone, or VEGF-directed)	Median OS 19 mo overall; *BRAF cohort median OS 43 mo*; met primary endpoint
Zafereo et al. ASCO 2025 [55]	NCT04675710	Phase II	BRAF V600E-mutant ATC (neoadjuvant)	Pembrolizumab + dabrafenib + trametinib	>80% surgical conversion; high R0/R1 rate; 1-yr OS ~70%
Hamidi et al. 2024 [56]	—	Phase II cohort	BRAF-mutant ATC	Dabrafenib + trametinib + PD-1 inhibitor	Improved durability of response vs BRAF/MEK alone
Dual ICI studies, ASCO 2024–25 [57]	NCT03246958	Phase II	Advanced ATC	Nivolumab + ipilimumab	Responses in subset; higher immune toxicity
Adjuvant pembrolizumab update, 2025 [58]	—	Phase II (non-randomized)	Stage IVB ATC post-CRT	Pembrolizumab (adjuvant)	Sustained relapse-free survival; OS not reached

Conclusion

Anaplastic thyroid carcinoma remains one of the most challenging malignancies, with a historically grim outlook. Incremental improvements are being achieved through a combination of vigilant multidisciplinary care and novel therapies. Optimal management involves rapid diagnosis, accurate tumour genotyping, and a multimodal treatment plan tailored to the patient's disease extent and mutation profile. For localized disease, aggressive surgery followed by chemoradiotherapy offers the best chance of extending survival. For metastatic or driver-positive disease, targeted therapies can produce meaningful responses. Immunotherapy incorporating PD-1 inhibitors along with targeted therapy in the neoadjuvant and adjuvant setting may significantly improve outcomes.

However, despite the advances, we should not forget that most ATC patients will succumb to their disease, underscoring the importance of clinical trials and research. With these approaches, and with continued scientific advances, there is cautious optimism that the historically intractable prognosis of anaplastic thyroid carcinoma can be gradually improved.

References

1. Bible KC, et al. 2021 American Thyroid Association guidelines for Management of Patients with anaplastic thyroid cancer. Thyroid. 2021;31:337–86. https://doi.org/10.1089/thy.2020.0944.
2. Mathur P, et al. Cancer statistics, 2020: report from National Cancer Registry Programme, India. JCO Glob Oncol. 2020;6:1063–75. https://doi.org/10.1200/GO.20.00122.
3. Nagaiah G, Hossain A, Mooney CJ, Parmentier J, Remick SC. Anaplastic thyroid cancer: a review of epidemiology, pathogenesis, and treatment. J Oncol. 2011;2011:542358. https://doi.org/10.1155/2011/542358.
4. Smallridge RC, et al. American Thyroid Association guidelines for management of patients with anaplastic thyroid cancer. Thyroid. 2012;22:1104–39. https://doi.org/10.1089/thy.2012.0302.
5. Quiros RM, Ding HG, Gattuso P, Prinz RA, Xu X. Evidence that one subset of anaplastic thyroid carcinomas are derived from papillary carcinomas due to BRAF and p53 mutations. Cancer. 2005;103:2261–8. https://doi.org/10.1002/cncr.21073.
6. Oishi N, et al. Molecular alterations of coexisting thyroid papillary carcinoma and anaplastic carcinoma: identification of TERT mutation as an independent risk factor for transformation. Mod Pathol. 2017;30:1527–37. https://doi.org/10.1038/modpathol.2017.75.
7. Garcia-Rostan G, et al. Mutation of the PIK3CA gene in anaplastic thyroid cancer. Cancer Res. 2005;65:10199–207. https://doi.org/10.1158/0008-5472.CAN-04-4259.
8. Landa I, et al. Genomic and transcriptomic hallmarks of poorly differentiated and anaplastic thyroid cancers. J Clin Invest. 2016;126:1052–66. https://doi.org/10.1172/JCI85271.
9. Melo M, et al. TERT promoter mutations are a major indicator of poor outcome in differentiated thyroid carcinomas. J Clin Endocrinol Metab. 2014;99:E754–65. https://doi.org/10.1210/jc.2013-3734.
10. Pozdeyev N, et al. Genetic analysis of 779 advanced differentiated and anaplastic thyroid cancers. Clin Cancer Res. 2018;24:3059–68. https://doi.org/10.1158/1078-0432.CCR-18-0373.
11. Santarpia L, El-Naggar AK, Cote GJ, Myers JN, Sherman SI. Phosphatidylinositol 3-kinase/akt and ras/raf-mitogen-activated protein kinase pathway mutations in anaplastic thyroid cancer. J Clin Endocrinol Metab. 2008;93:278–84. https://doi.org/10.1210/jc.2007-1076.

12. Cabanillas ME, et al. Acquired secondary RAS mutation in BRAF(V600E)-mutated thyroid cancer patients treated with BRAF inhibitors. Thyroid. 2020;30:1288–96. https://doi.org/10.1089/thy.2019.0514.
13. Podany P, et al. Anaplastic thyroid carcinoma: Cytomorphologic features on fine-needle aspiration and associated diagnostic challenges. Am J Clin Pathol. 2022;157:608–19. https://doi.org/10.1093/ajcp/aqab159.
14. Ha EJ, et al. Core needle biopsy could reduce diagnostic surgery in patients with anaplastic thyroid cancer or thyroid lymphoma. Eur Radiol. 2016;26:1031–6. https://doi.org/10.1007/s00330-015-3921-y.
15. Matrone A, et al. Core needle biopsy can early and precisely identify large thyroid masses. Front Oncol. 2022;12:854755. https://doi.org/10.3389/fonc.2022.854755.
16. Abe I, Lam AK. Anaplastic thyroid carcinoma: updates on WHO classification, clinicopathological features and staging. Histol Histopathol. 2021;36:239–48. https://doi.org/10.14670/HH-18-277.
17. Crescenzi A, Baloch Z. Immunohistochemistry in the pathologic diagnosis and management of thyroid neoplasms. Front Endocrinol (Lausanne). 2023;14:1198099. https://doi.org/10.3389/fendo.2023.1198099.
18. Tuttle RM, Haugen B, Perrier ND. Updated American joint committee on cancer/tumor-node-metastasis staging system for differentiated and anaplastic thyroid cancer (eighth edition): what changed and why? Thyroid. 2017;27:751–6. https://doi.org/10.1089/thy.2017.0102.
19. Glaser SM, Mandish SF, Gill BS, Balasubramani GK, Clump DA, Beriwal S. Anaplastic thyroid cancer: prognostic factors, patterns of care, and overall survival. Head Neck. 2016;38(Suppl 1):E2083–90. https://doi.org/10.1002/hed.24384.
20. Maniakas A, et al. Evaluation of overall survival in patients with anaplastic thyroid carcinoma, 2000-2019. JAMA Oncol. 2020;6:1397–404. https://doi.org/10.1001/jamaoncol.2020.3362.
21. Zivaljevic V, et al. Age as a prognostic factor in anaplastic thyroid cancer. Int J Endocrinol. 2014;2014:240513. https://doi.org/10.1155/2014/240513.
22. Wang JR, et al. Impact of somatic mutations on survival outcomes in patients with anaplastic thyroid carcinoma. JCO Precis Oncol. 2022;6:e2100504. https://doi.org/10.1200/PO.21.00504.
23. Chen J, Tward JD, Shrieve DC, Hitchcock YJ. Surgery and radiotherapy improves survival in patients with anaplastic thyroid carcinoma: analysis of the surveillance, epidemiology, and end results 1983-2002. Am J Clin Oncol. 2008;31:460–4. https://doi.org/10.1097/COC.0b013e31816a61f3.
24. Lin B, et al. The incidence and survival analysis for anaplastic thyroid cancer: a SEER database analysis. Am J Transl Res. 2019;11:5888–96.
25. Troch M, et al. High efficacy of concomitant treatment of undifferentiated (anaplastic) thyroid cancer with radiation and docetaxel. J Clin Endocrinol Metab. 2010;95:E54–7. https://doi.org/10.1210/jc.2009-2827.
26. Hu S, Helman SN, Hanly E, Likhterov I. The role of surgery in anaplastic thyroid cancer: a systematic review. Am J Otolaryngol. 2017;38:337–50. https://doi.org/10.1016/j.amjoto.2017.02.005.
27. Prasongsook N, et al. Survival in response to multimodal therapy in anaplastic thyroid cancer. J Clin Endocrinol Metab. 2017;102:4506–14. https://doi.org/10.1210/jc.2017-01180.
28. Agrawal AK, et al. Systemic therapy in thyroid cancer. Indian J Surg Oncol. 2022;13:68–80. https://doi.org/10.1007/s13193-021-01398-2.
29. Kanteti APK, et al. Anaplastic cancer: our experience. Indian J Surg Oncol. 2022;13:789–96. https://doi.org/10.1007/s13193-022-01576-w.
30. Perri F, Lorenzo GD, Scarpati GD, Buonerba C. Anaplastic thyroid carcinoma: a comprehensive review of current and future therapeutic options. World J Clin Oncol. 2011;2:150–7. https://doi.org/10.5306/wjco.v2.i3.150.
31. Raab GT, et al. Clinical and surgical outcomes of neoadjuvant targeted therapy in anaplastic and differentiated thyroid cancer. J Clin Oncol. 2025;43:e18143. https://doi.org/10.1200/JCO.2025.43.16_suppl.e18143.

32. Zafereo M, et al. Neoadjuvant pembrolizumab in combination with dabrafenib and trametinib (DTP) for *BRAF* V600E-mutated anaplastic thyroid cancer (*BRAF*m-ATC): a multicenter phase 2 trial. J Clin Oncol. 2025;43:6008. https://doi.org/10.1200/JCO.2025.43.16_suppl.6008.
33. Cabanillas ME, et al. Neoadjuvant BRAF- and immune-directed therapy for anaplastic thyroid carcinoma. Thyroid. 2018;28:945–51. https://doi.org/10.1089/thy.2018.0060.
34. Subbiah V, et al. Dabrafenib and Trametinib treatment in patients with locally advanced or metastatic BRAF V600-mutant anaplastic thyroid cancer. J Clin Oncol. 2018;36:7–13. https://doi.org/10.1200/JCO.2017.73.6785.
35. Capdevila J, et al. PD-1 blockade in anaplastic thyroid carcinoma. J Clin Oncol. 2020;38:2620–7. https://doi.org/10.1200/JCO.19.02727.
36. Wirth LJ, et al. Open-label, single-arm, multicenter, phase II trial of Lenvatinib for the treatment of patients with anaplastic thyroid cancer. J Clin Oncol. 2021;39:2359–66. https://doi.org/10.1200/JCO.20.03093.
37. Dierks C, et al. Combination of Lenvatinib and Pembrolizumab is an effective treatment option for anaplastic and poorly differentiated thyroid carcinoma. Thyroid. 2021;31:1076–85. https://doi.org/10.1089/thy.2020.0322.
38. Drilon A, et al. Efficacy of Larotrectinib in TRK fusion-positive cancers in adults and children. N Engl J Med. 2018;378:731–9. https://doi.org/10.1056/NEJMoa1714448.
39. Wirth LJ, et al. Efficacy of Selpercatinib in RET-altered thyroid cancers. N Engl J Med. 2020;383:825–35. https://doi.org/10.1056/NEJMoa2005651.
40. Godbert Y, et al. Remarkable response to Crizotinib in woman with anaplastic lymphoma kinase-rearranged anaplastic thyroid carcinoma. J Clin Oncol. 2015;33:e84–7. https://doi.org/10.1200/JCO.2013.49.6596.
41. Takahashi S, et al. A phase II study of the safety and efficacy of lenvatinib in patients with advanced thyroid cancer. Future Oncol. 2019;15:717–26. https://doi.org/10.2217/fon-2018-0557.
42. Savvides P, et al. Phase II trial of sorafenib in patients with advanced anaplastic carcinoma of the thyroid. Thyroid. 2013;23:600–4. https://doi.org/10.1089/thy.2012.0103.
43. Hamidi S, et al. Checkpoint inhibition in addition to Dabrafenib/Trametinib for BRAF(V600E)-mutated anaplastic thyroid carcinoma. Thyroid. 2024;34:336–46. https://doi.org/10.1089/thy.2023.0573.
44. Cabanillas ME, et al. Adjuvant Pembrolizumab after upfront multimodal therapy for stage IVB anaplastic thyroid cancer. Thyroid. 2025;35:763–70. https://doi.org/10.1089/thy.2025.0194.
45. Shaha AR. Airway management in anaplastic thyroid carcinoma. Laryngoscope. 2008;118:1195–8. https://doi.org/10.1097/MLG.0b013e3181726d36.
46. Pan Z, et al. Integrative proteogenomic characterization reveals therapeutic targets in poorly differentiated and anaplastic thyroid cancers. Nat Commun. 2025;16:3601. https://doi.org/10.1038/s41467-025-58910-3.
47. Ain KB, Egorin MJ, DeSimone PA. Treatment of anaplastic thyroid carcinoma with paclitaxel: phase 2 trial using ninety-six-hour infusion. Collaborative Anaplastic Thyroid Cancer Health Intervention Trials (CATCHIT) Group. Thyroid. 2000;10:587–94. https://doi.org/10.1089/thy.2000.10.587.
48. Paz-Ares L, et al. Patient-reported outcomes from STARTRK-2: a global phase II basket study of entrectinib for ROS1 fusion-positive non-small-cell lung cancer and NTRK fusion-positive solid tumours. ESMO Open. 2021;6:100113. https://doi.org/10.1016/j.esmoop.2021.100113.
49. Lopes-Ventura S, et al. The efficacy of HRAS and CDK4/6 inhibitors in anaplastic thyroid cancer cell lines. J Endocrinol Investig. 2019;42:527–40. https://doi.org/10.1007/s40618-018-0947-4.
50. Untch BR, et al. Tipifarnib inhibits HRAS-driven dedifferentiated thyroid cancers. Cancer Res. 2018;78:4642–57. https://doi.org/10.1158/0008-5472.CAN-17-1925.
51. Passaro C, Somma SD, Malfitano AM, Portella G. Oncolytic virotherapy for anaplastic and poorly differentiated thyroid cancer: a promise or a clinical reality? Int J Endocrine Oncol. 2018;5:IJE10. https://doi.org/10.2217/ije-2017-0028.

52. Marcus L, Lemery SJ, Keegan P, Pazdur R. FDA approval summary: Pembrolizumab for the treatment of microsatellite instability-high solid tumors. Clin Cancer Res. 2019;25:3753–8. https://doi.org/10.1158/1078-0432.CCR-18-4070.
53. Srour SA, et al. Safety and efficacy of AIC100 chimeric antigen receptor (CAR) T-cell therapy in patients with advanced thyroid cancers: results from the phase 1 study. J Clin Oncol. 2024;42:6112. https://doi.org/10.1200/JCO.2024.42.16_suppl.6112.
54. Cabanillas ME, Dadu R, Ferrarotto R, et al. Anti–PD-L1 plus targeted therapy in anaplastic thyroid carcinoma: a nonrandomized clinical trial. JAMA Oncol. 2024;10:1672–80. https://doi.org/10.1001/jamaoncol.2024.4729.
55. Zafereo M, et al. Neoadjuvant pembrolizumab with dabrafenib and trametinib for BRAF V600E–mutated anaplastic thyroid cancer. J Clin Oncol. 2025;43(suppl):6008.
56. Hamidi S, et al. Checkpoint inhibition in addition to dabrafenib/trametinib for BRAF-mutant ATC. Thyroid. 2024;34:336–46. https://doi.org/10.1089/thy.2023.0573.
57. Sehgal K, et al. Dual immune checkpoint inhibition in aggressive thyroid carcinoma. J Clin Oncol. 2024–2025 ASCO abstracts.
58. Cabanillas ME, et al. Adjuvant pembrolizumab following multimodal therapy for stage IVB ATC. Thyroid. 2025;35:763–70. https://doi.org/10.1089/thy.2025.0194.

Pathology Updates in Cancer of the Thyroid and Its Clinical Implications

20

Tomohiro Chiba

Abbreviations

ATC	Anaplastic thyroid carcinoma
BLTs	*BRAF* p.V600E-like tumors
CC-PTC	clear cell PTC
CRC	Cribriform-morular carcinoma
HGDTC	High-grade differentiated thyroid carcinoma
DS-PTC	Diffuse sclerosing PTC
ea.	Encapsulated angioinvasive
EFVPTC	Encapsulated follicular variant
FAP	Familial adenomatous polyposis
FNs	Follicular neoplasms
FTC	Follicular thyroid carcinoma
FT-UMP	Follicular tumour of uncertain malignant potential
FV-PTC	Follicular variant of PTC
HD	Hashimoto's disease
HN-PTC	Hobnail PTC
HTT	Hyalinizing trabecular tumor
IEFVPTC	Invasive encapsulated follicular variant PTC
ITC	Intrathyroidal thymic carcinoma
MASC	Mammary analogue secretory carcinoma
MEC	Mucoepidermoid carcinoma
mi	minimally invasive
MTC	Medullary thyroid carcinoma

T. Chiba (✉)
Department of Cytology and Department of Pathology, Cancer Institute Hospital of Japanese Foundation for Cancer Research (JFCR), Tokyo, Japan
e-mail: tomohiro.chiba@jfcr.or.jp

P. S. Pai et al. (eds.), *Controversies in Cancer of the Thyroid and Parathyroid Glands*, https://doi.org/10.1007/978-3-032-13130-0_20

NENs	Neuroendocrine neoplasms
NIFTP	Noninvasive follicular thyroid neoplasm with papillary-like nuclear features
OA	Oncocytic adenoma of the thyroid
OCA	Oncocytic carcinoma of the thyroid
O-PTC	Oncocytic PTC
PDTC	Poorly differentiated thyroid carcinoma
PTC	Papillary thyroid carcinoma
PTC, FA	follicular thyroid adenoma
RLTs	*RAS*-like tumors
SC	secretory carcinoma
SCC	Squamous cell carcinoma
SETTLE	Spindle cell tumor with thymus-like differentiation
SMECE	sclerosing mucoepidermoid carcinoma with eosinophilia
STI	Solid, trabecular, or insular
ST-PTC	Solid/trabecular PTC
TC-PTC	Tall cell PTC
TFND	Thyroid follicular nodular disease
TSH	Thyroid-stimulating hormone
TSHR	TSH receptor
TT-UMP	thyroid tumor of uncertain malignant potential
WDT-UMP	Well-differentiated tumors of uncertain malignant potential
WHO fifth	WHO classification of endocrine/neuroendocrine tumours fifth edition
WHO fourth	WHO classification of endocrine tumors fourth edition
wi	widely invasive

Editorial

Pathological diagnosis is very important for management and therapy of thyroid carcinoma. Papillary carcinoma has many variants which include some aggressive variants while follicular carcinoma vary depending on the degree of vascular invasion. Clinicians have come to expect an exact diagnosis as it significantly affects therapeutic strategies such as second surgery, adjuvant therapies and postoperative follow-up. Even among the "low-risk" tumours the histopathologic diagnosis is important and helpful for clinicians. Additional surgery (completion total thyroidectomy) in a NIFTP without BRAF p.V600E mutation can be avoided. Although a few metastatic cases were reported, HTT can generally be regarded as "almost" benign, and if it is accurately diagnosed on cytology (assisted by cytological/membranous MIB-1 staining), it may be a candidate for active surveillance (personal experience). Recently, not only morphological but also molecular findings have clarified thyroid pathology. This chapter covers all these aspects in a lucid manner which will increase readers' knowledge of thyroid pathology.

Yasuhiro Ito

Introduction

Thyroid cancer is the most common endocrine malignancy. Generally, it has a good prognosis, and the primary treatment is surgical resection. For high-risk cases, radioactive iodine therapy (RAI) is added. Chemotherapy is not effective, and drug therapy options were limited. However, in recent years, the advent of molecular targeted drugs, such as tyrosine kinase inhibitors, has expanded treatment options. Therefore, it is important to appropriately evaluate the pathology and predict the clinical risk.

Thyroid tumors were traditionally classified by listing the major histologic types: follicular thyroid adenoma (FA), papillary thyroid carcinoma (PTC), follicular thyroid carcinoma (FTC), anaplastic thyroid carcinoma (ATC), and medullary thyroid carcinoma (MTC) (1,2). Through large-scale unbiased genome analysis, the current WHO classification of thyroid tumors [1–3] has been fundamentally revised, based on tumor-specific molecular genetic information (Table 20.1).

Table 20.1 WHO classification of endocrine and neuroendocrine tumours, fifth edition (2022)

Developmental abnormalities
Follicular cell-derived neoplasms
Benign tumors Thyroid follicular nodular disease, FA, Oncocytic adenoma
Low risk neoplasm NIFTP, Thyroid tumours-UMP, Hyalinizing trabecular tumour
Malignant neoplasms FTC, IEFVPTC, PTC, Oncocytic carcinoma, High-grade follicular cell-derived carcinoma (PDTC and HGDTC), ATC (including SCC)
Thyroid C-cell derived carcinoma Medullary thyroid carcinoma
Mixed medullary and follicular-cell derived carcinomas Mixed medullary and follicular cell derived thyroid carcinoma
Salivary gland-type carcinomas of the thyroid Mucoepidermoid carcinoma, Secretory carcinoma of salivary gland type
Thyroid tumours of uncertain histogenesis Sclerosing mucoepidermoid carcinoma with eosinophilia, Cribriform morular thyroid carcinoma
Thymic tumours within the thyroid Thymoma family, SETTLE, ITC
Embryonal thyroid neoplasms Thyroblastoma

This section highlights the new WHO classification of thyroid tumors and the significance of genetic alterations. It also discusses clinical risk prediction based on histomorphology and genetic information.

Overview of the New WHO Classification of Endocrine and Neuroendocrine Tumors, Fifth Edition

In 2022, the new WHO Classification of Endocrine and Neuroendocrine Tumors, fifth edition (beta version) (WHO fifth) [1], was published (Table 20.1). Advances in large-scale genomic studies, such as The Cancer Genome Atlas (TCGA), have highlighted the significance of molecular genetics in thyroid tumor classification. As a result, the WHO fifth underwent fundamental revisions, leading to a systematic classification based on the cellular origin of tumors (cellular differentiation) and their clinical risk [1–3]. Specifically, tumors are now classified into follicular cell-derived neoplasms (FDNs), C-cell-derived carcinoma, and other tumors. FDNs are further subdivided into three risk categories: benign, low-risk, and malignant. Immunohistochemically, FDNs are positive for follicular cell markers such as thyroglobulin (TG), TTF-1, and PAX8. Key updates in the WHO fifth include the following:

1. *Revised framework for benign lesions*

WHO fifth introduces a new category: "developmental abnormalities." Benign FDNs comprise "thyroid follicular nodular disease (TFND)," follicular thyroid adenoma (FA), FA with papillary architecture (FAPA), and oncocytic adenoma (OA). "Hürthle cell adenoma/carcinoma" in WHO fourth has been renamed "oncocytic adenoma/oncocytic carcinoma of the thyroid (OA/OCA)" in WHO fifth based on its unique genetic background [4, 5].

2. *Low-risk tumors.*

This category comprises noninvasive follicular thyroid neoplasm with papillary-like nuclear features (NIFTP), thyroid tumors of uncertain malignant potential (TT-UMP), and hyalinizing trabecular tumor (HTT), all of which exhibit extremely low or uncertain malignant potential.

3. *Reordering based on differentiation*

FTC is listed first before PTC to reflect differentiation. Additionally, invasive encapsulated follicular variant of PTC (IEFVPTC) has been assigned its own classification, considering its driver gene profile.

4. *Renaming of histological "variants"*

Histological "variants" are now referred to as "subtypes" to distinguish them from genetic "variants."

5. *Introduction of high-grade carcinomas*

The new category of high-grade thyroid carcinomas includes poorly differentiated thyroid carcinoma (PDTC), high-grade differentiated thyroid carcinoma (HGDTC), and high-grade medullary thyroid carcinoma (MTC).

6. *Inclusion of squamous cell carcinoma in ATC*

Squamous cell carcinoma is grouped under anaplastic thyroid carcinoma (ATC) due to shared genetic and prognostic features.

7. *Miscellaneous tumor categories*

Other tumors are classified into categories such as salivary-gland-type carcinomas of the thyroid, thyroid tumors of uncertain histogenesis, thymic tumors within the thyroid, and embryonal thyroid neoplasms based on their cellular origin.

Thus, WHO fifth emphasizes the integration of genetic abnormalities and histomorphological features in tumor classification. This comprehensive approach enhances diagnostic accuracy and facilitates the early selection of appropriate treatment options, including molecular-targeted therapies.

Genetic Basis of the Differentiated Thyroid Follicular Cell-Derived Neoplasms (FDNs)

In FDNs, genetic alterations in the MAP kinase pathway, such as mutations or rearrangements in *RET*, *RAS*, and *BRAF*, act as key drivers of carcinogenesis (Fig. 20.1) [3, 6]. Since the 2000s, analyses of driver genes in PTC and FTC have revealed the following: *BRAF* p.V600E mutations and *RET* gene rearrangements (e.g., *CCDC6::RET*, *NCOA4::RET*) were prevalent in PTC, while *H/K/NRAS* mutations (e.g., *NRAS* p.Q61R) and *PAX8::PPARG* fusion genes are commonly found in FTC.

The 2014 TCGA analysis of PTC [7] provided several key insights:

(i) Most PTC cases harbor a single, mutually exclusive driver gene mutation.
(ii) The number of driver genes is relatively small, including pathogenic variants in *BRAF*, *N/H/KRAS*, *EIF1AX*, *PPM1D*, and *CHEK2*, as well as fusion genes involving *RET*, *PPARG*, *BRAF*, *NTRK1/3*, and *ALK*.
(iii) PTC exhibits a relatively low mutational burden compared to other cancer types.

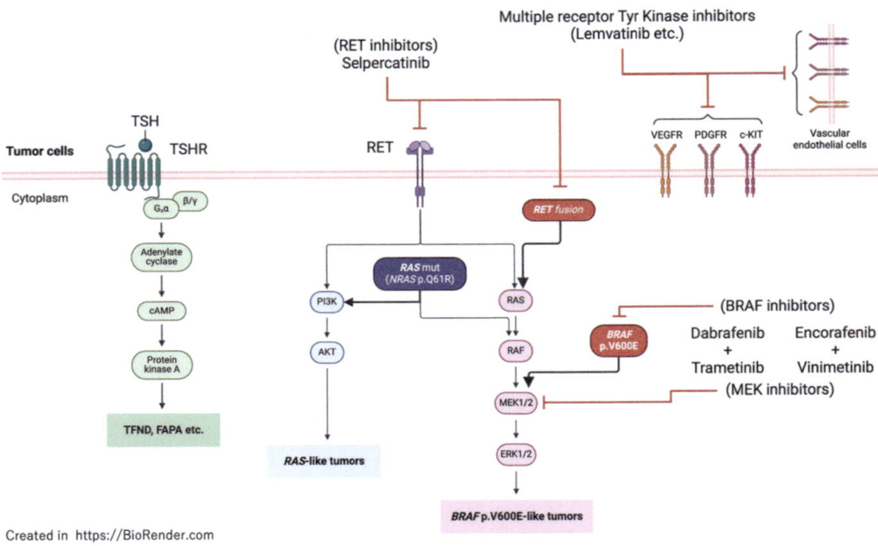

Fig. 20.1 Intracellular signaling pathways in differentiated thyroid tumors. Many driver gene mutations in differentiated thyroid cancer contribute to activation of the MAPK and PI3K/Akt pathways. The *BRAF* p.V600E mutation strongly activates the MAPK pathway, leading to highly proliferative activity. Tumors with the mutation are termed as *BRAF* p.V600E-like tumors (BLTs). Conversely, *N/H/KRAS* mutations activate both the MAPK and PI3K pathways. However, CRAF-mediated feedback inhibition reduces MAPK activity, resulting in a predominance of the anti-apoptotic effect via the PI3K pathway. These tumors are termed as *RAS*-like tumors (RLTs). In very well-differentiated thyroid tumors or tumorlike lesion such as thyroid follicular nodular disease (or functional nodule), the TSH receptor-mediated cAMP pathway is predominantly activated. This leads to mild proliferation, iodine metabolism, and expression of hormone-related genes. In addition to proliferation, there may be an increase in hormonal functions, such as iodine metabolism and expression of hormone-related genes

Additionally, PTCs were reclassified genetically using the BRAF-RAS score, which evaluates gene expression patterns resembling either *BRAF* p.V600E or *RAS* mutations. It was found that tumors with *BRAF* p.V600E-like genetic abnormalities exhibited the classical PTC morphology (*BRAF* p.V600E-like tumors: BLTs), while cases with *RAS*-like genetic abnormalities exhibited the follicular variant of PTC (FV-PTC) morphology (*RAS*-like tumors: RLTs). Subsequent studies [8, 9] have shown that FA and FTC primarily harbor *RAS* mutations as their main drivers. RLTs thus span a spectrum from follicular neoplasms (FNs) to FV-PTC, while BLTs encompass the majority of PTC cases.

RLTs retain a follicular structure and exhibit expansile, compressible growth within a fibrous capsule (Fig. 20.2). These tumors are driven by *H/K/NRAS* mutations, *PAX8::PPARG* translocations, *EIF1AX* mutations, and *BRAF* mutations other than p.V600E (e.g., *BRAF* p.K601E and *BRAF* rearrangements). They show high expression of iodine metabolism and hormone-related genes, maintaining a high degree of thyroid follicular cell differentiation.

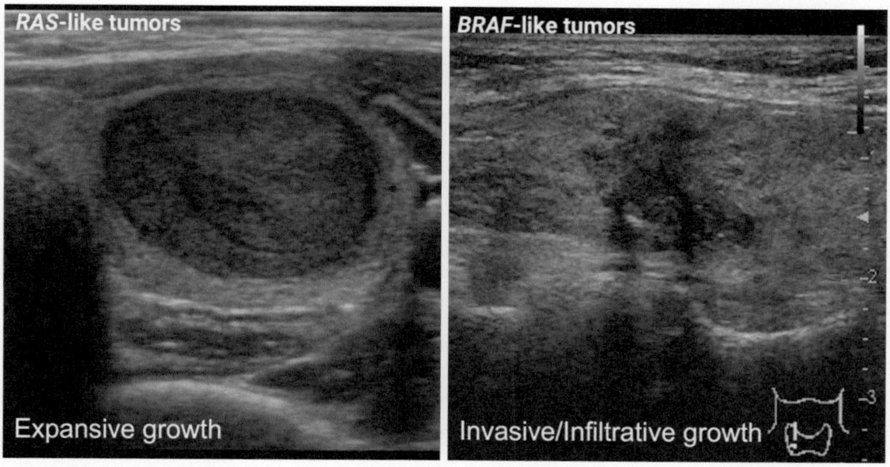

Fig. 20.2 Typical ultrasound images of *RAS*-like tumors and *BRAF* p.V600E-like tumors. Well-differentiated thyroid carcinomas can be broadly classified into *RAS*-like tumors (RLTs) (left panel) and *BRAF* p.V600E-like tumors (BLTs) (right panel). RLTs include follicular neoplasms and invasive encapsulated follicular variant of papillary thyroid carcinoma. They typically present as single encapsulated nodules with thick fibrous capsules, indicative of expansive growth patterns. Lesions with irregular margins may suggest infiltrative growth and potential malignancy. BLTs, such as classic papillary thyroid carcinoma, exhibit spiculated or lobulated masses with irregular margins, reflecting infiltrative or invasive growth patterns. Microcalcifications can be often found in BLTs

On the other hand, BLTs are characterized by papillary growth and nuclear atypia with classic "papillary-like nuclear features," such as ground-glass nuclei (chromatin clearing), nuclear grooves, intranuclear cytoplasmic inclusions, and overlapping nuclei (Fig. 20.2). BLTs often grow invasively and are driven by *BRAF* p.V600E mutations, *RET* fusion genes (e.g., *CCDC6::RET* and *NCOA4::RET*), and *NTRK1/3* fusions. These tumors exhibit reduced iodine metabolic capacity and lower hormone differentiation compared to RLTs. A small subset of tumors does not fit neatly into the BLT or RLT categories. It should be noted that a small portion of tumors are difficult to classify as either BLTs or RLTs (non-*BRAF*/non-*RAS* tumors).

Genetic Alterations Detected in Benign Thyroid Nodules: Hyperplasia or Neoplasm?

In WHO fourth [4], FA and Hürthle cell adenoma (renamed as oncocytic adenoma in WHO fifth) were categorized as benign lesions. WHO fifth expands the benign category to include "developmental abnormalities" (e.g., thyroglossal duct cysts and dyshormonogenetic goiter) and "thyroid follicular nodular disease (TFND)" (Table 20.1). TFND encompasses lesions formerly known as nodular hyperplasia or multinodular goiter. Clonality has been demonstrated in some TFND lesions, suggesting a potential neoplastic origin in certain cases [10, 11]. To reflect this uncertainty, the term "TFND" was adopted without explicitly designating these lesions as tumor or non-tumor entities.

While most FAs are classified as RLTs, TFND is associated with a distinct set of genetic alterations predominantly affecting the thyroid-stimulating hormone (TSH) signaling pathway. The most common mutation in TFND is in the *TSH receptor* (*TSHR*), occurring up to 70% of cases [1, 2, 10, 11]. Other mutations frequently reported include *GNAS*, *EZH1*, *ZNF148*, *SPOP*, and *DICER*1. In the Carney complex, mutations in *PRKAR1A*, a downstream component of the TSH signaling pathway, have been identified. Similarly, FAPA is often associated with hyperthyroidism and shares genetic alterations with TFND, including mutations in *TSHR*, *GNAS*, *PRKAR1A*, and *EZH1*. These findings highlight the molecular overlap and distinctions between benign thyroid nodules and their potential for neoplastic transformation.

"Low-Risk" Tumors and Evaluation of Capsular and Vascular Invasion

"Low-risk" tumors are defined as those that are morphologically and clinically intermediate between benign and malignant neoplasms in the category of FDNs. While these tumors possess the potential to metastasize, they do so infrequently. WHO fifth classifies NIFTP, TT-UMP, and HTT as low-risk tumors.

NIFTP

NIFTP is an encapsulated nodular lesion lacking capsular invasion. It exhibits a follicular architecture resembling FA but shows nuclear atypia characteristic of PTC. Previously diagnosed as FA or FV-PTC, NIFTP was reclassified as a distinct entity following recognition of its favorable prognosis.

WHO fifth has expanded the definition of NIFTP to include tumors smaller than 1 cm and oncocytic variants, which were previously excluded. However, the presence of the *BRAF* p.V600E mutation precludes a diagnosis of NIFTP, as these tumors are included in the RLTs. A standardized scoring system ("nuclear score") has been introduced to evaluate papillary-like nuclear features in NIFTP [12]. This system ensures consistent diagnostic criteria across institutions and pathologists.

Among follicular PTCs, those with obvious infiltrative growth remain classified as the PTC subtype (follicular variant of PTC: FV-PTC), while encapsulated tumors, including NIFTP and IEFVPTC, have become distinct entities (Fig. 20.3). Most FV-PTC belong to BLTs, while NIFTP and IEFVPTC predominantly exhibit a genetic background consistent with RLTs. If a tumor otherwise meeting the morphological criteria for NIFTP harbors the *BRAF* p.V600E mutation, it is diagnosed as encapsulated follicular variant PTC (EFVPTC). This differentiation underscores the critical role of molecular profiling in refining thyroid tumor classifications.

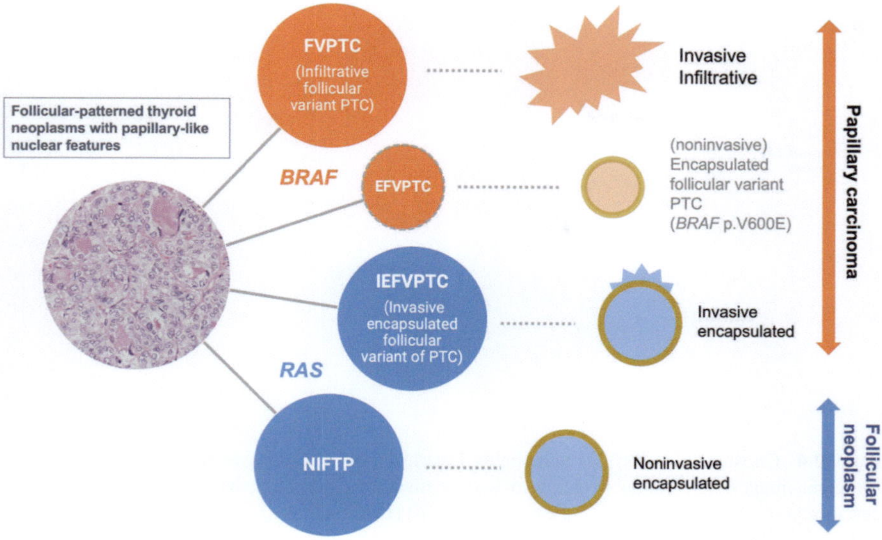

Fig. 20.3 Differential diagnosis of follicular-patterned thyroid neoplasms with papillary-like nuclear features. Noninvasive follicular neoplasms with papillary-like nuclear features (NIFTP) are genetically classified in the *RAS*-like tumors (RLTs, blue). Follicular variants of PTC can be subdivided into three types. Invasive encapsulated follicular variant of papillary thyroid carcinoma (IEFVPTC) has its own classification because it generally harbors *N/H/KRAS* mutations (RLTs). Follicular PTC with infiltrative growth (FV-PTC) remains in the PTC category, as it is classified as *BRAF* p.V600E-like tumors (BLTs, orange). Tumors meeting NIFTP criteria but harboring the *BRAF* p.V600E mutation are diagnosed as encapsulated follicular variant PTC (EFVPTC). This underscores the importance of molecular profiling in thyroid tumor classification

TT-UMP

TT-UMP are well-differentiated, well-circumscribed thyroid tumors with follicular architecture in which the presence of invasion remains "questionable" despite thorough sampling and exhaustive examination. TT-UMP without PTC-like nuclear atypia are classified as follicular tumor of uncertain malignant potential (FT-UMP), while those with PTC-like nuclear atypia are categorized as well-differentiated tumor of uncertain malignant potential (WDT-UMP). Some TT-UMP also exhibit oncocytic features. When high mitotic activity or tumor necrosis is observed in TT-UMP, WHO fifth recommends diagnosing the lesion as a high-grade encapsulated thyroid carcinoma with questionable invasion.

Capsular invasion is considered "questionable" when broad tumor cell protrusions reach, but do not unequivocally penetrate, the capsule [13] (Fig. 20.4). In well-circumscribed nodules with thin or incomplete capsules, irregular tumor contours or outpouching may be inconsistently interpreted as invasion. "Questionable" vascular invasion is more concerning than capsular invasion due to its higher risk for tumor dissemination. Early vascular invasion can be particularly challenging to confirm, especially when tumor cells undermine the vascular endothelium in the tumor

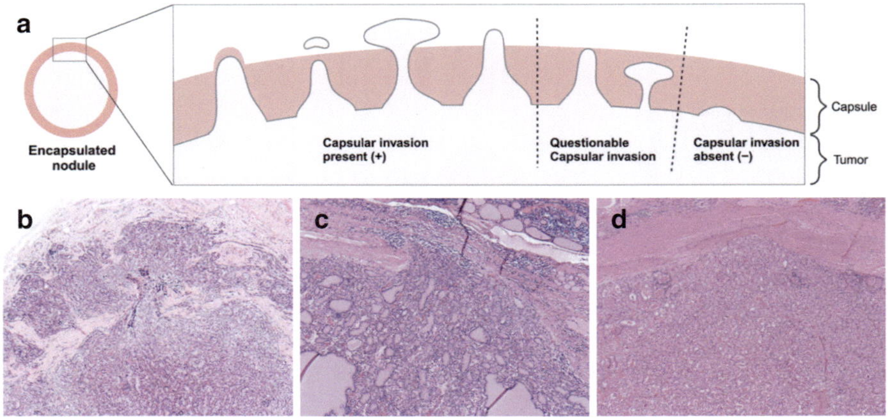

Fig. 20.4 Capsular invasion. (**a**) Schematic illustration of capsular invasion. Representative histological images of capsular invasion in widely invasive carcinoma (**b**) and minimally invasive carcinoma (**c**), as well as the absence of invasion (**d**) (H&E staining)

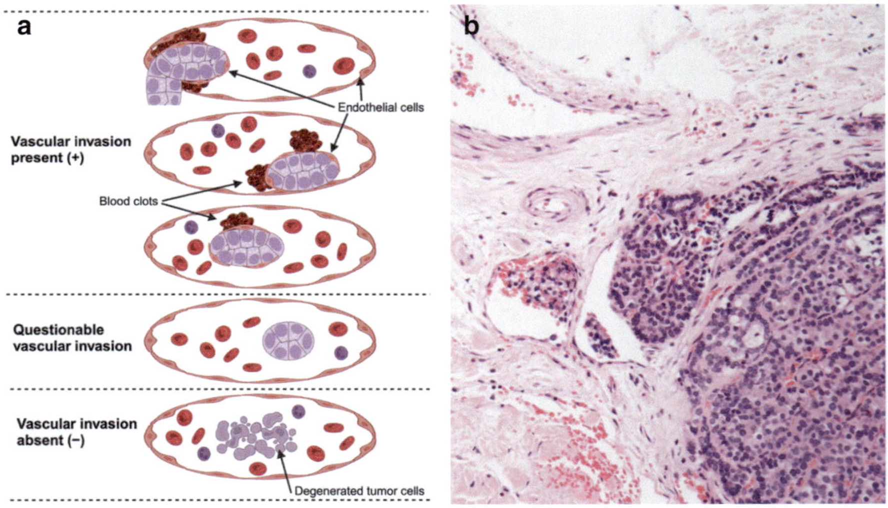

Fig. 20.5 Vascular invasion. (**a**) Schematic illustration of vascular invasion. Viable carcinoma cells in vessels with surface lining of endothelial cells should be evaluated as positive vascular invasion. Viable carcinoma cells without surface endothelial cells are defined as "questionable vascular invasion." Degenerated or necrotic tumor cells in vessels are evaluated as negative. (**b**) A representative histological image of vascular invasion (H&E staining)

capsule or variably protrude into vessels (Fig. 20.5). The presence of tumor cell nests with endothelial lining or thrombus in vascular spaces confirms the vascular invasion.

HTT

HTT is a well-circumscribed or encapsulated FDN composed of polygonal cells arranged in wide trabeculae or small nests interspersed with intra-trabecular hyaline material. HTT exhibits nuclear features including prominent grooves, vacuoles (cytoplasmic inclusions), and membrane irregularities. First described by Carney et al. in 1987 as a benign lesion (hyalinizing trabecular adenoma) [14], HTT was later renamed following reports of malignancy-related findings, such as lymph node metastases, in a small number of cases [15].

The diagnosis of HTT is supported by the presence of PTC-like nuclear features and distinct immunohistochemical staining of the cell membrane (but not the nucleus) with the Ki-67 (MIB-1) antibody. Genetically, HTT is strongly associated with translocations involving *PAX8::GLIS3* (93%) or *PAX8::GLIS1* (7%), which underpin its unique molecular profile [16].

Subtypes of Differentiated Thyroid Cancer and Their Clinical Relevance (Subtypes of PTC and FTC)

Subtypes of PTC (Table 20.2)

Significant changes in WHO fifth include the exclusion of the cribriform-morular variant from PTC subtypes, with cribriform-morular carcinoma now reclassified under thyroid tumors of uncertain histogenesis. Additionally, IEFVPTC has been designated as a separate classification, distinct from PTC subtypes.

Classic PTC, also referred to as typical or conventional PTC, is characterized by papillary structures with a central fibrovascular core and distinct nuclear features. These nuclear features include enlargement, elongation, irregular contours with intranuclear grooves and pseudoinclusions and a characteristic “ground-glass” or nuclear clearing appearance. Purely papillary growth is rare with most classic PTC cases also displaying neoplastic follicles. Tumor cell cytoplasm is typically slightly eosinophilic, and mitotic figures are rare, except in reactive conditions. Psammoma bodies, observed in 40–50% of cases, are laminated calcifications present within the tumor, stroma, or lymphatic vessels [1]. Additional features include squamous differentiation (15–45%), desmoplasia, lymphocyte infiltration at invasive edges, and variable cyst formation. Cystic PTC often retains identifiable papillae, though some cases show benign-appearing flattened epithelium.

PTC lesions measuring ≤10 mm are classified as PTC-microcarcinomas. These are often incidental findings during autopsies or surgeries performed for unrelated conditions. The prognosis for PTC-microcarcinoma is excellent, with minimal risk of progression [17].

Subtypes associated with a poorer prognosis include tall cell PTC (TC-PTC), hobnail PTC (HN-PTC), and columnar cell PTC (CC-PTC) [1, 18–21]. TC-PTC is defined by tumor cells whose height is at least three times their width. It exhibits a

Table 20.2 Subtypes of papillary thyroid carcinoma

PTC subtypes	Required propotion	Pathogenic variants	Prognosis
Classic PTC	–	*BRAF* p.V600E, *CCDC6::RET*, *NCOA4::RET*	–
(infiltrative) follicular PTC	≥90%	*BRAF* p.V600E, *NRAS*, reconstitution of *RET*, *NTRK*, *ALK*	Favorable
Tall cell PTC	≥30%	*BRAF* p.V600E, miR-21, *TERT* promoter, *TP53*	High-risk
Columnar cell PTC	NA	*BRAF* p.V600E, *BRAF* fusion, *CDKN2A* loss, gain of ch.1	High-risk
Hobnail PTC	≥30%	*BRAF* p.V600E, *TERT* promoter, *TP53*, *PIK3CA*	High-risk
Solid/trabecular PTC	>50%	*CCDC6::RET*, *NCOA4::RET*, *ETV6::NTRK3*, *BRAF* p.V600E(rare)	Int-high risk
Diffuse sclerosing PTC	100%	*NCOA4::RET*, *BRAF* p.V600E(20%), *ALK* rearrangement (10%)	Int-high risk
PTC with fibromatosis/ fasciitis- like/desmoid-type stroma	NA	*CTNNB1* mutations, *BRAF* p.V600E (frequent)	Unknown
Oncocytic PTC	NA (>75%?)	*BRAF* p.V600E, *GRIM-19*, *RET* rearrangement	Int risk
Warthin-like PTC	NA	*BRAF* p.V600E	Unknown

NA not available, *Int* intermediate

tightly packed growth pattern, often forming elongated trabecular structures described as having a "tram track" appearance. HN-PTC is named for its enlarged nuclear morphology, where nuclei bulge from the apical surface of papillary structures, resembling hobnails. These subtypes are strongly associated with *BRAF* p.V600E mutations, and some cases fulfill the diagnostic criteria for HGDTC. Solid/trabecular PTC (ST-PTC), which occurs more frequently in children than adults, demonstrates a higher risk of recurrence and a greater frequency of *RET* gene translocations.

TC-PTC and HN-PTC are diagnosed when they represent more than 30% of the tumor, and ST-PTC when it represents more than half of the tumor. CC-PTC is not specified in terms of proportion, but CDX2 positivity in immunostaining is a characteristic feature.

Diffuse sclerosing PTC (DS-PTC) is characterized by diffuse involvement of a single or bilateral lobe with extensive lymphatic permeation, dense sclerosis, and numerous psammoma bodies. DS-PTC may have a somewhat higher risk [22].

These prognostic distinctions emphasize the importance of accurate subtype identification for tailoring patient management and therapeutic strategies (Fig. 20.6).

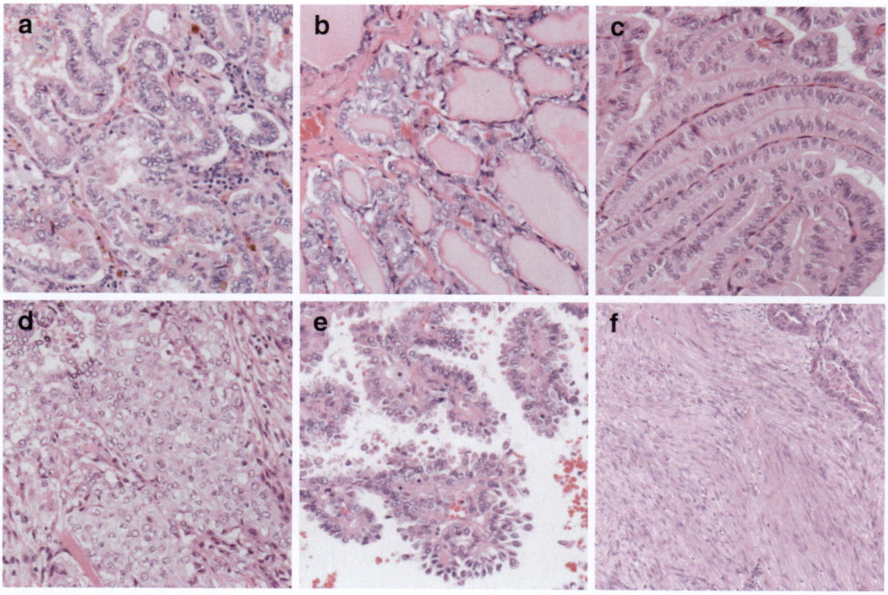

Fig. 20.6 Histological images of papillary carcinoma subtypes (H&E staining). Representative histological images of classical or conventional PTC (**a**), follicular PTC (**b**), tall cell PTC (**c**), solid/trabecular PTC (**d**), and hobnail PTC (**e**)

Subtypes of FTC

The distinction between FA and FTC is based on the presence of capsular and/or vascular invasion, not on the cellular atypia. FTC is further classified into three subtypes based on the extent of invasion: (i) minimally invasive FTC (miFTC) is characterized by limited capsular invasion without vascular invasion, (ii) encapsulated angioinvasive FTC (ea-FTC) is defined by encapsulation with evidence of vascular invasion, (iii) widely invasive FTC (wiFTC) is marked by extensive invasion into both the capsule and surrounding tissues, often accompanied by significant vascular involvement. In FTC, vascular invasion is a critical prognostic factor. The Armed Forces Institute of Pathology (AFIP) classification [23] further stratifies vascular invasion into limited (fewer than four sites) and extensive (four or more sites), emphasizing its prognostic significance.

Unlike PTC, FNs display minimal cytomorphological variation, and morphological subtypes are infrequently defined. Nevertheless, a few rare subtypes are recognized, including the clear cell subtype, signet-ring cell subtype, and spindle cell subtype, each distinguished by unique histological features.

Oncocytic Tumors

Oncocytic tumors, such as oncocytic adenoma and oncocytic carcinoma of the thyroid (OA/OTC), were previously referred to as the oxyphilic cell variant (subtype) of FA and FTC. However, in WHO fifth, these tumors are now recognized as distinct entities based on their characteristic morphology and unique genetic background [1, 5, 24]. The tumor cells exhibit abundant eosinophilic granular cytoplasm, round nuclei with prominent central nucleoli. Nuclear atypia, such as multinucleated giant cells, can be observed. Unlike FNs, which frequently harbor *RAS* mutations or *PAX8::PPARG* translocations, oncocytic tumors exhibit a higher prevalence of mutations in mitochondrial biosynthesis genes, including *Complex I*, *ESRRA*, and *PPARGC1A*, as well as characteristic genetic abnormalities such as a near-monoploid (hemiploid) karyotype. Interestingly, microinvasive oncocytic tumors often display a diploid karyotype, whereas widely invasive tumors frequently exhibit a hemiploid karyotype. The oncocytic subtype of papillary thyroid carcinoma (O-PTC) is not included in the category of oncocytic neoplasms, as O-PTC is rare and its genetic alterations remain poorly understood.

The criteria for differentiating OA from OTC are consistent with those for FNs and rely on the presence or absence of capsular and/or vascular invasion. Similar to FTC, oncocytic tumors are subdivided into three categories such as minimally invasive, encapsulated angioinvasive, and widely invasive OTC.

A key distinction between oncocytic tumors and FNs is the clear correlation between tumor size and the risk of capsular invasion. As a result, oncocytic tumors shows higher frequency of widely invasive OCA [25]. The best cutoff US tumor size for predicting malignancy in oncocytic tumors was 3.35 cm (sensitivity, 53.1%; specificity, 87.9%) [26].

Additional prognostic factors include features such as a cord-like or dense growth pattern with scant cytoplasm, the presence of necrosis, and mitotic activity, all of which are associated with a worse prognosis.

High-Risk Thyroid Carcinomas: High-Grade Carcinoma and Anaplastic Carcinoma

ATC and PDTC are high-risk thyroid cancers. In WHO fifth, a new category, high-grade differentiated thyroid carcinoma (HGDTC), was introduced as an additional high-risk classification (Table 20.3). This category includes well-differentiated thyroid carcinomas, such as FTC, PTC, and OTC, exhibiting prominent mitotic activity or necrosis, which are features indicative of aggressive behavior.

Table 20.3 High-grade thyroid carcinoma

	Poorly differentiated thyroid carcinoma (PDTC)	High-grade differentiated thyroid carcinoma (HGDTC)	High-grade MTC
Cell-of-origin	Follicular cell-derived tumors		C cell-derived tumors
Architectural pattern	Solid/trabecular/insular	Papillary, follicular, (solid)	Any
Nuclear features	No papillary-like features	Any	Any
Other conditions	(At least one of the following features)		
	1. Mitosis ≥3/2 mm² **2. Necrosis** **3. Convoluted nuclei**	**4. Mitosis ≥5/2 mm²** **5. Necrosis**	**6. Mitosis ≥5/2 mm²** **7. MIB1 index ≥5%** **8. Necrosis**
Anaplastic features	None	None	None

For MTC, which encompasses cases with varying clinical risks, a two-tiered grading system—low-grade and high-grade—has been recommended. This system aligns with the grading approach used for neuroendocrine neoplasms (NENs) in other organs and is based on key pathological features such as mitotic activity, the presence of necrosis, and the MIB-1 labeling index.

High-Grade Follicular Cell-Derived Non-anaplastic Thyroid Carcinoma

PDTC is diagnosed according to the Turin consensus criteria [27], which include (i) solid, trabecular, or insular proliferation patterns (STI patterns), (ii) absence of conventional papillary-like nuclear features, and (iii) the presence of at least one of the following: convoluted (raisin-like) nuclei, a mitotic count of ≥3 cells per 2 mm^2, or tumor necrosis.

In highly differentiated carcinomas such as FTC, PTC, and OTC, some high-risk cases exhibit characteristics comparable to PDTC. These cases can be identified by elevated mitotic activity (≥5 cells per 2 mm^2) and/or the presence of tumor necrosis and are classified as HGDTC. This classification underscores that a diagnosis of well-differentiated carcinoma can no longer rely solely on histological type in WHO fifth. Importantly, even a small area of increased mitotic activity or necrosis qualifies a tumor as HGDTC, necessitating careful pathological evaluation.

In both PDTC and HGDTC, *RAS* and *BRAF* p.V600E mutations occur at frequencies similar to those in well-differentiated carcinomas. *RAS* mutations are more common in PDTC, while *BRAF* mutations are more frequently observed in HGDTC, suggesting closer associations between PDTC and RLTs and between HGDTC and BLTs. Additional mutations implicated in malignant transformation include *TP53*,

CDKN2A, *PIK3CA*, and *AKT1* [28]. Furthermore, promoter mutations in *TERT* (C228T and C250T) are recognized as significant poor prognostic factors [29, 30].

Changes in the Definition of ATC

Previously, squamous cell carcinoma (SCC) of the thyroid without a component of well-differentiated thyroid carcinoma was considered a distinct histological entity. However, WHO fifth has incorporated SCC into ATC. This change reflects findings that thyroid SCCs frequently harbor *BRAF* p.V600E mutations (87%) and show immunohistochemical positivity for PAX8 (91%) and TTF-1 (38%) [1]. These molecular and immunohistological features support the follicular epithelial origin of thyroid SCCs, raising questions about the existence of "true" SCCs as a separate entity in the thyroid. Additionally, SCC was integrated into ATC because it has a poor prognosis comparable to that of other ATCs. Squamous metaplasia of the follicular epithelium and squamous differentiation of PTC are frequently observed changes that sometimes require careful differentiation. Furthermore, thyroid involvement by primary SCCs originating in the head and neck region must be carefully excluded (Fig. 20.7).

High-Grade MTC

As mentioned above, the concept of high-grade tumors has also been applied to MTC, a C-cell-derived, calcitonin-producing carcinoma. MTC exhibits neuroendocrine differentiation and can be regarded as a primary NEN of the thyroid gland. Similar to NENs in other organs, MTC encompasses cases with varying risk profiles. Recent studies reviewing the clinicopathological features and long-term outcomes of MTC have demonstrated that risk assessment can be effectively based on mitotic count, the presence of necrosis, and the Ki-67 labeling index [31, 32]. WHO fifth has recommended a two-tiered risk assessment system by proliferative activity and tumor necrosis: (1) mitosis, ≥5 cells/2 mm^2; (2) Ki67 labeling index, ≥5%; and (3) presence of tumor necrosis.

In MTC, *RET* mutations are common in both sporadic and hereditary forms. While nearly all hereditary and approximately half of sporadic MTCs harbor *RET* mutations, the associated risk varies by the type of mutation. The *RET* p.M918T mutation, which is frequently observed, is particularly associated with a high-risk profile [33, 34].

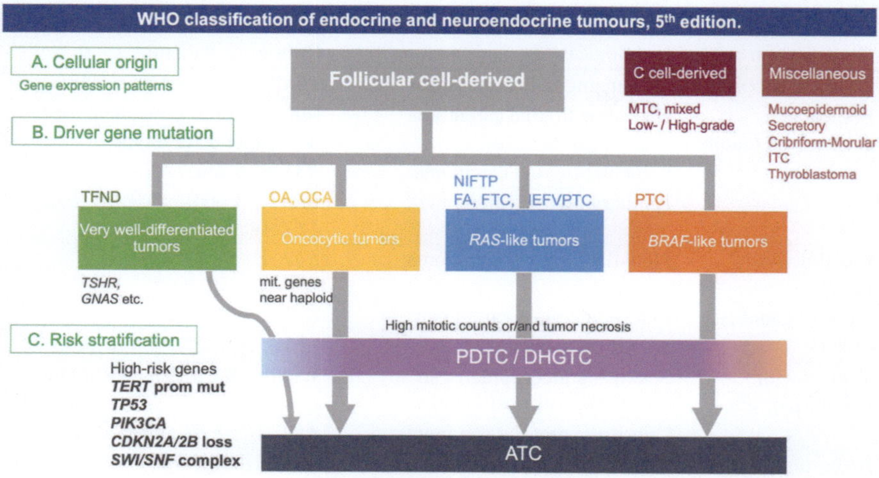

Fig. 20.7 A three-step diagnostic approach for classifying thyroid neoplasms. To classify thyroid neoplasms, the first step involves evaluating the cellular origin or differentiation of the tumor through histomorphological observations and the use of differentiation markers such as TTF1, PAX8, thyroglobulin, calcitonin, CD5, and SALL4. Next, tumors are classified into four types based on driver gene mutations: oncocytic tumors, very well-differentiated tumors, *RAS*-like tumors (RLTs), and *BRAF* p.V600E-like tumors (BLTs). This classification can be achieved by morphological observation. Finally, clinical risks of the tumor are stratified. A thorough evaluation of histomorphological features and genetic mutations is essential for confirming diagnoses and determining the clinical risks. High-risk gene alterations, such as *TERT* promoter mutations and *TP53* mutations, are associated with aggressive tumors like PDTC, HGDTC, and ATC. Early diagnosis of high-grade carcinomas is crucial for initiating molecular targeted therapies. *TFND thyroid follicular nodular disease, OA oncocytic adenoma of the thyroid, OCA oncocytic carcinoma of the thyroid, FA follicular thyroid adenoma, FTC follicular thyroid carcinoma, NIFTP, noninvasive follicular thyroid neoplasm with papillary-like nuclear features, IEFVPTC invasive encapsulated follicular papillary carcinoma, PTC papillary thyroid carcinoma, PDTC poorly differentiated thyroid carcinoma, ATC anaplastic thyroid carcinoma, HGDTC differentiated high-grade thyroid carcinoma, MTC medullary thyroid carcinoma, ITC intrathyroidal thymic carcinoma

Miscellaneous Tumors

Thyroid tumors with unusual histologies are categorized into four groups based on cellular origin: salivary gland-type carcinomas, thymic tumors within the thyroid, thyroid tumors of uncertain histogenesis, and embryonal thyroid neoplasms (Table 20.1). While these tumors are extremely rare, they warrant attention during the differential diagnosis of thyroid lesions. Key driver mutations and immunohistochemical profiles aiding in their differentiation are summarized in Tables 20.4 and 20.5. Lymphomas and mesenchymal tumors have been removed from the classification of thyroid tumors because they are now grouped together as endocrine tumors.

Table 20.4 Thyroid tumors and their characteristic gene alterations

Classification	Histological type	Pathogenic variants
Low-risk neoplasm	Hyalinizing trabecular tumor	*PAX8::GLIS3, PAX8::GLIS1*
Follicular cell-derived tumors	Oncocytic thyroid carcinoma	Mitochondrial gene alteration, near haploid karyotype
	Follicular thyroid carcinoma	*RAS* mutation, *PAX8::PPARG*
	Papillary thyroid carcinoma	*BRAF* p.V600E, *CCDC6::RET*, *NCOA4::RET*
C cell-derived tumors	Medullary thyroid carcinoma	*RET* mutation
Salivary gland-type tumors	Mucoepidermoid carcinoma	*CRTC1::MAML2*
	Secretory carcinoma	*ETV6::NTRK3*
Tumors with unknown origin	Sclerosing mucoepidermoid carcinoma with eosinophilia	Without *MAML2* reconstitution
	Cribriform morular carcinoma	*APC, CTNNB1* mutation
Embryonal tumors	Thyroblastoma	*DICER1* mutation

Salivary Gland-Type Tumors

This group includes mucoepidermoid carcinoma of the thyroid (MEC) and secretory carcinoma of salivary gland type (SC), also known as mammary analogue secretory carcinoma (MASC).

MEC is characterized histologically by large nests of epidermoid cells mixed with mucocytes, surrounded by fibrotic stroma. It often exhibits mild nuclear pleomorphism, rare mitotic figures, and occasional keratin formation. Immunohistochemically, MEC is positive for cytokeratins and p63. In some cases, it may coexist with PTC and can transform into ATC. A subset of MEC cases harbors the *CRTC1::MAML2* fusion gene, a molecular hallmark of salivary gland MEC.

SC typically presents as a solitary thyroid nodule and closely resembles secretory carcinomas found in other anatomical sites. SC is notable for its eosinophilic "bubbly" luminal secretions, highlighted by periodic acid-Schiff (PAS) and mucicarmine staining. Immunohistochemically, SC is positive for S100, mammaglobin, GATA3, and often GCDFP-15, but negative for thyroglobulin (TG) and TTF1. SC harbors the *ETV6::NTRK3* translocation, a hallmark genetic alteration.

Thyroid Tumors of Uncertain Histogenesis

Two notable tumors in this category are sclerosing mucoepidermoid carcinoma with eosinophilia (SMECE) and cribriform morular thyroid carcinoma (CMTC).

SMECE was initially considered a subtype of MEC, but became an independent histologic entity due to its frequent association with Hashimoto's disease (HD) and the absence of *MAML2* fusion gene. Women are predominantly affected with SMECE (female to male ratio, 13:1).

Table 20.5 Immunohistological markers for differential diagnosis in thyroid tumors

Cellular origin	Histology	TTF1	PAX8	Tg	CEA	Calci-tonin	CD5	P63	Other markers
Follicular cell-derived tumors	Oncocytic thyroid carcinoma, Follicular thyroid carcinoma	+	+	+	–	–	–	– (+)	
	Poorly diff. thyroid carcinoma	+/–	+	+/–	–	–	–	–	
	Anaplastic thyroid carcinoma	–/+	+/–	–	–	–	–	–/+	
C cell-derived tumors	Medullary carcinoma	+/–	–	–	+	+	–	–	Neuroendocrine markers
Salivary-gland type tumors	Mucoepidermoid carcinoma	+/–	+	+/–	+ (Muc.)[a]	–	–	+ (Ep.)[a]	
	Secretory carcinoma	–	+/–	–	NA[a]	–	–	–	S100, GATA3, mammaglobin, GCDFP15
Tumors with unknown origin	Sclerosing mucoepidermoid carcinoma with eosinophilia	+ (Sq.)	– (~+)	–	+ (Muc.)	–	–	+ (Ep.)	
	Cribriform morular carcinoma	+	– (~+)	–	NA	–	+ (Morula)	–	β-catenin, ER, PgR
Thymic tumors within thyroid	ITC	–	–	–	+	–	+	+	CD117(c-KIT), Bcl-2
	SETTLE	–	–	–	–	–	–	NA	Vimentin, Bcl-2
Embryonal tumors	Thyroblastoma	+/–	+/–	+/–	NA	–	–	–/+ (+ in Fol.)	SALL4

[a]*NA* not available, *Muc* mucocytes, *Ep* epidermoid cells, *Fol* follicular cells

CMTC is associated with the constitutive activation of the WNT/β-catenin pathway and is frequently linked to familial adenomatous polyposis (FAP), typically caused by mutations in the *APC* gene [35]. CMTC almost exclusively occurs in young women (female to male ratio, 31–61:1). CMTC is an encapsulated tumor, often lobulated with fibrous septa and frequent capsular and/or vascular invasion. It exhibits a diverse mix of growth patterns including cribriform, follicular, papillary, and solid architectures, often accompanied by squamoid morulae. The cribriform structures, which lack colloid, are composed of anastomosing bars and arches of tumor cells without intervening fibrous stroma. Squamoid morulae are whorls of spindle to ovoid cells that lack keratinization and exhibit nuclear clearing due to biotin accumulation. Aberrant strong nuclear and cytoplasmic β-catenin staining is a hallmark of CMTC. CMTC is positive for TTF1, estrogen, and progesterone receptors and negative for TG, PAX8, and calcitonin.

Thymic Tumors Within the Thyroid

Intrathyroid thymic tumors include the thymoma family, intrathyroidal thymic carcinoma (ITC), and spindle cell tumor with thymus-like differentiation (SETTLE). These tumors are thought to originate from ectopic thymic tissue or embryonic thymic rest in or adjacent to the thyroid. It commonly involves the lower poles of thyroid lobes or is attached to the thyroid. Histological and immunophenotypic analyses confirm their thymic differentiation.

Intrathyroidal thymomas exhibit histopathological features similar to thymomas in the mediastinum and are classified into subtypes analogous to those seen in the thymus [36]. SETTLE is a rare malignant tumor primarily affecting children and young adults, with a median age of 19 years. It is characterized by a lobulated architecture and biphasic cellular composition, with spindle epithelial cells transitioning into glandular structures. SETTLE is distinguished from synovial sarcoma by its lobulated architecture, specific cytokeratin and p63 expression, and the absence of the *SS18::SSX* gene fusion.

ITC is a rare carcinoma with thymic differentiation arising within or adjacent to the thyroid gland. Grossly, ITC appears as a hard, solid, and lobulated tumor, typically without calcifications or cystic features. Histologically, it resembles thymic squamous cell carcinoma, displaying irregular lobules and cords of epithelial cells within a sclerohyaline to desmoplastic stroma infiltrated by lymphocytes and plasma cells. The tumor cells are squamoid or syncytial in appearance, with mild to moderate nuclear atypia, rare mitotic figures, and occasional keratinization. Immunohistochemically, ITC cells are positive for pan-cytokeratin, CK19, p63, p40, CD5, and CD117 (c-kit) [1, 37]. They are negative for TTF1, TG, monoclonal PAX8, and calcitonin. The Ki-67 proliferation index ranges from 2% to 40%. Scattered cells may also show positivity for chromogranin A or synaptophysin.

Embryonal Thyroid Neoplasms

Thyroblastoma is a rare, high-grade embryonal thyroid neoplasm associated with *DICER1* gene mutations, resembling first-trimester thyroid parenchyma [38]. Most cases have been included in the spectrum of so-called malignant thyroid teratoma. Thyroblastoma comprises primitive thyroid-like follicles ($TTF1^+$, $PAX8^+$), small round to oval cells ($TTF1^-$, $PAX8^-$, $SALL4^+$) with areas of necrosis and high mitotic activity, and spindle cell stroma showing rhabdomyoblastic differentiation. Cartilaginous foci are commonly observed, while mature adult-like structures are notably absent. The differential diagnosis includes malignant thyroid teratoma, immature teratoma, carcinosarcoma, teratocarcinosarcoma, and PDTC.

Tumors Not Listed in the WHO Classification

Several thyroid tumors of uncertain histogenesis are either not clearly defined or have been recently recognized. These include thyroid teratoma/immature teratoma and carcinosarcoma [39, 40], NUT carcinoma [41], and calcitonin-negative MTC [42, 43]. Some of these may be included in the next edition of the WHO classification.

Pathological Factors Predicting the Clinical Risk of Thyroid Cancers

Thyroid cancer typically has a favorable prognosis, but some cases can have poor outcomes. Surgical decisions are primarily based on fine-needle aspiration cytology, while definitive diagnoses are made from resected specimens, guiding subsequent treatment and follow-up. Prognostic evaluation of surgical specimens follows established frameworks, such as the UICC TNM classification, ICCR guidelines, and the general rules for the description of thyroid cancer by the Japanese Society of Thyroid Pathology and Japan Association of Endocrine Surgery (ref). The prognostic significance of pathological findings varies by histological subtype, emphasizing the importance of accurate pathological interpretation.

Pathological Prognostic Factors in PTC

PTC generally has an excellent prognosis, although 5–10% of cases result in poor outcomes, accounting for most PTC-related deaths. Certain subtypes of PTC are associated with either a better or worse prognosis compared to classic PTC.

The prognostic significance of lymphovascular invasion in PTC remains controversial. PTC frequently invades lymphatic vessels, leading to a high incidence of regional lymph node metastases (≥80%). PTC can present as multifocal tumors within the thyroid gland, either from intrathyroidal lymphatic spread or multiple primary tumors. While some studies report vascular invasion as a prognostic factor [44], others do not find it to be an independent determinant of outcomes [45]. Clinically, lymphatic metastasis is common in PTC, yet morphological studies paradoxically indicate a higher frequency of vascular invasion compared to lymphatic invasion.

Surgical margin status is another critical prognostic factor. Analysis of large US databases shows that positive surgical margins are associated with an increased mortality risk [46]. However, other studies suggest that microscopic positive margins may not significantly affect prognosis [47–49], highlighting the need for careful evaluation of margin positivity.

Chronic thyroiditis (Hashimoto's disease (HD)) is commonly found in PTC. However, its impact on prognosis remains unclear. Some studies report a higher incidence of lymph node metastases in PTC cases with HD [50], while others suggest improved outcomes [51] or no significant clinicopathological differences, including prognosis [52]. In other cancers, such as breast cancer, tumor-infiltrating lymphocytes (TILs) are gaining attention for their prognostic and therapeutic implications. Evaluating TILs in PTC, considering the presence or absence of HD, may provide valuable insights.

Pathological Prognostic Factors in FTC

In FNs, malignancy is determined by the presence of capsular invasion, vascular invasion, or metastasis. The prognostic significance of vascular invasion is discussed above. Regarding capsular invasion, previous studies suggested a poor prognosis for widely invasive FTC (wiFTC). However, an analysis of 523 FTC cases by Ito et al. [53] revealed that wiFTC without vascular invasion had a prognosis comparable to miFTC. This finding may reflect unique characteristics of FTC in Asian populations.

The Impact of PDTC and ATC Components in Well-Differentiated Carcinomas

PDTC or ATC components can sometimes be identified in surgical specimens initially diagnosed as well-differentiated carcinoma such as PTC and FTC. When ATC components are present, even in small amounts, it is recommended to diagnose the tumor as ATC owing to its extremely poor prognosis. The proportion of ATC components should also be documented in such cases.

The definition of PDTC follows the WHO classification and the Turin proposal, although neither specifies the proportion of solid, trabecular, or insular (STI) growth patterns required for diagnosis. In Japan, PDTC is typically diagnosed when it constitutes more than 50% of the tumor.

Mitotic counts and tumor necrosis are critical criteria for diagnosing thyroid carcinomas. While the MIB-1 labeling index is not officially included in the diagnostic criteria, it is generally observed to range from 10% to 30% in DHGTC and PDTC, and it often exceeds 30% in ATC. Mitotic counts should be assessed in hotspots for accuracy. However, interobserver variability remains a challenge for consistent diagnosis.

Diagnosis of Thyroid Neoplasms: A Molecular Pathological Approach

WHO fifth outlines a simple three-step diagnostic approach for classifying thyroid neoplasms (Fig. 20.5). The first step involves considering the cellular origin or differentiation of the tumor cells. The second step involves an assessment of driver gene mutations, while the third step entails a risk assessment based on both genetic and histomorphological features.

Cellular Origin or Differentiation

Thyroid tumor diagnosis primarily relies on determining the cellular origin or differentiation through histomorphological observation and differentiation markers. Markers include TTF1, PAX8, and thyroglobulin for follicular cell differentiation, calcitonin for C-cell differentiation, CD5 for thymus-like differentiation, and SALL4 for embryonal features.

Categorization by Driver Gene Alterations

FDNs are classified into four types based on genetic alterations: oncocytic tumors, well-differentiated tumors (or tumorlike nodules), RLTs, and BLTs. This classification can be achieved through gene expression analysis or morphological observation. Immunostaining for mitochondria helps differentiate oncocytic tumors, which require more than 75% oncocytes for diagnosis. Tumors display solid growth patterns such as PDTC and ATC, and HGDTC will be discussed in the third step. Solid growing tumor with PTC-like nuclear features is classified as BLTs (solid/trabecular subtype of PTC).

For tumors other than FDNs, genetic analyses can identify unique or pathognomonic driver gene mutations like *APC*, *CRTC1::MAML2*, and *ETV6::NTRK3*.

Histomorphological and Genetic Risk Stratification

A thorough histomorphological evaluation is essential for confirming the diagnosis of FDNs. Oncocytic tumors and RLTs typically present as encapsulated nodular lesions. The assessment of capsular and vascular invasion is crucial in determining their benign or malignant status. For RLTs, evaluating the presence of PTC-like nuclear features is also necessary. FTA is diagnosed when there are no PTC-like nuclear features or capsular/vascular invasion, while FTC is diagnosed with capsular/vascular invasion but no PTC-like nuclear features. *RAS* mutation alone is insufficient to determine malignancy. Tumors with PTC-like nuclear features without capsular/vascular invasion are classified as NIFTP, whereas those with invasion are classified as IEFVPTC. Diagnosing PDTC, HGDTC, and ATC requires appropriate evaluation of mitotic counts and/or tumor necrosis, which can be aided by the MIB-1 labeling index. These histopathological features are also important in risk stratification of MTC.

Clinical risk can also be evaluated genetically. PDTC, HGDTC, and ATC are associated with gene mutations such as *TERT* promoter mutations, *TP53* mutations, *PIK3CA* mutations, and *CDKN2A/2B* loss, and loss of *SWI/SNF* chromatin remodeling complex genes, which are considered high-risk gene alterations [54, 55]. Tumors harboring these high-risk gene alterations exhibit morphological features such as brisk mitotic activity and tumor necrosis, leading to a diagnosis of high-grade carcinoma such as PDTC and HGDTC or ATC. However, the specific number or combination of genetic alterations required to transform a tumor into ATC remains unclear. Diagnosing high-grade carcinomas and ATC is crucial for the early initiation of molecular targeted therapies. A range of drugs, including selpercatinib, entrectinib, dabrafenib, and trametinib, are now available to treat radioactive iodine-resistant thyroid carcinomas effectively [56].

Conclusion

In WHO fifth, the classification of thyroid tumors has been revamped to a systematic approach based on cellular origin, genetic alterations, and clinical risks. In FDNs, there is a close relationship between driver gene mutations and morphological features, allowing for the estimation of driver genes through morphological observation. Distinguishing between RLTs and BLTs is essential for differentiated thyroid carcinomas. Knowledge of genetic abnormalities, including gene mutations related to malignancy, is now indispensable for pathological diagnosis. This classification system facilitates the standardization of pathological diagnosis for thyroid tumors, enabling early intervention for high-grade tumors. Understanding genetic alterations has become essential not only for the pathological diagnosis of thyroid tumors but also for selecting appropriate treatment options.

References

1. Asa SL, Baloch ZW, de Krijger RR, et al. WHO classification of tumours of endocrine organs (5th edition, β version). Lyon: IARC; 2022.
2. Baloch ZW, Asa SL, Barletta JA, et al. Overview of the 2022 WHO classification of thyroid neoplasms. Endocr Pathol. 2022;33:27–63.
3. Chiba T. Molecular pathology of thyroid tumors: essential points to comprehend regarding the latest WHO classification. Biomedicine. 2024;12:712.

4. Lloyd RV, Osamura RY, Klöppel G, et al. WHO classification of tumours of endocrine organs (4th edition). Lyon: IARC; 2017.
5. Ganly I, Makarov V, Deraje S, et al. Integrated genomic analysis of Hürthle cell cancer reveals oncogenic drivers, recurrent mitochondrial mutations, and unique chromosomal landscapes. Cancer Cell. 2018;34:256–70.
6. Nikiforov YE, Biddinger PW, Thompson LDR. Diagnostic pathology and molecular genetics of the thyroid. 3rd ed. Wolters Kluwer; 2020. p. 347–87.
7. The Cancer Genome Atlas Research Network. Integrated genomic characterization of papillary thyroid carcinoma. Cell. 2014;159:676.
8. Yoo SK, Lee S, Kim SJ, et al. Comprehensive analysis of the transcriptional and mutational landscape of follicular and papillary thyroid cancers. PLoS Genet. 2016;12:e1006239.
9. Chen H, Luthra R, Routbort MJ, et al. Molecular profile of advanced thyroid carcinomas by next-generation sequencing: characterizing tumors beyond diagnosis for targeted therapy. Mol Cancer Ther. 2018;17:1575–84.
10. Palos-Paz F, Perez-Guerra O, Cameselle-Teijeiro J, et al. Prevalence of mutations in TSHR, GNAS, PRKAR1A and RAS genes in a large series of toxic thyroid adenomas from Galicia, an iodine-deficient area in NW Spain. Eur J Endocrinol. 2008;159:623.
11. Ye L, Zhou X, Huan F, et al. The genetic landscape of benign thyroid nodules revealed by whole exome and transcriptome sequencing. Nat Commun. 2017;8(8):15533.
12. Nikiforov YE, Seethala RR, Tallini G, et al. Nomenclature revision for encapsulated follicular variant of papillary thyroid carcinoma: a paradigm shift to reduce over- treatment of indolent tumors. JAMA Oncol. 2016;2:1023.
13. Kamma H, Kameyama K, Kondo, et al. Pathological diagnosis of general rules for the description of thyroid cancer by Japanese Society of Thyroid Pathology and Japan Association of Endocrine Surgery. Endocr J. 2022;69:139–54.
14. Carney JA, Ryan J, Goellner JR. Hyalinizing trabecular adenoma of the thyroid gland. Am J Surg Pathol. 1987;11:583–91.
15. Carney JA, Hirokawa M, Lloyd RV, et al. Hyalinizing trabecular tumors of the thyroid gland are almost all benign. Am J Surg Pathol. 2008;32:1877–89.
16. Nikiforova MN, Nikitski AV, Panebianco F, et al. GLIS rearrangement is a genomic hallmark of hyalinizing trabecular tumors of the thyroid gland. Thyroid. 2019;29:161–73.
17. Ito Y, Miyauchi A, Oda H. Low-risk papillary microcarcinoma of the thyroid: a review of active surveillance trials. Eur J Surg Oncol. 2018;44:307–15.
18. Ito Y, Hirokawa M, Fukushima M, et al. Prevalence and prognostic significance of poor differentiation and tall cell variant in papillary carcinoma. World J Surg. 2008;32:1535–43.
19. Ganly I, Ibrahimpasic T, Rivera M, et al. Prognostic implications of papillary thyroid carcinoma with tall-cell features. Thyroid. 2014;24:662–70.
20. Ambrosi F, Righi A, Ricci C, et al. Hobnail variant of papillary thyroid carcinoma: a literature review. Endocr Pathol. 2017;28:293–301.
21. Wang S, Xiong Y, Zhao Q, et al. Columnar cell papillary thyroid carcinoma prognosis: findings from the SEER database using propensity score matching analysis. Am J Transl Res. 2019;11:6262–70.
22. Vuong HG, Kondo T, Pham TQ, et al. Prognostic significance of diffuse sclerosing variant papillary thyroid carcinoma: a systematic review and meta- analysis. Eur J Endocrinol. 2017;176:433–41.
23. Rosai J, Delellis RA, Carcangiu ML, et al. Tumors of the thyroid and parathyroid glands. In: AFIP Atlas of tumor pathology, 4th Series, No. 21. Washington, DC: American Registry of Pathology Press; 2016.
24. Kure S, Ohashi R. Thyroid Hurthle cell carcinoma: clinical, pathological, and molecular features. Cancers (Basel). 2020;13:26.
25. Sugino K, Kameyama K, Ito K, et al. Does Hürthle cell carcinoma of the thyroid have a poorer prognosis than ordinary follicular thyroid carcinoma? Ann Surg Oncol. 2013;20:2944–50.
26. Kim MJ, Shin JH, Hahn SY, et al. Ultrasonographic characteristics of Hürthle cell neoplasms: prediction of malignancy. Ultrasonography. 2022;41:689–97.

27. Volante M, Collini P, Nikiforov YE, et al. Poorly differentiated thyroid carcinoma: the Turin proposal for the use of uniform diagnostic criteria and an algorithmic diagnostic approach. Am J Surg Pathol. 2007;31:1256–64.
28. Ibrahimpasic T, Ghossein R, Shah JP, et al. Poorly differentiated carcinoma of the thyroid gland: current status and future prospects. Thyroid. 2019;29:311–21.
29. Xing M, Liu R, Liu X, et al. BRAF V600E and TERT promoter mutations cooperatively identify the most aggressive papillary thyroid cancer with highest recurrence. J Clin Oncol. 2014;32:2718–26.
30. Ebina A, Togashi Y, Baba S, et al. *TERT* promoter mutation and extent of thyroidectomy in patients with 1-4 cm Intrathyroidal papillary carcinoma. Cancers (Basel). 2020;12:2115.
31. Alzumaili B, Xu B, Spanheimer PM, et al. Grading of medullary thyroid carcinoma on the basis of tumor necrosis and high mitotic rate is an independent. Mod Pathol. 2020;33:1690–701.
32. Fuchs TL, Nassour AJ, Glover A, et al. A proposed grading scheme for medullary thyroid carcinoma based on proliferative activity (Ki-67 and Mitotic) and coagulative necrosis. Am J Surg Pathol. 2020;44:1419–28.
33. Wells SA Jr, Asa SL, Dralle H, et al. Revised American Thyroid Association guidelines for the management of medullary thyroid carcinoma. Thyroid. 2015;25:567–610.
34. Krampitz GW, Norton JA. RET gene mutations (genotype and phenotype) of multiple endocrine neoplasia type 2 and familial medullary thyroid carcinoma. Cancer. 2014;120:1920–31.
35. Cameselle-García S, Abdulkader-Nallib I, Sánchez-Ares M, et al. Cribriform morular thyroid carcinoma: Clinicopathological and molecular basis for both a preventive and therapeutic approach for a rare tumor (review). Oncol Rep. 2024;52:119.
36. Folpe AL, Lloyd RV, Bacchi CE, et al. Spindle epithelial tumor with thymus-like differentiation: a morphologic, immunohistochemical, and molecular genetic study of 11 cases. Am J Surg Pathol. 2009;33:1179–86.
37. Reimann JDR, Dorfman DM, Nosé V. Carcinoma showing thymus-like differentiation of the thyroid (CASTLE): a comparative study: evidence of thymic differentiation and solid cell nest origin. Am J Surg Pathol. 2006;30:994–1001.
38. Agaimy A, Witkowski L, Stoehr R, et al. Malignant teratoid tumor of the thyroid gland: an aggressive primitive multiphenotypic malignancy showing organotypical elements and frequent DICER1 alterations-is the term "thyroblastoma" more appropriate? Virchows Arch. 2020;477:787–98.
39. Ting J, Bell D, Ahmed S, et al. Primary malignant thyroid Teratoma: an institutional experience. Thyroid. 2019;29:229–36.
40. Abayie AO, Nyarko KM, Bährle M, et al. The first case report of primary thyroid teratocarcinosarcoma: an analog to sinonasal teratocarcinosarcoma. Rare Tumors. 2021;13:20363613211043662.
41. Barletta JA, Gilday SD, Afkhami M, et al. NUTM1 -rearranged carcinoma of the thyroid: a distinct subset of NUT carcinoma characterized by frequent NSD3 – NUTM1 fusions. Am J Surg Pathol. 2022;46:1706–15.
42. Chernyavsky VS, Farghani S, Davidov T, et al. Calcitonin-negative neuroendocrine tumor of the thyroid: a distinct clinical entity. Thyroid. 2011;21:193–6.
43. Kim GY, Park CY, Cho CH, et al. A calcitonin-negative neuroendocrine tumor derived from follicular lesions of the thyroid. Endocrinol Metab (Seoul). 2015;30:221–5.
44. Pontius LN, Youngwirth LM, Thomas SM, et al. Lymphovascular invasion is associated with survival for papillary thyroid cancer. Endocr Relat Cancer. 2016;23:555–62.
45. Wagner K, Abraham E, Tran B, et al. Lymphovascular invasion and risk of recurrence in papillary thyroid carcinoma. ANZ J Surg. 2020;90:1727–32.
46. Lee CI, Kutlu O, Khan ZF, et al. Margin positivity and survival in papillary thyroid microcarcinoma: a National Cancer Database Analysis. J Am Coll Surg. 2021;233:537–44.
47. Kluijfhout WP, Pasternak JD, Kwon JS, et al. Microscopic positive tumor margin does not increase the risk of recurrence in patients with T1-T2 well-differentiated thyroid cancer. Ann Surg Oncol. 2016;23:1446–51.

48. Lang BHH, Shek TWH, Wan KY. Does microscopically involved margin increase disease recurrence after curative surgery in papillary thyroid carcinoma? J Surg Oncol. 2016;113:635–539.
49. Back K, Kim SK, Chai YJ, et al. Does microscopic positive tumor margin in papillary thyroid cancer really matter? Surgery. 2019;166:1160–7.
50. Jara SM, Carson KA, Pai SI, et al. The relationship between chronic lymphocytic thyroiditis and central neck lymph node metastasis in North American patients with papillary thyroid carcinoma. Surgery. 2013;154:1272–80.
51. Kebebew E, Treseler PA, Ituarte PH, et al. Coexisting chronic lymphocytic thyroiditis and papillary thyroid cancer revisited. World J Surg. 2001;25:632–7.
52. Sakiz D, Sencar ME, Calapkulu M, et al. The effects of chronic lymphocytic thyroiditis on Clinicopathologic factors in papillary thyroid cancer. Endocr Pract. 2021;27:1199–204.
53. Ito Y, Hirokawa M, Matsuoka H, et al. Prognostic factors for follicular thyroid carcinoma: the importance of vascular invasion. Endocr J. 2022;69:1149–56.
54. Pozdeyev N, Gay LM, Sokol ES, et al. Genetic analysis of 779 advanced differentiated and anaplastic thyroid cancers. Clin Cancer Res. 2018;24:3059–68.
55. Landa I, Ibrahimpasic T, Boucai L, et al. Genomic and transcriptomic hallmarks of poorly differentiated and anaplastic thyroid cancers. J Clin Invest. 2016;126:1052–66.
56. Zhang L, Feng Q, Wang J, et al. Molecular basis and targeted therapy in thyroid cancer: Progress and opportunities. Biochim Biophys Acta Rev Cancer. 2023;1878:188928.

Quality of Life Following Cancer of the Thyroid Gland

21

Diane Bijou, Christopher de Souza, Vishal N. Tyagi, Preeti Dhingra, Rosemarie de Souza, Aishan Patil, and Anish Patil

Editorial

With few exceptions, thyroid carcinoma harbours a very good prognosis and patients live a very long life. Although survival rate is excellent, patients have a possibility of carcinoma recurrence even 40 years after surgery. Though recent guidelines do not recommend total thyroidectomy as an initial surgery for thyroid carcinoma a large proportion of patients still undergo completion thyroidectomy for follicular carcinoma. Such patients require administration of levothyroxine and in some, vitamin D and calcium. Although the incidence is low, they may suffer hoarseness and due to invasion by disease or iatrogenic injury to the RLN. RAI administration is very popular both in the adjuvant setting and for therapy for metastatic lesions. These increase stress in patients, and affect fertility in young female patients. This

D. Bijou (✉)
Holy Spirit Hospital, Mumbai, Maharashtra, India

C. de Souza
Lilavati Hospital, Holy Family Hospital, Holy Spirit Hospital, Mumbai, Maharashtra, India

V. N. Tyagi
ENT Department V N Desai Hospital (Santacruz), Fortis Hospital (Mulund), Holy Family Hospital (Bandra, West), Holy Spirit Hospital (Andheri East), P D Hinduja Hospital (Khar), Mumbai, Maharashtra, India

P. Dhingra
Lilavati Hospital, Mumbai, Maharashtra, India

R. de Souza
Department of Internal Medicine, and Medical Intensive Care, TN Medical College and Nair Hospital, Mumbai, Maharashtra, India

A. Patil
Spr, Vascular Surgery, Scotland, UK

A. Patil
GP Trainee, Manchester, UK

P. S. Pai et al. (eds.), *Controversies in Cancer of the Thyroid and Parathyroid Glands*, https://doi.org/10.1007/978-3-032-13130-0_21

chapter reiterates the need to assess factors affecting patients' QoL and the importance of QoL evaluation addressing the special needs of thyroid carcinoma survivors. These aspects tend to be neglected in the process of treatment and follow up, but are very important.

Yasuhiro Ito

Introduction

The patient's perspective for a treatment modality, especially when it concerns cancer, both before and after treatment, must be considered [1]. The quality of life (QoL) is an important consideration, and patient care continues long after the primary treatment modality has been concluded. Thyroid cancer patients can likely experience multiple health-related problems and disease-specific symptoms following primary treatment.

Thus, it becomes essential to take notice of these problems and provide relief to these sufferers. This is an ongoing, continuous process. This approach goes a long way to ensure patient compliance as well as determining the effectiveness of treatment along with minimizing the deleterious side effects. This also ensures that doctor-patient relationships remain robust and compassionate.

Thyroid cancer ranks as the ninth most common cause of cancer worldwide. This gives impetus to the concern for the QoL for patients suffering from cancer of the thyroid gland.

Definition

The World Health Organization (WHO) [2] defines QoL as an "individuals' perception of their position in life within the context of the culture and value systems in which they live and in relation to their goals, expectations, standards and concerns." The available literature on the subject frequently uses health-related quality of life (HRQoL) with QoL in an interchangeable manner. QoL is a multidimensional apparatus that looks at physical, social, psychological, disease, and treatment-related symptoms.

The widely accepted definition of QoL in cancer treatment is "a state of well-being." This has two components: (1) the ability to perform everyday activities that reflect physical, social, and psychological well-being and (2) assessment of the patients' own satisfaction with their own level of functioning, the control of the disease, and ability to cope with treatment-related symptoms. The first component can be assessed more objectively, while the second is more subjective and therefore relies on the patient's level of satisfaction. The Centers for Disease Control and Prevention defines HRQoL as "either an individual or groups perceived physical and mental health."

Using the HRQoL as a measuring standard has proved uniquely useful and important in assessing the effectiveness of treatment. The HRQoL has been of great help in revealing the burden of disease and helps explore the relationships between HRQoL and different risk factors, monitoring the progression/regression of disease and can be used to determine multiple indicators of a patient's health.

The European Organization for the Research and Treatment of Cancer (EORTC)

The EORTC designed one of the commonly used instruments termed the *Core Quality of Life Questionnaire (QLQ-C30)*. It was designed and developed to assess the QoL of cancer patients [3]. It is considered as being one of the most comprehensive instruments designed and has been validated and translated into over 100 languages and is used in many countries. It has also been used in numerous studies to assess the QoL in patients suffering from thyroid cancer all across the world.

The importance of using this platform to assess the QoL provides healthcare workers a validated insight into the problems that thyroid cancer sufferers go through and then helps them provide measures to cope with these problems. This has been proven to be extremely useful again and again in many studies using this instrument, thus validating its usefulness across various cultures.

It was, however, found that there were very few disease-specific instruments designed for patients suffering from thyroid cancer. It was also found that none of the instruments designed had been tested for responsiveness, that is to say the instrument was not designed to demonstrate changes in QoL over time. This would lead to obvious problems such as under-reporting of side effects of radioactive iodine, hormonal imbalances, and the like.

Therefore, to overcome these shortcomings and make it a useful tool, the EORTC Quality of Life Group designed a new instrument for thyroid cancer. The EORTC designed an instrument with an extensive Phase I to ensure content validity.

Phase II was generated with a response format (4-point Likert scale) and time frame (1 week). In Phase III, the new thyroid cancer module termed EORTC QLQ THY34 was pilot tested internationally. Its psychometric properties were tested prospectively in a large group of clinically, culturally, and linguistically diverse patients who were suffering from thyroid cancer.

Phase IV validation study [4] included two different groups of patients for different purposes. The first group looked at determining and measuring the instruments sensitivity to responsiveness/change over time. This group included patients who were about to undergo initial, additional treatment or supportive care.

The second group was set up to determine test–retest reliability especially in survivors in whom no quick changes in QoL were expected based on their clinical assessment. A representative for the patient was involved all through the entire module development process.

The European Organization for Research and Treatment of Cancer Quality of Life questionnaire version 3 (EORTC QLQ-C30) consists of multi-item scales and single-item measures. These include five functional scales (physical, role, cognitive, emotional, and social), three symptom scales (fatigue, pain, and nausea with or without vomiting), Global Health Status (GHS) subscales, and six single-item common symptoms (dyspnea, loss of appetite, constipation, diarrhea, sleep disturbance, and financial difficulty). The time frame of these questionnaires is the preceding week. After linear transformation, all scales range from 0 to 100. Therefore, the lower the score, the worse the QoL. Decreased QoL was defined as EORTC QLQC30 less than 60 points.

All items have four response categories (not at all, a little, quite a bit, very much). GHS contains just two questions that are scored on a 7-point Likert scale, which range from poor scored 1 to excellent score 7. After linear transformation, all subscales range from 0 to 100. A high score in the functional subscales and GHS indicates better functioning and good HRQoL. A high score in the symptom subscales is indicative of increased discomfort and complaints. The QLQ-C30 summary score is used to measure the overall HRQoL, and it is calculated with the means of all subscales except the GHS and the financial difficulty subscales. It can range from 0 to 100; thus, the lower the score, the poorer the HRQoL. When compared to the individual QLQ-C30 scales and the GHS, the QLQ-C30 summary score demonstrates equal to or even superior validity and responsiveness over time. This makes it a very good instrument for evaluating the QoL for thyroid cancer patients.

Other Modules

There are quite a few questionnaires to assess the QoL for patients suffering from thyroid cancer [5]. There are some specigic questionaires like the City of Hope version. These were designed to be used in conjunction with the EORTC QLQ-C30 questionnaire. The thyroid module of the MD Anderson Inventory consisted of just 25 items. It was devised and developed in the USA exclusively without the participation of other countries.

The THYPRO questionnaire was designed exclusively for benign thyroid disease. The THYCA-QoL was designed and developed to be used with the EORTC QLQ THY34. It contained just 24 items and was developed in the Netherlands, and it was found to be difficult to apply universally. THYCA-QoL is a very specific thyroid cancer QoL questionnaire. It has 24 items. It consists of seven symptoms (voice, concentration, sympathetic, neuromuscular, throat/mouth, psychological, and sensory problems) and six single-item subscales, which include (1) problems with the scar, (2) chills, (3) tingling of hands and feet, (4) weight gain, (5) headache, and (6) interest in sex. Each of these items is scored in the following manner: (a) not at all, (b) a little, (c) quite a bit, and (d) very much. It measures symptoms from the previous week excluding interest in sex, which is over 4 weeks. Subscales are then summed up. The higher the score indicates worse symptoms.

The EORTC QLQ THY34 scales were found to have very many useful characteristics, including reliability and validity.

Many studies have found the EORTC QoL module for thyroid cancer to be very useful. It has 34 items, is reliable, and is able to differentiate between clinically relevant groups. It is also able to capture changes over time. The scale and item characteristics are relevant and very good. All patients and survivors found all the items relevant.

The module can be obtained along with the scoring instructions from the EORTC (https://qol.eortc.org.form/#1).

Factors Affecting a Patient's QoL

The incidence of differentiated thyroid cancer (DTC) has been steadily rising over the past few years [6]. Cancer sufferers are known to suffer from depression. Since there is a potential risk of pain, hypocalcemia, dysphonia, and dysphagia [7], it is important that such patients be given focused attention to address these concerns. This is addressed through the EORTC QLY-C30. It is well known that radioactive iodine treatment is associated with a second malignancy [8, 9]. This affects the patients' QoL adversely. Metastases and hypocalcemia were also found to be associated with a lower QoL. Concerns regarding financial distress/difficulties following thyroid cancer treatment need consideration [10].

DTC usually has favorable prognoses, and these patents need to be followed up and their QoL checked regularly [11].

The most common cited complaints were fatigue and depression and are treatable [12]. Once these concerns are addressed, it has been found that the patients' QoL improved significantly [13].

Among the 14 domains of the general QoL scale, social and role functioning were the most affected. Insomnia, fatigue, and financial difficulty were the commonest symptoms reported across all cultures. Low serum TSH was associated with a low QoL. Neck dissection was also associated with low QoL scores [14].

The number of thyroid cancer survivors is steadily increasing. This is because of increasing incidence, higher survival rates, and younger persons are being diagnosed with cancer. DTC has a 95% survival rate. Thus, patients require prolonged periods of surveillance since relapse can occur much later. Patients on whom a total thyroidectomy has been performed require lifelong thyroxine replacement and will need to check their serum TSH and serum thyroglobulin levels frequently. This seemingly simple monitoring can cause anxiety and at times financial distress. Frequent adjustments of thyroxine replacement [15], which require repeated blood checking, may place additional burdens upon cancer survivors. These are valid concerns, and the healthcare givers need to keep this mind when dealing with thyroid cancer survivors. The elderly and the poorer educated suffer the most from this. Fatigue and insomnia are health issues most associated with thyroid cancer sufferers cross-culturally. Unemployment was significantly associated with a very poor QoL. Employment, on the other hand, was associated with a much better QoL. Many cancer survivors often find it difficult to return to work following a diagnosis of cancer of the thyroid gland. Concomitant psychiatric illnesses have been frequently associated with the diagnosis of cancer, and these need to be treated appropriately and effectively.

Why Are QoLs Important? [16]

1. The incidence of thyroid cancer is increasing globally.
2. In the QoL for thyroid cancer, many survivors report a similar quality of life similar to cancers with a not very good prognosis.
3. Females, younger the age of diagnosis of cancer of the thyroid, and lower educational status are all predictive of a lower QoL.
4. Patients on long-term levothyroxine therapy are more likely to experience sleep disorders, increased anxiety, and depression.
5. Radioactive iodine treatment is associated with impaired physical functioning and reproductive dysfunction, which in turn lead to lower QoL scores. It is also associated with secondary malignancies later on.
6. Financial burden is worsened by unemployment and bankruptcy.

For the reasons listed above, it behooves the healthcare givers to consider all these factors when treating patients suffering from thyroid cancer. QoLs represent a moment in time and can change over time as the patient is being monitored. These changes allow the healthcare givers to identify areas where and when support needs to be given to the survivor, thus allowing the persons' quality of life to improve. Should the healthcare giver after evaluating the recent QoL find that the scores are worsening, they can initiate timely intervention to alleviate suffering and prevent it from escalating.

What Are the Special Needs of Thyroid Cancer Survivors? [17]

Papillary cancer of the thyroid is associated with a 5-year survival rate of 98%. Recurrence can occur 40 years later. Thus, it is imperative to keep all thyroid cancer sufferers under surveillance. This will help timely detection of recurrences and offer treatment at the earliest possible time.

The overall incidence of secondary primary malignancies in thyroid cancer patients such as leukemia, prostate cancer, and breast cancer is higher than the general population. These risks are further raised when patients are subjected to radioactive iodine (RAI) therapy. RAI treatment is associated with an increased risk for malignancies of the salivary gland tumors, leukemia, soft tissue cancers, and colorectal cancers.

Thyroid cancer patients who have gone through total thyroidectomy will require lifelong thyroid hormone replacement [18]. Most patients who have undergone total thyroidectomy experience difficulty in maintaining laboratory-evaluated euthyroid levels. They experience a financial burden, which gets exacerbated by unemployment. Such patients also experience sleep disturbance, low energy levels, impaired social functioning, increased anxiety levels, and depression.

RAI can adversely affect fertility and can cause irregular menstrual cycles, transient amenorrhea, and menopause in young females. In males, it can cause a decrease in sperm counts.

Nutritional advice is particularly important, and the American Thyroid Association recommends a low iodine diet prior to undergoing body scans.

Thyroid Survivorship

A thyroid survivorship program includes a multidisciplinary team that plays a key role in definite management. This team includes a skilled thyroid cancer surgeon, dedicated nursing care, experienced genetic counsellor, endocrinologist, radiation oncologist along with a competent medical social worker, and a dietician. The entire team needs to function in an integrated manner for the patient to cope well. Patient education and a faithful adherence to a regular follow-up will attribute to a positive approach in quality of life and patient care.

Are There Any Controversies Surrounding the QoLs?

There are however a vast plethora of instruments assessing the QoLs of patients who are thyroid cancer sufferers. This could cause confusion among treating physicians as to which QoL they should select in order to continue to care for their patients over time. The QoL devised by the EORTC, the QLQ-C30, in the literature seems to be the one that is popular. Still a universal, uniform QoL questionnaire would help evaluate the QoLs of thyroid cancer survivors in such a way that it would make adjustments for all the geographical and cultural differences that exist. The EORTC QLQ-C30 appears to be one such instrument.

Conclusion

A holistic approach is essential to deal with the issues in regard to QoL. This prerequisite is necessary to accomplish the objectives of the QoL. The ultimate goal is to ensure that thyroid cancer survivors cope well socially, mentally, and physically. When we reflect on the goals, only then will the purpose of the protocol for QoL will have true meaning and relevance. The core truth is every thyroid cancer survivor's experience is unique, and a personalized approach is essential in addressing and overcoming challenges in the quality of life.

References

1. Alsaud JS, Alharbi MS, Aldekhail AI, et al. Quality of life in thyroid cancer patients. Cureus. 2023;15(9):e45222. https://doi.org/10.7759/cureus45222.
2. The WHOQOL group. The World Health Organization quality of life assessment (WHOQOL); position paper from the World Health Organization. Soc Sci Med. 1995;41:1403–9. https://doi.org/10.1016/0277-9536(95)00112-k.
3. Aaronson NK, Ahmedzai S, Bergman B, et al. The European Organization for Research and Treatment of Cancer QLQ-C30; a quality of life instrument for use in international clinical trials in oncology. J Natl Cancer Inst. 1995;85:365–76.
4. Singer S, Al- Ibraheem A, Pinto M, Lakovou I, et al. International phase IV field study for the reliability and validity the European Organization for Research and Treatment of Cancer Thyroid Cancer Module EORTC QLQ_THY34. Thyroid. 2023;33(9):1078–89. https://doi.org/10.1089/thy.2023.0221.
5. Thiagarajan S, Fateh K, Menon N, Sawant A. Assessment of quality of life in thyroid cancer patients using the EORTC thyroid specific questionnaire: a prospective cross-sectional study. Eur Arch Otorhinolaryngol. 2024;281:1953–60.
6. Dow KH, Ferell BR, Anello C. Quality of life changes in patients with thyroid cancer after withdrawal of thyroid hormone therapy. Thyroid. 1997;7(4):613–9.
7. Schroeder PR, Haugen BR, Pacini F, et al. A comparison of short term changes in health related quality of life in thyroid carcinoma patients undergoing diagnostic evaluation with recombinant human thyrotropin compared with thyroid hormone withdrawal. J Clin Endocrinol Metab. 2006;91(3):878–84.
8. Iyer NG, Morris LGT, Tuttle RM, Shaha AR, Ganly I. Rising incidence of second cancers in patients with low risk (T1N0) thyroid cancer who receive radioiodine therapy. Cancer. 2011;117(19):4439–46.
9. Aschebrook- Kilfoy B, James B, Nagar S, et al. Risk factors for decreased quality of life in thyroid cancer survivors: initial findings from the North American Thyroid Cancer Survivorship Study. Thyroid. 2015;25(12):1313–21.
10. Lubiitz CC, Kong CY, McMahon PM, et al. Annual financial impact of well differentiated thyroid cancer in the United States. Cancer. 2014;120(9):1345–52.
11. Koot A, Soares P, Robenshtok E, Locati LD, et al. Position paper from the endocrine task force of the European Organization for Research and Treatment of Cacer (EORTC) on the management and shared decision making I patients with low risk micropapillary thyroid cancer. Eur J Cancer. 2023;179:98–112.
12. Chan WL, Choi HCW, Lang B, et al. Health related quality of life in Asian differentiated thyroid cancer survivors. Cancer Control. 2021;28:1–8.
13. Chen C, Cao J, Wang Y, Han X, Zhang Y, Zhuang S. Health related quality of life and thyroid cancer specific symptoms in patients treated for differentiated thyroid cancer: a single center cross sectional survey from mainland China. Thyroid. 2023;33(4):474–83.
14. Locati LD, Colombo E, Dedecius M, et al. Current picture of anaplastic thyroid cancer patients care and meetable needs. A survey of 94 institutions from the EORTC Endocrine and Head and Neck Groups. Eur J Cancer. 2023;180:146–54.
15. Liu YH, Jin J, Liu YJ. Machine learning based random forest for predicting decreased quality of life in thyroid cancer patients after thyroidectomy. Support Care Cancer. 2022;30:2507–13.
16. Yang X, Yang Q, Tang Y, Ma J, Ye H. Impact of the extent of thyroidectomy on quality of life in differentiated thyroid ancer survivors: a propensity score matched analysis. Cancer Manag Res. 2021;13:6953–67.

17. Oerlemans S, Schagen SB, van den Hurk CJ, et al. Self perceived cognitive functioning and quality of life among cancer survivors: results from the PROFILES registry. J Cancer Surviv. 2022;16:303–13.
18. Musoro JZ, Coens C, Mirjam AG, Brandberg SY, et al. Minimally important differences for interpreting EORTC QLQ-C30 change scores over time. A synthesis across 21 clinical trials involving nine different cancer types. Eur J Cancer. 2023;188:171–82.

Surgical Management of Medullary Thyroid Cancer

22

Andreas Machens and Henning Dralle

Editorial

Machens and Dralle have done a fantastic job of discussing important controversies in the surgical management of medullary cancer in this chapter. Their contributions to the field of medullary thyroid cancer are well known from their large number of publications and their influence on the revision of ATA guidelines on medullary thyroid cancer. The authors have selected four controversial subjects in the surgical management of medullary thyroid cancer and described their conclusions extremely well. The first subject discussed relates to selective or routine calcitonin screening. There appears to be geographical differences between practices in Europe and the United States. Routine calcitonin-level screenings are not commonly performed in the United States as the incidence is probably quite low and may not be cost-effective.

The second controversy discussed in this chapter relates to the results of hemithyroidectomy or total thyroidectomy for sporadic medullary cancer. This has become a subject of great debate in the recent literature, and the authors have alluded to their experience with tumor desmoplasia. They have used desmoplasia on frozen sections as a decision-maker. However, this has not been practiced routinely around the world. The data is quite strong in relation to the impact of tumor desmoplasia.

The next controversy discussed in the chapter relates to the role of prophylactic thyroidectomy for hereditary medullary thyroid cancer. They have given the general guidelines as to the best timing of prophylactic thyroidectomy with consideration

A. Machens (✉)
Medical Faculty, Department of Visceral, Vascular and Endocrine Surgery, Martin Luther University Halle-Wittenberg, Halle (Saale), Germany

H. Dralle
Department of General, Visceral and Transplantation Surgery, Division of Endocrine Surgery, University of Duisburg-Essen, Essen, Germany

P. S. Pai et al. (eds.), *Controversies in Cancer of the Thyroid and Parathyroid Glands*, https://doi.org/10.1007/978-3-032-13130-0_22

for complications and, more importantly, monitoring in the low-risk mutations. This subject always brings debate: it may not be easy to convince the parents of a young child to undergo total thyroidectomy, which requires a lifetime of thyroid medication replacement and may have a small number of complications.

The last controversial subject relates to lateral neck dissection. The general consensus has been not to consider prophylactic lateral neck dissection if there are no suspicious lymph nodes in the imaging studies. Calcitonin is an important tumor marker, which should be used in the follow-up of these patients and to suspect recurrent disease. Calcitonin doubling time is an important consideration for the long-term prognosis.

Recently, there has been considerable interest in RET-directed targeted therapy, both preoperatively in advanced medullary thyroid cancer and in recurrent medullary thyroid cancer. The positive results shown with targeted therapy have brought in an entirely new approach of using neoadjuvant therapies in locally advanced medullary thyroid cancer.

Ashok R. Shaha

Introduction

Medullary thyroid cancer (MTC) is a slow-growing neuroendocrine malignancy originating from the parafollicular C cells of the thyroid gland that synthesize, store, and release calcitonin into the bloodstream [1]. Another key feature of MTC is its proclivity for early metastatic spread, which needs years to manifest clinically.

With an annual incidence of 0.19 per 100,000 and a prevalence of 3.8 per 100,000 [2], MTC is considerably rarer than papillary or follicular thyroid cancer, both of which derive from the thyrocyte and represent the predominant cell type within the thyroid gland. Unlike thyrocyte-derived cancers, which typically enrich iodine, MTC cells do not express the sodium-iodine transporter and thus do not concentrate iodine, which limits treatment options for MTC.

Parafollicular C cells cluster in the upper dorsolateral thyroid portions of the thyroid gland. As a corollary, the majority of MTCs arise in the upper dorsolateral thyroid lobe [3, 4]. From there, MTC spreads first via lymphatic channels running alongside thyroid veins to the central and lateral neck before crossing the midline to invade the contralateral neck [5].

MTC comes in a sporadic (~75%) and a hereditary (~25%) variant, which is characterized by the absence versus presence of a pathogenic germline mutation in the *rearranged during transfection (ret)* proto-oncogene mapping to chromosome 10 (10q11.2).

The ret proto-oncogene encodes a transmembrane tyrosine kinase receptor that mediates downstream signaling in parafollicular C cells, adrenal medullary, and parathyroid chief cells [6].

Except for earlier development and more frequent multifocal growth of hereditary MTC, p.Met918Thr-driven tumor development and progression is similar in hereditary and sporadic MTC [7]. Whether this concept applies equally to other acquired and inherited, but otherwise identical RET mutations is unclear.

When acquired, which may take many decades to occur, patients develop sporadic MTCs, 93–95% of which are unifocal [8–10], typically in their 50s. This explains why sporadic MTC is exceptional in infancy and childhood, and infrequent in adolescence, affecting fewer than <4% of patients aged <18 years [11].

When inherited, the constant growth stimulus from the mutated RET receptor produces C cell hyperplasia, adrenal medullary hyperplasia, and/or parathyroid hyperplasia in a genotype-specific manner, with subsequent progression to MTC, pheochromocytoma, and/or primary hyperparathyroidism [12]. These three neoplastic conditions collectively are subsumed under the umbrella of multiple endocrine neoplasia type 2 (MEN 2). At the time of thyroidectomy, ≥60% of hereditary MTCs are multifocal due to constitutive activation of the mutated RET receptor in the absence of a substrate [9]. This genetic background provides a framework within which the respective neoplasms emerge, without being able to predict tumor development precisely [13]. This is where biochemical screening, which is more sensitive than high-resolution imaging [14], comes into play.

Serum calcitonin levels and serum procalcitonin levels (in the absence of infection) are strong predictive biomarkers of tumor load and clinical outcome [15, 16] and more powerful than serum carcinoembryonic antigen (CEA) levels [17].

CEA levels, and putatively procalcitonin levels as well [18], are useful in particular for diagnosis and monitoring of the <1% subset of nonsecretory MTCs that fail to produce increased serum calcitonin levels [19].

Elevated levels of serum carbohydrate antigen 19.9 identify patients with advanced MTC who run a higher risk of mortality in the short run [20]. Sporadic and hereditary MTC, sharing similar tumor biology [21, 22], have similar disease-specific survival and clinical outcome when comparative tumor stages are evaluated [23]. Postoperative normalization and/or disappearance of serum calcitonin levels, usually within a fortnight [24], confirms the oncologic adequacy of the operation, barring rare exceptions [25, 26].

Technological progress has begun transforming medical practice over the past three decades, ushering in the era of precision medicine. The advent of high-resolution imaging, married with biochemical and genetic screening using highly sensitive calcitonin assays and advanced genomic technologies, has enlarged the pool of patients with occult MTC for whom the former "one-size-fits-all" approach would be downright overtreatment. Refined surgical techniques, specifically compartment-oriented microdissection [27] guided by intraoperative nerve monitoring [28], have enhanced patient safety while reducing locoregional tumor recurrence in node-positive disease.

These advances, widening treatment corridors, have sparked controversies that are awaiting reconciliation.

Controversy 1: Selective or Routine Calcitonin Screening for Early Diagnosis of Sporadic Medullary Thyroid Cancer?

For any medical intervention, there is a continuum of benefit versus harm [29].

For MTC, the cost-effectiveness of calcitonin screening for MTC is determined by the following:

- The prevalence of the target disease (*moderately low*, approximately 2.6–3.2 MTC per 1000 patients with nodular thyroid disease [30, 31])
- The coincidence ("background noise") with other thyroid disease (*likely high* in iodine insufficient countries; *less high* in iodine sufficient countries)
- The predictive value of the screening test (*likely high*, contingent on the calcitonin threshold selected for women vs. men who have a larger C cell mass to start with [32])
- The availability of effective treatment options (*likely high* for MTC confined to the thyroid gland that is curable by thyroidectomy alone; *moderately high* for node positive MTC that is more often curable by compartment-oriented node dissection in experienced hands depending on the number of node metastases [33], which portends distant metastases [34] and increasingly worse survival [35, 36].

Depending on the respective weights attached to the above items, cost-effectiveness analyses can differ a great deal. Various professional bodies and medical societies, interpreting essentially the same evidence, have arrived at discordant risk-benefit assessments.

In Europe where nodular thyroid disease is more widespread than in the United States, calcitonin screening has been greeted with a lot of enthusiasm [37, 38], whereas routine measurement of serum calcitonin in patients with thyroid nodules is neither recommended for nor against in the United States [39–41].

Controversies surrounding cost-effectiveness issues typically revolve around inclusion-exclusion criteria for calcitonin screening and absolute calcitonin thresholds for MTC.

As the threshold for intervention is lowered, medical interventions provide continuously diminishing returns [29].

This makes it imperative to define absolute calcitonin thresholds above which benefit clearly outweighs harm, such as 20–26 pg/ml for women and 68–80 pg/ml for men [32, 42] or 50–100 pg/ml for both [31, 43, 44]. Below absolute thresholds, a value judgment is needed as to where to set the relative calcitonin thresholds below which concern about harm prevails. Between these two thresholds lies the gray area of indeterminate net benefits where deference to the patient's personal preferences comes in given the absence of a societal consensus [29].

Not all calcitonin assays are created equal so that the respective upper normal limits vary somewhat [45, 46]. This inter-assay variability needs to be factored into the calculation when setting institution-specific action thresholds. That said, thyroidectomy may still be required for other thyroid diseases that triggered the biochemical work-up in the very beginning.

Systematic calcitonin screening programs work to raise the prevalence of the target disease, mainly by unearthing clinically occult disease that is asymptomatic and often, but not always, confined to the thyroid gland at the time of diagnosis. Whether incidental MTC represents an innocuous disease, as frequently portrayed by critics drawing analogies to papillary thyroid microcarcinoma, or invasive disease stalled on its growth trajectory before spreading to the neck and beyond remains unsettled.

Unless a cohort is followed over time, the probability that a subclinical abnormality such as node-negative sporadic MTC will result in an adverse outcome cannot be determined reliably [47]. This limitation is inherent in any screening program. Disease identified incidentally on testing may advance more slowly than symptomatic, clinically manifest disease. Incidental disease left untreated may regress, remain stable, or progress too slowly to manifest clinically during the patient's lifetime [47].

Although some of these issues remain contentious, routine screening of patients with thyroid nodular disease by high-resolution ultrasound and serum calcitonin screening have helped move the diagnosis of MTC forward in time [48–51].

Controversy 2: Hemithyroidectomy or Total Thyroidectomy for Clinically Node-Negative Sporadic Medullary Thyroid Cancer?

Owing to augmented interstitial matrix deposition and remodeling of fibrillar collagens, many solid cancer types, including MTC [52–56], are fibrotic. Tumor fibrosis, also referred to as "desmoplastic tumor reaction" or "desmoplasia," is critical for initiation, progression, and clinical outcome of many types of cancer [57].

For sporadic MTC, recent research uncovered a close relationship between the intensity of primary tumor desmoplasia and nodal status and the number of node metastases [58–60], outperforming serum calcitonin levels [60]. In all these studies, node metastases were absent when the primary thyroid tumor was desmoplasia negative (i.e., $\leq 5\%$ or $\leq 10\%$) (Fig. 22.1a). The greater the intensity of primary tumor desmoplasia, the more node metastases appeared on the scene (Fig. 22.1b) [58–60].

Because they present as unifocal tumors confined to a single thyroid lobe [9], desmoplasia-negative sporadic MTCs are curable by hemithyroidectomy alone [59]. Conversely, multifocal sporadic MTCs, affecting some 5% of sporadic MTCs, are marked by extensive lymphatic dissemination and node metastases [9] from a desmoplasia-positive MTC [59].

Representing a biological continuum, the concept of desmoplasia is somewhat fluid on a fibrous tissue scale, compounding utilization of absolute clinical cutoffs [60]. Appreciation of desmoplasia negativity in a primary thyroid tumor and feeding of this information quickly back to the operating surgeon necessitates an experienced pathology team working from a frozen section unit in close proximity to the operating room. These organizational requirements limit the applicability of the

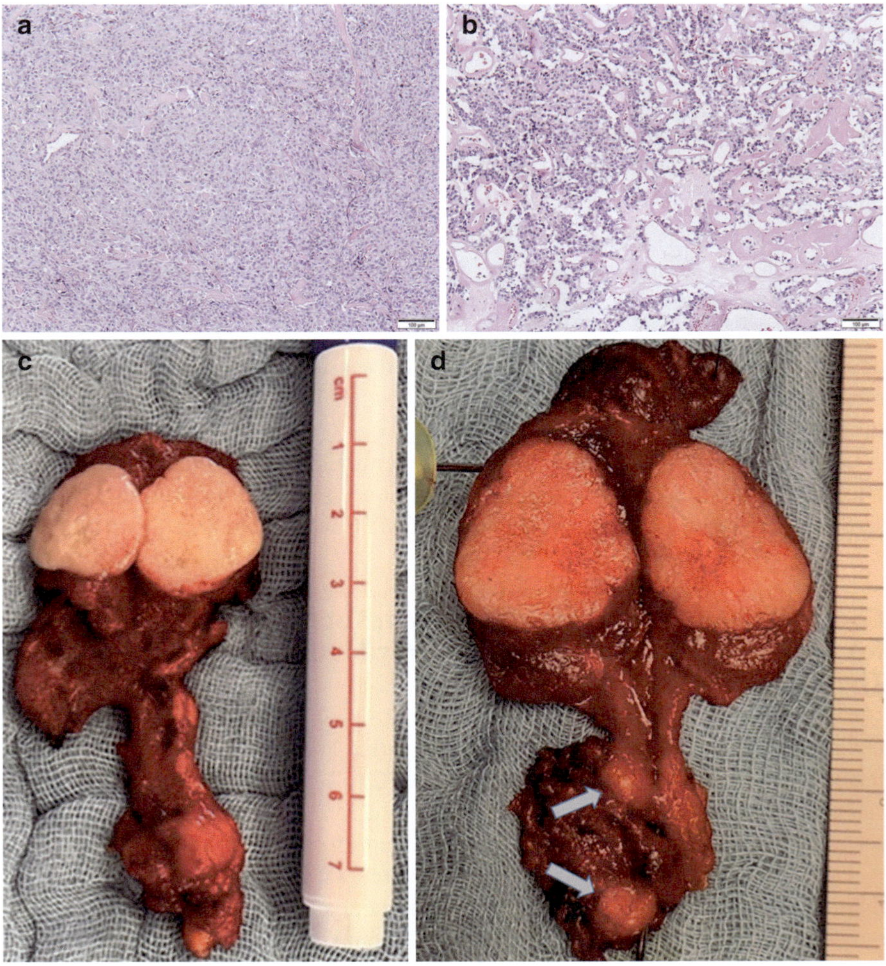

Fig. 22.1 Desmoplasia-negative and desmoplasia-positive sporadic medullary thyroid neoplasms. (**a**) Desmoplasia-negative medullary thyroid neoplasm (H&E 100×; extent of desmoplasia < 1%; surgical grade A). (**b**) Desmoplasia-positive medullary thyroid cancer (H&E 100×; extent of desmoplasia 21–32%; surgical grade C). (Courtesy of Prof. Kurt Werner Schmid, Department of Pathology, University of Duisburg-Essen, University Hospital Essen, Germany). (**c**) Surgical specimen of a 23 mm large desmoplasia-negative nonmetastatic thyroid tumor with sharp circumscribed margins. (**d**) Surgical specimen of a 22 mm large desmoplasia-positive, invasive thyroid tumor with inhomogeneous cut surface and blurred margins, displaying two macroscopic central node metastases (arrows). (Reproduced from [61] under a Creative Commons Attribution (CC BY) license)

frozen section-guided approach to high-volume tertiary surgical centers for thyroid cancer with frozen section units nearby.

Frozen section analysis provides useful information that enables intraoperative distinction between node-negative disease, for which node dissection is

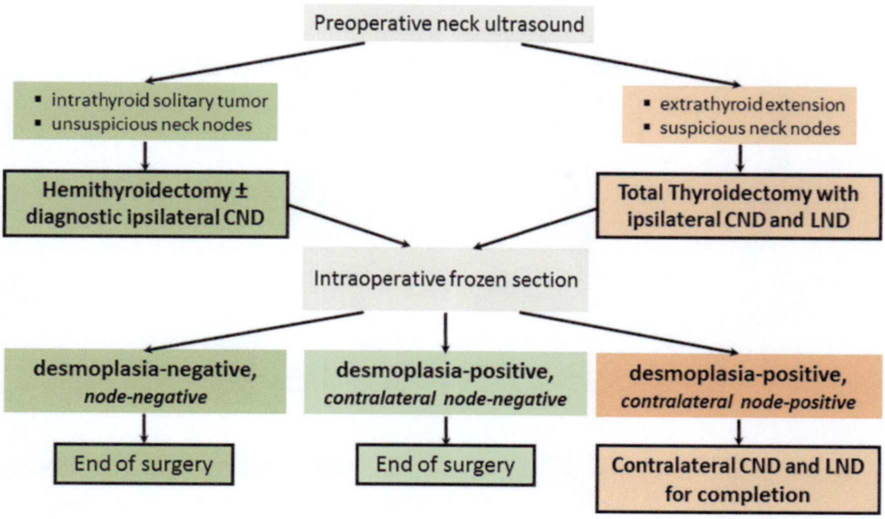

Fig. 22.2 Risk-adapted surgical algorithm for sporadic medullary thyroid cancer. CND central node dissection, LND lateral node dissection. (Reproduced from [61] under a Creative Commons Attribution (CC BY) license)

unnecessary, and node-positive disease, for which node dissection is required (Fig. 22.2) [61]:

- For desmoplasia-negative thyroid tumors (Fig. 22.1a and c), hemithyroidectomy alone is oncologically adequate, sparing most patients thyroid hormone replacement therapy for life and additional morbidity that comes with total thyroidectomy and systematic node dissection (Fig. 22.3a).
- By way of contrast, desmoplasia-positive MTC (Fig. 22.1b and d) still requires compartment-oriented node dissection guided by imaging and/or frozen section (Fig. 22.3b and c).

Desmoplasia-negative indolent thyroid tumors, for which the term "sporadic noninvasive medullary thyroid neoplasm (SNIMTN)" has been coined [59], must not be confused with invasive MTC, which typically requires at least an ipsilateral central and ipsilateral lateral node dissection [27].

In clinical oncology, heterogeneity of cancer is the norm. As a natural consequence, variation in the distribution of desmoplasia within a thyroid primary can lead to discordant interpretations of the extent of desmoplasia depending on which part of the tumor has been sent for frozen section.

Cognitive factors, accounting for an intra-observer concordance of 0.883 and an inter-observer reliability of 0.758–0.837 on histopathologic examination of paraffin-embedded thyroid specimens [54, 55], may produce further variability that defies standardization.

It is noteworthy in this respect that those desmoplasia-positive MTCs that run the greatest risk of being misdiagnosed as node negative exhibit predominantly

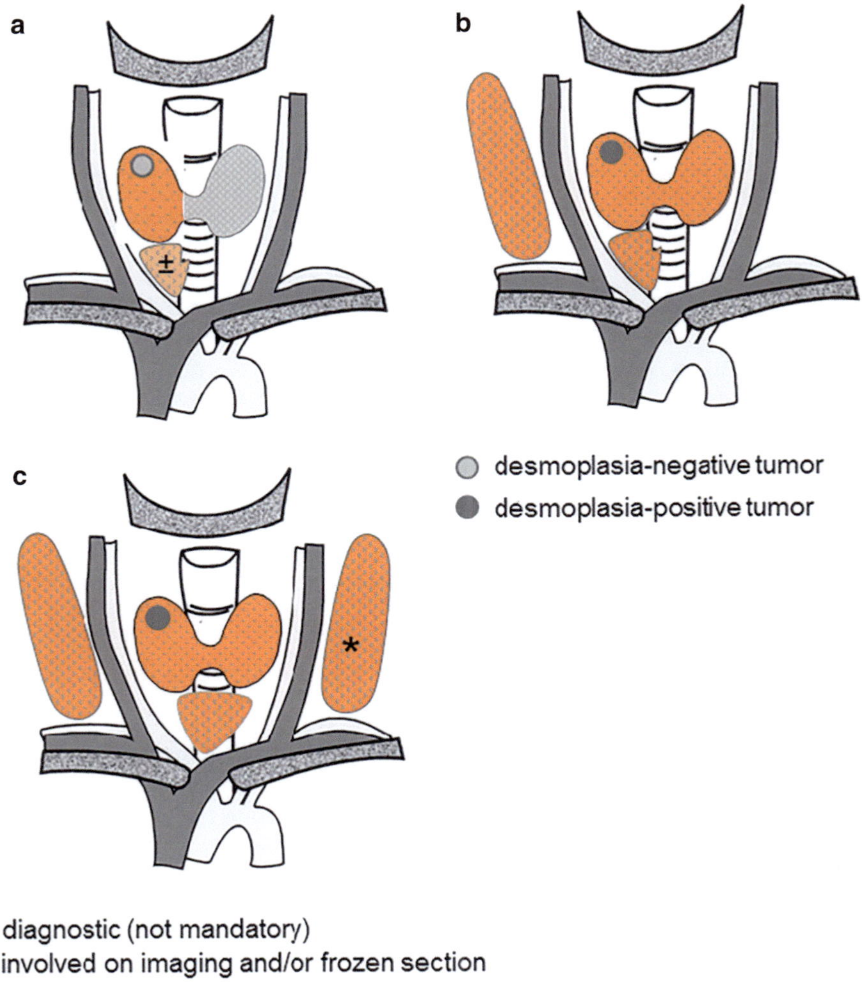

Fig. 22.3 Surgical de-escalation concept for sporadic medullary thyroid cancer. (**a**) Hemithyroidectomy, with or without diagnostic ipsilateral central node dissection, for a desmoplasia-negative medullary thyroid neoplasm. (**b**) Total thyroidectomy with concomitant ipsilateral central and lateral node dissection for a less advanced desmoplasia-positive medullary thyroid cancer. (**c**) Total thyroidectomy with concomitant bilateral central and lateral node dissection for an advanced desmoplasia-positive medullary thyroid cancer. (Reproduced from [61] under a Creative Commons Attribution (CC BY) license)

low-grade desmoplasia and mostly are node negative. For instance, when thyroid tumor desmoplasia ranged between 11 and 32%, ≤35% of patients revealed node-positive sporadic MTC [60]. If and when deemed necessary for risk mitigation, addition of a diagnostic ipsilateral central node dissection provides for an extra margin of safety. To make an informed decision, a competent patient, prepared to accept a small residual risk of completion surgery, needs to fully understand, and explicitly consent to, the frozen section-guided surgical approach.

An inherent limitation of any innovation is the absence of long-term outcome data demonstrating that the cure noted after a less extensive cancer operation is not short-lived.

Follow-up data on 19 patients with desmoplasia-negative sporadic MTC showed that the biochemical cure diagnosed postoperatively had been maintained for a median of 19.5 months [59], attesting to the high sensitivity of modern calcitonin assays.

This finding confirmed that the frozen section-guided surgical concept is safe in experienced hands.

High-resolution ultrasound screening of patients has become a mainstay of modern care because it reliably discriminates between clinically occult MTC, for which surgical de-escalation has become a viable option, and more advanced MTC, calling for standard compartment-oriented node dissection.

Absence of primary tumor desmoplasia on frozen section signifies absence of node metastases in sporadic MTC, prompting instant adjustment of the surgical treatment plan during the operation.

This competitive edge makes desmoplasia a strong surgical biomarker that outpaces conventional tumor classification systems depending on definitive histopathology [62, 63].

Controversy 3: Prophylactic Thyroidectomy for Hereditary Medullary Thyroid Cancer Without or With Central Neck Dissection?

Constitutive activation of the mutated RET receptor in the absence of the ligand is the hallmark of hereditary MTC. Constant lifelong stimulation and proliferation of parafollicular C cells, the intensity of which is encoded by the ret germline mutation, is driving nodular C cell hyperplasia, the predecessor of hereditary MTC [64].

When C cells breach the basement membrane, malignant transformation from C cell hyperplasia to early MTC (or "C cell cancer") has already taken place [65]. At that time, the MTC(s) may already have invaded lymphatic and/or venous vessels inside and outside the thyroid gland, which may result, or already have resulted, in node and/or distant metastases.

Serum calcitonin levels are more sensitive than high-resolution imaging [14]. Neck ultrasound tends to produce false-negative results more often in the central neck, which can be obscured by thyroid pathology, than in the lateral neck [66].

Although RET carriers undoubtedly need to have the thyroid gland removed as a whole, there is much less consensus in the medical community as to the timing of preemptive thyroidectomy or the need for concomitant central node dissection.

Proposed triggers for total thyroidectomy include age-specific thresholds, biochemical thresholds, and a combination of both.

Depending on their transforming activity, specifically the pace of malignant transformation, the 30+ RET mutations are grouped into four categories of highest-risk (codon 918 mutations), high-risk (codon 634 mutations), moderate-risk (codon 609, 611, 618, 620, and 630 mutations), and low-risk (codon 768, 790, 804, and 891 mutations) [12, 39, 64]). These tight genotype-phenotype correlations, exhibiting intrafamilial and interfamilial variability, prompted the American Thyroid Association (ATA) to issue the following recommendations in 2015 [39]:

Regarding preemptive ("prophylactic") total thyroidectomy:

- For highest-risk mutations ("ATA-HST," recommendation 34):
  "in the first year of life, perhaps even in the first months of life."
- For high-risk mutations ("ATA-H," recommendation 35):
  "at age 5 years, or earlier based on the detection of elevated serum calcitonin levels."
- For moderate-risk and low-risk mutations (combined into "ATA-MOD," (recommendation 36):
  "should be based on the detection of an elevated serum calcitonin level; however, 6-month or annual evaluations may extend to several years or decades. Parents who are concerned about a long-term evaluation program may opt to have their child's thyroid gland removed around 5 years of age."

Regarding concomitant central neck dissection:

- For highest-risk mutations ("ATA-HST," recommendation 34):
  "in the absence of suspicious lymph nodes … should be based on whether the parathyroid glands can be identified and left in situ or autotransplanted."
- For high-risk mutations ("ATA-H," recommendation 35):
  "central neck dissection should be performed in children with serum calcitonin levels above 40 pg/mL, or with evidence on imaging or direct observation of lymph node metastases."
- For moderate-risk and low-risk mutations (subsumed under "ATA-MOD"):

Whereas the use of carrier age as a surgical threshold is straightforward, the use of "elevated" serum calcitonin levels is not. Interpreting serum calcitonin levels correctly in a suckling or young infant carrying the trait requires experience and can be challenging. In the first and second year of life, serum calcitonin concentrations are inherently higher than in adulthood, and adult serum calcitonin levels are reached only from the third year of life onward [67].

Another crucial aspect, which perhaps is more relevant to carriers of moderate-risk and low-risk mutations observed expectantly beyond the above age thresholds, is the viability of the 40 pg/ml calcitonin threshold, below which central neck dissection was not advised in the 2015 revised ATA guidelines [39]. Conceptually, occult MTCs metastatic to a few neck nodes may be flying below the above biochemical radar screen and thus may not be considered for central neck dissection.

This important point was clarified in a recent study of 125 patients with previously untreated hereditary MTC who presented with preoperative basal calcitonin serum levels ≤100 pg/ml [68]. When preoperative basal calcitonin serum levels were ≤40 pg/ml, the incidence of node metastases was 5% (5 of 97 patients), as opposed to 14% (4 of 28 patients) with preoperative basal calcitonin serum levels of >40 pg/ml but ≤100 pg/ml. These five patients with preoperative basal calcitonin serum levels of ≤40 pg/ml made up 2.2% of all 225 patients with hereditary MTC referred for initial neck surgery during the study period.

Remarkably, five patients with hereditary MTC, carrying high-risk (RET p.Cys634Thr), moderate-risk (RET p.Cys611Phe and p.Cys611Tyr), and low-risk (RET p.Val804Leu and p.Ser891Ala) mutations, presented before initial neck surgery with serum calcitonin levels that ranged from 15.7 to 29.8 pg/ml. Intriguingly, one (20%) of these five patients, exhibiting a basal serum calcitonin of 15.7 pg/ml, harbored one solitary node metastasis in the ipsilateral lateral neck, whereas the central neck (16 negative nodes) had been spared (altogether 28 nodes dissected).

By way of contrast, two node-positive carriers of high-risk mutations (RET p.Cys634Tyr and p.Cys634Arg) presented with preoperative basal calcitonin serum levels of >40 pg/ml, i.e., 47.4 and 91.4 pg/ml. Two more index patients, carrying high-risk (RET p.Cys634Arg) and moderate-risk (RET p.Leu790Phe) mutations, revealed preoperative basal calcitonin serum levels of 91.4 and 99.8 pg/ml, respectively.

No node-positive carrier of a highest-risk mutation (RET p.Met918Thr) was encountered with a preoperative basal calcitonin serum level of ≤100 pg/ml [68]. These data convincingly showed that screening with subsequent surgical intervention preferentially intercepts slow-growing tumors driven by intermediate-risk and low-risk mutations early on their growth trajectories than fast-growing tumors powered by highest-risk or high-risk mutations [47].

Although node metastases do occur at any increased basal calcitonin serum level in the central and/or lateral neck, this risk is smallest for patients with basal calcitonin serum levels of ≤40 pg/ml. Whether a risk of 5% (with a basal serum calcitonin level of ≤40 pg/ml) or 14% (with basal serum calcitonin levels >40 and ≤100 pg/ml) justifies a central neck dissection to clear clinically inapparent node metastases is a point of controversy, which is influenced by surgeon experience and patient preference.

In experienced hands, to avoid missing occult node metastases in the central neck, it can be prudent to lower the 40 pg/ml threshold to the upper normal limit of the calcitonin assay in patients with tissue-proven MTC and, when serum calcitonin levels begin exceeding it, complement total thyroidectomy by a central node dissection [68].

In patients with MTCs that arise from the upper dorsolateral thyroid lobe, it may also be sensible to explore the ipsilateral lateral neck in addition [5, 68].

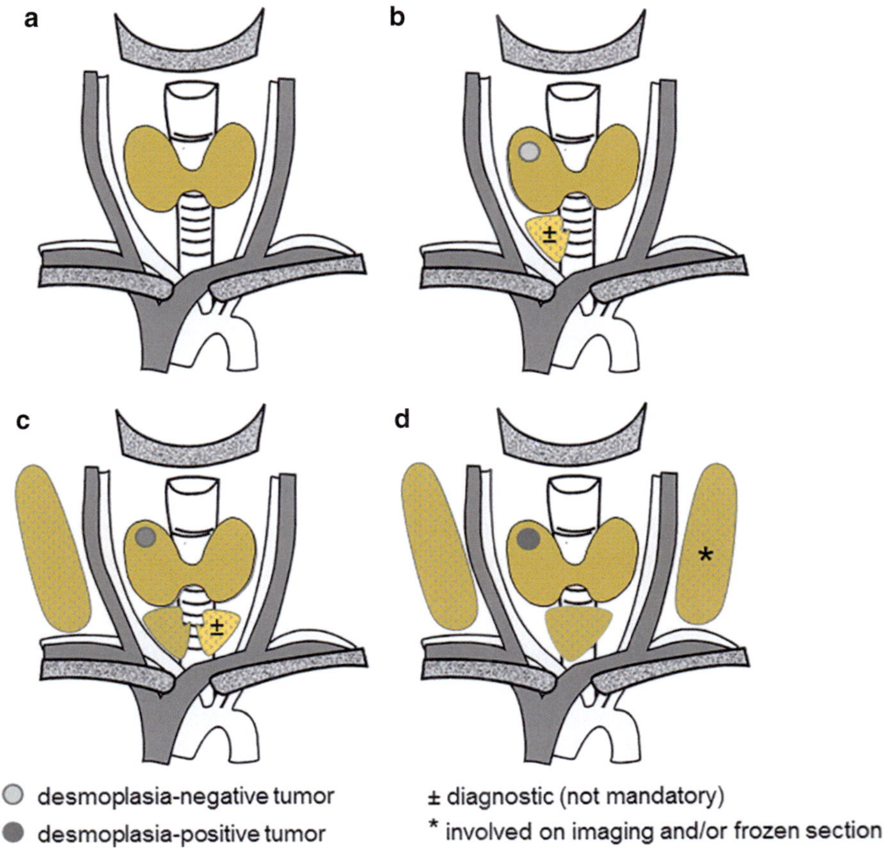

Fig. 22.4 Emerging surgical de-escalation concept for hereditary medullary thyroid cancer. (**a**) Total thyroidectomy, without node dissection, in the absence of an identifiable primary thyroid tumor. (**b**) Total thyroidectomy, with or without diagnostic ipsilateral central node dissection, for one (or more) desmoplasia-negative medullary thyroid cancer(s). (**c**) Total thyroidectomy with concomitant ipsilateral central and lateral node dissection, with or without diagnostic contralateral central node dissection, for one (or more ipsilateral) less advanced desmoplasia-positive medullary thyroid cancer(s). (**d**) Total thyroidectomy with concomitant bilateral central and lateral node dissection for one or more desmoplasia-positive medullary thyroid cancer(s), one of which is advanced. (Reproduced from [61] under a Creative Commons Attribution (CC BY) license)

Whether the extent of neck dissection can be further customized to the individual RET carriers, for instance, considering thyroid tumor desmoplasia (Fig. 22.4) [61], has become the subject of scientific inquiry.

Controversy 4: Selective or Routine Lateral Neck Dissection for Node Positive Medullary Thyroid Cancer?

Both *sporadic and hereditary MTCs* arise mostly from the central portions of the middle and upper dorsolateral thirds of the thyroid lobes, in which many parafollicular C cells cluster. From their site of origin, MTC cells migrate through the thyroid lymphatics primarily to the ipsilateral central and lateral neck nodes [5], which are both involved or both tumor-free in >75% of patients with unilateral MTC [5]:

- *From the upper thyroid* along the superior thyroid vein to the ipsilateral lateral neck
- *From the mid-thyroid* along the middle thyroid vein to the ipsilateral central and lateral neck
- *From the lower thyroid* along the inferior thyroid vein to the ipsilateral central neck

The *thyroid isthmus* very rarely, if at all, accommodates parafollicular C cells [69]. This is why tumor spread along the thyroid ima vein alone, leading to bilateral central node metastases in the absence of lateral node metastases, is exceptional.

The stronger the ipsilateral central neck involvement, the more frequent the involvement of the ipsilateral lateral neck (7–100%), the contralateral central neck (2–40%), and the contralateral lateral neck (1–6%), as illustrated in Fig. 22.5.

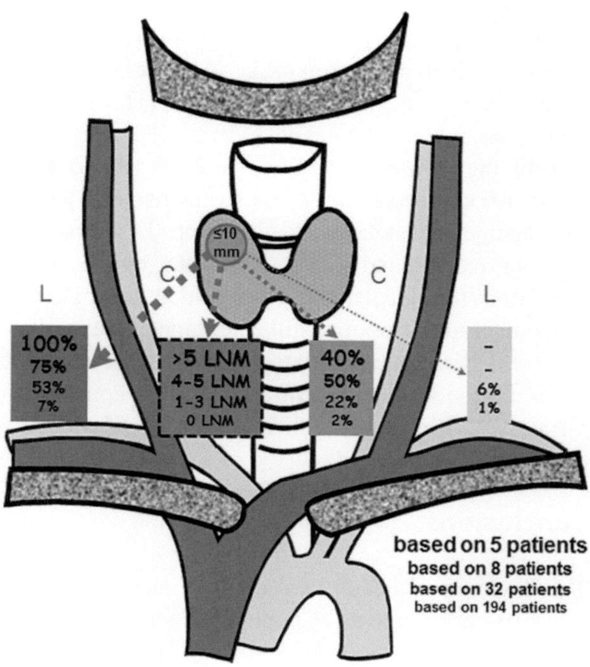

Fig. 22.5 Involvement of neck compartments by number of ipsilateral central node metastases in unilateral medullary thyroid cancer. C central, L lateral neck compartment (Building on data from [5])

Tumor diameter did not alter the patterns of nodal spread but rather intensified the magnitude of nodal spread [5].

For sporadic MTC, recent evidence supports a frozen section-guided approach [59], with ipsilateral central neck dissection as a starting point [5]:

- When the *ipsilateral central* neck specimen is *tumor-free* on frozen section, there is no need for prophylactic ipsilateral lateral neck dissection.
- When the *ipsilateral central* neck specimen is *tumor-free* on frozen section and the *MTC is located in the upper thyroid lobe*, it makes sense to explore the ipsilateral lateral neck.
- When the *ipsilateral central* neck is *node positive*, exploration of the ipsilateral lateral neck is worthwhile, in particular when imaging or fine needle aspiration cytology suggest nodal disease in the ipsilateral neck.
- When the *ipsilateral lateral* neck is *node positive*, so will be the ipsilateral central neck, which should be dissected in addition.
- When ipsilateral neck nodes are tumor-free, so will be the contralateral neck nodes.

For hereditary MTC, the patterns of nodal spread outlined above frequently are confounded by the concurrence of two and more independent thyroid cancers, each of which, if and when desmoplasia positive, may be capable of recruiting any of the above routes of lymphatic dissemination in its own right [70]. This makes it imperative to appraise all thyroid tumors in conjunction (Fig. 22.4) [61].

Despite these deliberations, performance of bilateral central and bilateral lateral neck dissections may be inevitable upon suspicion of bilateral neck involvement, erring on the safe side [27].

These metastatic patterns conflict somewhat with traditional concepts of nodal spread, in which the central neck used to be conceived as "the first echelon of lymph nodes in metastatic thyroid carcinoma" [71] from which takes off the tumor's metastatic journey to the lateral neck.

Building on this perception, the 2015 revised ATA guidelines [39] recommend central neck dissection for sporadic and hereditary MTC alike (recommendation 24) and therapeutic lateral neck dissection (based on a positive biopsy or suspicious imaging; recommendation 26) but differ on the need for prophylactic lateral neck dissection (serum calcitonin level guided; recommendation 25).

Counter to this notion, still entertained by a number of practice guidelines, runs the event of isolated ipsilateral lateral neck nodes that have spared (seemingly "leaped") the ipsilateral central neck. This constellation, incorrectly dubbed "skip metastases," is encountered in 11.3–14.1% of patients with unilateral MTC [5].

Conclusions

The direction of health care is clear: at one end, there is an emphasis on cost-effective improvements of population health and, at the other, increasing individualization of diagnosis and treatment [72].

Precision medicine, also called personalized medicine, focuses on prevention and treatment strategies that take individual variability into account [73].

Adoption of sensitive biochemical and genomic screening and high-resolution imaging has shifted the clinical landscape toward smaller tumors, opening "windows of opportunity" on the premise that early recognition of disease will ameliorate outcome because treatment initiated for occult disease will be more effective than later treatment for manifest disease. Indeed, smaller and more limited MTCs lend themselves more to de-escalating management approaches [74, 75] than advanced MTCs, which compartment-oriented neck surgery is geared at.

These trends resonate with the general philosophy in thyroid cancer that less is often more [76].

An important point in judging the benefits-to-harms trade-off for oncologic interventions is that many of the harms are front loaded and inversely proportional to the extent of surgery, and ultimately related to the experience of the operating surgeon [77]. These harms typically occur much earlier than the benefits (biochemical cure and progression-free survival), which are delayed by years. These issues call for operating teams that are skilled in extensive neck dissection at minimal surgical morbidity, flanked by pathologists within easy reach who are proficient in frozen section analysis.

The controversies outlined above beautifully illustrate how much familiarity with, and availability, take-up, and affordability of novel technologies emanating from translational research have revolutionized, and will continue to revolutionize, the practice of medicine.

Along these lines, the clinical corridors for MTC outlined above provide some leeway in favor of personalized treatments, moving away from a "one-size-fits-all" approach. The recent scientific advancements hold the hope that death and major morbidity from sporadic and hereditary MTC can be largely eliminated in the new millennium.

References

1. Machens A, Lorenz K, Dralle H. Progression of medullary thyroid cancer in RET carriers of ATA class A and C mutations. J Clin Endocrinol Metab. 2014;99(2):E286–92. https://doi.org/10.1210/jc.2013-3343.
2. Mathiesen JS, Kroustrup JP, Vestergaard P, Stochholm K, Poulsen PL, Rasmussen ÅK, Feldt-Rasmussen U, Schytte S, Londero SC, Pedersen HB, Hahn CH, Djurhuus BD, Bentzen J, Möller S, Gaustadnes M, Rossing M, Nielsen FC, Brixen K, Frederiksen AL, Godballe C, Danish Thyroid Cancer Group (DATHYRCA). Incidence and prevalence of sporadic and hereditary MTC in Denmark 1960-2014: a nationwide study. Endocr Connect. 2018;7(6):829–39. https://doi.org/10.1530/EC-18-0157.
3. Patel KN, Yip L, Lubitz CC, Grubbs EG, Miller BS, Shen W, Angelos P, Chen H, Doherty GM, Fahey TJ 3rd, Kebebew E, Livolsi VA, Perrier ND, Sipos JA, Sosa JA, Steward D, Tufano RP, McHenry CR, Carty SE. The American Association of Endocrine Surgeons guidelines for the definitive surgical management of thyroid disease in adults. Ann Surg. 2020;271(3):e21–93. https://doi.org/10.1097/SLA.0000000000003580.

4. Baloch ZW, Livolsi VA. Histopathology of the thyroid gland. In: Braverman LE, Cooper DS, Kopp P, editors. Werner & Ingbar's the thyroid. 11th ed. Wolters Kluwer; 2021. p. 332–51.
5. Machens A, Lorenz K, Weber F, Dralle H. Anatomical patterns of nodal spread in unilateral papillary and medullary thyroid cancer. Thyroid. 2024;34(7):871–9. https://doi.org/10.1089/thy.2024.0076.
6. Machens A, Dralle H. Multiple endocrine neoplasia type 2: towards a risk-based approach integrating molecular and biomarker results. Curr Opin Oncol. 2024;36(1):1–12. https://doi.org/10.1097/CCO.0000000000001009.
7. Machens A, Lorenz K, Weber F, Dralle H. Dissection of RET p.M918T-driven progression of hereditary vs. sporadic medullary thyroid cancer. Eur J Surg Oncol. 2025;51(3):109549. https://doi.org/10.1016/j.ejso.2024.109549.
8. Essig GF Jr, Porter K, Schneider D, Arpaia D, Lindsey SC, Busonero G, Fineberg D, Fruci B, Boelaert K, Smit JW, Meijer JA, Duntas LH, Sharma N, Costante G, Filetti S, Sippel RS, Biondi B, Topliss DJ, Pacini F, Maciel RM, Walz PC, Kloos RT. Multifocality in sporadic medullary thyroid carcinoma: an international multicenter study. Thyroid. 2016;26(11):1563–72. https://doi.org/10.1089/thy.2016.0255.
9. Machens A, Lorenz K, Weber F, Dralle H. Origin and impact of multifocal growth in sporadic vs. hereditary medullary thyroid cancer. Eur J Surg Oncol. 2024;50(11):108625. https://doi.org/10.1016/j.ejso.2024.108625.
10. Mao YV, Hughes EG, Steinmetz D, Troob S, Kim J, Tseng CH, Fishbein GA, Sajed DP, Livhits MJ, Yeh MW, Lee D, Angell TE, Wu JX. Extent of surgery for medullary thyroid cancer and prevalence of occult contralateral foci. JAMA Otolaryngol Head Neck Surg. 2024;150(3):209–14. https://doi.org/10.1001/jamaoto.2023.4376.
11. Machens A, Lorenz K, Weber F, Dralle H. Oncological features of sporadic vs. hereditary pediatric medullary thyroid cancer. Endocrine. 2024;85(3):1091–5. https://doi.org/10.1007/s12020-024-03959-1.
12. Machens A, Lorenz K, Weber F, Brandenburg T, Führer-Sakel D, Dralle H. Genotype-specific development of MEN 2 constituent components in 683 RET carriers. Endocr Relat Cancer. 2024;31(7):e240038. https://doi.org/10.1530/ERC-24-0038.
13. Machens A, Lorenz K, Dralle H. Individualization of lymph node dissection in RET (rearranged during transfection) carriers at risk for medullary thyroid cancer: value of pretherapeutic calcitonin levels. Ann Surg. 2009;250(2):305–10. https://doi.org/10.1097/SLA.0b013e3181ae333f.
14. Morris LF, Waguespack SG, Edeiken-Monroe BS, Lee JE, Rich TA, Ying AK, Warneke CL, Evans DB, Perrier ND, Grubbs EG. Ultrasonography should not guide the timing of thyroidectomy in pediatric patients diagnosed with multiple endocrine neoplasia syndrome 2A through genetic screening. Ann Surg Oncol. 2013;20(1):53–9. https://doi.org/10.1245/s10434-012-2589-7.
15. Machens A, Dralle H. Biomarker-based risk stratification for previously untreated medullary thyroid cancer. J Clin Endocrinol Metab. 2010;95(6):2655–63. https://doi.org/10.1210/jc.2009-2368.
16. Machens A, Lorenz K, Dralle H. Utility of serum procalcitonin for screening and risk stratification of medullary thyroid cancer. J Clin Endocrinol Metab. 2014;99(8):2986–94. https://doi.org/10.1210/jc.2014-1278.
17. Machens A, Ukkat J, Hauptmann S, Dralle H. Abnormal carcinoembryonic antigen levels and medullary thyroid cancer progression: a multivariate analysis. Arch Surg. 2007;142(3):289–93; discussion 294. https://doi.org/10.1001/archsurg.142.3.289.
18. Brutsaert EF, Gersten AJ, Tassler AB, Surks MI. Medullary thyroid cancer with undetectable serum calcitonin. J Clin Endocrinol Metab. 2015;100(2):337–41. https://doi.org/10.1210/jc.2014-3095.
19. Frank-Raue K, Machens A, Leidig-Bruckner G, Rondot S, Haag C, Schulze E, Lorenz A, Kreissl MC, Dralle H, Raue F, Schmid KW. Prevalence and clinical spectrum of nonsecretory medullary thyroid carcinoma in a series of 839 patients with sporadic medullary thyroid carcinoma. Thyroid. 2013;23(3):294–300. https://doi.org/10.1089/thy.2012.0236.

20. Elisei R, Lorusso L, Piaggi P, Torregrossa L, Pellegrini G, Molinaro E, Agate L, Bottici V, Pani F, Cacciato Insilla A, Casella F, Ciampi R, Tognetti I, Materazzi G, Basolo F, Romei C. Elevated level of serum carbohydrate antigen 19.9 as predictor of mortality in patients with advanced medullary thyroid cancer. Eur J Endocrinol. 2015;173(3):297–304. https://doi.org/10.1530/EJE-15-0304.
21. Machens A, Lorenz K, Weber F, Dralle H. Lymph node metastasis in hereditary medullary thyroid cancer is independent of the underlying RET germline mutation. Eur J Surg Oncol. 2021;47(4):920–3. https://doi.org/10.1016/j.ejso.2020.09.004.
22. Machens A, Lorenz K, Weber F, Dralle H. Exceptionality of distant metastasis in node-negative hereditary and sporadic medullary thyroid cancer: lessons learned. J Clin Endocrinol Metab. 2021;106(8):e2968–79. https://doi.org/10.1210/clinem/dgab214.
23. Raue F, Bruckner T, Frank-Raue K. Similar stage-dependent survival and outcome in sporadic and hereditary medullary thyroid carcinoma. J Clin Endocrinol Metab. 2021;106(9):e3582–91. https://doi.org/10.1210/clinem/dgab326.
24. Machens A, Lorenz K, Dralle H. Time to calcitonin normalization after surgery for node-negative and node-positive medullary thyroid cancer. Br J Surg. 2019;106(4):412–8. https://doi.org/10.1002/bjs.11071.
25. Fanget F, Demarchi MS, Maillard L, Lintis A, Decaussin M, Lifante JC. Medullary thyroid cancer outcomes in patients with undetectable versus normalized postoperative calcitonin levels. Br J Surg. 2021;108(9):1064–71. https://doi.org/10.1093/bjs/znab106.
26. Duval MADS, Ferreira CV, Marmitt L, Dora JM, Espíndola M, Benini AF, Camelier MV, Bulzico D, Andrade FA, Alves Júnior PA, Corbo R, Vaisman F, Zanella AB, Scheffel RS, Maia AL. An undetectable postoperative calcitonin level is associated with long-term disease-free survival in medullary thyroid carcinoma: results of a retrospective cohort study. Thyroid. 2023;33(1):82–90. https://doi.org/10.1089/thy.2022.0295.
27. Dralle H. Lymph node dissection and medullary thyroid carcinoma. Br J Surg. 2002;89(9):1073–5. https://doi.org/10.1046/j.1365-2168.2002.02160.x.
28. Schneider R, Machens A, Sekulla C, Lorenz K, Elwerr M, Dralle H. Superiority of continuous over intermittent intraoperative nerve monitoring in preventing vocal cord palsy. Br J Surg. 2021;108(5):566–73. https://doi.org/10.1002/bjs.11901.
29. Quanstrum KH, Hayward RA. Lessons from the mammography wars. N Engl J Med. 2010;363(11):1076–9. https://doi.org/10.1056/NEJMsb1002538.
30. Vierhapper H, Niederle B, Bieglmayer C, Kaserer K, Baumgartner-Parzer S. Early diagnosis and curative therapy of medullary thyroid carcinoma by routine measurement of serum calcitonin in patients with thyroid disorders. Thyroid. 2005;15(11):1267–72. https://doi.org/10.1089/thy.2005.15.1267.
31. Costante G, Meringolo D, Durante C, Bianchi D, Nocera M, Tumino S, Crocetti U, Attard M, Maranghi M, Torlontano M, Filetti S. Predictive value of serum calcitonin levels for preoperative diagnosis of medullary thyroid carcinoma in a cohort of 5817 consecutive patients with thyroid nodules. J Clin Endocrinol Metab. 2007;92(2):450–5. https://doi.org/10.1210/jc.2006-1590.
32. Machens A, Hoffmann F, Sekulla C, Dralle H. Importance of gender-specific calcitonin thresholds in screening for occult sporadic medullary thyroid cancer. Endocr Relat Cancer. 2009;16(4):1291–8. https://doi.org/10.1677/ERC-09-0136.
33. Machens A, Lorenz K, Dralle H. Prediction of biochemical cure in patients with medullary thyroid cancer. Br J Surg. 2020;107(6):695–704. https://doi.org/10.1002/bjs.11444.
34. Machens A, Dralle H. Prognostic impact of N staging in 715 medullary thyroid cancer patients: proposal for a revised staging system. Ann Surg. 2013;257(2):323–9. https://doi.org/10.1097/SLA.0b013e318268301d.
35. Moses LE, Oliver JR, Rotsides JM, Shao Q, Patel KN, Morris LGT, Givi B. Nodal disease burden and outcome of medullary thyroid carcinoma. Head Neck. 2021;43(2):577–84. https://doi.org/10.1002/hed.26511.
36. Wang Z, Tang C, Wang Y, Yin Z, Rixiati Y. Inclusion of the number of metastatic lymph nodes in the staging system for medullary thyroid cancer: validating a modified American Joint

Committee on cancer tumor-node-metastasis staging system. Thyroid. 2022;32(5):536–43. https://doi.org/10.1089/thy.2021.0571.
37. Karges W, Dralle H, Raue F, Mann K, Reiners C, Grussendorf M, Hüfner M, Niederle B, Brabant G, German Society for Endocrinology (DGE) - Thyroid Section. Calcitonin measurement to detect medullary thyroid carcinoma in nodular goiter: German evidence-based consensus recommendation. Exp Clin Endocrinol Diabetes. 2004;112(1):52–8. https://doi.org/10.1055/s-2004-815727.
38. Pacini F, Schlumberger M, Dralle H, Elisei R, Smit JW, Wiersinga W, European Thyroid Cancer Taskforce. European consensus for the management of patients with differentiated thyroid carcinoma of the follicular epithelium. Eur J Endocrinol. 2006;154(6):787–803. https://doi.org/10.1530/eje.1.02158.
39. Wells SA Jr, Asa SL, Dralle H, Elisei R, Evans DB, Gagel RF, Lee N, Machens A, Moley JF, Pacini F, Raue F, Frank-Raue K, Robinson B, Rosenthal MS, Santoro M, Schlumberger M, Shah M, Waguespack SG, American Thyroid Association Guidelines Task Force on Medullary Thyroid Carcinoma. Revised American Thyroid Association guidelines for the management of medullary thyroid carcinoma. Thyroid. 2015;25(6):567–610. https://doi.org/10.1089/thy.2014.0335.
40. Francis GL, Waguespack SG, Bauer AJ, Angelos P, Benvenga S, Cerutti JM, Dinauer CA, Hamilton J, Hay ID, Luster M, Parisi MT, Rachmiel M, Thompson GB, Yamashita S, American Thyroid Association Guidelines Task Force. Management guidelines for children with thyroid nodules and differentiated thyroid cancer. Thyroid. 2015;25(7):716–59. https://doi.org/10.1089/thy.2014.0460.
41. Haugen BR, Alexander EK, Bible KC, Doherty GM, Mandel SJ, Nikiforov YE, Pacini F, Randolph GW, Sawka AM, Schlumberger M, Schuff KG, Sherman SI, Sosa JA, Steward DL, Tuttle RM, Wartofsky L. 2015 American Thyroid Association Management guidelines for adult patients with thyroid nodules and differentiated thyroid cancer: the American Thyroid Association guidelines task force on thyroid nodules and differentiated thyroid cancer. Thyroid. 2016;26(1):1–133. https://doi.org/10.1089/thy.2015.0020.
42. Mian C, Perrino M, Colombo C, Cavedon E, Pennelli G, Ferrero S, De Leo S, Sarais C, Cacciatore C, Manfredi GI, Verga U, Iacobone M, De Pasquale L, Pelizzo MR, Vicentini L, Persani L, Fugazzola L. Refining calcium test for the diagnosis of medullary thyroid cancer: cutoffs, procedures, and safety. J Clin Endocrinol Metab. 2014;99(5):1656–64. https://doi.org/10.1210/jc.2013-4088.
43. Cheung K, Roman SA, Wang TS, Walker HD, Sosa JA. Calcitonin measurement in the evaluation of thyroid nodules in the United States: a cost-effectiveness and decision analysis. J Clin Endocrinol Metab. 2008;93(6):2173–80. https://doi.org/10.1210/jc.2007-2496.
44. Chambon G, Alovisetti C, Idoux-Louche C, Reynaud C, Rodier M, Guedj AM, Chapuis H, Lallemant JG, Lallemant B. The use of preoperative routine measurement of basal serum thyrocalcitonin in candidates for thyroidectomy due to nodular thyroid disorders: results from 2733 consecutive patients. J Clin Endocrinol Metab. 2011;96(1):75–81. https://doi.org/10.1210/jc.2010-0162.
45. Kratzsch J, Petzold A, Raue F, Reinhardt W, Bröcker-Preuss M, Görges R, Mann K, Karges W, Morgenthaler N, Luster M, Reiners C, Thiery J, Dralle H, Fuhrer D. Basal and stimulated calcitonin and procalcitonin by various assays in patients with and without medullary thyroid cancer. Clin Chem. 2011;57(3):467–74. https://doi.org/10.1373/clinchem.2010.151688.
46. Ito Y, Kaneko H, Sasaki Y, Ohana N, Ichijo M, Furuya F, Suzuki S, Suzuki S, Shimura H. Calcitonin levels by ECLIA correlate well with RIA values in higher range but are affected by sex, TgAb, and renal function in lower range. Endocr J. 2020;67(7):759–70. https://doi.org/10.1507/endocrj.EJ19-0610.
47. Black WC, Welch HG. Advances in diagnostic imaging and overestimations of disease prevalence and the benefits of therapy. N Engl J Med. 1993;328(17):1237–43. https://doi.org/10.1056/NEJM199304293281706.

48. Machens A, Dralle H. Surgical cure rates of sporadic medullary thyroid cancer in the era of calcitonin screening. Eur J Endocrinol. 2016;175(3):219–28. https://doi.org/10.1530/EJE-16-0325.
49. Randle RW, Balentine CJ, Leverson GE, Havlena JA, Sippel RS, Schneider DF, Pitt SC. Trends in the presentation, treatment, and survival of patients with medullary thyroid cancer over the past 30 years. Surgery. 2017;161(1):137–46. https://doi.org/10.1016/j.surg.2016.04.053.
50. Machens A, Lorenz K, Brandenburg T, Führer-Sakel D, Weber F, Dralle H. The changing face of multiple endocrine neoplasia 2A: from symptom-based to preventative medicine. J Clin Endocrinol Metab. 2023;108(9):e734–42. https://doi.org/10.1210/clinem/dgad156.
51. Weber T, Hummel R, Vorländer C, Zielke A, Hermann M, Krappitz A, Negele T, Dotzenrath C, Trupka A, Schabram J, Schmidtmann I, Klinger C, Lorenz K. Thyroid surgery in children and adolescents: results from a multi-institutional German and Austrian database. Br J Surg. 2023;110(12):1808–14. https://doi.org/10.1093/bjs/znad255.
52. Scheuba C, Kaserer K, Kaczirek K, Asari R, Niederle B. Desmoplastic stromal reaction in medullary thyroid cancer-an intraoperative "marker" for lymph node metastases. World J Surg. 2006;30(5):853–9. https://doi.org/10.1007/s00268-005-0391-4.
53. Koperek O, Scheuba C, Puri C, Birner P, Haslinger C, Rettig W, Niederle B, Kaserer K, Garin CP. Molecular characterization of the desmoplastic tumor stroma in medullary thyroid carcinoma. Int J Oncol. 2007;31(1):59–67. https://doi.org/10.3892/ijo.31.1.59.
54. Koperek O, Scheuba C, Cherenko M, Neuhold N, De Micco C, Schmid KW, Niederle B, Kaserer K. Desmoplasia in medullary thyroid carcinoma: a reliable indicator of metastatic potential. Histopathology. 2008;52(5):623–30. https://doi.org/10.1111/j.1365-2559.2008.03002.x.
55. Koperek O, Scheuba C, Cherenko M, Neuhold N, De Micco C, Schmid KW, Niederle B, Kaserer K. Clinical relevance of desmoplasia in medullary thyroid carcinoma. Histopathology. 2008;53(4):482–3. https://doi.org/10.1111/j.1365-2559.2008.03133.x.
56. Aubert S, Berdelou A, Gnemmi V, Behal H, Caiazzo R, D'herbomez M, Pigny P, Wemeau JL, Carnaille B, Renaud F, Bouchindhomme B, Leteurtre E, Perrais M, Pattou F, Do Cao C. Large sporadic thyroid medullary carcinomas: predictive factors for lymph node involvement. Virchows Arch. 2018;472(3):461–8. https://doi.org/10.1007/s00428-018-2303-7.
57. de Visser KE, Joyce JA. The evolving tumor microenvironment: from cancer initiation to metastatic outgrowth. Cancer Cell. 2023;41(3):374–403. https://doi.org/10.1016/j.ccell.2023.02.016.
58. Machens A, Kaatzsch P, Lorenz K, Horn LC, Wickenhauser C, Schmid KW, Dralle H, Siebolts U. Abandoning node dissection for desmoplasia-negative encapsulated unifocal sporadic medullary thyroid cancer. Surgery. 2022;171(2):360–7. https://doi.org/10.1016/j.surg.2021.07.035.
59. Dralle H, Brandenburg T, Weber F, Führer-Sakel D, Theurer S, Baba HA, Schmid KW, Machens A. Sporadic noninvasive medullary thyroid neoplasm: a desmoplasia-negative unifocal nonmetastatic tumor cured by hemithyroidectomy. Surgery. 2023;174(6):1356–62. https://doi.org/10.1016/j.surg.2023.09.003.
60. Machens A, Lorenz K, Bensch C, Wickenhauser C, Dralle H. Tumor desmoplasia outperforms preoperative serum calcitonin as surgical biomarker in sporadic medullary thyroid cancer. Head Neck. 2024;46(11):2843–52. https://doi.org/10.1002/hed.27827.
61. Machens A, Lorenz K, Brandenburg T, Führer D, Weber F, Dralle H. Latest progress in risk-adapted surgery for medullary thyroid cancer. Cancers (Basel). 2024;16(5):917. https://doi.org/10.3390/cancers16050917.
62. Xu B, Fuchs TL, Ahmadi S, Alghamdi M, Alzumaili B, Bani MA, Baudin E, Chou A, De Leo A, Fagin JA, Ganly I, Glover A, Hartl D, Kanaan C, Khneisser P, Najdawi F, Nigam A, Papachristos A, Repaci A, Spanheimer PM, Solaroli E, Untch BR, Barletta JA, Tallini G, Al Ghuzlan A, Gill AJ, Ghossein RA. International medullary thyroid carcinoma grading system: a validated grading system for medullary thyroid carcinoma. J Clin Oncol. 2022;40(1):96–104. https://doi.org/10.1200/JCO.21.01329.

63. Baloch ZW, Asa SL, Barletta JA, Ghossein RA, Juhlin CC, Jung CK, LiVolsi VA, Papotti MG, Sobrinho-Simões M, Tallini G, Mete O. Overview of the 2022 WHO classification of thyroid neoplasms. Endocr Pathol. 2022;33(1):27–63. https://doi.org/10.1007/s12022-022-09707-3.
64. Machens A, Lorenz K, Weber F, Dralle H. Genotype-specific progression of hereditary medullary thyroid cancer. Hum Mutat. 2018;39(6):860–9. https://doi.org/10.1002/humu.23430.
65. Machens A, Niccoli-Sire P, Hoegel J, Frank-Raue K, van Vroonhoven TJ, Roeher HD, Wahl RA, Lamesch P, Raue F, Conte-Devolx B, Dralle H, European Multiple Endocrine Neoplasia (EUROMEN) Study Group. Early malignant progression of hereditary medullary thyroid cancer. N Engl J Med. 2003;349(16):1517–25. https://doi.org/10.1056/NEJMoa012915.
66. Kouvaraki MA, Shapiro SE, Fornage BD, Edeiken-Monro BS, Sherman SI, Vassilopoulou-Sellin R, Lee JE, Evans DB. Role of preoperative ultrasonography in the surgical management of patients with thyroid cancer. Surgery. 2003;134(6):946–54; discussion 954–5. https://doi.org/10.1016/s0039-6060(03)00424-0.
67. Castagna MG, Fugazzola L, Maino F, Covelli D, Memmo S, Sestini F, Fioravanti C, Ferraris Fusarini C, Scapellato C, Macchini F, Cevenini G, Pacini F. Reference range of serum calcitonin in pediatric population. J Clin Endocrinol Metab. 2015;100(5):1780–4. https://doi.org/10.1210/jc.2014-4508.
68. Machens A, Lorenz K, Weber F, Dralle H. Incidence of neck node metastases in hereditary vs. sporadic medullary thyroid cancer at basal calcitonin serum levels ≤100 pg/ml: 30-year experience. Eur J Surg Oncol. 2025;51(7):109756. https://doi.org/10.1016/j.ejso.2025.109756.
69. LiVolsi VA. C cell hyperplasia/neoplasia. J Clin Endocrinol Metab. 1997;82(1):39–41. https://doi.org/10.1210/jcem.82.1.3707.
70. Machens A, Bensch C, Wickenhauser C, Dralle H, Lorenz K. Comparing nodal with primary tumor desmoplasia uncovers metastatic patterns in multiple endocrine neoplasia 2B. Eur J Endocrinol. 2024;190(1):K21–5. https://doi.org/10.1093/ejendo/lvad177.
71. Tang AL, Reid LM, Randolph GW, Steward DL. Central neck dissection: indications and technique. In: Randolph GW, editor. Surgery of the thyroid and parathyroid glands. 3rd ed. Philadelphia: Elsevier; 2021. p. 372–8.
72. Hill S. Introducing genomics into cancer care. Br J Surg. 2018;105:e14e5.
73. Bayer R, Galea S. Public health in the precision-medicine era. N Engl J Med. 2015;373(6):499–501. https://doi.org/10.1056/NEJMp1506241.
74. Machens A, Elwerr M, Lorenz K, Weber F, Dralle H. Long-term outcome of prophylactic thyroidectomy in children carrying RET germline mutations. Br J Surg. 2018;105(2):e150–7. https://doi.org/10.1002/bjs.10746.
75. Machens A, Lorenz K, Weber F, Dralle H. Prophylactic neck surgery for second-generation multiple endocrine neoplasia type 2B. Eur J Surg Oncol. 2021;47(4):924–7. https://doi.org/10.1016/j.ejso.2020.11.006.
76. Shaha AR, Davies L, Tuttle RM. Precision thyroidectomy in sporadic medullary thyroid cancer. JAMA Otolaryngol Head Neck Surg. 2024;150(3):215–6. https://doi.org/10.1001/jamaoto.2023.4600.
77. Shaha AR. Advances in the management of thyroid cancer. Int J Surg. 2005;3(3):213–20. https://doi.org/10.1016/j.ijsu.2005.03.012.

Mutational Testing in Advanced Thyroid Cancer and Its Implications on Targeted Treatments

23

Connor H. O'Meara and David C. Shonka Jr.

Editorial

David Shonka and O'Meara from the University of Virginia have reviewed the role of molecular testing in advanced thyroid cancer. The chapter is excellent, with up-to-date information regarding molecular testing and its implications on targeted treatment. There has been an explosion of molecular testing in all human tumors, and there appears to be enormous interest in targeted therapies for advanced or inoperable tumors. Clearly, this requires multi-institutional studies with a large number of patients evaluated and treated in a similar fashion to derive meaningful information. Individual institutions are unlikely to produce meaningful results, as there are many drugs available, with multiple mutational results.

Molecular testing has seen rapid expansion—not only in thyroid cancer but across all types of human cancers. However, many studies conducted at individual institutions involve relatively small patient cohorts, limiting the generalizability of their findings. To better understand the implications of molecular testing in both diagnostic evaluation and targeted treatment strategies, multi-institutional studies would be more appropriate and impactful.

The role of liquid biopsy remains unclear in the head and neck at this time, and its role in thyroid cancer also remains unclear. Once again, we would need to evaluate all advanced thyroid cancers before we can get definite information.

There is growing interest in neoadjuvant systemic therapy for patients with locally advanced tumors, particularly in cases where the surgeon anticipates that resection may be technically challenging or functionally suboptimal. The authors

C. H. O'Meara · D. C. Shonka Jr. (✉)
Division of Head & Neck Oncology and Microvascular Reconstruction, Department of Otolaryngology, Head & Neck Surgery, University of Virginia Health Services, Charlottesville, VA, USA
e-mail: connor.omeara@anu.edu.au; dcs5z@virginia.edu

P. S. Pai et al. (eds.), *Controversies in Cancer of the Thyroid and Parathyroid Glands*, https://doi.org/10.1007/978-3-032-13130-0_23

have done a splendid job in reviewing the current literature and its clinical application. I am sure the readers will enjoy this chapter.

Ashok R. Shaha

Introduction

Advanced thyroid cancers are characterized by their aggressiveness, propensity for recurrence, and increased disease specific mortality. Poorly differentiated thyroid carcinoma (PDTC), medullary thyroid carcinoma (MTC), and anaplastic thyroid carcinoma (ATC) are all aggressive sub-types of thyroid carcinoma, with PDTC and ATC arising from follicular cells and MTC deriving from neuroendocrine parafollicular cells within the thyroid gland.

Defining Advanced Thyroid Cancer

Unlike ATC, which is always defined as advanced thyroid cancer, defining criteria for advanced disease in DTC, PDTC, and MTC, benefiting from both somatic genomic testing and systemic targeted therapies, is both difficult and nuanced.

To aid stratification, criteria have been identified to clinically help define advanced thyroid disease. For simplification, these criteria can be grouped into specific categories, Structural and Surgical, Biochemical, and Histological, Molecular, and Concerning Features [1] (Fig. 23.1).

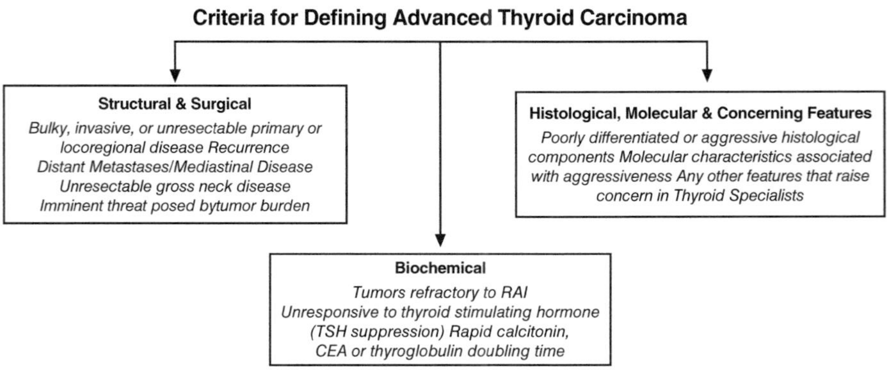

Fig. 23.1 Criteria for defining advanced thyroid cancer

Structural and Surgical

Invasive, Bulky, or Unresectable Primary or Locoregional Disease

Invasive disease and bulky cervical lymphadenopathy confer worse survival and elevated risk of locoregional recurrence, respectively [2, 3].

Where feasible, clinicians must aim to effectively treat locoregional disease with curative approaches prior to considering systemic targeted therapies as their potential efficacy and durability are limited [4, 5].

Given this, "resectability" is a critical factor within this criteria and can be influenced by multiple factors, including (a) the patient's ability to tolerate resection, (b) the surgeon's technical proficiency, (c) the treating team's access to additional subspecialty services (i.e., laryngology, cardiothoracic or reconstructive surgeons, radiation and medical oncology, and speech therapy), and (d) functional deficits associated with ablative surgery and the patient's subsequent quality of life.

These cases benefit from expert surgical or specialist thyroid center involvement optimizing patient outcomes in these complex cases.

The role of neoadjuvant targeted systemic therapies to reduce invasion and tumor bulk prior to surgical ablation is a rapidly evolving area of research and may play a key role in the management of this type of disease in the future [6].

Recurrence

Defined as Type 1, *easily treated* (i.e., with surgical ablation) *or monitored*, or Type 2, *advanced and refractory to treatment*. In this setting, somatic genetic testing should be considered in Type 2 patients, especially given these patients are at increased risk of persistent disease and further recurrence [7].

Distant Metastases/Mediastinal Disease

These types of metastatic disease portend a worse prognosis in DTC [8, 9]; this decrease in OS is exacerbated in the setting of metastatic disease derived from more aggressive PDTC or MTC [10, 11].

Unresectable Gross Residual Neck Disease

Somatic genetic testing is imperative in R2 resection of recurrent locoregional disease, especially when the anatomical or functional impact of additional ablative surgery would compromise quality of life or where medical comorbidities preclude further surgical intervention.

EBRT may afford locoregional control and symptom relief but does not confer either survival or a metastatic control advantage. It can cause additional morbidity and is associated with secondary radiation-induced malignancies, with recommendations against its use in patients <45 years [12]. Targeted systemic therapy represents a superior option over EBRT in these cases.

Imminent Threat Posed by Tumor Burden

Tumors associated with imminent neural, respiratory, or vascular compromise are aggressive and defined as advanced thyroid disease, benefiting from somatic genetic assessment and targeted systemic therapy, especially as a neoadjuvant strategy to reduce tumor burden and enable subsequent surgical ablation.

Biochemical

Tumors Refractory to RAI (RAIR)

RAIR thyroid cancers should be considered for somatic genetic testing and systemic targeted therapy in both DTC and PDTC [13]. DTC is considered RAIR when it (a) fails to concentrate RAI with initial treatment; (b) the tumor loses its previous ability to concentrate RAI; (c) RAI is concentrated in some tissues, but not others (RAI whole body scans vs ^{18}FDG-PET scans); or (d) there is metastatic disease progression in spite of an ability to concentrate RAI [14].

Unresectable and/or metastatic RAIR DTC confers a worse prognosis compared to RAI-sensitive follicular-derived thyroid cancers [15–17]. Prior to targeted systemic therapies, median 5-year disease specific survival rates in RAIR-DTC were 60–70%, while metastatic RAIR-DTC had a very poor prognosis with median 10-year survival of 10% [17, 18].

Tumors Unresponsive to Thyroid Stimulating Hormone (TSH) Suppression

Levothyroxine-mediated TSH suppression is an effective technique for inhibiting DTC cell growth, efficiently controlling disease, especially in the setting of recurrence or metastases [19, 20]. Therefore, disease refractory to TSH suppression less than 0.1mIU/L is a clinical indication for somatic genetic testing and systemic targeted therapy consideration [21].

Rapid Calcitonin, CEA, or Thyroglobulin Doubling Time

If thyroid tumor growth is aggressive and associated with either doubling of structural volume or biochemical markers (calcitonin, CEA or thyroglobulin) in less than a period of 6 months, then both genetic testing and targeted systemic therapy are warranted, given association with disease-specific outcomes, local and distant recurrence, and worse survival [22–25].

Histological, Molecular, and Concern Features

Poorly Differentiated or Aggressive Histological Components

Aggressive variants of PTC, namely, diffuse sclerosing, tall cell, columnar cell, solid, and hobnail, are associated with increased rates of recurrence, metastases, resistance to RAI, and reduced overall survival [26, 27]. Diagnosing these variants is imperative to ensure appropriate surgical and complementary treatment to improve prognosis.

These variants are also commonly associated with specific mutational drivers: diffuse sclerosing (RET/PTC1, RET/PTC3, *BRAF*^{V600E} 50–61%), tall (80–100%

BRAF^{V600E}, 35.8% *RET/PTC3*), columnar (33% *BRAF*^{V600E}) [28], solid (*RET/PTC3*) [29], and hobnail (72% *BRAF*-mutations, 55% *TP53*-mutations, 27.8% PIK3CA, 5% *NOTCH1*-mutations) [30]. In diffuse sclerosing, RET/PTC3 mutation is associated with advanced stage disease at presentation and worse outcomes [31–33].

They can be histologically characterized, especially PDTC and MTC, by increased mitotic activity, tumor necrosis, and elevated Ki67 index. Additionally, PDTC will demonstrate an STI (solid, trabecular, or insular growth pattern) with frequent mutation in *BRAF* (20%), *RAS* (20–40%), and *PIK3CA* (5–10%) [34].

Importantly, even in the presence of these histological features, small tumors confined to the thyroid do not require somatic genetic testing.

Differentiated Thyroid Cancer

Molecular Pathways

Technological advancement in high-throughput DNA sequencing techniques (DNA-seq) or "next-generation sequencing" (NGS) has enabled rapid and parallel assessment of DNA and has dramatically expanded our understanding of molecular pathways associated with thyroid cancer. Additionally, it has played an integral role in characterizing the tumor microenvironment (TME) and improving insight into the dynamic role of the immune system in tumor progression and metastases. Most importantly it has enabled the identification of actionable drivers and the development of targeted systemic therapies.

However, institutional access, cost, and test turnaround time remain rate limiting factors for NGS use. Immunohistochemistry (IHC) and polymerase chain reaction (PCR) provide low-cost, accessible, and rapid assessment of most known actionable drivers.

In the rapidly developing world of expedited, personalized, and minimally invasive diagnosis of malignancy, liquid biopsy represents the latest frontier. Derived from venous peripheral blood samples, liquid biopsy encompasses the analysis of circulating tumor cells (CTCs), circulating tumor DNA (ctDNA), and exosomes. Focusing upon liquid biopsy for driver mutations in thyroid cancer, research has demonstrated that quantifying ctDNA is sensitive and specific for ovarian, colorectal, lung, and breast cancers [35–37]. A single-center study using targeted Taqman PCR found that ctDNA could be utilized for detection of the BRAF^{V600E} mutation in plasma samples for patients with PTC, while also demonstrating that ctDNA levels of this mutation decreased after surgical ablation of the tumor [38].

Consequently, liquid biopsy may soon represent a more sensitive and specific mutational test for DTC.

The following sections will explore the genetic basis of DTC, MTC, and ATC, providing a molecular framework for approaching these tumors.

Papillary Thyroid Carcinoma

Papillary thyroid carcinoma (PTC) accounts for ~80% of all thyroid cancers [39]. Poor clinical prognostic factors include increased age at diagnosis, male gender, advanced stage, and extrathyroidal extension (ETE) [40]. Surgery is the treatment of choice for most presentations, the extent dependent upon the size of the primary thyroid tumor and the presence of locoregional nodal metastasis. RAI is recommended in high-risk cases or those associated with R1 residual disease, which attenuates recurrence and improves survival [41].

The classical variant of PTC (PTCC) is synonymous with mutation of the *RAS/RAF/MEK/ERK* (MAPK) signalling pathway. These mutations include point mutations in *BRAF (45%)* or *RAS* (10%) proto-oncogenes or chromosomal rearrangement of *RET* (20%) and are identified in around 70% of PTCC presentations. The driver mutations tend to be mutually exclusive and rarely overlap in the same tumor [42–45].

Nearly all point mutations in *BRAF* involve valine to glutamate substitution at residue 600 (V600E) [46, 47]. This mutation leads to constitutional activation of *BRAF* kinase, where V600E substitution disrupts the hydrophobic interactions of the dephosphorylated wild-type protein in its inactive conformation, promoting interactions that maintain the protein in a catalytically competent conformation, promoting continuous phosphorylation of the downstream kinase *MEK* [48].

In contrast to PTCC, follicular variant PTC (PTCFV) is predominately characterized by *RAS*- mutation and less frequently by $BRAF^{V600E}$ (23%). PTCFV is also associated with mutation in *TERT* (30%) and *ATM* (7%) and is associated with copy number variations (CNVs) [49].

The $BRAF^{V600E}$ mutation has also been observed in aggressive histological subtypes of PTC, specifically within 80–100% of TCV, 33% of CCV, and 25.3–57.1% of HV [27, 28, 50–52]. It is highly associated with specific aggressive tumor characteristics, including recurrence, advanced stage at presentation, ETE, and locoregional or distant metastases [53–55]. Notably, $BRAF^{V600E}$ mutation is also an independent predictor of recurrence in early-stage PTC [55, 56], confers resistance to ionizing radiation in preclinical models [57], and may also reduce tumor sensitivity to RAI [58].

Additionally, DNA-seq genetic profiling of more aggressive PTC cases identified mutations in *BRAF* (89%); the *PI3K/AKT/mTOR* (PAM) signalling pathway; tumor suppressor genes *ZFHX3*, *TP53*, and *CHEK2*; as well as *WNT*, epigenetic pathways, and *TERT-promoter* [59]. These mutations were associated with unfavorable clinical outcomes [59].

Both PTCC and PTCFV are usually associated with both low tumor mutational burden (TMB) and low PD-L1 expression [60, 61]. A recent study identified PD-L1 expression in 28.5% of PTCC cases and 0% of PTCFV cases [62], which suggests a potentially poor response to PD-1/PD-L1 axis immune checkpoint blockade therapy.

The given *BRAF* mutations and *RTK* gene rearrangements (including *RET* and *NTRK1/3* fusion products) are well characterized and actionable oncogenic drivers that are important when considering targeted systemic therapy in advanced DTC [63–65].

Follicular Thyroid Carcinoma

The second most common DTC histological type is follicular thyroid carcinoma (FTC) [66]. Reported in 10–56.9% of FTC [67, 68], *RAS* mutations are the most prevalent oncogenetic driver mutation, conferring worse survival and increased risk of distant metastasis [69–71]. *NRAS* is the most common, and the majority of *NRAS*/*HRAS* mutations are associated with codon 61, while *KRAS* mutations are associated with codons 12 and 13. Novel mutations aside from *RAS* include *EIF1AX*, *DICER1*, and *EZH1* [72].

PAX8/*PPARγ* rearrangements occur in ~30–35% of FTCs [73–75], the rearrangement producing a *PAX8*/*PPARγ* fusion oncoprotein that inhibits endogenous *PPARγ* activity [76]. Importantly, *PAX8*/*PPARγ* rearrangements have not been reported to worsen prognosis and are mutually exclusive from *RAS* mutations [77].

Additional chromosomal rearrangements involving *PPARγ* include fusion with *CREB3L2* [78]. *PI3K*/*AKT* pathway activation is also common in FTCs [79–81].

TERT-promoter mutations have been reported in ~15% of FTCs [60, 72, 82]. The prognostic influence of *TERT-promoter* mutations, especially C250T and C228T substitutions, can be attributed to the creation of de novo binding sites for transcription factors capable of enabling gene transcriptional activity and promoting telomerase activation [83]. *TERT-promoter* mutations are more common in older patients and associated with larger tumors and distant metastasis [84]. Studies have reported specific ultrasound characteristics associated with *TERT-promoter* mutations. Microlobulated margins and punctate echogenic foci were independent risk factors, while they were categorized more frequently as “highly suspicious” by the K-TIRADS and ACR-TIRADS scoring systems [85]. DNA copy number alterations and loss of heterozygosity are also attributed to playing a role in tumorigenesis in FTC.

TERT-promotor mutation, with TERT gene upregulation, encodes the telomerase catalytic subunit- maintaining telomere length and facilitates continuous replication of tumor cells [86].

PD-L1 is highly expressed in a subset of advanced DTC and is associated with greater recurrence risk and reduced DFS [87, 88]. Expressed in ~59.7% of FTC, its expression correlates with worse clinical and histological prognostic markers, specifically tumor size, multifocality, ETE, vascular invasion, and postoperative recurrence. PD-L1 expression is not correlated with lymph node or distant metastases.

Claudin-1 expression is also upregulated in FTC. Both PD-L1 and Claudin-1 have been identified to be highly expressed and associated with tumor aggressiveness in FTC. Claudin-1 is a key component of tight junctions between cells, and its overexpression is often associated with increased tumor aggressiveness, likely to play an integral role in tumor cell invasion, migration, and metastasis.

Diagnostically, FTC remains a challenge with FNA being insufficient for preoperative diagnosis, as it is morphologically impossible to distinguish FTC from benign follicular thyroid adenoma. Unfortunately, reports investigating the efficacy of liquid biopsy in FTC have not been as positive as those for PTC. A recent pilot study of 13 patients with diagnosed FTC found that peripheral blood contained low DNA yield and suboptimal material acquisition, failing to support this diagnostic technique in FTC [89].

Systemic Therapy

Given the high prevalence of $BRAF^{V600E}$ mutation in RAIR-DTC, the optimal sequence to utilize systemic therapy options arises commonly in the clinical environment. While lenvatinib is commonly commenced, there is also a trend to commencing *BRAF*-targeted therapies for specificity and reduced off-target side effects in $BRAF^{V600E}$ RAIR-PTC.

$BRAF^{V600E}$

MKIs

In DTC, the MKIs sorafenib (DECISION Trial) and lenvatinib (SELECT Trial) achieved FDA approval after improving PFS by 10–18.3 months, results which have been reflected in clinical practice [13, 90–92]. In both cases, the clinical anti-tumor activities do not correlate with the presence of specific mutations; therefore molecular testing does not predict clinical response [93]. As they are both MKIs, they both target multiple pathways, including *PDGF*, *RET*, *VEGFR*, and *MET/AXL*. Lenvatinib has mostly superseded sorafenib in the clinic [13], as it demonstrated improved PFS when compared to placebo (placebo vs sorafenib, 5.8 vs 10.8 months, placebo vs lenvatinib, 3.6 vs 18.3 months) and ORR (sorafenib, 12.2%; lenvatinib, 65%), although lenvatinib has been associated with greater adverse events [90]. Importantly, benefit in overall survival has not been clearly confirmed, potentially because patients who received placebo were permitted to cross-over to lenvatinib upon disease progression.

The FDA has approved a single agent as a second-line therapy in RAIR-DTC. The MKI cabozantinib (COSMIC-111 Trial, NCT03690388) has an ORR of 11% and mPFS of 11 months in patients already exposed to sorafenib and/or lenvatinib [94]. Adverse events associated with MKIs are not negligible and can include arterial hypertension, mucositis, skin lesions, and metabolic alterations [95–97].

In a randomized, double blind, placebo-controlled, phase III trial, patients aged over 16 were randomly assigned (2:1) to PO cabozantinib (60 mg OD) or matched placebo, stratified by previous lenvatinib treatment and age. CABO60 (n = 125) significantly improved PFS over placebo (n = 62), median not reached versus 1.9 months. Grade 3 or 4 AE occurred in 57% of patients. Serious treatment related AEs in 16% of patients. There were no treatment-related deaths. FDA approval was subsequently provided in 2021.

A recent systematic review and network meta-analysis investigating the efficacy and safety of MKIs for patients with refractory thyroid cancer (including RAIR-DTC) as well as advanced MTC identified that cabozantinib (60 mg/day) was superior when compared to lenvatinib (18–24 mg/day) and apatinib, for PFS in RAIR DTC. Overall survival also improves with increased dose of cabozantinib, lenvatinib, anlotinib, and sorafenib in RAIR-DTC. However, when compared with low-dose MKIs, higher doses exacerbate the incidence of adverse events [98].

Additionally, pazopanib, a new MKI targeting VEGFR 1–3, PDGFR a/b, FGFR, and c-Kit [99], has demonstrated 6-, 12-, and 18-month PFS of 55, 22, and 11%, respectively, after previous lenvatinib therapy, in 9 patients on retrospective analysis [100]. While it is FDA approved in advanced renal cell carcinoma and soft tissue sarcoma [101], it is not yet approved in thyroid carcinoma despite positive outcomes identified in a recent systematic review [102].

Second-generation competitive RAF kinase inhibitors that have specificity for $BRAF^{V600E}$ (i.e., dabrafenib and vemurafenib) have been studied in PTC [103]. Dabrafenib is a reversible and potent ATP competitive inhibitor of $BRAF^{V600E}$ activity and $BRAF^{V600K}$-mutated monomers [104], and there is now evidence that these molecules can restore sensitivity to RAI in RAIR-PTC, by extension facilitating thyroid-specific gene expression mediating iodine metabolism and active transport of iodine into thyrocytes [105, 106], a phenomenon known as re-differentiation. The addition of a histone deacetylase (vorinostat), which mediates histone deacetylation at the sodium/iodide symporter promoter, synergistically increased RAI uptake in preclinical studies, an affect further enhanced in the presence of TSH [107].

Interestingly the MKIs sorafenib and lenvatinib are not associated with elevated iodine avidity, which may be attributed to their receptor skew with their greater affinity toward VEGFR and PDGFR.

Of ten BRAF mutant patients, four patients demonstrated increased uptake in 124I, and subsequent treatment with 131I resulted in tumor regression at 6 months, with subsequent tumor biopsy assessment associated with increased thyroid gene expression and RAI uptake. Vemurafenib restores RAI uptake and efficacy in a subset of BRAF mutant PAIR patients, probably by upregulating thyroid-specific gene expression via MAPK pathway inhibition. Higher baseline thyroglobulin values among responders suggest that tumor differentiation status may be a predictor of vemurafenib benefit.

An additional potential benefit of this approach is data demonstrating that MAPK inhibition sensitizes $BRAF^{V600E}$ and *RAS* mutated thyroid cancer cells to radiation-induced DNA damage [108].

The BRAF-inhibitor vemurafenib sensitizes $BRAF^{V600E}$ thyroid cancer cells to radiation therapy in preclinical studies by inhibiting nonhomologous end-joining repair activity in these cancer cells, compromising their ability to repair DNA double strand breaks [57].

Importantly, although MKIs have demonstrated clinical efficacy despite mutational status, it is imperative to identify additional potentially actionable mutations to help guide optimal personalized therapeutic strategy in RAIR-DTC. These include RET and NTRK fusions.

Combination Targeted Therapy

A proportion of clinicians have moved toward combination targeted therapy, FDA-approved dabrafenib/trametinib (DT), for $BRAF^{V600E}$ mutated tumors based on efficacy demonstrated by ROAR and NCI-MATCH studies [109, 110]. These drugs work on the MAPK pathway. DT has demonstrated a response rate of 50–54% in patients with advanced BRAF-mutated PTC. Up to 44% of PTC patients have a BRAF mutation that can be specifically targeted. The challenge lies in the paucity of randomized trial data comparing BRAF targeted therapy to MKIs in RAIR-DTC. Dabrafenib/trametinib can be used in PTC that has a BRAF mutation. Interestingly, dabrafenib alone had similar efficacy to combination dabrafenib/trametinib in this trial.

When comparing non-generalizable trials, lenvatinib demonstrated an ORR of 65% in the SELECT Trial, while combination dabrafenib/trametinib was 30% [111]. Additionally, lenvatinib mPFS was 18.3 months, while combination dabrafenib/trametinib was 10–15 months.

A significant benefit of targeted therapy over MKI though is the attenuated adverse event profile. In the SELECT Trial, 76% of patients experienced greater than or equal to Grade 3 treatment-related AEs, when compared to 48–58% with dabrafenib and trametinib, respectively, although fewer people discontinued lenvatinib compared to combination dabrafenib/trametinib (14% vs ~20%) [90, 111].

NTRK Fusions

The NTRK family of genes (NTRK 1–3) code for receptors TRK-A-C, respectively. These receptors have intracellular kinase domains, transmembrane, and extracellular ligand binding. Fusions result from chromosomal rearrangements between the c-terminal domain of NTRK1, NTRK2, or NTRK3 and the 5′ region of a partner gene. These rearrangements act as oncogenic drivers for diverse cancer types, resulting in the uncontrolled ligand-independent activation of the TRK pathway [112–114]. The frequency of NTRK in thyroid cancer is 17.2% of all patients with thyroid cancer [115].

From 2019, the FDA has approved two agents for the treatment of NTRK fusion-positive cancer. Larotrectinib (Vitrakvi) was approved in 2018. It competitively blocks the ATP-binding site of the intracellular kinase domain of the TRK receptors, mitigating aberrant signaling and tumor regression [116, 117]. Its benefit has been identified in thyroid carcinoma. Additionally, entrectinib (Rozlytrek) was approved in 2019 for pediatric patients (>12 years) and adults with solid tumors that have a NTRK gene fusion. It has primary activity against TRKA-C, ROS1, and ALK [118, 119]. It has also shown benefit in thyroid cancer [120]. The second-generation TRK-inhibitor repotrectinib has also received accelerated FDA approval (2024) for the management of patients with NTRK fusions.

An analysis of patients treated with larotrectinib in 3 clinical trials ((a) phase II "basket" trial (NAVIGATE, NCT02576431), (b) a phase 1 trial in adults with advanced solid tumors (NCT02122913), and a phase I/II trial (SCOUT) in pediatric patients with advanced solid or primary CNS tumors (NCT026376687)) identified 21 eligible patients with either PTC (19) or FTC (2), demonstrating an ORR of 85%. Among patients with previous exposure to systemic therapy, the ORR was 92%, and mPFS at 12 months was 100% and 84% at 24 months [121].

TERT-Promoter

There are currently no FDA-approved targeted therapies specifically designed to directly target *TERT-promoter* mutations in FTC. Directly targeting the *TERT-promoter* is challenging due to the complex regulatory mechanisms involved in its transcription and the need for highly specific inhibitors to avoid disrupting normal telomerase activity in healthy cells. Potential therapeutic approaches include gene therapy and small molecule inhibitors. To date, most research on targeting TERT promoter mutations for FTC is in preclinical phase.

Immunotherapy

Immunotherapy alone has not been an effective therapeutic approach in clinical trials to date. NCT03246958, a non-randomized phase II clinical trial in RAIR-DTC, investigated combination PD-L1 and CTLA-4 (nivolumab/ipilimumab) immune checkpoint blockade in 49 patients. The study demonstrated an ORR of 9.4%, failed to meet its clinical end-points, and did not support further investigation in this patient population [122].

When combination lenvatinib with pembrolizumab (anti-PD-L1) was utilized in MKI naïve RAIR-DTC, the investigators identified an ORR of 65.5% (similar to lenvatinib alone), with a mPFS of 26.8% (Phase II, NCT02973997, $n = 30$). In the second cohort ("progressed on lenvatinib"), combination lenvatinib/pembrolizumab (patients continued on the lenvatinib dose they were receiving when tumor progression was noted), ORR was 16%, mPFS was 10 months, and 12-month OS was 76%. Ultimately, the study investigators noted that combination lenvatinib/pembrolizumab may increase durability in lenvatinib naïve patients over lenvatinib monotherapy alone [123]. Importantly, 19 (63.3%) of cohort 1 were classical PTC, 0% were FVPTC, 3 (10%) were FTC, 4 (13.3%) were oncocytic carcinoma, and 4 (13.3%) were PDTC. Twelve (48%) of cohort 2 were classical PTC, 2 (8.0%) were FVPTC, 1 (4%) was FTC, 6 (24%) were oncocytic carcinoma, and 4 (16%) were PDTC. PD-L1 expression (greater than or equal to 50%) was seen in 8/22 (36.4%) of tumors in cohort 1 and 6/19 (31.6%) of tumors in cohort 2. PD-L1 was not associated with PRS in either cohort [123] (Fig. 23.2).

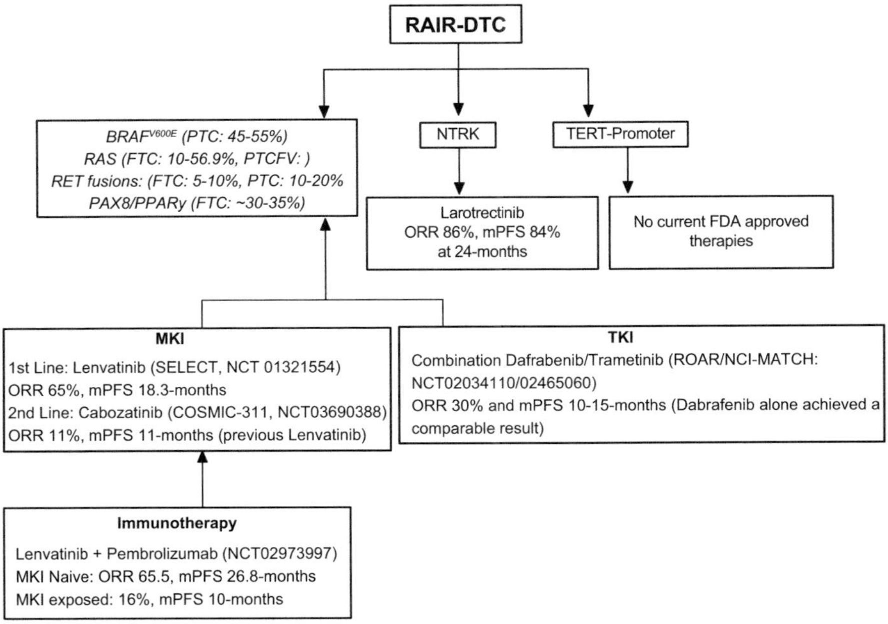

Fig. 23.2 *DTC therapeutic matrix*: Differentiated thyroid carcinoma refractory to radioactive iodine is defined as advanced thyroid carcinoma and represents a therapeutic challenge requiring systemic therapy. While the predominate molecular mutations for PTC and FTC are $BRAF^{V600E}$ and RAS, respectively, therapeutic strategy centers around either primary MKI or TKI. Immunotherapy provides marginal benefit to mPFS and in previously exposed patients. Although uncommon, NTRK mutations can be effectively treated with larotrectinib. There are currently no current FDA-approved therapies for TERT-promoter mutations

Medullary Thyroid Carcinoma

Introduction and Molecular Pathways

With an increasing incidence [124], especially in older patients [125, 126], medullary thyroid carcinoma (MTC) arises from neuroendocrine parafollicular c-cells and constitutes 2–5% of thyroid malignancies and confers a mortality risk of 8–13% [127, 128].

A total of 75–80% of MTC presentations are sporadic (sMTC), with 40–60% caused by somatic *RET* alterations, 80% being associated to Met918Thr (M918T), and 15% with a codon 634 mutation, both of which are more aggressive and confer a worse prognosis [129–131]. Consanguinity resulting in homozygous RET mutations is also linked to advanced presentations and early age of diagnosis [132]. Non-RET sMTC have demonstrated mutations in *RAS* (*HRAS*/*KRAS*), *BRAF*, *SF3B1*, and *NF1* [133–135]. A genetic mutation driver is yet to be identified in ~20% sMTC cases lacking either *RET* or *RAS* mutations (which are mutually exclusive).

With phenotypic variability and age-linked penetrance, 20–25% of MTC presentations are hereditary (hMTC) and linked to an autosomal dominant germline mutation in the *RET* proto-oncogene. This hereditary genotype is associated with the MEN2 phenotype, specifically MEN2A, MEN2B, and FMTC (considered to be a sub-type of MEN2A). Almost 100% of patients with this genotype will develop *h*MTC [136, 137], which is also more commonly associated with multifocal, bilateral, and younger age at diagnosis [138]. MEN2A is most frequently associated with a codon 634 mutation (exon 11) and less commonly in one of codons 609, 611, 618, and 620 (exon 10) and 630 (exon 11). It is recommended that MEN2A patients consider prophylactic thyroidectomy between the ages of 5–15 years, while MEN2B patients, nearly all of whom carry a M918T mutation on exon 16 (~95%), consider this surgery within the initial 12 months of life.

Therefore, advanced MTC is synonymous with mutation in the *RET* proto-oncogene. A total of 95–98% of *h*MTC and 91.4% of advanced and progressive sMTC demonstrate a *RET* mutation [139]. The American Thyroid Association (ATA) stratifies specific germline RET alterations into risk categories associated with disease aggressiveness. The "Highest" risk category specifically contains the MET918Thr (M918T) *RET* mutation and MEN2B [140].

The *RET*-gene (chromosome 10q11.21), encoding for a single-pass transmembrane glycoprotein receptor tyrosine kinase, is a proto-oncogene that has the capacity to become constitutively activated with mutation in either its structural elements resulting in fusion with a 5′-upstream partner or its cysteine-rich kinase domains, affording ligand-independent signalling and oncogenesis [141]. RET-kinase is key for cell growth, migration, proliferation, differentiation, and survival [142]. Embryonic development of the human enteric nervous system, central nervous system, and genitourinary tract is dependent upon RET [143, 144]. Specifically, codon mutations seen in MEN2A affect the extracellular domain of the RET TKR, which are involved in conformational stability and kinase activity via intramolecular disulfide bridges. These mutations result in covalent dimerization of RET, precipitating ligand-independent kinase activation [145–147]. Comparatively, M918T mutation increases the ATP bonding affinity to RET monomers with resultant autophosphorylation without the need of dimerization [148].

Recently, a proportion of MTCs have been demonstrated to overexpress the Notch signalling ligand Delta-like ligand 3 (DLL3), which confers worse DFS and OS. Desmoplastic MTCs are more likely to over-express DLL3. Consequently, DLL3 may also aid in risk stratification as a predictor of aggressive disease and worse clinical outcomes [149]. Several therapies targeting DLL3 are, or have been, in clinical trial in other neuroendocrine cancers (viz., small cell lung cancer (SLSC)) with limited success and significant off-target adverse reactions to date [150].

MTC expresses somatostatin receptors. Somatostatin analogs have been utilized in an attempt to modify disease progression. Results have not demonstrated disease control or significant reduction in tumor or tumor markers [151].

All newly diagnosed hMTC patients should be tested for germline RET mutations and receive genetic counselling, while sMTC patients with advanced stage disease should be offered somatic RET mutation testing, especially given the potential benefit of targeted therapies on tumor volume with neoadjuvant regimes enabling surgery in previously unresectable disease [152, 153].

Molecular Testing

If a germline RET mutation is identified, genetic testing of family members, commencing with first-degree relatives, is recommended. This is imperative to identify carriers that would benefit from prophylactic thyroidectomy prior to the development of MTC where possible [154].

DNA-seq can be utilized to test the entire *RET* gene or alternative focus upon regions of common mutations, namely, exons 10, 11, 13, 14, 15, and 16, noting that FMTC is usually associated with *RET* point mutations in exons 13 (codons 768, 790, and 791) and 14 (codons 804 and 844) [155].

Liquid Biopsy

Currently, there is a paucity of evidence to support liquid biopsy in the diagnosis or surveillance of MTC. In a recent study, peripheral ctDNA sampling identified less than half of the tumor confirmed RET M918T mutation cases (32%); however they did identify that detection of RET M918T ctDNA correlated with worse OS and more effectively identified worse prognostic outcomes than calcitonin doubling time [156], which may suggest a test-based threshold issue which may be overcome with improved diagnostic test sensitivity.

Systemic Therapy

Multikinase Inhibitors (MKIs)

Several MKIs are FDA approved for MTC, specifically cabozantinib (Cometriq), lenvatinib (Lenvima), and vandetanib (Caprelsa).

Phase III clinical trials, ZETA (NCT00410761, vandetanib) and EXAM (NCT0070430, cabozantinib), drove approval for treatment of locally recurrent or metastatic MTC, regardless of tumor genotype. Placebo compared cabozantinib increased median PFS by 7.2 months (ORR 28%) and vandetanib by 11.2 months (ORR 45%). When specifically stratified for M918T mutation, both conferred an advantage in PFS. Although cabozantinib improved mOS by 5.5 months, this failed to achieve statistical significance, while vandetanib mOS was not achieved secondary to placebo to active treatment cross-over confounding [157, 158].

Unfortunately, their clinical efficacy is limited by their specificity to RET, as these MKIs were designed to target alternate TKRs, namely, EGFR, MET, ALK, and VEGFR2 with significantly attenuated homology for RET-kinase. Primarily inhibitors of angiogenesis, vandetanib, lenvatinib, and cabozantinib, have the greatest specificity for VEGFR2 [159, 160]. High doses of these MKIs are subsequently required to overcome inferior pharmacokinetics; however this leads to increased drug-associated adverse events driven by suppression of VEGFR2, specifically hemorrhage, thrombosis, and compromise wound healing. This often leads to dose reduction or discontinuation, further compromising clinical efficacy [161].

Specific RET mutations also confer resistance to MKI therapy. V804L and V804M ($RET^{V804M/L}$) alter valine residues at the RET gatekeeper site, conferring steric hindrance to these three MKIs [162, 163].

RET-Specific Kinase Inhibitors (*R*sKIs)

High-affinity RET-tyrosine kinase inhibitors were a paradigm shift in treatment for advanced stage RET-variant MTC, overcoming gatekeeper mutations, decreasing drug-associated adverse events, and improving clinical outcomes.

Pralsetinib (Gavreto) was granted accelerated approval by the FDA in 2020, after preliminary results of the ARROW Phase I/II Clinical Trial (NCT03037385) for MKI naïve advanced or metastatic RET mutant MTC, and demonstrated an ORR of 65% (M918T, 61%; C634X, 28%; V804, 4%). Even in participants previously treated with MKI, ORR was 60%, regardless of gatekeeper mutations. Pralsetinib was well tolerated with few drug-associated adverse events [164]. Disappointingly, pralsetinib has been removed from the US market after issues with its Phase III Clinical Trial (AcceleRET-MTC, NCT 04760288).

During 2024, selpercatinib (Retevmo) received traditional approval for RET mutation associated advanced or metastatic MTC in patients aged ≥2. LIBRETTO-531(NCT04211337) was a Phase III PFS and OS superiority trial comparing selpercatinib to either cabozantinib or vandetanib in treatment naïve patients with progressive RET-mutant MTC ($n = 291$, M918T mutation equally distributed between groups). Comparison of PFS was not feasible as there was a paucity of disease progression in participants receiving selpercatinib at the interim endpoint. In contrast the MKIs attained a PFS of 16.8 months. Selpercatinib achieved a higher treatment response rate (69% vs 39%), with 12% of participants demonstrating complete response. OS estimates at 18 months for selpercatinib and control groups were 95.5% and 92.8%, respectively [165].

Interestingly, a neoadjuvant phase II clinical trial (NCT04759911) is recruiting to investigate the benefit of selpercatinib prior to ablative surgery in RET-mutant thyroid cancer after several case reports identified significant tumor reduction with this neoadjuvant strategy, subsequently enabling surgical resection of previously unresectable disease [166, 167].

Resistance remains a significant issue, compromising systemic targeted therapy efficacy and durability. *RET* mutation resistance mechanisms can be defined as either *on-target* (within the kinase domain) or *off-target* or bypass alterations [168].

On-Target

Steric inhibition of MKI binding can occur when the kinase gatekeeper limits access to the ATP binding pocket. In MTCs expressing a *RET* pVal804Met mutation, this type of resistance is well described for vandetinib. In this mutation there is replacement of valine 804 with longer hydrophobic side chain amino acids compromising vandetinib binding [169].

To overcome gatekeeper mutations like *RETp.VAL804M/L*, selective RET inhibitors like prasetinib and selpercatinib were developed. Unfortunately, prolonged exposure to both these agents has been reported to result in additional mutations, namely, solvent front (*p.PLY810*) or hinge region (*p.Tyr806*), that attenuate their efficacy in a proportion of patients [169].

Off-Target or Bypass Alterations

Long-term MKI use can result in the emergence of alternate oncogenic drivers, even though the primary oncogenic drivers are suppressed, known as "off-target" or "bypass alterations." Following selpercatinib and pralsetinib use, *MET* and *KRAS* amplifications have been identified in *RET*-driven NSCLC [170].

Resistance, durability, and variant RET mutations remain a challenge in the treatment of advanced or progressive MTC. The search for more effective "next-generation" RET inhibitors for RET-driven cancers continues.

Immune Checkpoint Inhibitors (ICIs)

RET mutation MTC tumors are commonly "cold," with low PD-L1 expression [171–173]. However, its expression has been associated with aggressive metastatic MTC disease and incurable recurrence [174]. An important cause of resistance to immunotherapy is "cold tumors" with an attenuated "tumor mutational burden (TMB)." This phenotype is characterized by a paucity of tumor microenvironment (TME) T cell infiltration and immune response [175]. A Phase II Clinical Trial evaluated nivolumab in combination with ipilimumab in patients with aggressive thyroid cancer (NCT03246958). Specifically seven patients with progressive MTC with previous TKI failure failed to demonstrate even a partial response [176]. In an additional Phase II Clinical Trial (NCT 03072160, pembrolizumab in advanced or metastatic MTC in whom surgery was not a curative option, ($n = 13$)), no enrolled patients achieved clinical response (defined as a 50% decrease in calcitonin levels) or imaging response (greater than or equal to 30% decrease in the sum of the largest diameter) [177] (Fig. 23.3).

Prognostication and management of medullary thyroid carcinoma (MTC) can be defined by mutational expression, with modifications [152].

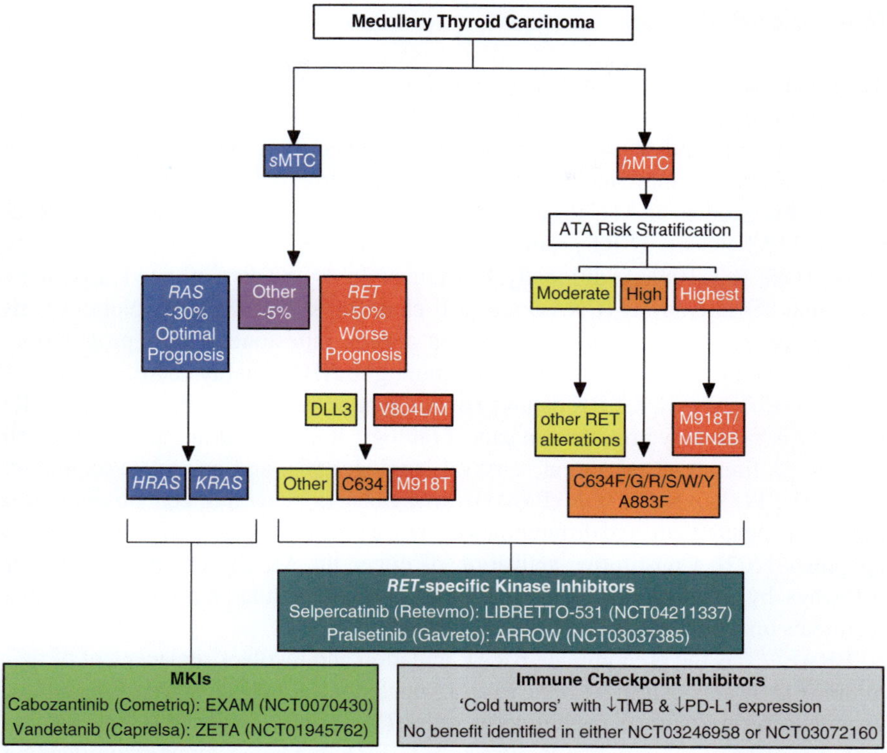

Fig. 23.3 MTC mutation risk stratification and associated kinase inhibitor therapies

Anaplastic Thyroid Carcinoma

ATC is a rare and aggressive cancer, acknowledged to represent the final stage of dedifferentiation from DTC [178, 179].

Accounting for 1–2% of all thyroid cancers [180], it has both a historical median OS of 5 months and 1-year OS of <20% [181, 182] and represents 14–50% of all thyroid mortality [183].

ATC is characterized by rapid locoregional invasion and early distant metastases, typically in patients approaching their seventh decade [184], with an age exceeding 70 years associated with worse prognosis [185].

Given its poor prognosis, any ATC is at least AJCC stage IV, with intrathyroidal disease classified as IVA, extrathyroidal extension or cervical lymph node metastases being classified as IVB, and IVC being associated with distant metastases [186].

Additionally, its diagnosis can be challenging, and expediting review by specialty services has been shown to improve survival [187].

Over the past decade, longer mOS has been achieved utilizing multimodal treatment regimens. These new strategies, especially targeted molecular therapy, have dramatically changed treatment paradigms and resultant outcomes [188–191].

Molecular Pathways

The mutational landscape of ATC is complex, demonstrating considerable interpatient tumor diversity, with mutations in multiple proto-oncogenes and tumor suppressors [179], and it is now generally accepted that ATC arises from the dedifferentiation of more indolent DTCs, secondary to extensive genomic alteration.

Genomic studies of ATC tissue have identified mutations in BRAF (45%), RAS (24%), TP53 (63%), TERT-promoter (75%), and within the PI3K/AKT pathway (18%) [188, 192–198]. Additionally, DNA aneuploidy and disseminated large-scale copy number alterations (CNAs) are also characteristic [198, 199]. Notably, this gain in aneuploidy represents a significant genetic milestone in ATC progression, with the given genome-wide CNAs contributing to ATC lethality [200].

The RAS/RAF/MEK/ERK pathway or mitogen-activated protein kinase (MAPK) pathway is extremely important in cancer biology. It is integral in regulation of cell growth, proliferation, migration, survival, angiogenesis, and cell cycle regulation [201]. The PI3K/AKT/mTOR (PAM) pathway is also integral to cell survival, proliferation, metabolism, and differentiation, with a primary function to protect against apoptosis [202]. Constitutive activation of either the MAPK or PAM molecular pathways by mutations in upstream kinases forces cellular reprogramming that facilitates uncontrolled growth.

$BRAF^{V600E}$ is the predominate BRAF mutation and involves replacement of thymidine (T) by adenosine (A) at the exon 15 nucleotide 1799 (T1799A) of the BRAF gene, which results in a substitution of valine (V) for glutamic acid (G) at position 600. The $BRAF^{V600E}$ mutation is refractory to ERK-mediated suppression, leading to unregulated MAPK signalling.

RAS mutations are less frequent; however, unlike $BRAF^{V600E}$, they can activate both MAPK and PI3K/Akt pathways. Upstream of RAF, RAS is a small G-protein, consisting of four GTPase isoforms (*KRAS4a, KRAS4b, HRAS, and NRAS: KRAS being the most frequent tumor driver*) that will bind to the intracellular section of the receptor tyrosine kinase ligand upon growth factor binding, subsequently activating downstream pathways via the RAF serine/threonine kinase [203].

$BRAF^{V600E}$ is the most common and actionable oncogenic driver in ATC. It confers optimal mOS (24 months), while RAS mutations carry a 2.5-fold greater risk of death and a mOS of 6 months [204]. The recognition that tumors can be phenotypically different has improved clinical awareness toward recurrence [205] and survival [206] and helped guide the development of targeted molecular therapies.

Tumor Microenvironment (TME)

NGS appraisal of the TME identified several distinct changes associated with ATC. Tumor-associated macrophages (TAMs) underwent phenotype switching from the anti-tumorigenic M1 to pro-tumorigenic M2 phenotype [207]. M2 phenotype TAMs can suppress T cell activity, promoting tumor progression, angiogenesis, invasion, motility, extracellular matrix remodeling, and metastasis [208, 209]. Cancer-associated fibroblasts (CAFs) differentiated to an inflammatory sub-type that supports tumor metabolism [210–212], progression, and metastasis [210, 213]. Generalized T cell exhaustion was noted, and RAS mutations were associated with aggressive TME phenotype change [200].

The ATC TME is characterized by T cell exhaustion. In keeping with this, there is significant upregulation of tumor PD-L1 expression, with 47–73.2% of ATCs demonstrating staining (TPS $\geq$ 1%) for this checkpoint ligand, with mTPS being 36% [214–217]. A TPS >50% was identified in 30.7–60% of cases. Interestingly, PD-L1 expression is strongly correlated with $BRAF^{V600E}$ mutation [218], with research demonstrating $BRAF^{V600E}$ activates signalling pathways that promote tumor cell PD-L1 expression [219].

Strong correlation between ATC and PD-L1 expression supports a role for ICI therapy targeting the PD-1/PD-L1 axis [220].

Molecular Testing

Given its rapid aggressive growth pattern and resistance to RAI, radiotherapy, and chemotherapy, upon diagnosis, comprehensive and expedited somatic mutational testing is imperative, aiding identification of potentially actionable tumor drivers. In addition, quantification of tumor tissue PD-L1 expression should be completed to determine the additional benefit of immune checkpoint blockade.

Time is always a rate-limiting step in the mutational testing of ATC. The median "turn-around" time for tissue-based DNA-seq was 21 days (range, 11–63 days) [221], potentially exacerbated by specialty services that may be required to acquire tissue samples. An expediated option is DNA-seq assessment of peripheral blood ctDNA (liquid biopsy). This technique provides a result in 11 days (range, 5–16), with a recent systematic review of this technique for $BRAF^{V600E}$ mutation identifying a sensitivity and specificity of 70–88.2% and 100%, respectively, with a tissue concordance of 83.7–92.9% [221]. A recent study demonstrated its effectiveness in identifying common somatic gene mutations in ATC. This approach may reduce biopsy geographical error and will support early implementation of appropriate therapeutic strategies. $BRAF^{V600E}$ immunohistochemistry can also expedite diagnosis; however this requires core biopsy, FNA cell block, or surgical specimens and may again be limited by access to specialty services and associated delays. However, a recent systematic review reported a sensitivity and specificity of 78.9% and 69.7%, respectively, for detecting $BRAF^{V600E}$ in ATC [222], and institutions have reported $BRAF^{V600E}$ results within 24 hours of the first hematoxylin and eosin slide being prepared [223], therefore providing a rapid turnaround time for this technique. TMB and PD-L1 tissue expression should also be completed. The ongoing discovery of new mutational drivers and the potential promise of matched targeted therapies support the benefit of comprehensive genomic profiling of all ATCs with DNA-seq.

Systemic Therapy

In patients with unresectable stage IVB disease, combination EBRT with radiosensitizing chemotherapy has previously been the standard of care. This treatment paradigm has changed with therapies targeting BRAF^{V600E} ATC mutation. Neoadjuvant BRAF-directed therapy, followed by surgical resection, with/without radiation can be an alternative considered to primary radiation in stage IVB or IVC disease. When an actionable mutational driver is absent in the setting of unresectable or stage IVC disease, palliative radiotherapy in conjunction with adjuvant systemic therapy is recommended. Genotoxic chemotherapy, including paclitaxel, docetaxel, carboplatin, and doxorubicin, although recommended by guidelines is largely ineffective. Paclitaxel is most effective; however, resistance is frequent and has been attributed to paracrine signalling in TAMs promoting tumor progression [224]. They can be considered as bridging therapy until the results of molecular testing return. In ATC, multikinase inhibitors (MKIs) and immune checkpoint inhibitors (ICIs) demonstrate promise [225, 226] and are recommended in patients with actionable target mutations.

Single agent MKIs do not confer a survival advantage in ATC. Lenvatinib failed to achieve a minimum threshold ORR of 15%, without improvement in mPFS or mOS in a ceased phase II clinical trial [227]. Additionally, lenvatinib is a potent inhibitor of VEGFRs 1–3, FGFR 1–4, PDGFR-a, RET, and KIT [228–230], and care should be applied with its use after reports of fistula formation and hemorrhage [231].

Although beneficial in preclinical models of ATC, sorafenib and pazopanib failed to improve either mPFS or mOS in phase II clinical trials [232, 233].

In contrast, combination *BRAF* and *MEK* inhibition with dabrafenib and trametinib, respectively, was more effective. Outcomes from the Phase II ROAR clinical trial (NCT02034110) informed FDA approval for BRAF^{V600E} mutant ATC in 2018, with results from the 36-participant trial demonstrating an ORR of 56%, including 3 complete responses. Compared to historical survival (mOS 5 months), mOS improved to 14 months, with a PFS of 6.7 months and 31.5% of patients were alive at 2 years [234].

Dabrafenib selectively inhibits mutated BRAF kinase, while trametinib provides reversible, highly specific, allosteric inhibition of MEK 1 and MEK 2 kinase activity [235]. Lenvatinib and anlotinib have also been approved for ATC [236].

The FDA approved the anti-PD-1/PD-L1 ICI pembrolizumab in 2017 for ATC cases associated with unresectable or metastatic microsatellite instability-high (MSI-H) or mismatch repair deficient (dMMR) solid tumors [237], extending this approval to unresectable or metastatic sold tumors of any tissue type expressing high tumor mutational burden (TMB).

Larger cohort studies have subsequently investigated the benefit of ICI monotherapy in ATC. One single institution study tested either pembrolizumab or nivolumab in 13 participants. In this study, 76.9% of participant tumors expressed PD-L1, with 70% of cases carrying a BRAF^{V600E} mutation. The ORR was 16% without improvement in mOS. However, two patients demonstrated a PR, and three had durable stable disease, and the 1-year survival was 38% [238]. A larger single arm Phase I/II clinical trial (NCT02404441) recruited 42 participants to test the ICI spartalizumab as monotherapy in ATC. An ORR of 19%, PFS of 1.7 months, and mOS of 5.6 months were achieved, with a PR and CR in five and three participants, respectively. Sub-group analysis found that response was linked to PD-L1 expression, PD-L1$^-$ 0% (0/12) and PD-L1$^+$ 29% (8/28), while a tumor PD-L1$^+$ expression ≥50% was 35% (6/17). Additionally, mOS in PD-L1$^+$ participants wasn't reached at publication, and 52.1% of this sub-group were alive at 1 year [217].

There is evidence supporting the ability of kinase abilities to alter the TME, increasing TMB and improve ICI response [239–241]. Specifically, they can precipitate immunogenic tumor cell death, improving ICI effectiveness and stimulating a robust immune response against tumor cells.

Certainly, combination kinase inhibitor and ICI therapy has proven effective in BRAF^{V600E} mutated advanced melanoma. The IMpsire 150 phase III superiority trial (NCT02908672) tested combination vemurafenib, cobimetinib, and atezolizumab against vemurafenib, cobimetinib, and placebo, identifying the addition of immune checkpoint blockade improved mPFS from 10.6 to 15.1 months [242].

Retrospective cohort studies have also accessed combination targeted kinase inhibitors with ICIs, demonstrating benefit in this therapeutic strategy [243]. A single arm study of combination kinase inhibitor (either combination dabrafenib/trametinib, lenvatinib, or anlotinib) with ICI (either sintilimab, camrelizumab, or pembrolizumab) in 18 participants with stage IVB or IVC disease improved mOS and 1-year OS to 14 months and 55.6%, respectively [243].

Another retrospective *BRAF*-mutation study was of particular interest as it in part explored the potential benefit of T cell mediated immunological memory [244]. Twenty-three participants received neoadjuvant dabrafenib/trametinib prior to surgical intervention, with pembrolizumab being delivered either prior to or after surgery. A mOS of 63 months was achieved in this group [245], far exceeding the benefit of any other treatment regime to date.

A prospective, non-randomized, phase II clinical trial (NCT03181100) allocated treatment according to tumor mutation. Forty-three participants were allocated to either combination vemurafenib/cobimetinib/atezolizumab with tumor BRAF^{V600E} expression, cobimetinib/atezolizumab with RAS or NF1/2 tumor mutation, or bevacizumab/atezolizumab ($n = 3$) if their tumor didn't express these mutations. Results supported the use of targeted systemic therapy regimes in ATC with dramatic response and mOS achieved in tumors with known driver mutations. BRAF^{V600E} mOS and mPFS were 43 months and 13.9 months, respectively, while RAS/NF1/NF2 achieved a mPFS of 4.8 months and 8.7 months [246].

Case studies have reported benefit utilizing ALK-inhibitors in ALK-mutation ATC, specifically brigatinib, crizotinib, and ceritinib [247], while mutation of PIK3CA of the PI3K/AKT/mTOR (PAM) pathway may represent another actionable tumor driver [194]. Infrequently present with BRAF^{V600E} mutation, PIK3CA mutation commonly occurs in ATC without another actionable driver. The mTOR inhibitor everolimus has demonstrated some benefit in these cases [248], while also potentially demonstrating benefit in TSC2-associated ATC mutations [249, 250].

There is new evidence that targeting the PI3K/AKT/mTOR (PAM) pathway can decrease the production of immunosuppressive cytokines and reduce TME immunosuppressive Treg and MDSCs, improving ICI efficacy [251–253]. Agents targeting PAM and upstream kinase signalling attenuate tumor PD-L1 expression [254]. This has been demonstrated in multiple preclinical cancer models [253, 255, 256]. Early phase clinical trials have attempted to capitalize on this phenomenon, testing the efficacy and tolerability of combination ICI and PAM inhibition in advanced solid tumors [254]. NCT03131908 is studying combination pembrolizumab with PI3Kbeta inhibitor GSK2636771 in PD-1 refractory patients with metastatic melanoma and loss of PTEN [257], while MCT04688658 is investigating combination nivolumab and the PI3K-inhibitor duvelisib in patients with unresectable melanoma demonstrating progression on PD-1 therapy [258].

NCT03181100 treated three patients without BRAF/RAS/NF1/NF2 mutation with combination bevacizumab and atezolizumab, achieving an ORR of 33% minimal improvement in mPFS and mOS, 1.35 months and 6.21 months, respectively [246]. Interestingly, in *BRAF*^{V600E} patients that progressed in this study, this progression was associated with a new *RAS* mutation. This has also been noted in an additional ATC patient and implies these tumors find a molecular pathway around the kinase inhibitor blocked MAPK pathway [259].

Upon confirmation of BRAF^{V600E} mutation, *consideration* should be given to neoadjuvant combination MKI therapy, either dabrafenib/trametinib or vemurafenib/cobimetinib, in conjunction with an ICI (pembrolizumab, nivolumab or atezolizumab) in ATC amenable to surgical resection; however combination MKI and ICI is *recommended* and should be promptly commenced in patients presenting with unresectable disease (Fig. 23.4).

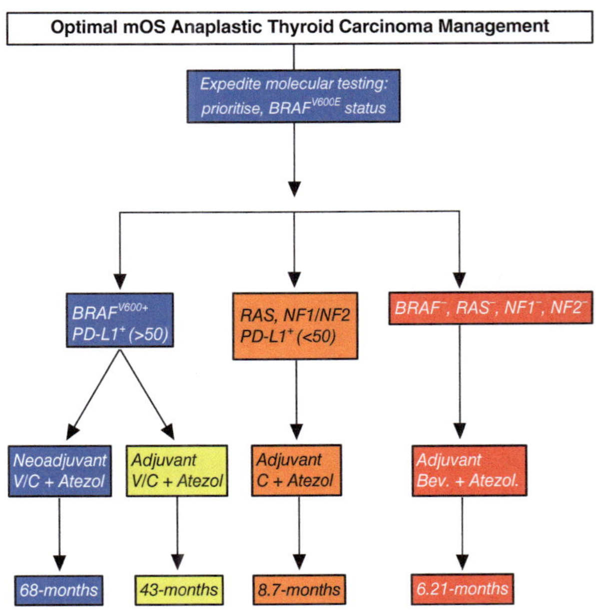

Fig. 23.4 ATC mutation risk stratification and associated kinase inhibitor therapies

Targeted systemic therapy approach to anaplastic thyroid carcinoma, by mutation status, to achieve optimal mOS [246].

Conclusion

Advanced thyroid cancers remain a therapeutic challenge. However, the rapidly developing landscape of mutation testing and targeted therapeutic strategies has created a paradigm shift in our approach to managing these malignancies, promising continued improvements in DFS and OS. Of note, appraisal of developing preclinical "next-generation" targeted therapies demonstrates that the future of targeted therapeutic approaches holds great promise for improved patient outcomes.

References

1. Shonka DC Jr, et al. American Head and Neck Society Endocrine Surgery Section and International Thyroid Oncology Group consensus statement on mutational testing in thyroid cancer: defining advanced thyroid cancer and its targeted treatment. Head Neck. 2022;44:1277–300. https://doi.org/10.1002/hed.27025.
2. Song E, et al. A relook at the T stage of differentiated thyroid carcinoma with a focus on gross extrathyroidal extension. Thyroid. 2019;29:202–8. https://doi.org/10.1089/thy.2018.0300.
3. Urken ML, Haser GC, Likhterov I, Wenig BM. The impact of metastatic lymph nodes on risk stratification in differentiated thyroid cancer: have we reached a higher level of understanding? Thyroid. 2016;26:481–8. https://doi.org/10.1089/thy.2015.0544.
4. Shah MD, et al. Clinical course of thyroid carcinoma after neck dissection. Laryngoscope. 2003;113:2102–7. https://doi.org/10.1097/00005537-200312000-00008.
5. Yun KM, Cohen EEW. An era of advances in systemic therapies for advanced thyroid cancer. JCO Oncol Pract. 2024;20:899–906. https://doi.org/10.1200/op.23.00747.
6. Zhao X, et al. Surgery after BRAF-directed therapy is associated with improved survival in BRAF(V600E) mutant anaplastic thyroid cancer: a single-center retrospective cohort study. Thyroid. 2023;33:484–91. https://doi.org/10.1089/thy.2022.0504.
7. Lamartina L, et al. Surgery for neck recurrence of differentiated thyroid cancer: outcomes and risk factors. J Clin Endocrinol Metab. 2017;102:1020–31. https://doi.org/10.1210/jc.2016-3284.
8. Verburg FA, et al. Life expectancy is reduced in differentiated thyroid cancer patients ≥ 45 years old with extensive local tumor invasion, lateral lymph node, or distant metastases at diagnosis and normal in all other DTC patients. J Clin Endocrinol Metab. 2013;98:172–80. https://doi.org/10.1210/jc.2012-2458.
9. Moritani S. Impact of superior mediastinal metastasis on the prognosis of papillary thyroid carcinoma. Endocr J. 2016;63:349–57. https://doi.org/10.1507/endocrj.EJ15-0677.
10. Scollo C, et al. Rationale for central and bilateral lymph node dissection in sporadic and hereditary medullary thyroid cancer. J Clin Endocrinol Metab. 2003;88:2070–5. https://doi.org/10.1210/jc.2002-021713.
11. Ibrahimpasic T, Ghossein R, Shah JP, Ganly I. Poorly differentiated carcinoma of the thyroid gland: current status and future prospects. Thyroid. 2019;29:311–21. https://doi.org/10.1089/thy.2018.0509.
12. Kiess AP, et al. External-beam radiotherapy for differentiated thyroid cancer locoregional control: a statement of the American Head and Neck Society. Head Neck. 2016;38:493–8. https://doi.org/10.1002/hed.24357.

13. Brose MS, et al. Sorafenib in radioactive iodine-refractory, locally advanced or metastatic differentiated thyroid cancer: a randomised, double-blind, phase 3 trial. Lancet. 2014;384:319–28. https://doi.org/10.1016/s0140-6736(14)60421-9.
14. Haugen BR, et al. 2015 American Thyroid Association management guidelines for adult patients with thyroid nodules and differentiated thyroid cancer: the American Thyroid Association guidelines task force on thyroid nodules and differentiated thyroid cancer. Thyroid. 2016;26:1–133. https://doi.org/10.1089/thy.2015.0020.
15. Tuttle RM, et al. Controversies, consensus, and collaboration in the use of (131)I therapy in differentiated thyroid cancer: a joint statement from the American Thyroid Association, the European Association of Nuclear Medicine, the Society of Nuclear Medicine and Molecular Imaging, and the European Thyroid Association. Thyroid. 2019;29:461–70. https://doi.org/10.1089/thy.2018.0597.
16. Schlumberger M, et al. Definition and management of radioactive iodine-refractory differentiated thyroid cancer. Lancet Diabetes Endocrinol. 2014;2:356–8. https://doi.org/10.1016/s2213-8587(13)70215-8.
17. Durante C, et al. Long-term outcome of 444 patients with distant metastases from papillary and follicular thyroid carcinoma: benefits and limits of radioiodine therapy. J Clin Endocrinol Metab. 2006;91:2892–9. https://doi.org/10.1210/jc.2005-2838.
18. Nixon IJ, et al. The impact of distant metastases at presentation on prognosis in patients with differentiated carcinoma of the thyroid gland. Thyroid. 2012;22:884–9. https://doi.org/10.1089/thy.2011.0535.
19. Cooper DS, et al. Thyrotropin suppression and disease progression in patients with differentiated thyroid cancer: results from the National Thyroid Cancer Treatment Cooperative Registry. Thyroid. 1998;8:737–44. https://doi.org/10.1089/thy.1998.8.737.
20. Jonklaas J, et al. Outcomes of patients with differentiated thyroid carcinoma following initial therapy. Thyroid. 2006;16:1229–42. https://doi.org/10.1089/thy.2006.16.1229.
21. Carhill AA, et al. Long-term outcomes following therapy in differentiated thyroid carcinoma: NTCTCS registry analysis 1987-2012. J Clin Endocrinol Metab. 2015;100:3270–9. https://doi.org/10.1210/jc.2015-1346.
22. Yeh T, Yeung M, Sherman EJ, Tuttle RM, Sabra MM. Structural doubling time predicts overall survival in patients with medullary thyroid cancer in patients with rapidly progressive metastatic medullary thyroid cancer treated with molecular targeted therapies. Thyroid. 2020;30:1112–9. https://doi.org/10.1089/thy.2019.0579.
23. Barbet J, Campion L, Kraeber-Bodéré F, Chatal JF. Prognostic impact of serum calcitonin and carcinoembryonic antigen doubling-times in patients with medullary thyroid carcinoma. J Clin Endocrinol Metab. 2005;90:6077–84. https://doi.org/10.1210/jc.2005-0044.
24. Laure Giraudet A, et al. Progression of medullary thyroid carcinoma: assessment with calcitonin and carcinoembryonic antigen doubling times. Eur J Endocrinol. 2008;158:239–46. https://doi.org/10.1530/eje-07-0667.
25. Miyauchi A, et al. Prognostic impact of serum thyroglobulin doubling-time under thyrotropin suppression in patients with papillary thyroid carcinoma who underwent total thyroidectomy. Thyroid. 2011;21:707–16. https://doi.org/10.1089/thy.2010.0355.
26. Lam AK, Lo CY, Lam KS. Papillary carcinoma of thyroid: a 30-yr clinicopathological review of the histological variants. Endocr Pathol. 2005;16:323–30. https://doi.org/10.1385/ep:16:4:323.
27. Coca-Pelaz A, et al. Papillary thyroid cancer-aggressive variants and impact on management: a narrative review. Adv Ther. 2020;37:3112–28. https://doi.org/10.1007/s12325-020-01391-1.
28. Chen JH, Faquin WC, Lloyd RV, Nosé V. Clinicopathological and molecular characterization of nine cases of columnar cell variant of papillary thyroid carcinoma. Mod Pathol. 2011;24:739–49. https://doi.org/10.1038/modpathol.2011.2.
29. Vander Poorten V, Hens G, Delaere P. Thyroid cancer in children and adolescents. Curr Opin Otolaryngol Head Neck Surg. 2013;21:135–42. https://doi.org/10.1097/MOO.0b013e32835e15d9.

30. Morandi L, et al. Somatic mutation profiling of hobnail variant of papillary thyroid carcinoma. Endocr Relat Cancer. 2017;24:107–17. https://doi.org/10.1530/erc-16-0546.
31. Silver CE, et al. Aggressive variants of papillary thyroid carcinoma. Head Neck. 2011;33:1052–9. https://doi.org/10.1002/hed.21494.
32. Sheu SY, Schwertheim S, Worm K, Grabellus F, Schmid KW. Diffuse sclerosing variant of papillary thyroid carcinoma: lack of BRAF mutation but occurrence of RET/PTC rearrangements. Mod Pathol. 2007;20:779–87. https://doi.org/10.1038/modpathol.3800797.
33. Joung JY, et al. Diffuse sclerosing variant of papillary thyroid carcinoma: major genetic alterations and prognostic implications. Histopathology. 2016;69:45–53. https://doi.org/10.1111/his.12902.
34. Dettmer MS, Schmitt A, Komminoth P, Perren A. Poorly differentiated thyroid carcinoma: an underdiagnosed entity. Pathologe. 2020;41:1–8. https://doi.org/10.1007/s00292-019-0600-9.
35. Uchida J, et al. Diagnostic accuracy of noninvasive genotyping of EGFR in lung cancer patients by deep sequencing of plasma cell-free DNA. Clin Chem. 2015;61:1191–6. https://doi.org/10.1373/clinchem.2015.241414.
36. Bettegowda C, et al. Detection of circulating tumor DNA in early- and late-stage human malignancies. Sci Transl Med. 2014;6:224ra224. https://doi.org/10.1126/scitranslmed.3007094.
37. Forshew T, et al. Noninvasive identification and monitoring of cancer mutations by targeted deep sequencing of plasma DNA. Sci Transl Med. 2012;4:136ra168. https://doi.org/10.1126/scitranslmed.3003726.
38. Pupilli C, et al. Circulating BRAFV600E in the diagnosis and follow-up of differentiated papillary thyroid carcinoma. J Clin Endocrinol Metab. 2013;98:3359–65. https://doi.org/10.1210/jc.2013-1072.
39. Zhu X, Yao J, Tian W. Microarray technology to investigate genes associated with papillary thyroid carcinoma. Mol Med Rep. 2015;11:3729–33. https://doi.org/10.3892/mmr.2015.3180.
40. LiVolsi VA. Papillary thyroid carcinoma: an update. Mod Pathol. 2011;24(Suppl 2):S1–9. https://doi.org/10.1038/modpathol.2010.129.
41. Ruel E, et al. Adjuvant radioactive iodine therapy is associated with improved survival for patients with intermediate-risk papillary thyroid cancer. J Clin Endocrinol Metab. 2015;100:1529–36. https://doi.org/10.1210/jc.2014-4332.
42. Nikiforova MN, Tseng GC, Steward D, Diorio D, Nikiforov YE. MicroRNA expression profiling of thyroid tumors: biological significance and diagnostic utility. J Clin Endocrinol Metab. 2008;93:1600–8. https://doi.org/10.1210/jc.2007-2696.
43. Kimura ET, et al. High prevalence of BRAF mutations in thyroid cancer: genetic evidence for constitutive activation of the RET/PTC-RAS-BRAF signaling pathway in papillary thyroid carcinoma. Cancer Res. 2003;63:1454–7.
44. Fagin JA. Genetics of papillary thyroid cancer initiation: implications for therapy. Trans Am Clin Climatol Assoc. 2005;116:259-269; discussion 269-271.
45. Kondo T, Ezzat S, Asa SL. Pathogenetic mechanisms in thyroid follicular-cell neoplasia. Nat Rev Cancer. 2006;6:292–306. https://doi.org/10.1038/nrc1836.
46. Xing M. BRAF mutation in thyroid cancer. Endocr Relat Cancer. 2005;12:245–62. https://doi.org/10.1677/erc.1.0978.
47. Ciampi R, Nikiforov YE. Alterations of the BRAF gene in thyroid tumors. Endocr Pathol. 2005;16:163–72. https://doi.org/10.1385/ep:16:3:163.
48. Wan PT, et al. Mechanism of activation of the RAF-ERK signaling pathway by oncogenic mutations of B-RAF. Cell. 2004;116:855–67. https://doi.org/10.1016/s0092-8674(04)00215-6.
49. Zhu Z, Gandhi M, Nikiforova MN, Fischer AH, Nikiforov YE. Molecular profile and clinical-pathologic features of the follicular variant of papillary thyroid carcinoma. An unusually high prevalence of ras mutations. Am J Clin Pathol. 2003;120:71–7. https://doi.org/10.1309/nd8d-9laj-trct-g6qd.
50. Lubitz CC, et al. Hobnail variant of papillary thyroid carcinoma: an institutional case series and molecular profile. Thyroid. 2014;24:958–65. https://doi.org/10.1089/thy.2013.0573.

51. Wong KS, et al. Tall cell variant of papillary thyroid carcinoma: impact of change in WHO definition and molecular analysis. Endocr Pathol. 2019;30:43–8. https://doi.org/10.1007/s12022-018-9561-4.
52. Asioli S, et al. Papillary thyroid carcinoma with prominent hobnail features: a new aggressive variant of moderately differentiated papillary carcinoma. A clinicopathologic, immunohistochemical, and molecular study of eight cases. Am J Surg Pathol. 2010;34:44–52. https://doi.org/10.1097/PAS.0b013e3181c46677.
53. Nikiforova MN, et al. BRAF mutations in thyroid tumors are restricted to papillary carcinomas and anaplastic or poorly differentiated carcinomas arising from papillary carcinomas. J Clin Endocrinol Metab. 2003;88:5399–404. https://doi.org/10.1210/jc.2003-030838.
54. Namba H, et al. Clinical implication of hot spot BRAF mutation, V599E, in papillary thyroid cancers. J Clin Endocrinol Metab. 2003;88:4393–7. https://doi.org/10.1210/jc.2003-030305.
55. Xing M, et al. BRAF mutation predicts a poorer clinical prognosis for papillary thyroid cancer. J Clin Endocrinol Metab. 2005;90:6373–9. https://doi.org/10.1210/jc.2005-0987.
56. Kim TY, et al. The BRAF mutation is useful for prediction of clinical recurrence in low-risk patients with conventional papillary thyroid carcinoma. Clin Endocrinol. 2006;65:364–8. https://doi.org/10.1111/j.1365-2265.2006.02605.x.
57. Robb R, et al. Inhibiting BRAF oncogene–mediated radioresistance effectively radiosensitizes BRAFV600E-mutant thyroid cancer cells by constraining DNA double-strand break repair. Clin Cancer Res. 2019;25:4749–60. https://doi.org/10.1158/1078-0432.Ccr-18-3625.
58. Crispo F, et al. BRAF inhibitors in thyroid cancer: clinical impact, mechanisms of resistance and future perspectives. Cancers (Basel). 2019;11:1388. https://doi.org/10.3390/cancers11091388.
59. Jin M, et al. Genetic profiles of aggressive variants of papillary thyroid carcinomas. Cancers (Basel). 2021;13:892. https://doi.org/10.3390/cancers13040892.
60. Integrated genomic characterization of papillary thyroid carcinoma. Cell. 2014;159:676–90. https://doi.org/10.1016/j.cell.2014.09.050.
61. Lawrence MS, et al. Mutational heterogeneity in cancer and the search for new cancer-associated genes. Nature. 2013;499:214–8. https://doi.org/10.1038/nature12213.
62. Shobab L, et al. PD-L1 expression varies in thyroid cancer types and is associated with decreased progression free survival (PFS) in patients with anaplastic thyroid cancer. Cancers (Basel). 2024;16:3632. https://doi.org/10.3390/cancers16213632.
63. Drilon A, et al. Efficacy of larotrectinib in TRK fusion-positive cancers in adults and children. N Engl J Med. 2018;378:731–9. https://doi.org/10.1056/NEJMoa1714448.
64. Doebele RC, et al. Entrectinib in patients with advanced or metastatic NTRK fusion-positive solid tumours: integrated analysis of three phase 1-2 trials. Lancet Oncol. 2020;21:271–82. https://doi.org/10.1016/s1470-2045(19)30691-6.
65. Hong DS, et al. Larotrectinib in patients with TRK fusion-positive solid tumours: a pooled analysis of three phase 1/2 clinical trials. Lancet Oncol. 2020;21:531–40. https://doi.org/10.1016/s1470-2045(19)30856-3.
66. Megwalu UC, Moon PK. Thyroid cancer incidence and mortality trends in the United States: 2000-2018. Thyroid. 2022;32:560–70. https://doi.org/10.1089/thy.2021.0662.
67. Song YS, Lim JA, Park YJ. Mutation profile of well-differentiated thyroid cancer in Asians. Endocrinol Metab (Seoul). 2015;30:252–62. https://doi.org/10.3803/EnM.2015.30.3.252.
68. Howell GM, Hodak SP, Yip L. RAS mutations in thyroid cancer. Oncologist. 2013;18:926–32. https://doi.org/10.1634/theoncologist.2013-0072.
69. Cabanillas ME, McFadden DG, Durante C. Thyroid cancer. Lancet. 2016;388:2783–95. https://doi.org/10.1016/s0140-6736(16)30172-6.
70. Fukahori M, et al. The associations between RAS mutations and clinical characteristics in follicular thyroid tumors: new insights from a single center and a large patient cohort. Thyroid. 2012;22:683–9. https://doi.org/10.1089/thy.2011.0261.
71. Jang EK, et al. NRAS codon 61 mutation is associated with distant metastasis in patients with follicular thyroid carcinoma. Thyroid. 2014;24:1275–81. https://doi.org/10.1089/thy.2014.0053.

72. Yoo SK, et al. Comprehensive analysis of the transcriptional and mutational landscape of follicular and papillary thyroid cancers. PLoS Genet. 2016;12:e1006239. https://doi.org/10.1371/journal.pgen.1006239.
73. French CA, et al. Genetic and biological subgroups of low-stage follicular thyroid cancer. Am J Pathol. 2003;162:1053–60. https://doi.org/10.1016/s0002-9440(10)63902-8.
74. Nikiforova MN, et al. RAS point mutations and PAX8-PPAR gamma rearrangement in thyroid tumors: evidence for distinct molecular pathways in thyroid follicular carcinoma. J Clin Endocrinol Metab. 2003;88:2318–26. https://doi.org/10.1210/jc.2002-021907.
75. Marques AR, et al. Expression of PAX8-PPAR gamma 1 rearrangements in both follicular thyroid carcinomas and adenomas. J Clin Endocrinol Metab. 2002;87:3947–52. https://doi.org/10.1210/jcem.87.8.8756.
76. Raman P, Koenig RJ. Pax-8-PPAR-γ fusion protein in thyroid carcinoma. Nat Rev Endocrinol. 2014;10:616–23. https://doi.org/10.1038/nrendo.2014.115.
77. Boos LA, et al. Diagnostic and prognostic implications of the PAX8-PPARγ translocation in thyroid carcinomas-a TMA-based study of 226 cases. Histopathology. 2013;63:234–41. https://doi.org/10.1111/his.12150.
78. Lui WO, et al. CREB3L2-PPARgamma fusion mutation identifies a thyroid signaling pathway regulated by intramembrane proteolysis. Cancer Res. 2008;68:7156–64. https://doi.org/10.1158/0008-5472.Can-08-1085.
79. Hou P, et al. Genetic alterations and their relationship in the phosphatidylinositol 3-kinase/Akt pathway in thyroid cancer. Clin Cancer Res. 2007;13:1161–70. https://doi.org/10.1158/1078-0432.Ccr-06-1125.
80. Kim CS, et al. AKT activation promotes metastasis in a mouse model of follicular thyroid carcinoma. Endocrinology. 2005;146:4456–63. https://doi.org/10.1210/en.2005-0172.
81. Saito J, et al. Regulation of FRTL-5 thyroid cell growth by phosphatidylinositol (OH) 3 kinase-dependent Akt-mediated signaling. Thyroid. 2001;11:339–51. https://doi.org/10.1089/10507250152039073.
82. Liu R, Xing M. TERT promoter mutations in thyroid cancer. Endocr Relat Cancer. 2016;23:R143–55. https://doi.org/10.1530/erc-15-0533.
83. Gaspar TB, et al. Telomere maintenance mechanisms in cancer. Genes (Basel). 2018;9:241. https://doi.org/10.3390/genes9050241.
84. Melo M, et al. TERT promoter mutations are a major indicator of poor outcome in differentiated thyroid carcinomas. J Clin Endocrinol Metabol. 2014;99:E754–65. https://doi.org/10.1210/jc.2013-3734.
85. Kim MK, et al. Role of ultrasound in predicting telomerase reverse transcriptase (TERT) promoter mutation in follicular thyroid carcinoma. Sci Rep. 2024;14:15323. https://doi.org/10.1038/s41598-024-66351-z.
86. Park H, et al. Molecular classification of follicular thyroid carcinoma based on TERT promoter mutations. Mod Pathol. 2022;35:186–92. https://doi.org/10.1038/s41379-021-00907-6.
87. Ahn S, et al. Comprehensive screening for PD-L1 expression in thyroid cancer. Endocr Relat Cancer. 2017;24:97–106. https://doi.org/10.1530/erc-16-0421.
88. Shi RL, et al. Programmed death-ligand 1 expression in papillary thyroid cancer and its correlation with clinicopathologic factors and recurrence. Thyroid. 2017;27:537–45. https://doi.org/10.1089/thy.2016.0228.
89. Hansen MU, et al. Liquid biopsies in follicular thyroid carcinomas-a brief report. Diagnostics (Basel). 2024;14:1577. https://doi.org/10.3390/diagnostics14141577.
90. Schlumberger M, et al. Lenvatinib versus placebo in radioiodine-refractory thyroid cancer. N Engl J Med. 2015;372:621–30. https://doi.org/10.1056/NEJMoa1406470.
91. Fleeman N, et al. A systematic review of lenvatinib and sorafenib for treating progressive, locally advanced or metastatic, differentiated thyroid cancer after treatment with radioactive iodine. BMC Cancer. 2019;19:1209. https://doi.org/10.1186/s12885-019-6369-7.
92. Kish JK, et al. Lenvatinib and subsequent therapy for radioactive iodine-refractory differentiated thyroid cancer: a real-world study of clinical effectiveness in the United States. Adv Ther. 2020;37:2841–52. https://doi.org/10.1007/s12325-020-01362-6.

93. Ringel MD. New horizons: emerging therapies and targets in thyroid cancer. J Clin Endocrinol Metab. 2021;106:e382–8. https://doi.org/10.1210/clinem/dgaa687.
94. Brose MS, et al. Cabozantinib for radioiodine-refractory differentiated thyroid cancer (COSMIC-311): a randomised, double-blind, placebo-controlled, phase 3 trial. Lancet Oncol. 2021;22:1126–38. https://doi.org/10.1016/s1470-2045(21)00332-6.
95. Cabanillas ME, Takahashi S. Managing the adverse events associated with lenvatinib therapy in radioiodine-refractory differentiated thyroid cancer. Semin Oncol. 2019;46:57–64. https://doi.org/10.1053/j.seminoncol.2018.11.004.
96. Colombo C, et al. Daily management of patients on multikinase inhibitors' treatment. Front Oncol. 2022;12:903532. https://doi.org/10.3389/fonc.2022.903532.
97. Acitelli E, Maiorca C, Grani G, Maranghi M. Metabolic adverse events of multitarget kinase inhibitors: a systematic review. Endocrine. 2023;81:16–29. https://doi.org/10.1007/s12020-023-03362-2.
98. Jing R, et al. Efficacy and safety of multikinase inhibitors for patients with refractory thyroid cancer: systematic review and network meta-analysis. J Clin Endocrinol Metab. 2024;109:2658–72. https://doi.org/10.1210/clinem/dgae454.
99. Bible KC, et al. A multicenter phase 2 trial of pazopanib in metastatic and progressive medullary thyroid carcinoma: MC057H. J Clin Endocrinol Metab. 2014;99:1687–93. https://doi.org/10.1210/jc.2013-3713.
100. Inampudi JV, et al. Retrospective analysis of the multikinase inhibitor (MKI) pazopanib in differentiated thyroid carcinoma (DTC) in the beyond-first-line setting. J Clin Oncol. 2023;41:e18097. https://doi.org/10.1200/JCO.2023.41.16_suppl.e18097.
101. Cella D, Beaumont JL. Pazopanib in the treatment of advanced renal cell carcinoma. Ther Adv Urol. 2016;8:61–9. https://doi.org/10.1177/1756287215614236.
102. Mederle AL, et al. Efficacy and safety of pazopanib in the treatment of thyroid cancer: a systematic review. Biomedicine. 2024;12:2820. https://doi.org/10.3390/biomedicines12122820.
103. Brose MS, et al. Vemurafenib in patients with BRAF(V600E)-positive metastatic or unresectable papillary thyroid cancer refractory to radioactive iodine: a non-randomised, multicentre, open-label, phase 2 trial. Lancet Oncol. 2016;17:1272–82. https://doi.org/10.1016/s1470-2045(16)30166-8.
104. Falchook GS, et al. Dabrafenib in patients with melanoma, untreated brain metastases, and other solid tumours: a phase 1 dose-escalation trial. Lancet. 2012;379:1893–901. https://doi.org/10.1016/s0140-6736(12)60398-5.
105. Liu D, et al. Suppression of BRAF/MEK/MAP kinase pathway restores expression of iodide-metabolizing genes in thyroid cells expressing the V600E BRAF mutant. Clin Cancer Res. 2007;13:1341–9. https://doi.org/10.1158/1078-0432.Ccr-06-1753.
106. Chakravarty D, et al. Small-molecule MAPK inhibitors restore radioiodine incorporation in mouse thyroid cancers with conditional BRAF activation. J Clin Invest. 2011;121:4700–11. https://doi.org/10.1172/jci46382.
107. Cheng W, Liu R, Zhu G, Wang H, Xing M. Robust thyroid gene expression and radioiodine uptake induced by simultaneous suppression of BRAF V600E and histone deacetylase in thyroid cancer cells. J Clin Endocrinol Metabol. 2016;101:962–71. https://doi.org/10.1210/jc.2015-3433.
108. Robb R, et al. Inhibiting BRAF oncogene-mediated radioresistance effectively radiosensitizes BRAF(V600E)-mutant thyroid cancer cells by constraining DNA double-strand break repair. Clin Cancer Res. 2019;25:4749–60. https://doi.org/10.1158/1078-0432.Ccr-18-3625.
109. Subbiah V, et al. Dabrafenib plus trametinib in BRAFV600E-mutated rare cancers: the phase 2 ROAR trial. Nat Med. 2023;29:1103–12. https://doi.org/10.1038/s41591-023-02321-8.
110. O'Dwyer PJ, et al. The NCI-MATCH trial: lessons for precision oncology. Nat Med. 2023;29:1349–57. https://doi.org/10.1038/s41591-023-02379-4.
111. Busaidy NL, et al. Dabrafenib versus Dabrafenib + Trametinib in BRAF-mutated radioactive iodine refractory differentiated thyroid cancer: results of a randomized, phase 2, open-label multicenter trial. Thyroid. 2022;32:1184–92. https://doi.org/10.1089/thy.2022.0115.

112. Amatu A, Sartore-Bianchi A, Siena S. NTRK gene fusions as novel targets of cancer therapy across multiple tumour types. ESMO Open. 2016;1:e000023. https://doi.org/10.1136/esmoopen-2015-000023.
113. Cocco E, Scaltriti M, Drilon A. NTRK fusion-positive cancers and TRK inhibitor therapy. Nat Rev Clin Oncol. 2018;15:731–47. https://doi.org/10.1038/s41571-018-0113-0.
114. Knezevich SR, McFadden DE, Tao W, Lim JF, Sorensen PH. A novel ETV6-NTRK3 gene fusion in congenital fibrosarcoma. Nat Genet. 1998;18:184–7. https://doi.org/10.1038/ng0298-184.
115. Gouda MA, Nelson BE, Buschhorn L, Wahida A, Subbiah V. Tumor-agnostic precision medicine from the AACR GENIE database: clinical implications. Clin Cancer Res. 2023;29:2753–60. https://doi.org/10.1158/1078-0432.Ccr-23-0090.
116. Filippi R, Depetris I, Satolli MA. Evaluating larotrectinib for the treatment of advanced solid tumors harboring an NTRK gene fusion. Expert Opin Pharmacother. 2021;22:677–84. https://doi.org/10.1080/14656566.2021.1876664.
117. Berger S, Martens UM, Bochum S. Larotrectinib (LOXO-101). Recent Results Cancer Res. 2018;211:141–51. https://doi.org/10.1007/978-3-319-91442-8_10.
118. Khotskaya YB, et al. Targeting TRK family proteins in cancer. Pharmacol Ther. 2017;173:58–66. https://doi.org/10.1016/j.pharmthera.2017.02.006.
119. Rolfo C, et al. Entrectinib: a potent new TRK, ROS1, and ALK inhibitor. Expert Opin Investig Drugs. 2015;24:1493–500. https://doi.org/10.1517/13543784.2015.1096344.
120. Theik NWY, et al. NTRK therapy among different types of cancers, review and future perspectives. Int J Mol Sci. 2024;25:2366. https://doi.org/10.3390/ijms25042366.
121. Waguespack SG, et al. Efficacy and safety of larotrectinib in patients with TRK fusion-positive thyroid carcinoma. Eur J Endocrinol. 2022;186:631–43. https://doi.org/10.1530/eje-21-1259.
122. Sehgal K, et al. Dual immune checkpoint inhibition in patients with aggressive thyroid carcinoma: a phase 2 nonrandomized clinical trial. JAMA Oncol. 2024;10:1663–71. https://doi.org/10.1001/jamaoncol.2024.4019.
123. French JD, et al. Combination targeted therapy with pembrolizumab and lenvatinib in progressive, radioiodine-refractory differentiated thyroid cancers. Clin Cancer Res. 2024;30:3757–67. https://doi.org/10.1158/1078-0432.Ccr-23-3417.
124. Caillé S, et al. Medullary thyroid cancer: epidemiology and characteristics according to data from the Marne-Ardennes register 1975-2018. J Endocr Soc. 2024;8:bvae084. https://doi.org/10.1210/jendso/bvae084.
125. Torresan F, Mian C, Cavedon E, Iacobone M. Cure and survival of sporadic medullary thyroid carcinoma following systematic preoperative calcitonin screening. Langenbeck's Arch Surg. 2019;404:411–9. https://doi.org/10.1007/s00423-019-01764-3.
126. Tao Z, Deng X, Guo B, Ding Z, Fan Y. Subgroup analysis of steadily increased trends in medullary thyroid carcinoma incidence and mortality in the USA, 2000-2020: a population-based retrospective cohort study. Endocr Relat Cancer. 2024;31. https://doi.org/10.1530/erc-23-0319.
127. Jaber T, Dadu R, Hu MI. Medullary thyroid carcinoma. Curr Opin Endocrinol Diabetes Obes. 2021;28:540–6. https://doi.org/10.1097/med.0000000000000662.
128. Matias-Guiu X, De Lellis R. Medullary thyroid carcinoma: a 25-year perspective. Endocr Pathol. 2014;25:21–9. https://doi.org/10.1007/s12022-013-9287-2.
129. Elisei R, et al. Prognostic significance of somatic RET oncogene mutations in sporadic medullary thyroid cancer: a 10-year follow-up study. J Clin Endocrinol Metab. 2008;93:682–7. https://doi.org/10.1210/jc.2007-1714.
130. Bai Y, Niu D, Yao Q, Lin D, Kakudo K. Updates in the advances of sporadic medullary thyroid carcinoma: from the molecules to the clinic. Gland Surg. 2020;9:1847–56. https://doi.org/10.21037/gs-2019-catp-21.
131. Mulligan LM. 65 YEARS OF THE DOUBLE HELIX: exploiting insights on the RET receptor for personalized cancer medicine. Endocr Relat Cancer. 2018;25:T189–t200. https://doi.org/10.1530/erc-18-0141.

132. Machens A, Dralle H. Accelerated MEN2A in homozygous RET carriers in the context of consanguinity. Eur J Endocrinol. 2024;190:K43–k46. https://doi.org/10.1093/ejendo/lvae025.
133. Castroneves LA, et al. Not only RET but NF1 and chromosomal instability are seen in young patients with sporadic medullary thyroid carcinoma. J Endocr Soc. 2024;8:bvae059. https://doi.org/10.1210/jendso/bvae059.
134. Ciampi R, et al. NF1 gene inactivation acts as tumor driver in RET/RAS negative medullary thyroid carcinomas. Eur J Endocrinol. 2023; https://doi.org/10.1093/ejendo/lvad051.
135. Prabhash K, et al. RET alterations differentiate molecular profile of medullary thyroid cancer. JCO Precis Oncol. 2024;8:e2300622. https://doi.org/10.1200/po.23.00622.
136. Al-Salameh A, Baudry C, Cohen R. Update on multiple endocrine neoplasia Type 1 and 2. Presse Med. 2018;47:722–31. https://doi.org/10.1016/j.lpm.2018.03.005.
137. Moline J, Eng C. Multiple endocrine neoplasia type 2: an overview. Genet Med. 2011;13:755–64. https://doi.org/10.1097/GIM.0b013e318216cc6d.
138. Prinzi A, et al. Sporadic and familial medullary thyroid carcinoma: a retrospective single center study on presentation and outcome. Endocr Res. 2024;49:179–85. https://doi.org/10.1080/07435800.2024.2344103.
139. Romei C, et al. New insights in the molecular signature of advanced medullary thyroid cancer: evidence of a bad outcome of cases with double RET mutations. J Med Genet. 2016;53:729–34. https://doi.org/10.1136/jmedgenet-2016-103833.
140. Wells SA Jr, et al. Revised American Thyroid Association guidelines for the management of medullary thyroid carcinoma. Thyroid. 2015;25:567–610. https://doi.org/10.1089/thy.2014.0335.
141. Masahide T. RET Proto-Oncogene. In: Piccaluga PP, editor. Molecular diagnostics of cancer. IntechOpen; 2024. https://www.intechopen.com/books/1003088. London. https://doi.org/10.5772/intechopen.111118.
142. Arighi E, Borrello MG, Sariola H. RET tyrosine kinase signaling in development and cancer. Cytokine Growth Factor Rev. 2005;16:441–67. https://doi.org/10.1016/j.cytogfr.2005.05.010.
143. Schuchardt A, D'Agati V, Larsson-Blomberg L, Costantini F, Pachnis V. Defects in the kidney and enteric nervous system of mice lacking the tyrosine kinase receptor Ret. Nature. 1994;367:380–3. https://doi.org/10.1038/367380a0.
144. Mahato AK, Sidorova YA. RET receptor tyrosine kinase: role in neurodegeneration, obesity, and cancer. Int J Mol Sci. 2020;21:7108. https://doi.org/10.3390/ijms21197108.
145. Plaza-Menacho I, Burzynski GM, de Groot JW, Eggen BJ, Hofstra RM. Current concepts in RET-related genetics, signaling and therapeutics. Trends Genet. 2006;22:627–36. https://doi.org/10.1016/j.tig.2006.09.005.
146. Mologni L. Development of RET kinase inhibitors for targeted cancer therapy. Curr Med Chem. 2011;18:162–75. https://doi.org/10.2174/092986711794088308.
147. Goodman KM, et al. RET recognition of GDNF-GFRα1 ligand by a composite binding site promotes membrane-proximal self-association. Cell Rep. 2014;8:1894–904. https://doi.org/10.1016/j.celrep.2014.08.040.
148. Laganà M, et al. The evolving treatment landscape of medullary thyroid cancer. Curr Treat Options in Oncol. 2023;24:1815–32. https://doi.org/10.1007/s11864-023-01145-5.
149. Ruz-Caracuel I, et al. Transcriptomic differences in medullary thyroid carcinoma according to grade. Endocr Pathol. 2024;35:207–18. https://doi.org/10.1007/s12022-024-09817-0.
150. Peddio A, et al. DLL3 as a potential diagnostic and therapeutic target in neuroendocrine neoplasms: a narrative review. Crit Rev Oncol Hematol. 2024;204:104524. https://doi.org/10.1016/j.critrevonc.2024.104524.
151. Díez JJ, Iglesias P. Somatostatin analogs in the treatment of medullary thyroid carcinoma. J Endocrinol Investig. 2002;25:773–8. https://doi.org/10.1007/bf03345511.
152. Zhang Y, et al. Molecular genetics, therapeutics and RET inhibitor resistance for medullary thyroid carcinoma and future perspectives. Cell Commun Signal. 2024;22:460. https://doi.org/10.1186/s12964-024-01837-x.
153. Segall G, et al. Real-world clinical profile, RET mutation testing, treatments, and PROs for MTC in Europe. Eur Thyroid J. 2024;13. https://doi.org/10.1530/etj-23-0172.

154. Torresan F, et al. Prophylactic and early thyroidectomy in RET germline mutation carriers in pediatric and adult population: long-term outcomes of a series of 63 patients. Cancers (Basel). 2022;14:6226. https://doi.org/10.3390/cancers14246226.
155. Kouvaraki MA, et al. RET proto-oncogene: a review and update of genotype-phenotype correlations in hereditary medullary thyroid cancer and associated endocrine tumors. Thyroid. 2005;15:531–44. https://doi.org/10.1089/thy.2005.15.531.
156. Cote GJ, et al. Prognostic significance of circulating RET M918T mutated tumor DNA in patients with advanced medullary thyroid carcinoma. J Clin Endocrinol Metab. 2017;102:3591–9. https://doi.org/10.1210/jc.2017-01039.
157. Wells SA Jr, et al. Vandetanib in patients with locally advanced or metastatic medullary thyroid cancer: a randomized, double-blind phase III trial. J Clin Oncol. 2012;30:134–41. https://doi.org/10.1200/jco.2011.35.5040.
158. Schlumberger M, et al. Overall survival analysis of EXAM, a phase III trial of cabozantinib in patients with radiographically progressive medullary thyroid carcinoma. Ann Oncol. 2017;28:2813–9. https://doi.org/10.1093/annonc/mdx479.
159. Yakes FM, et al. Cabozantinib (XL184), a novel MET and VEGFR2 inhibitor, simultaneously suppresses metastasis, angiogenesis, and tumor growth. Mol Cancer Ther. 2011;10:2298–308. https://doi.org/10.1158/1535-7163.Mct-11-0264.
160. Bentzien F, et al. In vitro and in vivo activity of cabozantinib (XL184), an inhibitor of RET, MET, and VEGFR2, in a model of medullary thyroid cancer. Thyroid. 2013;23:1569–77. https://doi.org/10.1089/thy.2013.0137.
161. Drilon A, et al. Cabozantinib in patients with advanced RET-rearranged non-small-cell lung cancer: an open-label, single-centre, phase 2, single-arm trial. Lancet Oncol. 2016;17:1653–60. https://doi.org/10.1016/s1470-2045(16)30562-9.
162. Carlomagno F, Santoro M. Identification of RET kinase inhibitors as potential new treatment for sporadic and inherited thyroid cancer. J Chemother. 2004;16(Suppl 4):49–51. https://doi.org/10.1179/joc.2004.16.Supplement-1.49.
163. Moccia M, et al. Identification of novel small molecule inhibitors of oncogenic RET kinase. PLoS One. 2015;10:e0128364. https://doi.org/10.1371/journal.pone.0128364.
164. Subbiah V, et al. Pralsetinib in patients with advanced/metastatic rearranged during transfection (RET)-altered thyroid cancer: updated efficacy and safety data from the ARROW study. Thyroid. 2024;34:26–40. https://doi.org/10.1089/thy.2023.0363.
165. Hadoux J, et al. Phase 3 trial of selpercatinib in advanced <i>RET</i>-mutant medullary thyroid cancer. N Engl J Med. 2023;389:1851–61. https://doi.org/10.1056/NEJMoa2309719.
166. Jozaghi Y, et al. Neoadjuvant selpercatinib for advanced medullary thyroid cancer. Head Neck. 2021;43:E7–e12. https://doi.org/10.1002/hed.26527.
167. Contrera KJ, et al. Neoadjuvant selective RET inhibitor for medullary thyroid cancer: a case series. Thyroid. 2023;33:129–32. https://doi.org/10.1089/thy.2022.0506.
168. Lin JJ, Gainor JF. An early look at selective RET inhibitor resistance: new challenges and opportunities. Br J Cancer. 2021;124:1757–8. https://doi.org/10.1038/s41416-021-01344-7.
169. Subbiah V, et al. Structural basis of acquired resistance to selpercatinib and pralsetinib mediated by non-gatekeeper RET mutations. Ann Oncol. 2021;32:261–8. https://doi.org/10.1016/j.annonc.2020.10.599.
170. Lin JJ, et al. Mechanisms of resistance to selective RET tyrosine kinase inhibitors in RET fusion-positive non-small-cell lung cancer. Ann Oncol. 2020;31:1725–33. https://doi.org/10.1016/j.annonc.2020.09.015.
171. Kemal Y, Çalişkan S, Gun S, Kefeli M. PD-L1 expression in medullary thyroid carcinoma and its association with clinicopathological findings. Turk Patoloji Derg. 2022;38:106–13. https://doi.org/10.5146/tjpath.2021.01558.
172. Bongiovanni M, et al. Very low expression of PD-L1 in medullary thyroid carcinoma. Endocr Relat Cancer. 2017;24:L35–l38. https://doi.org/10.1530/erc-17-0104.
173. Wusiman D, et al. Clinicopathological and prognostic significance of PD-L1 and TIM-3 expression in medullary thyroid carcinoma: a retrospective immunohistochemistry study. J Endocrinol Investig. 2024;47:91–100. https://doi.org/10.1007/s40618-023-02126-z.

174. Shi X, et al. Association between programmed death-ligand 1 expression and clinicopathological characteristics, structural recurrence, and biochemical recurrence/persistent disease in medullary thyroid carcinoma. Thyroid. 2019;29:1269–78. https://doi.org/10.1089/thy.2019.0079.
175. Wu B, Zhang B, Li B, Wu H, Jiang M. Cold and hot tumors: from molecular mechanisms to targeted therapy. Signal Transduct Target Ther. 2024;9:274. https://doi.org/10.1038/s41392-024-01979-x.
176. Sehgal K, et al. Dual immune checkpoint inhibition in patients with aggressive thyroid carcinoma: a phase 2 nonrandomized clinical trial. JAMA Oncol. 2024; https://doi.org/10.1001/jamaoncol.2024.4019.
177. Pinheiro Neto A, Lucchesi HL, Valsecchi V, Ward LS, Cunha LL. Immunotherapy for patients with thyroid cancer: a comprehensive appraisal. Chin Clin Oncol. 2024;13:36. https://doi.org/10.21037/cco-23-133.
178. Fagin JA, Krishnamoorthy GP, Landa I. Pathogenesis of cancers derived from thyroid follicular cells. Nat Rev Cancer. 2023;23:631–50. https://doi.org/10.1038/s41568-023-00598-y.
179. Zeng PYF, et al. The genomic and evolutionary landscapes of anaplastic thyroid carcinoma. Cell Rep. 2024;43:113826. https://doi.org/10.1016/j.celrep.2024.113826.
180. Molinaro E, et al. Anaplastic thyroid carcinoma: from clinicopathology to genetics and advanced therapies. Nat Rev Endocrinol. 2017;13:644–60. https://doi.org/10.1038/nrendo.2017.76.
181. Smallridge RC, Copland JA. Anaplastic thyroid carcinoma: pathogenesis and emerging therapies. Clin Oncol (R Coll Radiol). 2010;22:486–97. https://doi.org/10.1016/j.clon.2010.03.013.
182. Kebebew E, Greenspan FS, Clark OH, Woeber KA, McMillan A. Anaplastic thyroid carcinoma. Treatment outcome and prognostic factors. Cancer. 2005;103:1330–5. https://doi.org/10.1002/cncr.20936.
183. Nagaiah G, Hossain A, Mooney CJ, Parmentier J, Remick SC. Anaplastic thyroid cancer: a review of epidemiology, pathogenesis, and treatment. J Oncol. 2011;2011:542358. https://doi.org/10.1155/2011/542358.
184. Zivaljevic V, et al. Age as a prognostic factor in anaplastic thyroid cancer. Int J Endocrinol. 2014;2014:240513. https://doi.org/10.1155/2014/240513.
185. Kong N, et al. Age influences the prognosis of anaplastic thyroid cancer patients. Front Endocrinol (Lausanne). 2021;12:704596. https://doi.org/10.3389/fendo.2021.704596.
186. Tuttle RM, Haugen B, Perrier ND. Updated American Joint Committee on Cancer/tumor-node-metastasis staging system for differentiated and anaplastic thyroid cancer (eighth edition): what changed and why? Thyroid. 2017;27:751–6. https://doi.org/10.1089/thy.2017.0102.
187. Hvilsom GB, et al. Anaplastic thyroid carcinoma in Denmark 1996-2012: a national prospective study of 219 patients. Cancer Epidemiol. 2018;53:65–71. https://doi.org/10.1016/j.canep.2018.01.011.
188. Xu B, et al. Dissecting anaplastic thyroid carcinoma: a comprehensive clinical, histologic, immunophenotypic, and molecular study of 360 cases. Thyroid. 2020;30:1505–17. https://doi.org/10.1089/thy.2020.0086.
189. Cabanillas ME, et al. Facilitating anaplastic thyroid cancer specialized treatment: a model for improving access to multidisciplinary care for patients with anaplastic thyroid cancer. Head Neck. 2017;39:1291–5. https://doi.org/10.1002/hed.24784.
190. Bible KC, et al. 2021 American Thyroid Association guidelines for management of patients with anaplastic thyroid cancer. Thyroid. 2021;31:337–86. https://doi.org/10.1089/thy.2020.0944.
191. Maniakas A, et al. Evaluation of overall survival in patients with anaplastic thyroid carcinoma, 2000-2019. JAMA Oncol. 2020;6:1397–404. https://doi.org/10.1001/jamaoncol.2020.3362.
192. Kunstman JW, et al. Characterization of the mutational landscape of anaplastic thyroid cancer via whole-exome sequencing. Hum Mol Genet. 2015;24:2318–29. https://doi.org/10.1093/hmg/ddu749.

193. Sykorova V, et al. Search for new genetic biomarkers in poorly differentiated and anaplastic thyroid carcinomas using next generation sequencing. Anticancer Res. 2015;35:2029–36.
194. Landa I, et al. Genomic and transcriptomic hallmarks of poorly differentiated and anaplastic thyroid cancers. J Clin Invest. 2016;126:1052–66. https://doi.org/10.1172/jci85271.
195. Jeon MJ, et al. Genomic alterations of anaplastic thyroid carcinoma detected by targeted massive parallel sequencing in a BRAF(V600E) mutation-prevalent area. Thyroid. 2016;26:683–90. https://doi.org/10.1089/thy.2015.0506.
196. Tiedje V, et al. NGS based identification of mutational hotspots for targeted therapy in anaplastic thyroid carcinoma. Oncotarget. 2017;8:42613–20. https://doi.org/10.18632/oncotarget.17300.
197. Bonhomme B, et al. Molecular pathology of anaplastic thyroid carcinomas: a retrospective study of 144 cases. Thyroid. 2017;27:682–92. https://doi.org/10.1089/thy.2016.0254.
198. Pozdeyev N, et al. Genetic analysis of 779 advanced differentiated and anaplastic thyroid cancers. Clin Cancer Res. 2018;24:3059–68. https://doi.org/10.1158/1078-0432.Ccr-18-0373.
199. Yoo SK, et al. Integrative analysis of genomic and transcriptomic characteristics associated with progression of aggressive thyroid cancer. Nat Commun. 2019;10:2764. https://doi.org/10.1038/s41467-019-10680-5.
200. Lu L, et al. Anaplastic transformation in thyroid cancer revealed by single-cell transcriptomics. J Clin Invest. 2023;133. https://doi.org/10.1172/jci169653.
201. Friday BB, Adjei AA. Advances in targeting the Ras/Raf/MEK/Erk mitogen-activated protein kinase cascade with MEK inhibitors for cancer therapy. Clin Cancer Res. 2008;14:342–6. https://doi.org/10.1158/1078-0432.Ccr-07-4790.
202. Glaviano A, et al. PI3K/AKT/mTOR signaling transduction pathway and targeted therapies in cancer. Mol Cancer. 2023;22:138. https://doi.org/10.1186/s12943-023-01827-6.
203. Pratilas CA, et al. (V600E)BRAF is associated with disabled feedback inhibition of RAF-MEK signaling and elevated transcriptional output of the pathway. Proc Natl Acad Sci USA. 2009;106:4519–24. https://doi.org/10.1073/pnas.0900780106.
204. Wang JR, et al. Impact of somatic mutations on survival outcomes in patients with anaplastic thyroid carcinoma. JCO Precis Oncol. 2022;6:e2100504. https://doi.org/10.1200/po.21.00504.
205. O'Neill CJ, et al. BRAF(V600E) mutation is associated with an increased risk of nodal recurrence requiring reoperative surgery in patients with papillary thyroid cancer. Surgery. 2010;148:1139–45.; discussion 1145-1136,. https://doi.org/10.1016/j.surg.2010.09.005.
206. Xing M, et al. Association between BRAF V600E mutation and mortality in patients with papillary thyroid cancer. JAMA. 2013;309:1493–501. https://doi.org/10.1001/jama.2013.3190.
207. Noy R, Pollard JW. Tumor-associated macrophages: from mechanisms to therapy. Immunity. 2014;41:49–61. https://doi.org/10.1016/j.immuni.2014.06.010.
208. Qian BZ, Pollard JW. Macrophage diversity enhances tumor progression and metastasis. Cell. 2010;141:39–51. https://doi.org/10.1016/j.cell.2010.03.014.
209. Liu J, Geng X, Hou J, Wu G. New insights into M1/M2 macrophages: key modulators in cancer progression. Cancer Cell Int. 2021;21:389. https://doi.org/10.1186/s12935-021-02089-2.
210. Chen Y, McAndrews KM, Kalluri R. Clinical and therapeutic relevance of cancer-associated fibroblasts. Nat Rev Clin Oncol. 2021;18:792–804. https://doi.org/10.1038/s41571-021-00546-5.
211. Sanford-Crane H, Abrego J, Sherman MH. Fibroblasts as modulators of local and systemic cancer metabolism. Cancers (Basel). 2019;11. https://doi.org/10.3390/cancers11050619.
212. Nihashi Y, Song X, Yamamoto M, Setoyama D, Kida YS. Decoding metabolic symbiosis between pancreatic cancer cells and cancer-associated fibroblasts using cultured tumor microenvironment. Int J Mol Sci. 2023;24:11015. https://doi.org/10.3390/ijms241311015.
213. Hanahan D, Coussens LM. Accessories to the crime: functions of cells recruited to the tumor microenvironment. Cancer Cell. 2012;21:309–22. https://doi.org/10.1016/j.ccr.2012.02.022.
214. Chern B, Pinto D, Lum JH, Parameswaran R. Nearly half of patients with anaplastic thyroid cancer may be amenable to immunotherapy. Biomedicine. 2024;12. https://doi.org/10.3390/biomedicines12061304.

215. Boruah M, et al. PD-L1 expression in rare and aggressive thyroid cancers: a preliminary investigation for a role of immunotherapy. J Cancer Res Ther. 2023;19:312–20. https://doi.org/10.4103/jcrt.jcrt_1471_22.
216. Agarwal S, et al. PD-L1 expression and its modulating factors in anaplastic thyroid carcinoma: a multi-institutional study. Am J Surg Pathol. 2024;48:1233–44. https://doi.org/10.1097/pas.0000000000002284.
217. Capdevila J, et al. PD-1 blockade in anaplastic thyroid carcinoma. J Clin Oncol. 2020;38:2620–7. https://doi.org/10.1200/jco.19.02727.
218. Sekino M, et al. Analysis of expression of programmed cell death ligand 1 (PD-L1) and BRAFV600E mutation in thyroid cancer. Cancer. 2023;15:3449.
219. Feng D, et al. BRAF(V600E)-induced, tumor intrinsic PD-L1 can regulate chemotherapy-induced apoptosis in human colon cancer cells and in tumor xenografts. Oncogene. 2019;38:6752–66. https://doi.org/10.1038/s41388-019-0919-y.
220. Chintakuntlawar AV, et al. Expression of PD-1 and PD-L1 in anaplastic thyroid cancer patients treated with multimodal therapy: results from a retrospective study. J Clin Endocrinol Metabol. 2017;102:1943–50. https://doi.org/10.1210/jc.2016-3756.
221. Qin Y, et al. Clinical utility of circulating cell-free DNA mutations in anaplastic thyroid carcinoma. Thyroid. 2021;31:1235–43. https://doi.org/10.1089/thy.2020.0296.
222. Behnagh AK, et al. An overview on prevalence and detection approaches of BRAF V600E mutation in anaplastic thyroid carcinoma: a systematic review and meta-analysis. Iran J Public Health. 2024;53:1496–507. https://doi.org/10.18502/ijph.v53i7.16044.
223. Lawless AK, et al. Anaplastic thyroid cancer: a review of recent evidence and summary of an Australian institutional protocol. Asia Pac J Clin Oncol. 2024;20:681–9. https://doi.org/10.1111/ajco.14106.
224. Ryder M, et al. Genetic and pharmacological targeting of CSF-1/CSF-1R inhibits tumor-associated macrophages and impairs BRAF-induced thyroid cancer progression. PLoS One. 2013;8:e54302. https://doi.org/10.1371/journal.pone.0054302.
225. Sabra MM, et al. Clinical outcomes and molecular profile of differentiated thyroid cancers with radioiodine-avid distant metastases. J Clin Endocrinol Metab. 2013;98:E829–36. https://doi.org/10.1210/jc.2012-3933.
226. Durante C, et al. BRAF mutations in papillary thyroid carcinomas inhibit genes involved in iodine metabolism. J Clin Endocrinol Metab. 2007;92:2840–3. https://doi.org/10.1210/jc.2006-2707.
227. Wirth LJ, et al. Open-label, single-arm, multicenter, phase II trial of lenvatinib for the treatment of patients with anaplastic thyroid cancer. J Clin Oncol. 2021;39:2359–66. https://doi.org/10.1200/jco.20.03093.
228. Matsui J, et al. Multi-kinase inhibitor E7080 suppresses lymph node and lung metastases of human mammary breast tumor MDA-MB-231 via inhibition of vascular endothelial growth factor-receptor (VEGF-R) 2 and VEGF-R3 kinase. Clin Cancer Res. 2008;14:5459–65. https://doi.org/10.1158/1078-0432.Ccr-07-5270.
229. Matsui J, et al. E7080, a novel inhibitor that targets multiple kinases, has potent antitumor activities against stem cell factor producing human small cell lung cancer H146, based on angiogenesis inhibition. Int J Cancer. 2008;122:664–71. https://doi.org/10.1002/ijc.23131.
230. Okamoto K, et al. Antitumor activities of the targeted multi-tyrosine kinase inhibitor lenvatinib (E7080) against RET gene fusion-driven tumor models. Cancer Lett. 2013;340:97–103. https://doi.org/10.1016/j.canlet.2013.07.007.
231. Cabanillas ME, Ryder M, Jimenez C. Targeted therapy for advanced thyroid cancer: kinase inhibitors and beyond. Endocr Rev. 2019;40:1573–604. https://doi.org/10.1210/er.2019-00007.
232. Savvides P, et al. Phase II trial of sorafenib in patients with advanced anaplastic carcinoma of the thyroid. Thyroid. 2013;23:600–4. https://doi.org/10.1089/thy.2012.0103.
233. Bible KC, et al. A multiinstitutional phase 2 trial of pazopanib monotherapy in advanced anaplastic thyroid cancer. J Clin Endocrinol Metabol. 2012;97:3179–84. https://doi.org/10.1210/jc.2012-1520.

234. Subbiah V, et al. Dabrafenib plus trametinib in patients with BRAF V600E-mutant anaplastic thyroid cancer: updated analysis from the phase II ROAR basket study. Ann Oncol. 2022;33:406–15. https://doi.org/10.1016/j.annonc.2021.12.014.
235. Subbiah V, et al. Dabrafenib and trametinib treatment in patients with locally advanced or metastatic BRAF V600-mutant anaplastic thyroid cancer. J Clin Oncol. 2018;36:7–13. https://doi.org/10.1200/jco.2017.73.6785.
236. Ito Y, Onoda N, Okamoto T. The revised clinical practice guidelines on the management of thyroid tumors by the Japan associations of endocrine surgeons: core questions and recommendations for treatments of thyroid cancer. Endocr J. 2020;67:669–717. https://doi.org/10.1507/endocrj.EJ20-0025.
237. Marcus L, Lemery SJ, Keegan P, Pazdur R. FDA approval summary: pembrolizumab for the treatment of microsatellite instability-high solid Tumors. Clin Cancer Res. 2019;25:3753–8. https://doi.org/10.1158/1078-0432.Ccr-18-4070.
238. Hatashima A, et al. An evaluation of clinical efficacy of immune checkpoint inhibitors for patients with anaplastic thyroid carcinoma. Thyroid. 2022;32:926–36. https://doi.org/10.1089/thy.2022.0073.
239. Ni JJ, Zhang ZZ, Ge MJ, Chen JY, Zhuo W. Immune-based combination therapy to convert immunologically cold tumors into hot tumors: an update and new insights. Acta Pharmacol Sin. 2023;44:288–307. https://doi.org/10.1038/s41401-022-00953-z.
240. Brauner E, et al. Combining BRAF inhibitor and anti PD-L1 antibody dramatically improves tumor regression and anti tumor immunity in an immunocompetent murine model of anaplastic thyroid cancer. Oncotarget. 2016:7.
241. Gunda V, et al. Blocks to thyroid cancer cell apoptosis can be overcome by inhibition of the MAPK and PI3K/AKT pathways. Cell Death Dis. 2014;5:e1104. https://doi.org/10.1038/cddis.2014.78.
242. Gutzmer R, et al. Atezolizumab, vemurafenib, and cobimetinib as first-line treatment for unresectable advanced BRAF(V600) mutation-positive melanoma (IMspire150): primary analysis of the randomised, double-blind, placebo-controlled, phase 3 trial. Lancet. 2020;395:1835–44. https://doi.org/10.1016/s0140-6736(20)30934-x.
243. Song Y, et al. Combination kinase inhibitors and immunotherapy for unresectable anaplastic thyroid carcinoma: a retrospective single-center study. Oral Oncol. 2024;159:107067. https://doi.org/10.1016/j.oraloncology.2024.107067.
244. Wherry EJ, et al. Molecular signature of CD8+ T cell exhaustion during chronic viral infection. Immunity. 2007;27:670–84. https://doi.org/10.1016/j.immuni.2007.09.006.
245. Hamidi S, et al. Checkpoint inhibition in addition to dabrafenib/trametinib for BRAF(V600E)-mutated anaplastic thyroid carcinoma. Thyroid. 2024;34:336–46. https://doi.org/10.1089/thy.2023.0573.
246. Cabanillas ME, et al. Anti-programmed death ligand 1 plus targeted therapy in anaplastic thyroid carcinoma: a nonrandomized clinical trial. JAMA Oncol. 2024; https://doi.org/10.1001/jamaoncol.2024.4729.
247. Leroy L, et al. Remarkable response to ceritinib and brigatinib in an anaplastic lymphoma kinase-rearranged anaplastic thyroid carcinoma previously treated with crizotinib. Thyroid. 2020;30:343–4. https://doi.org/10.1089/thy.2019.0202.
248. Hanna GJ, et al. Genomic correlates of response to everolimus in aggressive radioiodine-refractory thyroid cancer: a phase II study. Clin Cancer Res. 2018;24:1546–53. https://doi.org/10.1158/1078-0432.Ccr-17-2297.
249. Lim SM, et al. Next-generation sequencing reveals somatic mutations that confer exceptional response to everolimus. Oncotarget. 2016;7:10547–56. https://doi.org/10.18632/oncotarget.7234.
250. Harris EJ, et al. Everolimus in anaplastic thyroid cancer: a case series. Front Oncol. 2019;9:106. https://doi.org/10.3389/fonc.2019.00106.
251. Schmid MC, et al. Receptor tyrosine kinases and TLR/IL1Rs unexpectedly activate myeloid cell PI3kγ, a single convergent point promoting tumor inflammation and progression. Cancer Cell. 2011;19:715–27. https://doi.org/10.1016/j.ccr.2011.04.016.

252. Hirsch E, Ciraolo E, Franco I, Ghigo A, Martini M. PI3K in cancer-stroma interactions: bad in seed and ugly in soil. Oncogene. 2014;33:3083–90. https://doi.org/10.1038/onc.2013.265.
253. Peng W, et al. Loss of PTEN promotes resistance to T cell-mediated immunotherapy. Cancer Discov. 2016;6:202–16. https://doi.org/10.1158/2159-8290.Cd-15-0283.
254. He Y, et al. Targeting PI3K/Akt signal transduction for cancer therapy. Signal Transduct Target Ther. 2021;6:425. https://doi.org/10.1038/s41392-021-00828-5.
255. Lastwika KJ, et al. Control of PD-L1 expression by oncogenic activation of the AKT-mTOR pathway in non-small cell lung cancer. Cancer Res. 2016;76:227–38. https://doi.org/10.1158/0008-5472.Can-14-3362.
256. Yan C, et al. Inhibition of the PI3K/mTOR pathway in breast cancer to enhance response to immune checkpoint inhibitors in breast cancer. Int J Mol Sci. 2021;22. https://doi.org/10.3390/ijms22105207.
257. Tawbi HA-H, et al. Phase I/II study of the PI3Kβ inhibitor GSK2636771 in combination with pembrolizumab (P) in patients (pts) with PD-1 refractory metastatic melanoma (MM) and PTEN loss. J Clin Oncol. 2018;36:TPS9596-TPS9596. https://doi.org/10.1200/JCO.2018.36.15_suppl.TPS9596.
258. Jin J, et al. Interim results from a phase I/II study of duvelisib PI3Kδγ inhibitor and nivolumab in patients with advanced unresectable melanoma who have progressed on anti-PD1 therapy. J Clin Oncol. 2023;41:9540. https://doi.org/10.1200/JCO.2023.41.16_suppl.9540.
259. Hofmann MC, et al. Molecular mechanisms of resistance to kinase inhibitors and redifferentiation in thyroid cancers. Endocr Relat Cancer. 2022;29:R173–r190. https://doi.org/10.1530/erc-22-0129.

Pediatric Thyroid Cancer

24

Chad K. Sudoko and Ken Kazahaya

Editorial Less is more. This is nowhere more relevant than in thyroid cancers, which are in majority a low-grade indolent disease with very good prognosis. Age is an important prognostic indicator. In well-differentiated thyroid cancers, those with metastatic disease and age less than 55 years have an excellent outcome and hence staged II.

Extremes of age warranted aggressive surgical resection at the primary and regional sites. Studies have shown 77% reduction in redo surgery and improved survival with radical surgery. The need for guideline-based management with total thyroidectomy and central nodal clearance in all is being debated. With a large majority of familial non-medullary thyroid cancers, having mutations and being part of syndromes indicate a rising need to assess the pathways at risk. High-risk patients need to be triaged out for aggressive treatment and adjuvant radioiodine therapy. The large majority might benefit from lesser surgery both at the primary and neck, reducing long-term morbidity and avoiding radioiodine therapy.

Medullary thyroid cancers limited to the thyroid, non-familial, and non-syndromic might merit from lesser surgery. These are dogmas which need to be challenged, and as the long-term data emerges, there will be more clarity on the extent of therapy.

C. K. Sudoko (✉) · K. Kazahaya
Division of Pediatric Otolaryngology, Children's Hospital of Philadelphia, Philadelphia, PA, USA

Department of Otorhinolaryngology-Head and Neck Surgery, University of Pennsylvania, Philadelphia, PA, USA
e-mail: sudokoc@chop.edu; kazahaya@chop.edu

P. S. Pai et al. (eds.), *Controversies in Cancer of the Thyroid and Parathyroid Glands*, https://doi.org/10.1007/978-3-032-13130-0_24

Systemic therapy in advanced thyroid cancers seems to reduce the volume, improve operability, and re-differentiate cancers which improve radio iodine efficacy. The last word on these indolent cancers is yet to be written.

Prathamesh S. Pai

Intro

Thyroid carcinoma currently represents up to 3% of all pediatric cancers and, over the last two decades, has been slowly increasing in incidence [1–3]. When compared to their adult counterparts, pediatric patients will present with more advanced disease including extrathyroidal extension, nodal involvement, and pulmonary metastasis [4, 5]. However, despite the advanced disease at presentation, the overall survival is greater than 90% at 30 years [6].

The majority of children and adolescents diagnosed with thyroid cancer are asymptomatic and have no identifiable risk factors. In a small cohort of patients, the most common risk factors are a history of exposure to radiation and genetic predisposition. The association between radiation and thyroid cancer has been seen from observations in Hiroshima and Nagasaki, patients who have had multiple CT scans, and childhood cancer survivors who received therapeutic radiation therapy [7–12]. Studies of childhood cancer survivors who have received radiation to the neck have demonstrated a standardized incidence ratio of thyroid cancer from 5- to 69-fold, with the dose of exposure and a younger age correlating with the highest risk and shortest latency for the development of thyroid cancer [13]. It is thought that the increased risk of both thyroid nodules and cancer is due to the increased cellular activity in the thyroid which is observed during childhood compared to during adulthood [14].

Genetic predisposition is the second most common identifiable risk factor and can be classified as non-syndromic and syndromic. Non-syndromic genetic predisposition is often referred to as familial non-medullary thyroid cancer (FNMTC) and is defined as two or more first-degree relatives with either papillary or follicular thyroid cancer. Although a single germline locus has not been identified, the method of inheritance most resembles an autosomal dominant pattern [15, 16]. Syndromic forms of thyroid cancer are associated with mutations in several genes that increases the risk of thyroid and non-thyroid malignancies, often associated with phenotypic findings on physical exam. For differentiated thyroid carcinoma (DTC), these syndromes include DICER1 syndrome, Carney complex, familial adenomatous polyposis (FAP), and PTEN hamartoma tumor syndrome. In medullary thyroid cancer (MTC), the familial syndrome is multiple endocrine neoplasia (MEN) type II.

Pediatric thyroid cancer is staged by the American Joint Committee on Cancer (AJCC) TNM classification system based on primary tumor size (T1–4), nodal involvement of the central (N1a) or cervical (N1b) lymph nodes, and the presence of distant metastasis (M1). In DTC, the American Thyroid Association (ATA) stratifies the patient's risk and defines three groups (low, intermediate, and high risk) in order to guide treatment [17].

Clinical Presentation and Evaluation

As previously mentioned, most pediatric patients are asymptomatic when first diagnosed with thyroid cancer. Smaller thyroid nodules can be incidentally found on imaging studies performed for a non-thyroid related indication, whereas larger lesions can present as a neck mass that was noted on examination by the primary care provider. A certain challenge in children is palpable level II lymph nodes are a common finding. However, the presence of a thyroid nodule with cervical lymphadenopathy in level III or IV is a finding that is concerning for malignancy [18].

Although thyroid nodules are relatively uncommon in children (<2% incidence), the incidence increases with age and is up to 13% in older adolescents [19]. There is also an increased incidence of thyroid nodules in children with iodine deficiency, prior radiation exposure, a history of thyroid disease, and various genetic syndromes. When compared to adults with thyroid nodules, there is an increased risk of malignancy in thyroid nodules of pediatric patients (25% vs 5%), emphasizing the need for appropriate workup and evaluation [20, 21]. Guidelines have been published on the appropriate evaluation and management of pediatric thyroid nodules including a focused and detailed history, physical exam, imaging, laboratory testing, need for fine needle aspiration (FNA), and an assessment of vocal cord mobility if malignancy is suspected [17].

Imaging

An ultrasound (US) of the thyroid is the best initial imaging modality to assess a thyroid nodule. An assessment of the central and lateral neck lymph nodes should also be performed in patients with moderate- to high-risk thyroid lesions [22, 23]. The thyroid nodule is then graded using the Thyroid Imaging Reporting and Data System (TI-RADS), in accordance with the ATA guidelines [17, 24]. The stratification and risk assessment of the nodule using TI-RADS will dictate the need for FNA. In many patients, an US will be sufficient; however, in those with large lesions or metastatic lymphadenopathy, cross-sectional imaging with a CT with contrast or MRI with contrast can provide useful information in the assessment of the mediastinum, retropharynx, and subclavicular regions [17, 22]. Chest imaging with a CT should also be considered to assess for pulmonary metastasis in patients with significant lymphadenopathy.

Fine-Needle Aspiration

If there is a concern for possible malignancy based off of characteristics of the thyroid nodule according to the TI-RADS score, an FNA should be performed. Similar to adults, the Bethesda System for Reporting Thyroid Cytopathology is used to characterize the results. Although the Bethesda System is dependent on the familiarity and experience of the provider performing the FNA and subsequently the pathologist, there does appear to be an increased risk of malignancy for pediatric patients with indeterminate cytology [25]. The increased risk is largely in part due to the Bethesda IV indeterminate nodules. When compared to adults, the risk for malignancy in Bethesda III is similar in pediatric patients, at approximately 15%. However, in Bethesda IV nodules, the risk for malignancy is 55% in children compared to 40% in adults [26].

Oncogenic Testing

In patients who have an indeterminant thyroid nodule, oncogenic testing may be helpful as the presence of a mutation or rearrangement is directly associated with malignancy [27]. However, the clinician should be cautious over a negative molecular test, as there is insufficient data on negative molecular studies to reliably exclude malignancy.

In adults, oncogenic testing is commonly performed, and the BRAF V600E mutation has been associated with a higher recurrence and mortality rate [28–31]. BRAF mutations are the most common molecular abnormality in adults with PTC; however, in children with PTC, these mutations are uncommon [32, 33]. Additionally, a correlation between a BRAF mutation and a more invasive phenotype has not been shown in the pediatric population [34–36]. Meanwhile, the presence of a fusion oncogene in a pediatric thyroid nodule has been shown to be associated with more extensive disease [37]. Depending on the clinical presentation, extent of disease, resources of the facility, and discussion of the potential impact or lack thereof, molecular testing can be considered in pediatric patients.

Vocal Cord Assessment

Assessment of the vocal cords is essential to the preoperative workup of thyroid cancer as invasive disease can lead to compromise of the recurrent laryngeal nerve (RLN), resulting in paresis of one or both of the vocal cords. As such, evaluation of the vocal cords should be performed on all patients undergoing thyroid surgery. The evaluation can be performed with a flexible fiberoptic laryngoscopy or laryngeal ultrasound [38]. Children may not be able to cooperate with passing a flexible scope through their nose; therefore, the option to US the larynx is particularly useful. In children, the thyroid cartilage may not be ossified and, therefore, permit sonographic imaging of the vocal cords. In older children where the thyroid cartilage may have started to become ossified, the probe may be angled up over the cricothyroid membrane to allow visualization of the vocal cord motion. If paresis is seen, then further discussion regarding the extent of disease, surgical approach, adjuvant treatment, and post-operative expectations should be had with the patient and their family.

Papillary Thyroid Carcinoma

Papillary thyroid carcinoma (PTC) is the most common form of pediatric thyroid cancer and makes up approximately 85–90% of all thyroid malignancies. The most common histologic subtypes are classic PTC (60%) and follicular variant PTC (20%). Other subtypes include diffuse sclerosing variant PTC (dsvPTC), widely invasive (diffuse) follicular variant PTC, solid-trabecular PTC (sPTC), and tall-cell variant PTC (tcvPTC). When compared to adults, pediatric PTC has a higher predilection to invade lymphatics resulting in regional lymph node involvement of 70–90% of patients in addition to an increased rate of multifocal disease (30–80%) and distant metastasis, most commonly to the lungs (8–20%) at the time of diagnosis [39].

Surgical Management

Is a Total Thyroidectomy Always Necessary?

PTC is initially treated with surgical resection. Due to the high rate of multifocality and bilateral involvement of the tumor, the current guidelines and most providers advocate for a total thyroidectomy [40]. Some studies have also shown an increased rate of local recurrence with a lobectomy compared to a total thyroidectomy [41]. Another benefit of performing a total thyroidectomy is that thyroglobulin can then be used a marker to detect persistent or recurrent disease and radioactive iodine (RAI) can also be used for whole body imaging and/or treatment [6, 42]. However, these guidelines have been criticized as overly aggressive for early-stage PTC as it likely does not influence patient survival and does result in life-long thyroid hormone replacement therapy. Additionally, many pediatric patients in these studies have advanced disease, potentially overshadowing the low T-stage patients who may benefit from a less aggressive surgical approach. Recent studies have looked at patients with limited disease and have shown that a cohort of pediatric patients with papillary thyroid microcarcinoma, low-stage PTC, or a low invasive potential PTC (encapsulated fvPTC) may benefit from a unilateral lobectomy [43–46].

What Is the Utility of a Prophylactic Central Neck Dissection?

When there is gross extrathyroidal extension of thyroid cancer or evidence of nodal disease, then a therapeutic neck dissection should be performed [17]. Otherwise, there is no consensus regarding the utility of a prophylactic neck dissection. There is evidence that a prophylactic central neck dissection has no impact on locoregional or distant metastasis [47]. There is also data suggesting that children who undergo a total thyroidectomy and a prophylactic central neck dissection have a reduced risk of reoperation and an increased disease-free survival at 5 and 10 years [48]. Additionally, another study showed that a total thyroidectomy with prophylactic central neck dissection may reduce the risk for reoperation by as much as 77% [49]. Overall, the data are mixed and potentially related to the use of adjuvant RAI ablation, as another study showed that in a large proportion of patients who underwent total thyroidectomy with RAI ablation, there was no association of the extent of neck dissection on the risk for locoregional or distant metastasis [47]. Despite the mixed data and given the higher rate of lymph node metastasis in the pediatric population, there is a growing agreement that a central neck dissection should be performed with a total thyroidectomy. With data on both sides, it stands to reason that removing the lymph nodes of the central neck, and the first drainage pathway for the thyroid, an improvement of the disease-free status and local recurrence could be expected. The pathologic status of the prophylactic central neck dissection also provides valuable information and is used to stratify patients into risk levels. The ATA categorizes patients into low-, intermediate-, and high-risk levels in order to balance the risk and benefits of post-operative radioactive iodine treatment [17]. The potential benefits for performing a prophylactic central neck dissection have been presented; however, the risks of a more extensive surgery should not be forgotten and must be weighed to achieve the best outcome for the patient.

When a neck dissection is performed, there is a consensus that node "plucking" is not appropriate, and a full compartment-oriented resection is the standard. Hematoma, vocal cord paralysis, and hypocalcemia due to hypoparathyroidism are the major complications associated with thyroid surgery, and unfortunately the complication rate is higher in children than adults. Due to these factors, the thyroid surgery and neck dissection should be performed by a surgeon highly experienced in the procedure in the pediatric population as there is an overall reduction in post-operative complications when performed at a high-volume pediatric thyroid surgery center [50–52].

Follicular Thyroid Carcinoma

Like PTC, follicular thyroid carcinoma (FTC) is a well-differentiated thyroid cancer. FTC is the second most common thyroid cancer in children, making up about 10% of cases. FTC has an increased incidence in iodine deficient areas of the world and is more commonly diagnosed in adolescents, than in younger children [53]. FTC metastasizes hematogenously, with the risk of metastasis mostly determined by the extent of angioinvasion into the peri- and intracapsular blood vessels [54, 55]. Depending on the extent of invasion, FTC can be classified as minimally invasive (invasion of tumor in <4 blood vessels) or widely invasive (invasion of tumor in ≥ 4 blood vessels). Widely invasive FTC carries an increased risk of distant metastasis, recurrence, and worse outcomes [40, 56]. Fortunately, most FTC in children is minimally invasive.

Surgical Management

FTC can be challenging to differentiate from a follicular adenoma as it is invasion through the capsule or the presence of angioinvasion that differentiates the cancer from the adenoma. Given this challenge, a thyroid lobectomy is recommended. If FTC is identified, then based on the presence and extent of angioinvasion, completion thyroidectomy is then considered [57, 58]. Unless there are clinically detectable lymph nodes, a neck dissection is not performed.

Medical Management for DTC

Radioactive Iodine

Radioactive iodine (RAI) is an effective therapy to treat persistent post-surgical disease in patients with DTC. The decision to treat with RAI is based on the ATA guidelines, which as previously mentioned stratify patients into low-, intermediate-, and high-risk levels. Given the extremely low mortality rate, the risk is defined as the likelihood of having persistent regional or distant disease following surgery rather than the mortality risk [17].

Those placed in the low-risk category will not receive RAI and are followed with a TSH-suppressed thyroglobulin and neck US [59]. For those in the intermediate- and high-risk categories, a TSH-stimulated thyroglobulin and I^{123} diagnostic whole-body scan (DxWBS) are performed. Depending on the findings, RAI therapy may be recommended.

Is Systemic Therapy Warranted?

Unfortunately, some patients will develop progressive DTC that is refractory to treatment with RAI. Patients with RAI refractory DTC are defined by four clinical scenarios: (1) metastatic disease with absence of initial RAI uptake, (2) metastatic disease that loses the ability to take up RAI after prior evidence of uptake, (3) presence of RAI uptake in some metastatic lesions but absence in others, and (4) progression of disease despite RAI uptake [60]. In patients with RAI refractory DTC, RAI should be discontinued, and systemic treatments may be considered. Additionally, suppressive levothyroxine treatment is administered in order to maintain a low TSH.

In the pediatric population, there are no criteria to define when to initiate or monitor the response of systemic therapy. The main criteria for initiating systemic therapy in adults include (1) large tumor burden (greater than 1–2 cm), (2) Response Evaluation Criteria in Solid Tumors (RECIST) progressive disease in less than 12 months, and (3) symptomatic disease and the risk of local complications [60]. Given the nature of pediatric DTC, a majority of patients with pulmonary metastasis have diffuse, micronodular disease that makes it challenging to apply the RECIST criteria to, as the lesions typically need to be at least 1 cm [61].

In many patients with DTC, there is abnormal activation of the mitogen-activated protein (MAP) kinase signaling cascade by a tyrosine-kinase receptor, encoded by the *RET* proto-oncogene and other point mutations [60, 62]. Two multitargeted tyrosine kinase inhibitors (MKIs) have been approved for treatment of RAI refractory DTC, lenvatinib and sorafenib [63, 64]. Additionally, there is a growing number of oncogenic-specific targeted inhibitors. These inhibitors tend to have an increased efficacy and decreased toxicity when compared to the MKIs. In patients with unresectable disease, discussion has been had over neoadjuvant therapy prior to surgical resection [65].

Medullary Thyroid Carcinoma

Medullary thyroid carcinoma (MTC) accounts for approximately 5% of pediatric thyroid cancers and originates from the parafollicular C cells. In contrast to adults, pediatric MTC is generally associated with MEN II. MEN II is transmitted in an autosomal dominant pattern and is caused by activating mutations in the *RET* proto-oncogene. The MEN II subtype and tumor phenotype is also associated with the specific *RET* proto-oncogene mutation [40, 54].

Surgical Management

Pediatric patients with MEN II are optimally managed by a prophylactic total thyroidectomy. MEN IIA is categorized into high- and moderate-risk mutations depending on the codon mutation and calcitonin level. In patients with high-risk mutations, a total thyroidectomy should be performed by 5 years of age. In patients with moderate-risk mutations, a total thyroidectomy should be performed in childhood or young adulthood, but it depends on the serum calcitonin levels and trend [66]. If there is a concern for nodal metastasis, then a neck dissection should be considered. However, if there is a low concern for nodal metastasis and the calcitonin level is less than 40 pg/mL, then a prophylactic central neck dissection is not required [66–69].

There is a growing recognition that familial MTC syndrome (FMTC) is a variant along the spectrum of disease in MEN IIA. Therefore, FMTC is treated similarly to MEN IIA with genetic testing, calcitonin levels, and timing over prophylactic thyroidectomy [66]. In patients with MEN IIB, ideally, a thyroidectomy should be performed before the age of 1 year [66]. The benefits of a central neck dissection must be weighed against the risk to the parathyroid glands and post-operative hypocalcemia.

Systemic Therapy

If initial or revision surgery is contraindicated, then systemic therapy can be considered. In patients with MTC, *RET* mutations are the most common oncogenic alteration, and the receptor tyrosine kinase inhibitors have shown a variety of response rates with most patients demonstrating stable disease [70, 71]. Some data has shown that selective *RET* inhibitors yield a favorable response; however there is a dearth of studies in the pediatric population [72].

Conclusion

Pediatric thyroid cancer is a disease with excellent survival outcomes but with an increasing incidence over the last two decades. As more data comes out, the recommendations, treatment, and guidelines will ultimately evolve. There is a consensus on a majority of the treatment approaches for pediatric thyroid cancer. However, there still remains a number of clinical scenarios for which there is no consensus. Is oncogenic testing worthwhile and what should the test include? Does a patient with a papillary thyroid microcarcinoma need a total thyroidectomy, or is a lobectomy enough? What is the utility of a prophylactic central neck dissection? At what point should the patient stop RAI and consider systemic treatment? These are all challenging questions in complex patients that require an open and nuanced discussion between all parties involved with the patient's care from the otolaryngologist, endocrinologist, oncologist, and pediatrician to align with the best treatment for the patient's disease.

References

1. Holmes L, Hossain J, Opara F. Pediatric thyroid carcinoma incidence and temporal trends in the USA (1973–2007): race or shifting diagnostic paradigm? ISRN Oncol. 2012;2012:1–10. https://doi.org/10.5402/2012/906197.
2. Millman B, Pellitteri P. Thyroid carcinoma in children and adolescents. JAMA Otolaryngol Head Neck Surg. 1995;121 https://doi.org/10.1016/B978-0-323-03454-8.50057-7.
3. Vergamini LB, Frazier AL, Abrantes FL, Ribeiro KB, Rodriguez-Galindo C. Increase in the incidence of differentiated thyroid carcinoma in children, adolescents, and young adults: a population-based study. J Pediatr. 2014;164(6):1481–5. https://doi.org/10.1016/j.jpeds.2014.01.059.
4. Al-Qurayshi Z, Hauch A, Srivastav S, Aslam R, Friedlander P, Kandil E. A national perspective of the risk, presentation, and outcomes of pediatric thyroid cancer. JAMA Otolaryngol Head Neck Surg. 2016;142(5):472–8. https://doi.org/10.1001/jamaoto.2016.0104.
5. Niedziela M. Best practice & research clinical endocrinology & metabolism thyroid nodules. Best Pract Res Clin Endocrinol Metab. 2014;28(2):245–77. https://doi.org/10.1016/j.beem.2013.08.007.
6. Hogan AR, Zhuge Y, Perez EA, Koniaris LG, Lew JI, Sola JE. Pediatric thyroid carcinoma: incidence and outcomes in 1753 patients. J Surg Res. 2009;156(1):167–72. https://doi.org/10.1016/j.jss.2009.03.098.
7. Yoshimoto Y, Ezaki H, Etoh R, Hiraoka T. Prevalence rate of thyroid diseases among autopsy cases of the atomic bomb survivors in Hiroshima, 1951-1985. Radiat Res. 1995;141(3):278–86.
8. Hamilton TE, Van Belle G, Logerfo JP. Thyroid neoplasia in Marshall islanders exposed to nuclear fallout. JAMA. 1987;258:629–35.
9. Schonfeld SJ, Lee C, Berrington de González A. Medical exposure to radiation and thyroid cancer. Clin Oncol. 2011;23(4):244–50. https://doi.org/10.1016/j.clon.2011.01.159.
10. Ronckers CM, Sigurdson AJ, Stovall M, et al. Thyroid cancer in childhood cancer survivors: a detailed evaluation of radiation dose response and its modifiers. Radiat Res. 2006;166(4):618–28. https://doi.org/10.1667/RR3605.1.
11. Meadows AT, Friedman DL, Neglia JP, et al. Second neoplasms in survivors of childhood cancer: findings from the childhood cancer survivor study cohort. J Clin Oncol. 2009:2356–62. https://doi.org/10.1200/JCO.2008.21.1920.

12. Morton LM, Karyadi DM, Stewart C, et al. Radiation-related genomic profile of papillary thyroid carcinoma after the Chernobyl accident. Science (1979). 2021;372(6543):eabg2538. https://doi.org/10.1126/science.abg2538.
13. Clement SC, Kremer LCM, Verburg FA, et al. Balancing the benefits and harms of thyroid cancer surveillance in survivors of childhood, adolescent and young adult cancer: recommendations from the International Late Effects of Childhood Cancer Guideline Harmonization Group in collaboration with the PanCareSurFup consortium. Cancer Treat Rev. 2018:28–39. https://doi.org/10.1016/j.ctrv.2017.11.005.
14. Saad AG, Kumar S, Ron E, et al. Proliferative activity of human thyroid cells in various age groups and its correlation with the risk of thyroid cancer after radiation exposure. J Clin Endocrinol Metab. 2006;91(7):2672–7. https://doi.org/10.1210/jc.2006-0417.
15. Klubo-Gwiezdzinska J, Yang L, Merkel R, et al. Results of screening in familial non-medullary thyroid cancer. Thyroid. 2017;27(8):1017–24. https://doi.org/10.1089/thy.2016.0668.
16. Bauer AJ. Clinical behavior and genetics of nonsyndromic, familial nonmedullary thyroid cancer. Frontiers Hormone Res. 2013;41:141–8.
17. Francis GL, Waguespack SG, Bauer AJ, et al. Management guidelines for children with thyroid nodules and differentiated thyroid cancer. Thyroid. 2015;25(7):716–59. https://doi.org/10.1089/thy.2014.0460.
18. Buryk MA, Simons JP, Picarsic J, et al. Can malignant thyroid nodules be distinguished from benign thyroid nodules in children and adolescents by clinical characteristics? A review of 89 pediatric patients with thyroid nodules. Thyroid. 2015;25(4):392–400. https://doi.org/10.1089/thy.2014.0312.
19. Rallison ML, Brown DM, Keating R, Rall JE, Tyler FH. Thyroid nodularity in children. JAMA. 1975;233(10):1069–72.
20. Niedziela M. Pathogenesis, diagnosis and management of thyroid nodules in children. Endocr Relat Cancer. 2006:427–53. https://doi.org/10.1677/erc.1.00882.
21. Gupta A, Ly S, Castroneves LA, et al. A standardized assessment of thyroid nodules in children confirms higher cancer prevalence than in adults. J Clin Endocrinol Metab. 2013;98(8):3238–45. https://doi.org/10.1210/jc.2013-1796.
22. Yeh MW, Bauer AJ, Bernet VA, et al. American thyroid association statement on preoperative imaging for thyroid cancer surgery. Thyroid. 2015;25(1):3–14. https://doi.org/10.1089/thy.2014.0096.
23. Navallas M, Daneman A, Amirabadi A, Ngan B-Y, Wasserman J. Utility of sonography for identifying metastatic cervical adenopathy in children with differentiated thyroid carcinoma at presentation. Pediatr Radiol. 2021;51(2):273–81. https://doi.org/10.1007/s00247-020-04804-z.
24. Martinez-Rios C, Daneman A, Bajno L, van der Kaay DCM, Moineddin R, Wasserman JD. Utility of adult-based ultrasound malignancy risk stratifications in pediatric thyroid nodules. Pediatr Radiol. 2018;48(1):74–84. https://doi.org/10.1007/s00247-017-3974-y.
25. Bauer AJ. Thyroid nodules in children and adolescents. Curr Opin Endocrinol Diabetes Obes. 2019:266–74. https://doi.org/10.1097/MED.0000000000000495.
26. Jia MR, Baran JA, Bauer AJ, et al. Utility of fine-needle aspirations to diagnose pediatric thyroid nodules. Horm Res Paediatr. 2021;94(7–8):263–74. https://doi.org/10.1159/000519307.
27. Monaco SE, Pantanowitz L, Khalbuss WE, et al. Cytomorphological and molecular genetic findings in pediatric thyroid fine-needle aspiration. Cancer Cytopathol. 2012;120(5):342–50. https://doi.org/10.1002/cncy.21199.
28. Xing M, Liu R, Liu X, et al. BRAF V600E and TERT promoter mutations cooperatively identify the most aggressive papillary thyroid cancer with highest recurrence. J Clin Oncol. 2014;32(25):2718–26. https://doi.org/10.1200/JCO.2014.55.5094.
29. Chen Y, Sadow PM, Suh H, et al. BRAFV600E is correlated with recurrence of papillary thyroid microcarcinoma: a systematic review, multi-institutional primary data analysis, and meta-analysis. Thyroid. 2016;26(2):248–55. https://doi.org/10.1089/thy.2015.0391.
30. Xing MM, Alzahrani AS, Carson KA, et al. Association between BRAF V600E mutation and mortality in patients with papillary thyroid cancer. JAMA. 2013;309(14):1493–501. https://doi.org/10.1001/jama.2013.3190.

31. Xing M, Alzahrani AS, Carson KA, et al. Association between BRAF V600E mutation and recurrence of papillary thyroid cancer. J Clin Oncol. 2015;33(1):42–50. https://doi.org/10.1200/JCO.2014.56.8253.
32. Sobrinho-Simões M, Máximo V, Rocha AS, et al. Intragenic mutations in thyroid cancer. Endocrinol Metab Clin North Am. 2008:333–62. https://doi.org/10.1016/j.ecl.2008.02.004.
33. Penko K, Livezey J, Fenton C, et al. BRAF mutations are uncommon in papillary thyroid cancer of young patients. Thyroid. 2005;15(4):320–5. https://doi.org/10.1089/thy.2005.15.320.
34. Mostoufi-Moab S, Labourier E, Sullivan L, et al. Molecular testing for oncogenic gene alterations in pediatric thyroid lesions. Thyroid. 2018;28(1):60–7. https://doi.org/10.1089/thy.2017.0059.
35. Givens DJ, Buchmann LO, Agarwal AM, Grimmer JF, Hunt JP. BRAF V600E does not predict aggressive features of pediatric papillary thyroid carcinoma. Laryngoscope. 2014;124(9):E389. https://doi.org/10.1002/lary.24668.
36. Chakraborty D, Shakya S, Ballal S, Agarwal S, Bal C. BRAF V600Eand TERT promoter mutations in paediatric and young adult papillary thyroid cancer and clinicopathological correlation. J Pediatr Endocrinol Metab. 2020;33(11):1465–74. https://doi.org/10.1515/jpem-2020-0174.
37. Prasad ML, Vyas M, Horne MJ, et al. NTRK fusion oncogenes in pediatric papillary thyroid carcinoma in Northeast United States. Cancer. 2016;122(7):1097–107. https://doi.org/10.1002/cncr.29887.
38. Hamilton CE, Su E, Tawfik D, et al. Assessment of vocal cord motion using laryngeal ultrasound in children: a systematic review and meta-analysis. Pediatr Crit Care Med. 2021;22(10):e532–9. https://doi.org/10.1097/PCC.0000000000002734.
39. Golpanian S, Perez EA, Tashiro J, Lew JI, Sola JE, Hogan AR. Pediatric papillary thyroid carcinoma: outcomes and survival predictors in 2504 surgical patients. Pediatr Surg Int. 2016;32(3):201–8. https://doi.org/10.1007/s00383-015-3855-0.
40. Haugen BR, Alexander EK, Bible KC, et al. 2015 American Thyroid Association management guidelines for adult patients with thyroid nodules and differentiated thyroid cancer: the American Thyroid Association guidelines task force on thyroid nodules and differentiated thyroid cancer. Thyroid. 2016;26(1):1–133. https://doi.org/10.1089/thy.2015.0020.
41. Hay ID, Gonzalez-Losada T, Reinalda MS, Honetschlager JA, Richards ML, Thompson GB. Long-term outcome in 215 children and adolescents with papillary thyroid cancer treated during 1940 through 2008. World J Surg. 2010;34(6):1192–202. https://doi.org/10.1007/s00268-009-0364-0.
42. Jarząb B, Handkiewicz-Junak D, Włoch J. Juvenile differentiated thyroid carcinoma and the role of radioiodine in its treatment: a qualitative review. Endocr Relat Cancer. 2005:773–803. https://doi.org/10.1677/erc.1.00880.
43. Memeh K, Ruhle B, Alsafran S, et al. Total thyroidectomy vs thyroid lobectomy for localized papillary thyroid cancer in children: a propensity-matched survival analysis. J Am Coll Surg (Elsevier Inc.). 2021;233:39–49.
44. Sudoko CK, Jenks CM, Bauer AJ, et al. Thyroid lobectomy for T1 papillary thyroid carcinoma in pediatric patients. JAMA Otolaryngol Head Neck Surg. 2021;147(11):943–50. https://doi.org/10.1001/jamaoto.2021.2359.
45. Kluijfhout WP, Pasternak JD, van der Kaay D, Vriens MR, Propst EJ, Wasserman JD. Is it time to reconsider lobectomy in low-risk paediatric thyroid cancer? Clin Endocrinol. 2017;86(4):591–6. https://doi.org/10.1111/cen.13287.
46. Sugino K, Nagahama M, Kitagawa W, et al. Risk stratification of pediatric patients with differentiated thyroid cancer: is total thyroidectomy necessary for patients at any risk? Thyroid. 2020;30(4):548–56. https://doi.org/10.1089/thy.2019.0231.
47. Popovtzer A, Shpitzer T, Bahar G, Feinmesser R, Segal K. Thyroid cancer in children: management and outcome experience of a referral center. Otolaryngol Head Neck Surg. 2006;135(4):581–4. https://doi.org/10.1016/j.otohns.2006.04.004.
48. Savio R, Gosnell J, Palazzo FF, et al. The role of a more extensive surgical approach in the initial multimodality management of papillary thyroid cancer in children. J Pediatr Surg. 2005;40(11):1696–700. https://doi.org/10.1016/j.jpedsurg.2005.07.029.

49. MacHens A, Lorenz K, Nguyen TP, Brauckhoff M, Dralle H. Papillary thyroid cancer in children and adolescents does not differ in growth pattern and metastatic behavior. J Pediatr. 2010;157(4):648–52. https://doi.org/10.1016/j.jpeds.2010.04.026.
50. Yu YR, Fallon SC, Carpenter JL, et al. Perioperative determinants of transient hypocalcemia after pediatric total thyroidectomy. J Pediatr Surg. 2017;52(5):684–8. https://doi.org/10.1016/j.jpedsurg.2017.01.011.
51. Hanba C, Svider PF, Siegel B, et al. Pediatric thyroidectomy: hospital course and perioperative complications. Otolaryngol Head Neck Surg (United States). 2017;156(2):360–7. https://doi.org/10.1177/0194599816677527.
52. Baumgarten HD, Bauer AJ, Isaza A, Mostoufi-Moab S, Kazahaya K, Adzick NS. Surgical management of pediatric thyroid disease: complication rates after thyroidectomy at the Children's Hospital of Philadelphia high-volume Pediatric Thyroid Center. J Pediatr Surg. 2019;54(10):1969–75. https://doi.org/10.1016/j.jpedsurg.2019.02.009.
53. Nettore IC, Colao A, Macchia PE. Nutritional and environmental factors in thyroid carcinogenesis. Int J Environ Res Public Health. 2018; https://doi.org/10.3390/ijerph15081735.
54. Bauer AJ. Pediatric thyroid cancer: genetics, therapeutics and outcome. Endocrinol Metab Clin North Am. 2020:589–611. https://doi.org/10.1016/j.ecl.2020.08.001.
55. Lin X, Zhu B, Liu Y, Silverman JF. Follicular thyroid carcinoma invades venous rather than lymphatic vessels. Diagn Pathol. 2010;5(1):8.
56. Dionigi G, Kraimps J-L, Schmid KW, et al. Minimally invasive follicular thyroid cancer(MIFTC)—a consensus report of the European Society of Endocrine Surgeons (ESES). Langenbecks Arch Surg. 2014;399:165–84.
57. Leong D, Gill AJ, Turchini J, et al. The prognostic impact of extent of vascular invasion in follicular thyroid carcinoma. World J Surg. 2023;47(2):412–20. https://doi.org/10.1007/s00268-022-06696-6.
58. Mete O, Asa SL. Pathological definition and clinical significance of vascular invasion in thyroid carcinomas of follicular epithelial derivation. Mod Pathol. 2011;24(12):1545–52. https://doi.org/10.1038/modpathol.2011.119.
59. Bojarsky M, Baran JA, Halada S, et al. Outcomes of ATA low-risk pediatric thyroid cancer patients not treated with radioactive iodine therapy. J Clin Endocrinol Metab. 2023;108(12):3338–44. https://doi.org/10.1210/clinem/dgad322.
60. Berdelou A, Lamartina L, Klain M, Leboulleux S, Schlumberger M. Treatment of refractory thyroid cancer. Endocr Relat Cancer. 2018:R209–23. https://doi.org/10.1530/ERC-17-0542.
61. Eisenhauer EA, Therasse P, Bogaerts J, et al. New response evaluation criteria in solid tumours: revised RECIST guideline (version 1.1). Eur J Cancer. 2009;45(2):228–47. https://doi.org/10.1016/j.ejca.2008.10.026.
62. Covell LL, Ganti AK. Treatment of advanced thyroid cancer: role of molecularly targeted therapies. Target Oncol. 2015:311–24. https://doi.org/10.1007/s11523-014-0331-z.
63. Waguespack SG, Sherman SI, Williams MD, Clayman GL, Herzog CE. The successful use of Sorafenib to treat pediatric papillary thyroid carcinoma. Thyroid. 2009;19(4):407–12.
64. Mahajan P, Dawrant J, Kheradpour A, et al. Response to lenvatinib in children with papillary thyroid carcinoma. Thyroid. 2018;28(11):1450–4. https://doi.org/10.1089/thy.2018.0064.
65. Kazahaya K, Prickett KK, Paulson VA, et al. Targeted oncogene therapy before surgery in pediatric patients with advanced invasive thyroid cancer at initial presentation: is it time for a paradigm shift? JAMA Otolaryngol Head Neck Surg. 2020;146(8):748–53. https://doi.org/10.1001/jamaoto.2020.1340.
66. Wells SA, Asa SL, Dralle H, et al. Revised American thyroid association guidelines for the management of medullary thyroid carcinoma. Thyroid. 2015;25(6):567–610. https://doi.org/10.1089/thy.2014.0335.
67. Rohmer V, Vidal-Trecan G, Bourdelot A, et al. Prognostic factors of disease-free survival after thyroidectomy in 170 young patients with a RET germline mutation: a multicenter study of the Groupe Français d'Etude des Tumeurs Endocrines. J Clin Endocrinol Metab. 2011;96(3):E509. https://doi.org/10.1210/jc.2010-1234.

68. Niccoli-Sire P, Murat A, Rohmer V, et al. When should thyroidectomy be performed in familial medullary thyroid carcinoma gene carriers with non-cysteine RET mutations? n.d. https://doi.org/10.1016/S0039-6060(03)00490-2.
69. Machens A, Schneyer U, Holzhausen HJ, Dralle H. Prospects of remission in medullary thyroid carcinoma according to basal calcitonin level. J Clin Endocrinol Metab. 2005;90(4):2029–34. https://doi.org/10.1210/jc.2004-1836.
70. Weitzman SP, Cabanillas ME. The treatment landscape in thyroid cancer: a focus on cabozantinib. Cancer Manag Res. 2015;7:265–78. https://doi.org/10.2147/CMAR.S68373.
71. Fox E, Widemann BC, Chuk MK, et al. Vandetanib in children and adolescents with multiple endocrine neoplasia type 2b associated medullary thyroid carcinoma. Clin Cancer Res. 2013;19(15):4239–48. https://doi.org/10.1158/1078-0432.CCR-13-0071.
72. Thein KZ, Velcheti V, Mooers BHM, Wu J, Subbiah V. Precision therapy for RET-altered cancers with RET inhibitors. Trends Cancer. 2021:1074–88. https://doi.org/10.1016/j.trecan.2021.07.003.

25 History of Parathyroid Disorders and Management

Natasha Quraishi and Muhammad S. Quraishi

The parathyroid glands have been described as the last endocrine organs to be discovered. The eventful journey of these tiny glands from the discovery of their existence to uncovering their function and linking them with disease to the development of cutting-edge technology in disease management spans less than two centuries.

Prathamesh Pai

Discovering the Parathyroid Glands

The first description of the parathyroid glands is often cited as that by Sir Richard Owen, after he observed them during the dissection of a rhinoceros at London Zoo during the mid-nineteenth century [1]. However, the story of this discovery is not so simple, and the credit to Owen came nearly a century later.

The London Zoological Society purchased a male Indian rhinoceros on 24th May 1834 for 1000 guineas. This had been requested by Sir Richard Owen who was Hunterian Professor at the Royal College of Surgeons. The rhinoceros died 15 years later on 19th November 1849, and Owen subsequently performed an autopsy over a period of months [2]. During this autopsy, he wrote of finding that "a small compact yellow glandular body was attached to the thyroid at the point where the veins emerge" [1–3]. Owen did not describe or examine this gland further, and so there was no microscopic analysis at this stage. The gland was included in a specimen

N. Quraishi
Bradford Royal Infirmary, Bradford, UK
e-mail: natasha.quraishi@nhs.net

M. S. Quraishi (✉)
Doncaster Royal Infirmary, Doncaster, UK
e-mail: muhamad.quraishi@nhs.net

P. S. Pai et al. (eds.), *Controversies in Cancer of the Thyroid and Parathyroid Glands*, https://doi.org/10.1007/978-3-032-13130-0_25

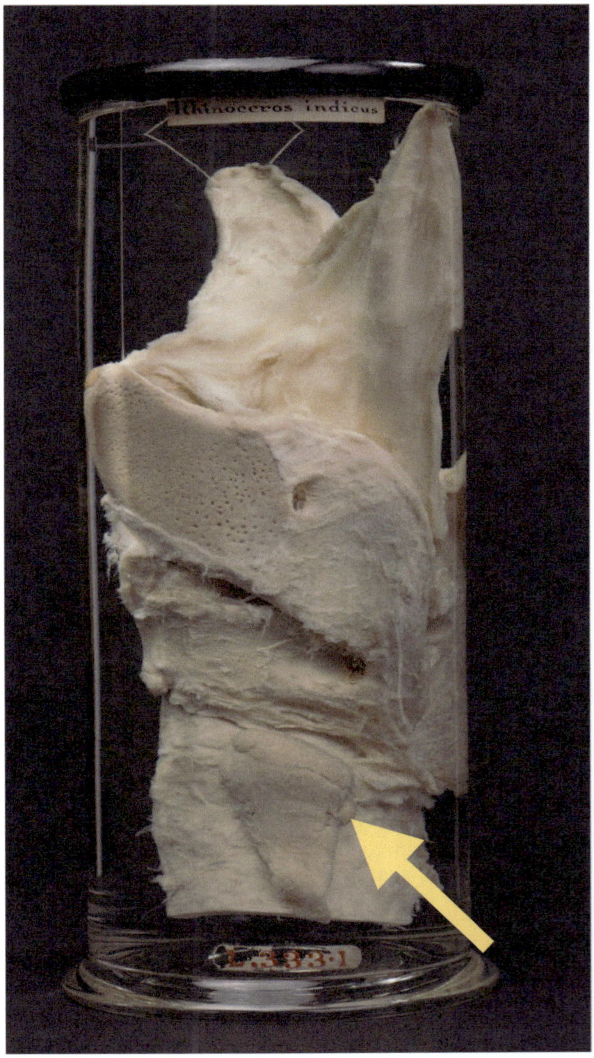

Image 25.1 Yellow arrow indicating the parathyroid gland observed in an Indian rhinoceros by Sir Richard Owen. (Image by kind permission of the Royal College of Surgeons of England)

with the larynx, trachea and thyroid of the rhinoceros which remains at the Hunterian Museum at the Royal College of Surgeons of England [1, 2] (Image 25.1).

Owen presented his findings in a lecture at the Zoological Society on 12th February 1850. In 1852 his work was then accepted for publication as a journal article [2]. Initially it was thought that this paper was published as part of volume in 1862; however, this changed in 1953. Professor AJE Cave, the man who followed Owen to become Professor of Anatomy at the Royal College of Surgeons, discovered that Owen's paper had been published separately 10 years earlier in March 1852, and thus he termed the parathyroid glands "the glands of Owen", cementing Owen's status as the first person to describe the parathyroid glands [4, 5].

Owen was followed by others in Europe who gave descriptions that are felt to have been of the parathyroid gland such as Robert Remak in Berlin in 1855 who described a corresponding tissue in a cat [6, 7]. Remak was followed by the renowned German pathologist, Rudolf Virchow, who noted a structure in the neck that may have been the parathyroid gland as early as 1863. However, he did not give it a name or attribute any importance to it at that time [7–9].

The next commonly lauded description of the parathyroid glands was by Ivar Sandström who detailed the glands in human cadavers while a medical student in 1880 in his monograph "On a New Gland in Man and Fellow Animals" [1, 10]. Sandström is commonly described as the first person to report the parathyroid glands in humans. It has been suggested that in 1881 Cresswell Baber observed the parathyroid glands as well [11]. Sandström initially identified the gland in animals. He then dissected 50 human cadavers, of which in 43 he found two glands, one on either side. He then took the further step of examining these glands under the microscope, naming them "glandulae parathyroidea" [7, 10, 12].

However, Sandström's discovery was hampered by difficulties he faced in publishing his findings. He initially submitted his report to Rudolf Virchow's German journal, but his paper was rejected. The given reason was the length of paper (there are varying reports of a length of 30–50 pages), although it has been suggested that the real cause for the rebuff was that Virchow may have realised that Sandström was describing what Virchow himself had observed earlier in 1863 and did not wish for the credit to go to another [9, 13]. Ultimately, Sandström's findings were published in a local Swedish journal, the *Upsala Läkareförenings Förhandlingar*, and so did not receive any immediate recognition [5].

Much later, in 1907, William Halsted and Herbert Evans would describe and illustrate the blood supply to human parathyroid glands [14]. Furthermore, the work of John Gilmour in 1938 would illustrate the presence of four parathyroid glands in 87% of 400 cases that he autopsied [15].

Understanding the Function of the Parathyroid Glands

In order to appreciate the development of mankind's understanding of the function of the parathyroid glands, it is important to begin with the history of tetany. This term describes patients experiencing a range of neuromuscular symptoms such as cramps, spasms and perioral paraesthesia and is now known to be caused by electrolyte derangements such as hypocalcaemia which in turn could be induced by parathyroidectomy. The term was thought to have been coined by Lucien Corvisart in 1852 [16]. This notion was further developed in 1862 by Trousseau's description of carpal spasm resulting from brachial artery occlusion in the presence of tetany [17]. Chvostek then noted in 1876 that in tetany, percussion of the facial nerve elicited facial spasms [18]. While Trousseau and Chvostek described clinical signs of tetany which have carried their names to the present day, they did not advance the understanding of what caused tetany.

Further seeds in the understanding of tetany were sown in 1879 when Anton Wölfler noted its symptoms in a patient following total thyroidectomy by Theodor Billroth [19]. Wölfler posited that the cause of the patient's symptoms was "hyperaemia" of the brain. It has been suggested that the link between tetany and thyroidectomy may have been discerned by William Halsted who compared the post-operative outcomes of Theodor Billroth and Theodor Kocher. He contrasted Billroth's rapid surgical technique with Kocher's more careful and painstaking approach which involved subcapsular dissection. He observed that Billroth had greater post-operative rates of tetany and voice change than Kocher [7, 9]. Halsted did not publish his findings until 1920 [7, 20].

Ultimately the linking of tetany to the parathyroid glands has been attributed to Eugene Gley, a French physiologist and endocrinologist, who became acquainted with Sandström's work in 1890 [11]. In 1891, Gley described tetany induced by the removal of parathyroid glands during a thyroidectomy in a dog [21]. His series of animal experiments where thyroidectomy and parathyroidectomy were performed together resulted in a tetany rate of 90% [22]. Subsequently Gley discovered that removal of the parathyroids also led to tetany [9]. It should also be noted that it was thanks to Gley's reference to Sandström's earlier work that Sandström finally achieved recognition for his identification of the human parathyroid gland [5].

Alfred Kohn of Prague established the presence of four parathyroid glands in animal subjects between 1895 and 1896 [23, 24]. Also in 1896, Francesco Generali and Giulio Vassale reported they had found tetany to occur following the removal of all the parathyroid glands alone which they felt highlighted the parathyroid glands to have their own unique function separate to the thyroid gland [25]. They found death to occur sooner than in animals who had undergone parathyroidectomy only in comparison with those who had undergone thyroidectomy combined with parathyroidectomy. These findings lead to the theory that the parathyroids were involved in detoxification of the circulation [7, 26, 27]. Walter Edmunds further demonstrated that following a thyroidectomy, the parathyroid glands do not transform into thyroid tissue [28].

Connecting the Parathyroid Gland to Calcium

The function of the parathyroid gland remained linked to the theory of detoxification into the early twentieth century. However, work was afoot to further understand the parathyroid gland. Firstly in 1898, Meusseu reported remedying tetany in dogs caused by removal of the parathyroid gland by the administration of parathyroid gland extract derived from horses [29]. Subsequently, in 1901 Jacques Loeb found that by administering salts that rendered calcium insoluble, he could induce tetany in animal subject [30]. In 1907, William Halsted described the use of parathyroid extract to treat tetany [14].

The suggestion of a link between the parathyroid glands and calcium finally came in 1909. In 1905 William George MacCallum had established that tetany was alleviated by injections of parathyroid extract but believed this to be due to the extract neutralising a toxin [11, 31]. Then in 1909 he and Carl Voegtlin linked tetany to hypocalcaemia which was could be remedied through injections of calcium or parathyroid tissue (they also found that potassium and sodium did not treat tetany)

[32]. Then in 1914 McCallum found that by causing hypocalcaemia in dogs via dialysis, he was able to induce tetany which he could then alleviate with injections of normal blood but not with blood without calcium. From this he concluded that the mechanism by which removal of the parathyroid glands led to tetany was through hypocalcaemia [33]. Later in 1923, Harald Salvesen also posited that parathyroidectomy caused hypocalcaemia and felt this was what caused tetany [34].

Similarly, also in 1909, Berkeley and Beebe demonstrated treatment of parathyroidectomy-induced tetany using bovine parathyroid extract. Specifically, from this extract they were able to isolate a nucleoprotein which appeared to remedy the tetany [35]. In 1911 Isidor Greenwald reported noting the decrease in urinary excretion of phosphate in dogs who had undergone parathyroid removal [36]. Further development in the understanding of parathyroid function was aided by Adolf Hanson's work as a student at the University of Minnesota in 1923. Hanson used bovine parathyroid to cultivate a parathyroid extract that was stable and could be reproduced [37].

By 1925, James Bertram Collip had formulated a strong variety of the parathyroid extract which he found normalised calcium level in animals without parathyroid glands and was prophylactic against tetany [38]. This extract was used by Greenwald and Gross to induce hypercalcaemia in dogs. This further demonstrated the action of the parathyroid gland on calcium [27].

Linking the Parathyroid Gland to Disease

In parallel to the developments on understanding the function of the parathyroid gland, events were also underway that would lead to the link between the parathyroid gland and disease. Indeed, as early as 1864, Gerhard Engel discussed a case where a patient was noted to have what may have been parathyroid adenoma in addition to bony disease [39]. However, the more famous precipitating event occurred in 1891 when Friedrich von Recklinghausen published a case series of patients with skeletal abnormalities, namely, decalcification of the bone. At that time this condition was termed von Recklinghausen's disease of bone; however it is now known as osteitis fibrosa cystica, the skeletal changes that occur in hyperparathryroidism. Interestingly, von Recklinghausen reported a cervical nodule found at post-mortem in one of these patients [40]. This finding was echoed in 1903 in Geneva by Swiss pathologist Max Askanazy who noted a nodule in the neck of patient with osteitis fibrosa cystica upon whom he was performing an autopsy. He did not, however, link these two findings [41]. There were further reports of similar findings from others such as Schmorl (1907), Molineus and Poltaf (1913) and Harbits (1915) [7, 27].

This connection between skeletal disease and parathyroid malfunction was established through the work of Jakob Erdheim in Vienna in 1906. He eliminated the parathyroid gland tissue in rats following which he observed not only tetany but also demineralisation of the incisors which he was then able to reverse through the grafting of parathyroid tissue obtained from another rat [42]. Erdheim furthered this by noting enlarged parathyroid glands when studying patients who died with skeletal disease in 1907 [43]. Sadly, the conclusion drawn from this work was that the parathyroid glands became enlarged due to the skeletal disease which later proved to be incorrect [7, 27, 44].

The correct theory of parathyroid enlargement causing bony changes was first posited by Friedrich Schlagenhaufer of Vienna in 1915, following post-mortems on patients who were found to have bony disease and an enlarged parathyroid gland. Based on this theory, Schlagenhaufer advocated parathyroidectomy to treat skeletal disease. However, it is believed that a decade passed before this was done [5, 7, 27, 44, 45].

The First Parathyroidectomy

The achievement of the first parathyroidectomy is most commonly attributed to Felix Mandl in 1925 [46]. Mandl was assistant to Julius von Hochenegg, Professor of Surgery at the University Clinic in Vienna. The patient was a 38-year-old man named Albert Gahne. At the age of 34, Gahne had experienced musculoskeletal pains in his lower limbs in addition to fatigue. A radiograph 2 years later was deemed to show osteopenia and cystic changes characteristic of osteitis fibrosa cystica. He later developed a bony fracture. When Mandl initially reviewed him, he noted hypercalcaemia and raised urinary calcium excretion. Mandl attempted to treat this with a cadaveric parathyroid gland transplant based on the detoxification theory; however this was to no avail.

Mandl then attempted to approach the issue using Schlagenhaufer's theory and so on 30th July performed surgical exploration of the neck under local anaesthesia. During the procedure he found and removed a 21 × 15 × 12 mm mass in close proximity to the inferior thyroid artery. This mass was subsequently examined under the microscope and was found to be a parathyroid adenoma. Following the procedure, Gahne experienced a significant improvement in his condition such that a radiograph 4 months post-operatively showed an increase in his bone density and his bony pain had resolved within 6 months of the operation.

Gahne remained asymptomatic for 6 years, after which he developed renal calculi. Mandl repeated a surgical exploration of the neck and removed further parathyroid glands including one in thyroid tissue excised as part of a subtotal thyroidectomy. However, the parathyroid glands appeared normal microscopically, and Gahne's symptoms persisted. Following Gahne's death 3 years later, no parathyroid abnormality was found at post-mortem. However, despite this sad ending, Gahne had afforded Mandl the opportunity to prove that parathyroidectomy was a valid treatment [1, 5, 7, 9, 12, 44].

Some months prior to Mandl's success, parathyroidectomy had been attempted unsuccessfully by Oscar Hirsch also in Vienna in April 1925. Hirsch had performed a neck exploration in a patient with bony disease but, however, was unable to find any parathyroid pathology [5, 7].

Some have argued that the first parathyroidectomy was actually performed earlier than Mandl's much feted case, by Sir John Bland-Sutton, as he described the procedure in the sixth edition of his book *Tumours: Innocent and Malignant* published in 1917 [47]. Bland-Sutton described a case of a woman on board a ship who began to experience difficulty breathing and who was noted to have a neck lump. She underwent a tracheotomy on board the ship, and when she returned to England, Bland-Sutton removed the neck mass stating "it had the microscopic features of a parathyroid" [48].

The first parathyroidectomy performed in the USA was reportedly performed at the Cook Hospital in Chicago by E. J. Lewis, less than 6 months after Mandl [11].

Four months later, another famous example of parathyroid disease and early parathyroid surgery is the case of Captain Charles E Martell which provided ample opportunity for further learning. Fuller Albright presented Martell's case of hyperparathyroidism while he was President of the American Society for Endocrinology [5].

A merchant seaman, Martell began to develop symptoms of hyperparathyroidism at the age of 22 in 1918. He experienced right loin pain after a fall and then developed further pain around the body over the next year. Martell's colleagues noted that his build was changing and he also began to develop urinary calculi. He began to feel lethargic as well despite continuing to work until 1922. Unfortunately, Martell then suffered a fracture of his left radius and ulna in 1923. Subsequent radiographs of these bones revealed osteomalacia. In 1924 Martell trialled a number of unsuccessful treatments while admitted at Marine Hospital on Statton Island. Then in 1926 he was treated by Eugene Dubois at the Bellevue Hospital in New York. During this admission, Martell underwent tests which revealed hypercalcaemia, hypophosphataemia and hypercalciuria which Dubois observed to be akin to the results seen in trials where excessive amounts of Collip's parathyroid extract had been given. Dubois also noted that Collip's extract caused Martell to experience a worsening of his symptoms. Therefore, Dubois inferred "a search for some abnormality of the parathyroid glands was the next step indicated" [49].

Martell was then shifted to Massachusetts General Hospital where he underwent numerous failed explorations where normal parathyroid glands had been excised [50]. Edward D. Churchill and Oliver Cope successfully found a 3 cm by 3 cm parathyroid tumour in the mediastinum during a repeat exploration in 1932. In order to access the tumour, a sternal split was required. In an attempt to stave off post-operative tetany, 10% of the gland was re-implanted. Regardless, Martell experienced post-operative tetany 3 days after the procedure which required treatment with intravenous calcium chloride and Collip's extract. He then developed a renal calculus that was impacted and necessitated operative management. Following this procedure, Martell experienced laryngospasm and sadly passed away [7].

Cope and Churchill dealt with 343 cases of hyperparathyroidism between 1930 and 1965, of which they gave detailed accounts [51]. They would also publish papers discussing post-operative complications such as tetany and renal calculi [52]. Churchill and Cope's expertise provided pearls of wisdom that still ring true with Churchill advising "the success of parathyroid surgery must lie in the ability of the surgeon to know a parathyroid when he sees one, to know the distribution of the glands, where they hide, and also be delicate enough in technique to be able to use this knowledge" [51]. In 1931, James Walton, of London, advised "wide exposure is essential, for not only is it necessary to explore all the parathyroid glands, but also sometimes to search behind the trachea and in the mediastinum" [11].

Another notable early case of parathyroid surgery was that of Elva Dawkins in the USA. Dawkins experienced urinary and musculoskeletal symptoms resulting in a presentation to Barnes Hospital in St Louis, Missouri, in 1927. David Barr and Harold Bulger observed that her case appeared to be similar to the findings in experiments where excessive doses of Collip's extract had been given to dogs. In 1928 neck exploration was performed revealing a parathyroid mass approximately 3 cm in size. Unfortunately, Dawkins developed tetany following the procedure and so was treated with "heroic doses of parathormone and oral calcium" [53]. With time Dawkins's symptoms improved. Barr and Bulger's work with their colleague Henry Dixon contributed to the understanding of hyperparathyroidism as they advocated that it caused osteitis fibrosa cystica. Indeed, they are thought to have coined the term "hyperparathyroidism" and delineated five key features of this condition (hypercalcaemia, hypercalciuria and urinary calcium stones, muscular weakness and reduced tone, reduced bone density and cystic tumours of the bone) [54].

Better Understanding of Parathyroid Disease

In 1925 James Collip confirmed the role of parathyroid hormone in calcium regulation when he found that parathyroidectomy-induced tetany was alleviated by parathyroid hormone extract [55]. Initially hyperparathyroidism was considered to be a condition that was diagnosed on clinical presentation characterised by bony disease and urinary calculi [44].

Fuller Albright's work in the 1930s was a crucial period in the understanding of hyperparathyroidism [28]. He described the presence of renal calculi due to hyperparathyroidism in 80% of his patients and was amongst the first surgeons to screen for primary hyperparathyroidism in patients suffering from renal calculi [27]. He and Bloomberg and colleagues advocated that single or multigland parathyroid adenoma, parathyroid hyperplasia and parathyroid carcinoma caused primary hyperparathyroidism [5]. Albright also discriminated between primary, secondary and tertiary hyperparathyroidism in the book *The Parathyroid Glands and Metabolic Bone Disease: Selected Studies* which he wrote in 1948 with Reifenstein [5]. This text was regarded as a classic [56].

In 1932 Fuller Albright became amongst the first to describe the excision of a parathyroid adenoma in a patient with renal calculi and significant hypercalcaemia. He went on to describe how serum calcium levels normalised post-operatively [12]. Understanding of the effects of hyperparathyroidism was furthered in 1946 by Milton Rofers and Raymond Keating who described a link between peptic ulcer disease and parathyroid disease [27]. In 1948, Barnicott reported how parathyroid hormone caused resorption of bone [28]. Jahan and Pitts also detailed its effect of reducing urinary excretion of calcium and magnesium in 1948 [28]. The now classic phrase "bones, stones and abdominal groans" was coined by Walter St Goar [27]. In 1957 Cope and colleagues also observed a link between pancreatitis and hyperparathyroidism [27].

Advancements in Testing

In 1951 in the USA, Leonard Skeggs invented an autoanalyser to perform diagnostic testing. In 1954 this model was acquired by the Technician company. 1959 saw the development of reliable and reproducible extraction of parathyroid hormone. Popularity increased over subsequent years, and with further innovation, analysis of serum levels became quicker and less expensive [44]. In 1959 Rasmussen and Craig isolated and purified parathyroid hormone, going on to delineate its polypeptide structure in 1962 [57, 58].

In 1963 Solomon Berson and Rosalyn Yalow developed the immunoassay of parathyroid hormone [59], and the latter received the Nobel Prize for Medicine and Physiology for her work on radioimmunoassays of peptide hormones in 1977. Then in 1987 Samuel Nussbaum at Massachusetts General Hospital formulated a method for the rapid detection of parathyroid hormone which enabled the technique of intraoperative testing to confirm successful parathyroid exploration [60]. Alongst the earliest use of intraoperative parathyroid hormone assay was that reported in early 1990s by Irvin and colleagues [61].

The Age of Asymptomatic Hyperparathyroidism

These technological advancements led to the rise of the diagnosis of asymptomatic hyperparathyroidism through the incidental finding of hypercalcaemia where hyperparathyroidism less frequently presented with end organ damage [44]. An apparent increase in the incidence of asymptomatic hyperparathyroidism was described over the twentieth century. In Washington DC, in 1977, Robert Coffey compared an incidence of asymptomatic hyperparathyroidism of 5% prior to 1970 with 40% after 1970 [62]. The Mayo Clinic reinforced this impression, reporting of all their cases of hyperparathyroidism between 1974 and 1980, 64% were asymptomatic [27].

Alongside the increase in asymptomatic hyperparathyroidism, the rates of parathyroidectomy also increased to the extent that in the 1970s all asymptomatic hyperparathyroidism patients were reportedly offered parathyroidectomy [63].

Progression of Parathyroid Surgery and Pathology

Initial surgical methods included identifying all 4 glands [64] and then removing 3.5 glands, the rationale being that this technique would reduce the changes of recurrence [65]. This procedure was complicated by a 10% tetany rate [44]. From the 1920s until the 1970s, the technique utilised was the exploration of the neck through the transverse cervical skin crease Kocher incision. The subsequent exploration could take varying amounts of time depending on what was found and if frozen section analysis by histopathologists confirmed parathyroid adenoma [1].

As previously described, at Massachusetts General Hospital, Cope and colleagues had built extensive experience from the 1930s. In a case series of 200 cases published in 1958. They described 158 (79%) of cases having single gland adenoma, 10 cases (5%) having double adenomas, 14 cases (7%) having water clear-cell type parathyroid hyperplasia and 10 cases (5%) having chief-cell type hyperplasia [66]. Case series of parathyroid surgery were published not only by Cope and colleagues at Massachusetts General Hospital but also by Marden Black at the Mayo Clinic, John Hellstrom in Stockholm and Ernest Morrison in Northern Ireland [27].

Alongside surgical advances, appreciation for the variety of different underlying pathological entities which would cause hyperparathyroidism arose [44]. Chiu-an Wang of Massachusetts General Hospital published a paper following up Cope's double adenoma cases and noted that many had had recurrences, and therefore it was concluded that double adenomas may actually be hyperplasia [67]. Subtotal parathyroidectomy was a technique utilised for multigland disease and involved the sparing of 60 mg of a gland [27].

Secondary Hyperparathyroidism

Secondary hyperparathyroidism describes hyperparathyroidism due to a stimulus that is external to the parathyroid glands, e.g. impaired renal function. Surgical management of this condition grew with subtotal parathyroidectomy being advocated to treat this form of hyperparathyroidism [68].

Parathyroid Cancer

Malignancy of the parathyroid glands is extremely rare. It was initially described in 1929 by Russell Wilder [69]. By 1973, diagnostic histopathological criteria had been developed [70, 71]. Surgery in the form of an en bloc resection has become the established approach to parathyroid cancer [44].

Multiple Endocrine Neoplasia

Parathyroid hyperplasia is now known to be associated with multiple endocrine neoplasia type 1 (MEN1) and type 2A (MEN2A). The traits common to MEN1 were first described by Paul Wermer in 1954 where he observed them in a family where the father and four of the nine children had these characteristics [72]. Thompson described his approach to MEN1 cases involving total parathyroidectomy and cervical thymectomy [27]. MEN2A was then described John H Sipple in

1961 when he observed a patient with parathyroid hyperplasia, thyroid carcinoma and bilateral phaeochromocytomas [73]. Since then, a greater understanding of MEN and its associated hyperparathyroidism has developed, and it is considered that hyperparathyroidism associated with MEN1 is more severe than that associated with MEN2A and so the management differs according to the underlying MEN type [74].

Parathyroid Localisation

Chiu-an Wang of Massachusetts General Hospital was an early advocate of minimally invasive parathyroidectomy, undertaking unilateral neck explorations under the guidance of USS as early as 1981. He would excise the apparent parathyroid adenoma and take a biopsy of the other ipsilateral parathyroid gland and then performed a mannitol density test on the table to compare the fat content of the two glands to confirm that an adenoma had been removed. Where there was a significant difference, he could consider the procedure to be successful and complete; where there was no difference, Wang would then undertake exploration of the contralateral neck considering multigland hyperplasia to be the possible diagnosis. His re-operation rate using this method was 1–2% [11]. As there was a shift towards single gland resection, there also began an interest in gland localisation.

Since the 1950s there had been various techniques described for the localisation of the culprit parathyroid glands such as cine-oesophagoscopy and arteriography [44]. During the 1960s toluidine blue was utilised in dogs and then in humans [75]. Methylene blue quickly superseded due to cardiotoxicity associated with toluidine blue [76]. Methylene blue, however, is not completely without risk as it has been associated with adverse reactions in patients who take serotonergic medication. Its use is not widespread [77]. Ellis describes his first use of methylene blue during parathyroid surgery in 1975. He described how following induction of anaesthesia the methylene blue was injected intravenously and then would be preferentially taken up by the parathyroid glands, thus highlighting them to the naked eye. The surgeon would then remove the largest one as this was considered to be the adenoma. He went to explain how when he utilised methylene blue the patient may also go blue post-operatively [1].

Selective venous catheterisation was described by John Potts at Massachusetts General [78] and is where a catheter is placed through the femoral vein, inferior vena cava, right heart and neck veins. Blood samples are taken to pinpoint the area where there is the highest level of parathyroid hormone and in this way locates the parathyroid gland that is overactive. This technique was initially considered helpful in revision cases [79]; however due to the possibility of significant morbidity, it is currently only performed in certain centres [44].

Since the 1970s, ultrasonography (USS) has been considered a helpful tool in identifying culprit glands with parathyroid adenoma especially with Doppler enabling distinction from other tissues through its illustration of circulation [44]. Around this time computerised tomography (CT) also began to be utilised for parathyroid gland localisation [27]. In the 1980s, Coakley and colleagues were responsible for introducing what has become the stalwart of parathyroid assessment: the Tc 99 sestamibi (MIBI) scanning [80]. Contemporary practice often consists of both USS and sestamibi to localise parathyroid glands and facilitate a focussed parathyroid exploration that is minimally invasive [44].

Parathyroid Transplantation

In 1885 the first parathyroid transplant was alleged to have been performed by Schift and Horsley [5]. Then in 1892 von Eiselberg carried out autotransplantation of the parathyroids in the abdomen of cats. Following this he demonstrated that there was no tetany in his subjects until the parathyroids were removed [81]. He also demonstrated the formation of new blood vessels after this operation [9]. It has been proposed that Herman Pfeiffer and Otto Meyer first performed parathyroid autograft successfully in puppies in 1907 [11]. In 1909 William Halsted successfully performed a parathyroid autotransplant in a canine subject, finding it to be lifesaving as a treatment for tetany [82].

Over time, as an appreciation for the link between parathyroid glands and tetany developed, there were further attempts to perform autotransplantation of the parathyroid glands [11]. In 1926, Frank Howard Lahey reported autotransplanting parathyroid tissue into sternocleidomastoid [83]. Then in 1976, Sam Wells published descriptions of his practice of autotransplanting parathyroid into the forearm after excising all the glands as opposed to simply performing a subtotal parathyroidectomy, with the rationale being that should the patient develop hyperparathyroidism once more, the autotransplanted tissue could be excised [84, 85].

Conclusion

Due to the efforts of numerous people across the world over a short couple of centuries, our understanding of the parathyroid glands has rapidly developed from acknowledging their existence to uncovering their function to the innovative technological advances that now inform the assessment and management of their numerous pathologies.

References

1. Ellis H. The story of parathyroid surgery. J Perioper Pract. 2020;30(7–8):240–1.
2. Felger EA, Zeiger MA. The death of an Indian rhinoceros. World J Surg. 2010;34(8):1805–10.
3. Owen R III. On the anatomy of the Indian rhinoceros (Rh. unicornis, L.). Trans Zool Soc Lond [Internet]. 1852;4(2):31–58. https://doi.org/10.1111/j.1469-7998.1862.tb08046.x.
4. Cave A. Richard Owen and the discovery of the parathyroid glands. In: Underwood EA, editor. Science, medicine and history, essays of the evolution of scientific thought and medical practice, written in honour of Charles Singer. London: Oxford University Press; 1953. p. 217–22.

5. Kafetzis ID, Diamantopoulos A, Christakis I, Leoutsakos B. The history of the parathyroid glands historical note. Hormones (Athens). 2011;10
6. Remak R. Untersuchungen über die Entwickelung der Wirbelthiere. Berlin: Reimer; 1855.
7. Giddings CEB, Rimmer J, Weir N. History of parathyroid gland surgery: an historical case series. J Laryngol Otol. 2009;123:1075–81.
8. Virchow R. Die krankhaften Geschwülste: dressig Volesungen gehalten während des Wintersemesters 1862–1863 an der Universität zu Berlin. Berlin: A. Hirschwald; 1863.
9. Toneto MG, Prill S, Debon LM, Furlan FZ, Steffen N. A história da cirurgia das paratireoides. Rev Col Bras Cir. 2016;43(3):214–22.
10. Sandstrom I. Om en ny Kortl has menniskan och atskilliga daggdjur. Upsala lakarforening Forh [Internet]. 1880 [cited 2024 Nov 2];15:441. Available from: https://cir.nii.ac.jp/crid/1572824499155949184.bib?lang=en
11. Slough CM, Liddy W, Brooks J, Kaplan EL, Bura M, Romanchisen AF, et al. History of thyroid and parathyroid surgery. In: Randolph GW, editor. Surgery of the thyroid and parathyroid glands. 3rd ed. Philadelphia: Elsevier; 2021. p. 2–14.
12. Ellis H. The early days of parathyroid surgery. J Perioper Pract. 2011;21(3):106–7.
13. Johansson H. The uppsala anatomist ivar sandström and the parathyroid gland. Ups J Med Sci. 2015;120(2):72–7.
14. Halsted WS, Evans HM. The parathyroid glandules. Their blood supply, and their preservation in operation upon the thyroid gland. Ann Surg. 1907;46(4):489–506.
15. Gilmour JR. The gross anatomy of the parathyroid glands. J Pathol Bacteriol. 1938;46(1):133–49.
16. Corvisart L. De la contracture idiopathique des extrémités ou tétanie, vol. 5. Paris: Faculte de Médecine de Paris; 1852.
17. Trousseau A. Clinique médicale de l'Hôtel-Dieu de Paris, vol. 2. Paris/Londres/New York: Baillière; 1862. p. 112–4.
18. Chvostek F. Beitrag zur Tetanie, vol. 17. Wiener medizinische Presse; 1876. p. 1201–4.
19. Wölfler A. Die Kropfextirpationen an Hofr. Billroth's Klinik von 1877 bis 1881, vol. 32. Wiener Medizinische Wochenschrift; 1882. p. 5–7.
20. Halsted W. The operative story of goitre: the author's operation. In: Johns Hopkins hospital reports. Baltimore: The Johns Hopkins Press; 1919.
21. Gley E. Sur Les fonctions du corps thyroide. CR Soc Biol. 1891;43:841.
22. Vermeulen AHM. The birth of endocrine pathology: how Erdheim misunderstood parathyroids. Virchows Arch. 2010;457:283–90.
23. Kohn A. Studien über die Schilddrüse. Archiv für mikroskopische Anatomie [Internet]. 1895;44(1):366–422. https://doi.org/10.1007/BF02934024.
24. Kohn A. Studien über die Schildrüse II. Archiv für mikroskopische Anatomie [Internet]. 1896;48(1):398–429. https://doi.org/10.1007/BF02977439.
25. Vassale G, Generali F. Sur les effets de l'extirpation des glandes parathyréoïdes. Arch Ital Biol. 1896;25:459–64.
26. Vassale G, Generale F. Fonction parathyroidienne et fonction thyroïdienne. Arch Ital Biol. 1900;33:154–6.
27. Dorairajan N, Pradeep PV. Vignette hyperparathyroidism: glimpse into its history. Int Surg. 2014;99:528–33. International College of Surgeons
28. Kalra S, Baruah M, Sahay R, Sawhney K. The history of parathyroid endocrinology. Indian J Endocrinol Metab. 2013;17(2):320.
29. Meusseu G. Sur la fonction parathyroïdienne. CR Biol. 1898;50
30. Loeb J. On an apparently new form of muscular irritability (contact irritability?) produced by solution of salts (preferably sodium salts) whose anions are liable to form insoluble calcium compound. Am J Physiol Legacy Content. 1901;5(6):362–73.
31. Dolev E. The parathyroid glands and the explanations of tetany 1903–1926 [Internet]; 1987. Available from: https://about.jstor.org/terms
32. MacCallum WG, Voegtlin C. On the relation of tetany to the parathyroid glands and to calcium metabolism. J Exp Med. 1909;11(1):118–51.

33. MacCallum WG, Lambert RA, Vogel KM. The removal of calcium from the blood by dialysis in the study of tetany. J Exp Med. 1914;20(2):149–68.
34. Salvesen HA. The function of the parathyroids. J Biol Chem [Internet]. 1923;56(2):443–56. Available from: https://www.sciencedirect.com/science/article/pii/S0021925818855818
35. Berkeley WN, Beebe SP. A contribution to the physiology and chemistry of the parathyroid gland. J Med Res. 1909;20(2):149–73.
36. Greenwald I. The effect of parathyroidectomy upon metabolism. Am J Physiol. 1911;28(2):103.
37. Li AJB. Collip, Hanson and the isolation of the parathyroid hormone, or endocrines and enterprise. J Hist Med Allied Sci. 1992;47(4):405–38.
38. Collip JB. The extraction of a parathyroid hormone which will prevent or control parathyroid tetany which regulates the level of blood calcium. J Biol Chem. 1925;63:395–438.
39. Engel G. Über einen Fall von cystoider Entartung des ganzen Skelletes. Giessen FC, Pietsch; 1864.
40. von Recklinghausen F. The mutual relations of the fibrous or deformative osteitis, osteomalacia and osteoplastic carcinoma [in German]. Festschrift fur Rudolph Virchow. 1891:295–89.
41. Askanazy M. On osteitis deformans without bony tissue [in German]. Arbeiten aus dem pathologisch-anato- mischen Institut zu Tu¨bingen. 1903;4:398–422.
42. Erdheim J. Dental calcification in rodent front teeth after epithelial gland transplantation [in German]. Frankfurter Zeitschrift fu¨r Pathologie. 1911;7:295–342.
43. Erdheim J. Über Epithelkörperbefunde bei Osteomalacie. Sitzungsber d kais Akad d Wissensch in Wien, math naturw. Klasse Abt III. 1907;116:311–70.
44. Sethi N, England RJA. Parathyroid surgery: from inception to the modern day. Br J Hosp Med. 2017;78(6):333–7.
45. Schlagenhaufer F. Zwei Fälle von Parathyreoideatumoren. Offizielles Protokoll der k.k. Gesellschaft der Aerzte in Wien Sitzung von 3 Dezember 1915. Wien Klin Wochenschr. 1915;28:1362.
46. Mandl F. Therapeutischer Versuch bei Ostitis fibrosa generalisata mittels extirpation eines Epithelkörperchentumors. Wien Klin Wochenschr. 1925;38:1343–4.
47. Delbridge LW, Palazzo FF. First parathyroid surgeon: sir John Bland-Sutton and the parathyroids. ANZ J Surg. 2007;77:1058–61.
48. Bland-Sutton J. Tumours: innocent and malignant, their clinical characters and appropriate treatment. 1st–7th ed. London: Cassell 1893; 1922.
49. Hannon R, Shore E, McClellan S, DuBois E. A case of osteitis fibrosa cystica (osteomalacia?) with evidence of hyperactivity of the parathyroid bodies. Metabolic study I. J Clin Invest. 1930;8(2):215–27.
50. Spartalis ED, Kouriannidi E, Athanasiadis DI, Chrysikos DT, Makay Ö, Troupis T. Edward D. Churchill (1895-1972): an innovative surgeon, his work, and his contribution to parathyroid surgery. Surg Innov. 2021;28(1):159–62.
51. Oliver C. The story of hyperparathyroidism at the Massachusetts General Hospital. N Engl J Med [Internet]. 1966;274(21):1174–82. https://doi.org/10.1056/NEJM196605262742105.
52. Churchill ED, Cope O. The surgical treatment of hyperparathyroidism: based on 30 cases confirmed by operation. Ann Surg. 1936;104(1):9–35.
53. Barr D, Bulger H. The clinical syndrome of hyperparathyroidism. Am J Med Sci. 1930;179:449–76.
54. Barr D, Bulger H, Dixon H. Hyperparathyroidism. JAMA. 1929;92:951–2.
55. Collip JB, Leitch DB. A case of tetany treated with parathyrin. Can Med Assoc J. 1925;15(1):59–60.
56. Eknoyan G. A history of the parathyroid glands.
57. Rasmussen H, Craig LC. The parathyroid polypeptides. Recent Prog Horm Res. 1962;18:269–95.
58. Rasmussen H, Craig LC. Purification of parathyroid hormone by use of countercurrent distribution. J Am Chem Soc [Internet]. 1959;81(18):5003. https://doi.org/10.1021/ja01527a066.
59. Berson SA, Yalow RS, Aurbach GD, Potts JT. Immunoassay of bovine and human parathyroid hormone. Proc Natl Acad Sci USA. 1963;49(5):613–7.

60. Nussbaum SR, Zahradnik RJ, Lavigne JR, Brennan GL, Nozawa-Ung K, Kim LY, et al. Highly sensitive two-site immunoradiometric assay of parathyrin, and its clinical utility in evaluating patients with hypercalcemia. Clin Chem. 1987;33(8):1364–7.
61. Irvin GL, Dembrow VD, Prudhomme DL. Clinical usefulness of an intraoperative "quick parathyroid hormone" assay. Surgery. 1993;114(6):1019–22; discussion 1022–3
62. Coffey RJ, Lee TC, Canary JJ. The surgical treatment of primary hyperparathyroidism: a 20 year experience. Ann Surg [Internet]. 1977;185(5) Available from: https://journals.lww.com/annalsofsurgery/fulltext/1977/05000/the_surgical_treatment_of_primary.3.aspx
63. Russell CF, Edis AJ. Surgery for primary hyperparathyroidism: experience with 500 consecutive cases and evaluation of the role of surgery in the asymptomatic patient. Br J Surg [Internet]. 1982;69(5):244–7. https://doi.org/10.1002/bjs.1800690503.
64. Taylor S. Hyperparathyroidism: retrospect and prospect. Ann R Coll Surg Engl. 1976;58(4):255–65.
65. Block MA, Greenawald K, Horn RC, Frame B. Involvement of multiple parathyroids in hyperparathyroidism. Surgical aspects. Am J Surg. 1967;114(4):530–7.
66. Cope O, Keynes WM, Roth SI, Castleman B. Primary chief-cell hyperplasia of the parathyroid glands: a new entity in the surgery of hyperparathyroidism. Ann Surg. 1958;148(3):375–88.
67. Wang CA, Castleman B, Cope O. Surgical management of hyperparathyroidism due to primary hyperplasia. Ann Surg. 1982;195(4):384–92.
68. Katz AI, Hampers CL, Wilson RE, Bernstein DS, Wachman A, Merrill JP. The place of subtotal parathyroidectomy in the management of patients with chronic renal failure. Trans Am Soc Artif Intern Organs. 1968;14:376–84.
69. Wilder RM. Hyperparathyroidism: tumor of the parathyroid glands associated with osteitis fibrosa*. Endocrinology [Internet]. 1929;13(3):231–44. https://doi.org/10.1210/endo-13-3-231.
70. Schantz A, Castleman B. Parathyroid carcinoma. A study of 70 cases. Cancer. 1973;31(3):600–5.
71. Hundahl SA, Fleming ID, Fremgen AM, Menck HR. Two hundred eighty-six cases of parathyroid carcinoma treated in the U.S. between 1985-1995: a National Cancer Data Base Report. The American College of Surgeons Commission on Cancer and the American Cancer Society. Cancer. 1999;86(3):538–44.
72. Wermer P. Genetic aspects of adenomatosis of endocrine glands. Am J Med. 1954;16(3):363–71.
73. Sipple JH. The association of pheochromocytoma with carcinoma of the thyroid gland. Am J Med. 1961;31(1):163–6.
74. Li Y, Simonds WF. Endocrine neoplasms in familial syndromes of hyperparathyroidism. Endocr Relat Cancer. 2016;23(6):R229–47.
75. Klopper PJ, Moe RE. Demonstration of the parathyroids during surgery in dogs, with preliminary report of results in some clinical cases. Surgery. 1966;59(6):1101–7.
76. Dudley NE. Methylene blue for rapid identification of the parathyroids. Br Med J. 1971;3(5776):680–1.
77. Patel HP, Chadwick DR, Harrison BJ, Balasubramanian SP. Systematic review of intravenous methylene blue in parathyroid surgery. Br J Surg. 2012;99(10):1345–51.
78. E RR, J PJ, Chiu-An W, J FD, Oliver C, M MT, et al. Localization of parathyroid adenomas by selective venous catheterization and radioimmunoassay. N Engl J Med [Internet]. 1969;281(7):348–51. https://doi.org/10.1056/NEJM196908142810704.
79. O'Riordan JL, Kendall BE, Woodhead JS. Preoperative localisation of parathyroid tumours. Lancet. 1971;2(7735):1172–5.
80. Coakley AJ, Kettle AG, Wells CP, O'Doherty MJ, Collins RE. 99Tcm sestamibi--a new agent for parathyroid imaging. Nucl Med Commun. 1989;10(11):791–4.
81. Von Eiselberg A. Über erfolgreiche Einheilung der Katzen Schildrüse in die Baueehdecke und Auftreten von Tetanie nach der extirpation; 1892.
82. Halsted WS. Auto- and isotransplantation, in dogs, of the parathyroid glandules. J Exp Med. 1909;11(1):175–99.

83. Lahey FH. The transplantation of parathyroids in partial thyroidectomy. Surg Gynecol Obstet [Internet]. 1926 [cited 2024 Nov 29];42:508–9. Available from: https://cir.nii.ac.jp/crid/1572543024252493696.bib?lang=en
84. Wells SA, Ellis GJ, Gunnells JC, Schneider AB, Sherwood LM. Parathyroid autotransplantation in primary parathyroid hyperplasia. N Engl J Med. 1976;295(2):57–62.
85. Wells SA, Gunnells JC, Gutman RA, Shelburne JD, Schneider AB, Sherwood LM. The successful transplantation of frozen parathyroid tissue in man. Surgery. 1977;81(1):86–90.

Evaluation and Management of Hyperparathyroidism

26

Natasha Quraishi and Muhammad S. Quraishi

Editorial

The authors provide an overall insight into the management of parathyroid disorders. They stress on the importance of correct evaluation of parathyroid disorders in order to treat effectively.

Not only are the anatomy and physiology of parathyroid gland function discussed, but this chapter focusses on the modalities to investigate and localise the parathyroid gland that is malfunctioning.

Near-infrared autofluorescence (NIR-AF) is also discussed as the new exciting modality to correctly identify the parathyroid adenoma intra-operatively in real time.

Prathamesh S. Pai

Introduction

The parathyroid glands are usually two pairs of small endocrine glands found within the neck. Their function is to control calcium levels within the body through the excretion of parathyroid hormone (PTH). Hyperparathyroidism (HPT) is a condition characterised by increased levels of PTH resulting in hypercalcaemia, urinary tract calculi, osteoporosis, musculoskeletal pain, change in mood and fatigue. It may be classed as primary, secondary and tertiary depending on the cause for the raised

N. Quraishi
Bradford Royal Infirmary, Bradford, UK
e-mail: natasha.quraishi@nhs.net

M. S. Quraishi (✉)
Doncaster Royal Infirmary, Doncaster, UK
e-mail: muhamad.quraishi@nhs.net

P. S. Pai et al. (eds.), *Controversies in Cancer of the Thyroid and Parathyroid Glands*, https://doi.org/10.1007/978-3-032-13130-0_26

PTH level. Endocrine surgeons are predominantly involved in the management of primary HPT where the underlying pathology is frequently a parathyroid adenoma.

This chapter sets out to describe the embryology, anatomy and function of the parathyroid glands in order to facilitate an understanding of HPT including its aetiology, presentation, evaluation and management.

Anatomy and Embryology

The embryology of the parathyroid glands informs their anatomy. Typically, there are four parathyroid glands. Each gland is approximately 5–7 mm in size and weighs 30–40 mg. The parathyroid glands are an ovoid shape with a reddish-brown appearance in younger patients and a more yellow appearance in older patients. The colour is affected by the contents of the gland such as the quantity of oxyphil cells and fat.

The parathyroid glands are frequently described as the superior pair and the inferior pair and usually lie on the posterolateral aspect of each thyroid lobe. The distinction between the upper and lower pairs of parathyroid glands is not simply differing anatomical locations; they differ in their embryological origins. The superior parathyroid glands are derived from the endoderm of the fourth pharyngeal pouch, while the inferior parathyroid glands originate from the endoderm of the third pharyngeal pouch. As the parathyroid cells develop, they migrate from the neck to the mediastinum. However, this migration can arrest at any point. There have been reports of supernumerary glands in approximately 5% of cases [1], and these are often found in the thymic tissue.

The superior parathyroid glands lie deep to the recurrent laryngeal nerve in the coronal plane. The migration of the superior glands is more limited than that of the inferior glands, and this is reflected in the fact that their position is less variable than the inferior glands. The superior parathyroid glands are found posterolateral to the upper half of the thyroid lobes, adjacent to the cricothyroid junction and approximately 1 cm cephalic to the junction of the recurrent laryngeal nerve and the inferior thyroid artery in 80% of cases [2]. Less commonly the superior parathyroid glands can be located in other positions such as retropharyngeal, retro-oesophageal or retrolaryngeal (3–4% of cases) or in the posterior mediastinum or above the superior pole of the thyroid lobe (less than 1% of cases) [2]. In the majority of cases, the arterial blood supply for the superior parathyroid glands comes from the inferior thyroid artery; however, in 35–40% of cases, it may be from the superior thyroid artery [1].

By contrast the position of the inferior parathyroid glands is more variable. In up to 61% of cases, they are located 1 cm posterior, lateral or inferior to the lower pole of the thyroid lobe, lying superficially to the recurrent laryngeal nerve and caudal to the inferior thyroid artery where they cross the recurrent laryngeal nerve [2]. As the inferior parathyroid glands develop with the thymus, in 25% of cases, they may be found within the thyrothymic horn [2]. Other positions described include lateral to the thyroid gland or adjacent to the trachea. Rarely, they may be intrathyroidal (0.5–4%), subcapsular or even ectopic, sitting below the suprasternal notch in the mediastinal thymus or near the carotid sheath [2]. The inferior parathyroid glands are supplied by inferior thyroid artery.

The innervation of the parathyroid glands is derived from the superior and middle cervical sympathetic plexus or from the perivascular plexus of the thyroid. The parathyroid glands receive their venous drainage from the middle and superior thyroid veins.

Histopathology

The parathyroid glands are covered in a thin capsule of connective tissue which forms septations dividing the glands into lobules. Each gland is made up of adipose cells and an abundant network of sinusoidal capillaries within which are islands of parenchymal cells. There are four types of parenchymal cells within the parathyroid glands: chief or principal cells, oxyphil cells, transitional cells and clear cells. The chief cells produce PTH and in children are the predominant cell type in the gland. Over time, the proportion of chief cells fall, while the proportion of adipose increases to make up 20% of the gland by early adulthood [3]. The oxyphil cells are larger cells with plentiful mitochondria, and the number of these cells increases with age. Their function remains unclear. The transitional cells are intermediate cells between oxyphil and chief cells. The clear cells are named thus for their clear cytoplasm.

Various parathyroid pathologies are associated with altered histopathological appearance of the gland. In parathyroid adenomas, chief cells make up the adenomatous part of the gland which typically compresses the normal parathyroid tissue into a thin rim. In pHPT 15% of cases are caused by chief cell hyperplasia, while in 25% pHPT may be associated with a familial syndrome such as multiple endocrine neoplasia (MEN) [3].

Physiology

The parathyroid gland's main function is the regulation of serum calcium and phosphate levels through the secretion of PTH. PTH increases the serum calcium level through a number of actions when the parathyroid glands detect reduced serum calcium levels. PTH stimulates osteoclast activity resulting in resorption of bone and thus release of calcium into the blood. PTH acts on the kidney in three ways to increase serum calcium. Firstly, PTH increases serum calcium reabsorption at the distal tubules and renal collecting duct although this is considered less important than its other effects on the kidney. Secondly, PTH decreases phosphate reabsorption in the proximal tubule of the kidney, thus reducing serum phosphate levels which increases the amount of ionised calcium in blood plasma as phosphate ions combine with calcium ions to form salts that are insoluble in water. Thirdly PTH acts on the kidney to stimulate the production of calcitriol (1, 25-dihydroxy vitamin D) from 25-hydroxy vitamin D. Calcitriol then acts on the intestine to increase calcium uptake thus increasing serum calcium levels.

In addition to reduced serum calcium levels, secretion of PTH is also stimulated by mild reduction in serum magnesium levels and an increase in serum phosphate levels, adrenaline and histamine. The secretion of PTH is regulated through negative feedback as it is inhibited by increased serum calcium levels and calcitriol.

Hyperparathyroidism (HPT)

HPT is characterised by raised serum levels of PTH. It can be further categorised as primary (pHPT), secondary and tertiary. pHPT is where the raised PTH level is due to a disorder of the parathyroid glands themselves rather than being influenced by any other biochemical factors. This disorder may be due to hyperplasia of the parenchyma of the gland or by a neoplasm of the gland such as parathyroid adenoma or more rarely carcinoma.

In 75–85% of cases, pHPT is due to parathyroid adenoma, whereas 10–15% may have multigland hyperplasia and 2–12% may have a double adenoma [4]. Parathyroid adenomas can present at any age although they are frequently diagnosed in the fourth decade and show a preponderance for females [3]. While parathyroid adenomas are benign, typically histopathological confirmation is required for this diagnosis, and carcinoma should be excluded in any enlarged gland.

Parathyroid carcinoma is extremely rare, accounting for 1% of patients with pHPT [5]. It has a purported incidence of 10–13 cases per 10, 000, 000 per year in the USA [5]. It typically arises in patients in their fifth or sixth decades and has an equal sex incidence. It is unknown what causes parathyroid carcinoma. Typically, biochemical testing will demonstrate a serum calcium greater than 3.75 mmol/L, and the PTH level in these patients can be up to 50 times greater than the normal range. In addition to serum calcium and PTH assay, it has been suggested that for parathyroid cancer further investigations may include parafibromin, Galectin 3, PGP9.5, Ki67 and tissue expression of APC [6].

Secondary HPT is where the raised PTH level arises as a response to a stimulus beyond the parathyroid gland itself and then resolves on removal of said stimulus. Commonly secondary HPT is caused by chronic impaired renal function which causes low serum calcium and high phosphate which causes proliferation of the parathyroid gland tissue. Chronic renal failure also causes metabolic acidosis which impairs the response of calcium receptors to PTH secretion. Other causes of secondary HPT can include vitamin D deficiency and lithium.

Tertiary HPT occurs when the external stimulation of the parathyroid gland has been prolonged to the point that the hyperplastic gland no longer reverts back to its normal state on removal of the stimulus and so the gland has become autonomous.

HPT may also be familial when associated with a number of conditions including MEN1 and MEN2. MEN1 is associated with multigland HPT (resulting in nearly all patients having pHPT [3] in addition to pituitary tumours and gastrointestinal and pancreatic carcinoids. The MEN1 gene has a 95% penetrance. By contrast, MEN2 causes pHPT in 20–30% of patients [3], resulting in milder hypercalcaemia which may not necessitate any treatment. Both MEN1 and MEN2 are associated with phaeochromocytoma and medullary thyroid carcinoma. Other conditions associated with familial HPT include neonatal severe HPT, hyperparathyroidism-jaw tumour syndrome, familial isolated HPT and autosomal dominant mild HPT.

Clinical Assessment

While pHPT can present at any stage of life, it shows a preponderance towards women in their sixth and seventh decades of life. There are three presentations of pHPT: symptomatic, asymptomatic and normocalcaemic HPT.

The typical presentation of a HPT patient is an incidental finding of hypercalcaemia, with 80% of patients being asymptomatic [7]. These patients will typically present to otolaryngologists or endocrine surgeons having been referred by endocrine physicians who have diagnosed pHPT. The endocrinologists assess the patient using PTH assays, a 24-hour urinary collection for calcium level and creatinine clearance/glomerular filtration rate (GFR). They diagnose pHPT where there is a picture of hypercalcaemia, a raised PTH assay and hypercalciuria. Some patients have normocalcaemic pHPT which is characterised by patients with bony loss, increased PTH levels, normal vitamin D levels and a normal serum calcium in the absence of any other cause.

Traditionally the presentation of HPT was described as 'bones, stones, abdominal groans and psychic moans' which are essentially symptoms of the complications of this condition. While now the majority of pHPT present asymptomatically, there is still a proportion that are symptomatic at presentation. These symptoms include lethargy, fatigue, low mood and reduced concentration which may mimic dementia in older patients. Symptomatic patients may also complain of musculoskeletal pain or even reduced bone density and fractures. Even in patients who appear asymptomatic patients, bone densitometry is helpful in the monitoring the anabolic effect of pHPT at the lumbar spine, catabolic effect at the distal third of the radius and the mixed effect at the hip [8]. Patients may also experience gastrointestinal symptoms such as chronic constipation, abdominal pain, peptic ulcers and pancreatitis. Urinary complications such as nephrolithiasis (21–55%) and hypercalciuria are the commonest manifestations of pHPT [8].

In pHPT, physical examination is frequently unremarkable, as it is uncommon for the affected gland(s) to be palpable. If a palpable neck mass is present in a patient with apparent pHPT, parathyroid carcinoma should be considered. The most common symptoms of parathyroid carcinoma are musculoskeletal pain and weakness. The presentation may also include severe hypercalcaemia, fatigue, depression, nausea and polyuria [5]. On examination a neck mass or a vocal cord palsy may be found. Parathyroid carcinoma invades local structures such as the thyroid gland, recurrent laryngeal nerve, muscles, trachea or oesophagus. It can behave in an indolent manner.

Although the endocrinologists have usually performed a 'work-up' prior to referral, on review one should still enquired regarding risk factors for HPT such as lithium therapy and neck irradiation and consider investigating other causes of hypercalcaemia if this has not already been done. Another important aspect to consider is the possibility of MEN especially in younger patients with pHPT, particularly in the presence of a family history. In such scenarios, the patient should be investigated for MEN. The presentation of MEN-associated pHPT can differ, as these patients tend to have multiple gland disease. Their management is also different to that of solitary adenomas. pHPT may also be associated with metabolic and potential cardiovascular manifestations, including diabetes, hypertension and left ventricular hypertrophy.

Management

Management of HPT varies according to the type of HPT and the underlying pathology.

Medical Management of Primary Hyperparathyroidism (pHPT)

The management of pHPT can range from observation and lifestyle measures to medical treatment to surgery. Medical management can be offered to asymptomatic patients and usually consists of adequate hydration, avoidance of thiazide diuretics and control of calcium and PTH levels through the use of bisphosphonates. Denosumab and bisphosphonates reduce bone resorption as well as decreasing calcium levels in serum and urine. Calcimimetic drugs such as cinacalcet have been used to control serum PTH levels, often in secondary HPT, since 2004. Their mechanism of action is through their mimicry of calcium at parathyroid receptors, thus reducing the amount of PTH secreted.

Thermal Ablation for Primary Hyperparathyroidism

Thermal ablation may also have an emerging role in the management of pHPT in the form of radiofrequency or microwave ablation [9, 10].

Surgical Management of Primary Hyperparathyroidism

Parathyroidectomy for pHPT confers a greater cure rate than observation or medical management [11]. The definition of cure is often considered to be based on biochemical factors such as normocalcaemia. However, it is also important to consider quality of life, which is also reported to improve after parathyroidectomy [12]. Even asymptomatic patients have been noted to experience a worsening of their condition over time. For example, Rubin and colleagues undertook an observational study of pHPT patients over a period of 15 years where they found that approximately 37%

Table 26.1 Indications for parathyroidectomy made by the authors based on the American Association of Endocrine Surgeons Guidelines for Definitive Management of Primary Hyperparathyroidism [14]

Indications	Other
Symptomatic pHPT Serum calcium level > 1 mg/dL above normal Objective evidence of renal involvement[a] Osteoporosis, fragility fracture, or evidence of vertebral compression fracture seen on spine imaging Age 50 years or younger Clinical or biochemical evidence consistent with parathyroid cancer	*Preferred* – patients who cannot or do not wish to follow observation protocols *Recommended* – patients experiencing neurocognitive and/or neuropsychiatric symptoms that are attributable to pHPT

[a]Defined as including asymptomatic nephrolithiasis seen on imaging of the renal tract, nephrocalcinosis, hypercalciuria (24-hour urine calcium level > 400 mg/dL) with increased risk of developing stones or impaired renal function (glomerular filtration rate < 60 mL/min)

of asymptomatic patients demonstrated disease progression, especially in younger patients [13]. If opting for a nonsurgical approach, there should be yearly monitoring of calcium, PTH, renal function and bone mineral density. In cases of normocalcaemic pHPT, watchful waiting is advised, as some may develop hypercalcaemia (0.6–19%) [8].

Surgical management may be indicated in patients with HPT who are symptomatic or asymptomatic but with certain stipulations. There is guidance available describing when to consider parathyroidectomy from a number of professional bodies including the American Association of Endocrine Surgeons [14] (Table 26.1).

Pre-operative Localisation Investigations for Parathyroid Surgery

When planning surgical management of HPT, careful pre-operative planning with the use of localisation investigations is vital to reduce the risk of complications. Accurate and reliable parathyroid localisation investigations have permitted the growing trend of minimal access focussed parathyroid surgery. Pre-operative localisation investigations for patients with single gland adenomas typically involve cervical ultrasonography (USS) for anatomical details and sestamibi (MIBI) scans for functional details. Usual practice for solitary adenomas is to perform both USS and MIBI. Where the USS and MIBI scans have been concordant, parathyroidectomy has been associated with a 98.5% success rate [15].

Computed tomography (CT) or magnetic resonance imaging (MRI) is helpful in the localisation of ectopic glands. There is also a role for invasive procedures such as selective venous PTH sampling and image-guided fine needle aspiration (FNE) with PTH assay in revision surgery [16].

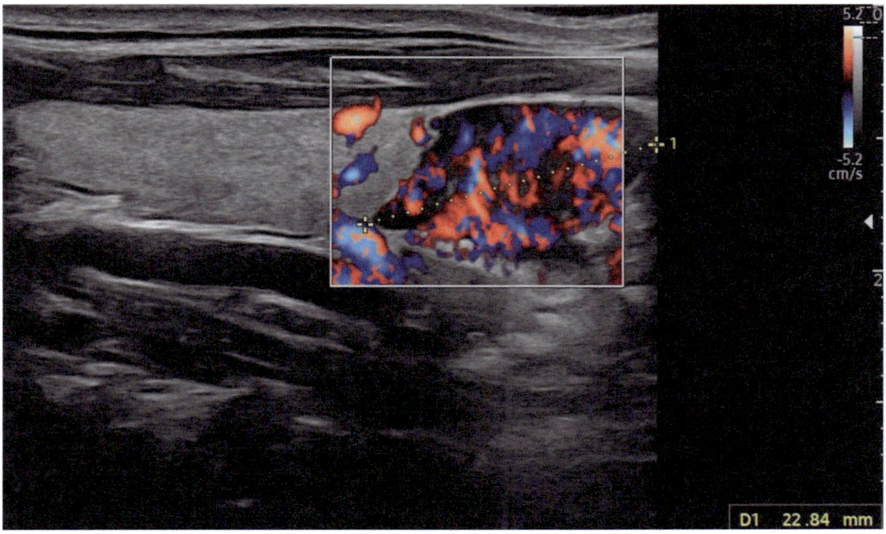

Image 26.1 USS Doppler showing the peripheral vasculature of the parathyroid gland

Ultrasound Scan

Cervical ultrasonography (USS) is a helpful tool in the localisation of solitary parathyroid adenomas, with a reported sensitivity between 51% and 96% and a positive predictive value (PPV) of 50–100% [17], although working with an experienced radiologists ensures outcomes in keeping with the higher limits of these ranges. On USS the abnormal gland is identified by its correct anatomical position, its homogeneously hypoechoic texture and its shape which may be oval, triangular or enlarged. The use of colour flow Doppler (CFD) is helpful in highlighting the peripheral blood flow of the abnormal parathyroid gland (Image 26.1) which distinguishes it from a lymph node which typically has a vascular pedicle. USS can supply further information on the anatomical relations of the abnormal gland including anatomical structures which could act as landmarks in surgery. Additional benefits include avoidance of ionising radiation and it is non-invasive and can be undertaken in clinic in some surgeons' practice.

The main disadvantage of USS is due to its limited tissue penetration; it may not identify adenomas that are deep-seated, retrotracheal, retro-oesophageal, superior mediastinal or in other ectopic positions. Furthermore, USS is operator dependent, and thyroid nodules may reduce its sensitivity.

Sestamibi Scintigraphy

Sestamibi scintigraphy (MIBI) is a metabolic scan that may be utilised to identify parathyroid adenomas. These scans involve the use of a radioisotope known as sestamibi (technetium-99 m methoxyisobutylisonitrile) which is taken up by

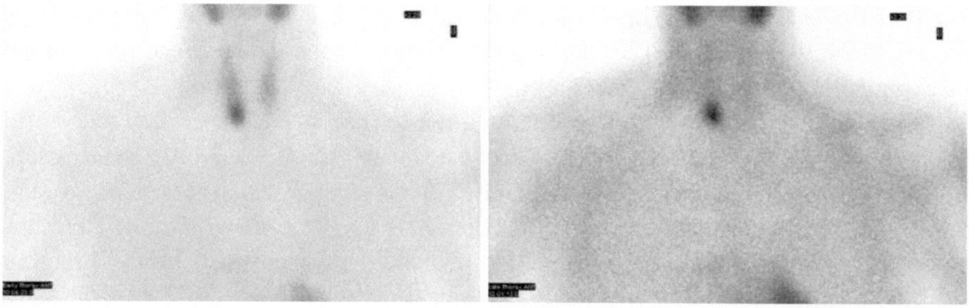

Image 26.2 Subtraction imaging showing late persistence at the right lower thyroid region, suggestive of right inferior parathyroid lesion

mitochondria within cells. It is a monovalent lipophilic cation and so can diffuse through cell membranes. This is specifically helpful in parathyroid tissue which has high levels of mitochondrial activity and so demonstrates high uptake of sestamibi especially when compared with thyroid tissue which has a lower volume of mitochondria. The sestamibi washes out more rapidly in tissues with lower mitochondrial content such as the thyroid than it does in parathyroid tissue, thus helping to distinguish the latter. The histopathological composition of a parathyroid adenoma may affect the findings as those with an oxyphil cell content greater than 20% are more likely to have a positive MIBI scan than an adenoma that comprises mainly of chief cells.

MIBIs with dual-phase imaging with double tracer (99 m-sestamibi and iodine-123) subtraction can improve the accuracy of localisation of scintigraphy and has a sensitivity of 89% [4]. Essentially the sestamibi is administered, and images are taken of the parathyroids at an early phase (20 minutes after administration) and a late phase (2 hours after administration). The iodine-123 is administered to enable imaging of the thyroid which can then be subtracted from the early and late-phase images of the parathyroid glands allowing better visualisation of parathyroid adenomas and improving sensitivity (Image 26.2). Pre-operative planning can be aided through the fusion of these images with CT image as this provides a three-dimensional view of the anatomy.

CT, MRI and PET

The use of conventional CT and MRI in parathyroid surgery is less common than MIBI or USS. Four-dimensional (4D) CT has been reported to have a better sensitivity than MIBI in pHPT and also in revision cases; however there is not sufficient evidence to ascertain the impact on cure rates [18]. 4D CT can be helpful in the identification of ectopic glands as the intravenous contrast used has a quicker update and washout in a parathyroid adenoma when compared with other local structures such as lymph nodes. It may also be helpful in cases where USS and MIBI scans have been discordant [19]. However, 4D CT entails greater radiation exposure than

MIBI. Conventional MRI has been reported to have a sensitivity ranging from 39.1% to 94.3% for pHPT [20] and may be helpful in the detection of mediastinal or ectopic glands.

While not used commonly, fluorodeoxyglucose (FDG)-PET scans can be helpful in cases where the MIBI and USS have been negative or equivocal or in cases where revision surgery is being considered. FDG-PET has an 86% sensitivity rate and 78% specificity rate for solitary parathyroid adenomas [21]. ^{18}F-fluorocholine-PET has also been reported to be helpful in cases of discordant or negative initial imaging [22], with some suggesting it to have a greater sensitivity than 4D CT [23].

Fine Needle Aspiration

Fine needle aspiration (FNA) can be performed under radiological guidance (US or CT) to test for PTH assay. This technique is suggested more for revision parathyroid surgery than primary surgery. Cytology from FNA should be regarded with caution as follicular thyroid neoplastic cells may mimic the appearance of parathyroid tissue making this test less sensitive.

Venous Sampling

Venous sampling is an invasive procedure that may be used as a pre-operative localisation technique, with a reported sensitivity of 74%, and has been considered beneficial when utilised where imaging has been negative or in revision surgery [24]. Targeted samples are taken from neck or mediastinal veins, and PTH assay from these is compared with PTH assay from peripheral venous samples. When PTH levels are 1.5–2 times higher in the targeted samples, this can assist surgeons in focussing their exploration in terms of side and region (neck versus mediastinum).

Intra-operative Localisation Techniques for Parathyroid Surgery

Intra-operative localisation techniques can be used to improve surgical outcomes and include:

1. Intra-operative PTH monitoring (IOPTH)
2. Radio-guided parathyroidectomy (RGP)
3. Frozen section (FS)
4. Near-infrared autofluorescence (NIR-AF)
5. Methylene blue (MB) injections

Intra-operative PTH Monitoring

IOPTH involves the use of PTH assay on venous samples which may be taken from peripheral or central sites (as long as it remains consistent for the entire procedure). It may be utilised in cases where the pre-operative localisation studies have been discordant and in revision cases. It can also be used intra-operatively to confirm the achievement of biochemical cure following excision of the target gland as PTH has a half-life of approximately 4–7 minutes. Typically, a sample will be taken prior to the gland excision (sometimes prior to the skin incision), and then an intra-operative sample is taken at least 10 minutes after the removal of the target gland. If there is a 50% or more decrease in PTH in the intra-operative sample compared with the pre-excision sample, biochemical cure can be considered to have been achieved. While the use of IOPTH may result in longer operating times, it has been associated with better cure rates in both minimally invasive parathyroidectomy and bilateral neck exploration as well as lower rates of re-operation and disease persistence [25]. It has been reported that success rate of minimally invasive parathyroidectomy (MIP) is between 97% and 99% when IOPTH is used [26].

Radio-Guided Parathyroidectomy

In this technique, MIBI is administered pre-operatively, and then during the procedure a gamma probe is used to localise parathyroid tissue. There is no single superior published protocol for the dose and timing of the administration of the MIBI. Its use is limited to cases where the pre-operative MIBI scan has been positive, and it may be beneficial in localising ectopic glands and in re-operative cases. However, it can prolong surgery and is contraindicated in patients with an allergy or sensitivity to MIBI and in pregnancy.

RGP may be considered an alternative to IOPTH monitoring and FS and is used mainly in North America. It is rarely employed in the UK as it is felt that the success rate of parathyroid surgery is related more to surgical skill and experience and that this technique does not usually provide any further information.

Frozen Section

This test is extremely helpful in confirming if the tissue removed by the surgeon intra-operatively is parathyroid tissue or non-parathyroid tissue such as thyroid tissue or a lymph node. It is considered to have a high degree of accuracy and with the cooperation of experienced histopathology colleagues can be done in 20 minutes. It may therefore be of use in patients whose pre-operative localisation imaging has been inconclusive or in revision surgery. One key limitation, however, is that FS may not distinguish between parathyroid adenoma and multigland dysplasia.

Near-Infrared Autofluorescence

This technology utilises the parathyroid glands' properties of autofluorescence which in vivo is 2–20 times greater than the thyroid gland. Therefore, when NIR-AF is used, the parathyroid glands appear brighter than surrounding anatomical structures and tissue. This is shown as a processed image which is generated in real time. Limitations of this technique include the fact that histological composition of a parathyroid adenoma and in parathyroid gland hyperplasia can vary and so affect the autofluorescence signal. NIR-AF may not detect parathyroid glands that are embedded in soft tissue due to limitation of the depth to which it can penetrate. Since its first description for parathyroid surgery in 2009, the role of NIR-AF has been debated as cure rates from parathyroidectomy for HPT can be up to 98% without its use.

Methylene Blue

Methylene blue (MB) acts as a dye to selectively stain parathyroid tissue. Therefore, it may be used to identify parathyroid glands intra-operatively by being infused intravenously about 60 minutes before surgery or just prior to the induction of general anaesthesia. The infusion typically consists of 5 mg/kg body weight of MB which is then diluted in 100 ml of 0.9% saline. However, MB is now rarely used as it can interfere with pulse oximetry monitoring and has also been associated with toxic encephalopathy.

Surgical Approaches to Primary Hyperparathyroidism

The gold standard surgical approach to HPT is considered to be the bilateral neck exploration (BNE). This approach is associated with a success rate of 95–98% of cases [27]. However there has been an increasing trend towards the use of minimally invasive parathyroidectomy (MIP) which involves a more focussed approach. Ultimately the decision as to approach must consider factors relating to the surgeon (e.g. experience) and to the patient (e.g. underlying pathology). BNE is utilised in cases of multigland disease, residual or recurrent disease (including as an extension of single gland surgery when intra-operative testing has not indicated biochemical cure has been achieved) or where pre-operative localisation imaging has been negative. Its other indications include suspected MEN syndromes, secondary or tertiary HPT with renal failure and surgeon's preference. By contrast, MIP is better placed in the management of single gland adenomas and can be performed under both general and local anaesthesia.

Minimally Invasive Parathyroidectomy (MIP)

MIP is an approach associated with less morbidity, less cost and a shorter operating time with a rate of success that is comparable to BNE [28]. The advancement of localisation imaging techniques such as USS and MIBI has arguably driven the increasing popularity of MIP as it underpins its likelihood of success [29]. Accurate imaging interpreted by a dedicated radiologist is key in precise pre-operative localisation which is required for a targeted approach.

There are various surgical techniques/access that may be used for MIP such as open mini-incision, video-assisted and endoscopic. Open mini-incision MIP (OMIP) involves the use of a small (less than 2.5 cm) horizontal cervical skin incision positioned according to the localisation of the gland on imaging. Video-assisted MIP (VAP) utilises a rigid endoscope without gas insufflation and can provide a magnified view of the operative field with optimal lighting. By contrast endoscopic MIP (EP) uses gas insufflation with a rigid endoscope. Access may be lateral through the para-carotid gutter or midline between the strap muscles. This technique also offers a magnified view with optimal lighting. Of these techniques, OMIP has been reported as being less complicated with less risk to the recurrent laryngeal nerve. MIP has been reported to have a low recurrence rate of 1.5% [29]. Robotic-assisted parathyroidectomy has also been described, but further evidence is required before this approach can be considered the gold-standard approach [30].

When performing OMIP, the patient is typically positioned supine with a sandbag beneath the shoulders to extend the neck and the head placed on a ring to stabilise it. The head is kept in a midline position to avoid distortion of anatomical landmarks. A skin crease incision is usually made over the area reported on USS to house the target gland (Image 26.3). Superior and inferior subplatysmal flaps are raised and retracted with Joll's self-retaining retractors (Image 26.2).

The medial border of the sternocleidomastoid is identified and separated from the strap muscles to enable it to be laterally retracted with a right-angled retractor (Image 26.4). Another retractor is deployed by the surgical assistant to rotate the ipsilateral thyroid lobe and thus expose its posterolateral edge. Using the pre-operative localisation imaging as a guide, the parathyroid adenoma can then be identified and removed (Image 26.5). To remove the gland, one uses a combination blunt dissection (with an artery clip and moist swab) as well as bipolar diathermy for painstaking haemostasis. The middle thyroid vein, if identified, can be preserved and retracted. By adopting the technique of staying as close to the gland as possible,

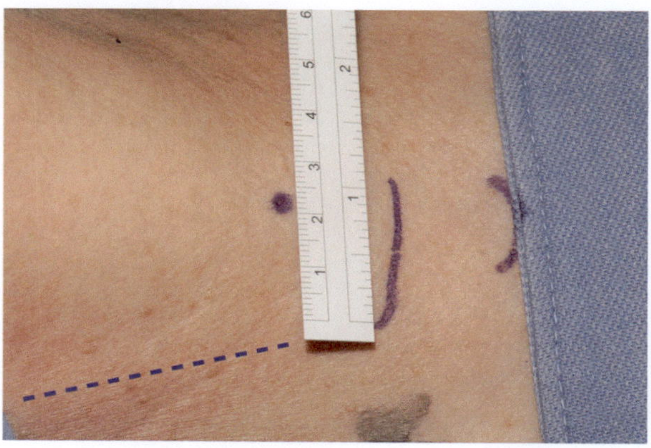

Image 26.3 Markings for landmarks (cricoid cartilage, sternal notch, sternocleidomastoid) and cervical skin crease incision

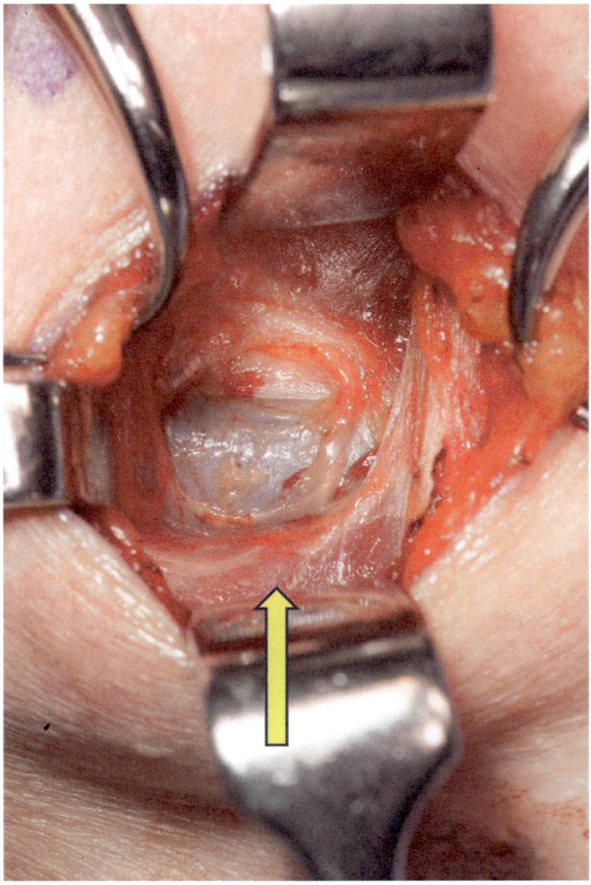

Image 26.4 Superior and inferior subplatysmal flaps are raised, and the medial border of the sternocleidomastoid is identified

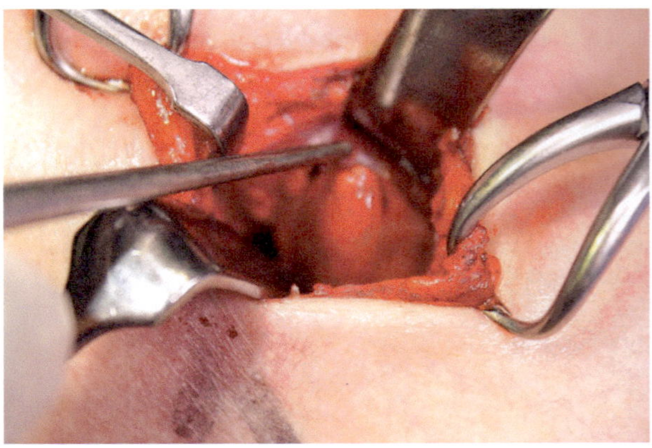

Image 26.5 The target parathyroid gland has been found and will be excised

one may avoid the recurrent laryngeal nerve. It is also important to consider the fragile nature of the gland and so avoid instrumentation of the gland where possible to avoid rupture.

Following the excision of the gland, the specimen may be sent for FS, and/or a post-excision intra-operative PTH assay may be performed depending on local practice. A surgical drain is not commonly required for this approach, and following haemostasis the wound is closed in two layers with some subcutaneous local anaesthetic being administered around the incision site. In general anaesthesia cases, laryngeal nerve monitoring is regularly used although some surgeons may only employ it for revision cases or for deeply located adenomas. Patient factors allowing single-gland exploration are typically a day-case procedure.

If the procedure has been successful, within 48 hours patients will return to normal serum calcium levels, and their symptoms should resolve. Over time, bone density may also improve; both asymptomatic and symptomatic patients have a reduced risk of fracture.

Bilateral Neck Exploration

In contrast to the targeted nature of MIP, BNE involves exploration of the neck through bilateral dissection and identification of all four parathyroid glands. Access may be open or using an endoscopic technique. Once all glands have been identified, the gland that appears abnormal macroscopically is excised. Again, this specimen can be sent for FS, and IOPTH can also be carried out to corroborate biochemical cure. Excision of further glands will be considered by the surgeon if these tests are negative.

Local Anaesthesia Considerations

Both local infiltration and regional block anaesthesia (such as a superficial or deep cervical block) may be used in MIP surgery with or without intravenous sedation. Specifically, local anaesthesia may enable parathyroid surgery in patients who are unsuitable for general anaesthesia due to comorbidities. It is also associated with a shorter recovery time and with fewer symptoms such as nausea or pain. When considering local anaesthesia, appropriate patient selection is key. Factors that will optimise the likelihood of success include positive localisation scans with target glands being non-ectopic, a long thin neck and, most importantly, a cooperative patient.

Failed Initial Exploration, Persistent and Recurrent Hyperparathyroidism and Re-exploration

Although the surgical management of sporadic pHPT has a success rate of over 95% and a very low morbidity rate (when performed by an experienced surgeon), it is important to be aware of the possibility of recurrence or a failed exploration.

Persistent HPT describes hypercalcaemia within 6 months of surgery. It has been suggested that lack of recognition of multigland disease is the main reason for failure of primary parathyroidectomy [31]. Other causes for persistent sporadic pHPT include inadequate neck exploration, failure to identify and excise ectopic parathyroid adenomas which may lie in alternate locations in the neck, superior or middle mediastinum or supernumerary parathyroid glands.

Recurrence is defined as HPT being diagnosed after 6-month period of normal calcium levels following the initial surgery. The estimated recurrence rate of sporadic pHPT following parathyroidectomy is 1.56% [32]. Long-term recurrence rates (5–10 years following the procedure) do not appear significantly different between different surgical approaches [32].

When re-exploration of the neck is to be considered, this should utilise a systematic approach and ideally should be performed at a tertiary referral centre. In expert centres, 84–98% of re-operative surgery cases achieve normocalcaemia [33].

Management of Other Pathologies Associated with Hyperparathyroidism

Management of Parathyroid Carcinoma

In parathyroid carcinoma, the aim of medical treatment is to control hypercalcaemia which may be severe enough to necessitate the use of intravenous bisphosphonates. The operative management of parathyroid carcinoma involves en bloc removal, i.e. hemithyroidectomy, excision of paratracheal nodes and fat, thymic tissue ± modified/radical neck dissection in gross nodal involvement which has been described as the gold standard of treatment [5]. Post-operatively patients must be monitoring closely for 'hungry bone syndrome' resulting in a reduction in serum calcium. There is unclear evidence for the role of radiotherapy and no role for chemotherapy or immunotherapy at present [5]. Parathyroid cancer is associated with a recurrence rate of about 50% [5]. In the majority of cases, recurrence is characterised by hypercalcaemia [34], which is then followed by physical evidence of recurrence and locoregional disease. The main cause of morbidity and mortality of parathyroid carcinoma is related to the metabolic consequences of the disease rather than from malignant growth itself. In a US database of 286 patients, a 10-year survival rate of 49% was reported in 1999 [35]. As recurrence may even occur up to 20 years following treatment, lifelong follow-up is recommended [5].

Management of Hyperparathyroidism Associated with MEN1

Due to the severe extent of parathyroid gland hyperplasia associated with MEN1, surgery for HPT in these patients is associated with a failure rate of up to 20% in experienced hands [36]. Surgery is prioritised in patients with Zollinger-Ellison syndrome or osteoporosis. The typical surgical method favoured is a subtotal parathyroidectomy and bilateral thymectomy [37, 38]. The subtotal parathyroidectomy involves preservation of 20–30 mg of the smallest parathyroid gland, which is marked with a non-absorbable suture. In the presence of significant four-gland enlargement, the favoured procedure is a total parathyroidectomy with 30–60 mg of the smallest gland being auto-transplanted in the patient's forearm. While subtotal parathyroidectomy has traditionally been considered the balance between avoiding hypoparathyroidism associated with total parathyroidectomy and HPT associated with less than subtotal parathyroidectomy, it has been suggested that the future advancement of pre-operative localisation techniques may reduce the risk of HPT following subtotal parathyroidectomy [39].

Management of Hyperparathyroidism Associated with MEN2A

In MEN2A patients, HPT is typically less severe, with many patients being asymptomatic. Even in MEN2A patients undergoing total thyroidectomy for medullary thyroid carcinoma, only parathyroid glands that are noted to be enlarged intra-operatively are excised in order to avoid hypoparathyroidism. Where it has been deemed that surgical management is required for HPT for MEN2A patients, MIP approach appears to be increasingly favoured over BNE [40].

Management of Secondary and Tertiary Hyperparathyroidism

The initial management of secondary and tertiary HPT is determined by nephrologists who may consider surgical intervention in the advent of failure of medical management. Indications for surgery in such cases are usually to alleviate symptoms as well as to correct biochemical derangement. In patients with four-gland enlargement, the recommended approach is total parathyroidectomy with autotransplantation, although some favour a subtotal parathyroidectomy to avoid hypoparathyroidism. In this approach, there is preservation of approximately 50% of the gland most normal in appearance with a vascular pedicle.

Secondary Hyperparathyroidism Approaches

In severe secondary HPT, parathyroidectomy has been reported to confer a greater survival advantage over medical management [41]. The literature describes a number of approaches to the surgical management of secondary HPT: subtotal parathyroidectomy, total parathyroidectomy alone and total parathyroidectomy with autotransplantation. Some have claimed that subtotal parathyroidectomy and total parathyroidectomy with autotransplantation do not show significantly differences in success rates [42]; however the latter has been found to have lower rates of re-operation and recurrence [43]. It is generally agreed that total parathyroidectomy alone is associated with lower rates of recurrence and re-operation than the other two approaches; however it has greater risk of post-operative hypoparathyroidism and hypocalcaemia [43, 44].

Tertiary Hyperparathyroidism Approaches

The main indication for surgical intervention for tertiary HPT is typically symptomatic hypercalcaemia [45] and is associated with greater rates of cure than medical management [46]. Operative management of tertiary HPT can include subtotal parathyroidectomy and total parathyroidectomy with the latter being reported to have slightly higher cure rates and slightly lower recurrence rates [46].

References

1. Cho NL, Doherty GM. Principles in surgical management of primary hyperparathyroidism. In: Randolph GW, editor. Surgery of the thyroid and parathyroid glands. 3rd ed. Elsevier; 2021. p. 502–16.
2. Pradhan R, Agarwal A, Lombardi CP, Raffaelli M. Applied embryology of the thyroid and parathyroid glands. In: Randolph GW, editor. Surgery of the thyroid and parathyroid glands. 3rd ed. Elsevier; 2021. p. 15–25.
3. Ahadi MS, Gill AJ. Surgical pathology of parathyroid glands. In: Randolph GW, editor. Surgery of the thyroid and parathyroid glands. 3rd ed. Elsevier; 2021. p. 597–604.
4. Lubitz CC, Duh QY. Guide to preoperative parathyroid localization testing. In: Randolph GW, editor. Surgery of the thyroid and parathyroid glands. 3rd ed. Elsevier; 2021. p. 494–501.
5. Roser P, Leca BM, Coelho C, Schulte KM, Gilbert J, Drakou EE, et al. Diagnosis and management of parathyroid carcinoma: a state-of-the-art review. Vol. 30, Endocrine-related cancer. BioScientifica Ltd.; 2023.
6. Davies MP, John Evans TW, Tahir F, Balasubramanian SP. Parathyroid cancer: a systematic review of diagnostic biomarkers. Surgeon [Internet]. 2021;19(6):e536–48. Available from: https://www.sciencedirect.com/science/article/pii/S1479666X21000329.
7. Silverberg S, Bilezikian J. The diagnosis and management of asymptomatic primary hyperparathyroidism. Nat Clin Pract Endocrinol Metab. 2006;2(9):494–503.
8. Silverberg SJ, Bilzekian JP. Primary hyperparathyroidism: pathophysiology, surgical indications and preoperative workup. In: Randolph GW, editor. Surgery of the thyroid and parathyroid glands. 3rd ed. Elsevier; 2021. p. 486–93.
9. Xu W, Li S, Cheng F, Gong L, Tang W, Lu J, et al. Microwave ablation versus radiofrequency ablation for patients with primary and secondary hyperparathyroidism: a meta-analysis, vol. 55. Int Urol Nephrol. Springer Science and Business Media B.V; 2023. p. 2237–47.
10. Issa PP, Kandil E, Lee GS. Radiofrequency ablation as a treatment modality for primary hyperparathyroidism: a systematic literature review. Vol. 13, Gland Surgery. AME Publishing Company; 2024. p. 87–99.
11. Pappachan JM, Lahart IM, Viswanath AK, Borumandi F, Sodi R, Metzendorf MI, et al. Parathyroidectomy for adults with primary hyperparathyroidism. Cochrane Database Syst Rev. 2023;2023(3).
12. Livschitz J, Yen TWF, Evans DB, Wang TS, Dream S. Long-term quality of life after arathyroidectomy for primary hyperparathyroidism: a systematic review. JAMA Surg [Internet]. 2022;157(11):1051–8. https://doi.org/10.1001/jamasurg.2022.4249.
13. Rubin MR, Bilezikian JP, McMahon DJ, Jacobs T, Shane E, Siris E, et al. The natural history of primary hyperparathyroidism with or without parathyroid surgery after 15 years. J Clin Endocrinol Metab [Internet]. 2008;93(9):3462–70. https://doi.org/10.1210/jc.2007-1215.
14. Wilhelm SM, Wang TS, Ruan DT, Lee JA, Asa SL, Duh QY, et al. The American Association of Endocrine Surgeons guidelines for definitive management of primary hyperparathyroidism. JAMA Surg [Internet]. 2016;151(10):959–68. https://doi.org/10.1001/jamasurg.2016.2310.
15. Kim WW, Lee YM, Sung TY, Chung KW, Hong SJ. Selection of parathyroidectomy methods for primary hyperparathyroidism according to concordance between ultrasonography and MIBI scan results. Gland Surg. 2021;10(1):298–306.

16. Mihai R, Simon D, Hellman P. Imaging for primary hyperparathyroidism—an evidence-based analysis. Langenbecks Arch Surg [Internet]. 2009;394(5):765–84. https://doi.org/10.1007/s00423-009-0534-4.
17. Wojtczak B, Syrycka J, Kaliszewski K, Rudnicki J, Bolanowski M, Barczynski M. Surgical implications of recent modalities for parathyroid imaging. Vol. 9, Gland surgery. AME Publishing Company; 2020. p. S86–94.
18. Kattar N, Migneron M, Debakey MS, Haidari M, Pou AM, McCoul ED. Advanced computed tomographic localization techniques for primary hyperparathyroidism: a systematic review and meta-analysis. JAMA Otolaryngol [Internet]. 2022;148(5):448–56. https://doi.org/10.1001/jamaoto.2022.0271.
19. Warshavsky A, Rubin R, Carmel-Neidermann NN, Brenner A, Shendler G, Kampel L, et al. 4DCT in discordant parathyroid adenoma scans: case series and meta-analysis. Laryngoscope. 2024;134(5):2198–205.
20. Scheepers MHMC, Al-Difaie Z, Brandts L, Peeters A, Winkens B, Al-Taher M, et al. Diagnostic performance of magnetic resonance imaging for parathyroid localization of primary hyperparathyroidism: a systematic review. Diagnostics [Internet]. 2024;14(1). Available from: https://www.mdpi.com/2075-4418/14/1/25.
21. Neumann DR, Esselstyn CB, MacIntyre WJ, Go RT, Obuchowski NA, Chen EQ, et al. Comparison of FDG-PET and Sestamibi-SPECT in primary hyperparathyroidism. J Nucl Med [Internet]. 1996;37(11):1809. Available from: http://jnm.snmjournals.org/content/37/11/1809.abstract
22. Boccalatte LA, Higuera F, Gómez NL, de la Torre AY, Mazzaro EL, Galich AM, et al. Usefulness of 18F-fluorocholine positron emission tomography–computed tomography in locating lesions in hyperparathyroidism: a systematic review. JAMA Otolaryngol [Internet]. 2019;145(8):743–50. https://doi.org/10.1001/jamaoto.2019.0574.
23. Patel DD, Bhattacharjee S, Pandey AK, Kopp CR, Ashwathanarayana AG, Patel HV, et al. Comparison of 4D computed tomography and F-18 fluorocholine PET for localisation of parathyroid lesions in primary hyperparathyroidism: a systematic review and meta-analysis. Clin Endocrinol (Oxf) [Internet]. 2023;99(3):262–71. https://doi.org/10.1111/cen.14875.
24. Ibraheem K, Toraih EA, Haddad AB, Farag M, Randolph GW, Kandil E. Selective parathyroid venous sampling in primary hyperparathyroidism: a systematic review and meta-analysis. Laryngoscope [Internet]. 2018;128(11):2662–7. https://doi.org/10.1002/lary.27213.
25. Quinn AJ, Ryan ÉJ, Garry S, James DL, Boland MR, Young O, et al. Use of intraoperative parathyroid hormone in minimally invasive Parathyroidectomy for primary hyperparathyroidism: a systematic review and meta-analysis. JAMA Otolaryngol [Internet]. 2021;147(2):135–43. https://doi.org/10.1001/jamaoto.2020.4021.
26. Carneiro-Pla D, Pellitteri PK. Intraoperative PTH monitoring during parathyroid surgery. In: Randolph GW, editor. Surgery of the thyroid and parathyroid glands. 3rd ed. Elsevier; 2021. p. 546–52.
27. Siperstein AE, Stephen AE, Milas M. Standard bilateral parathyroid exploration. In: Randolph GW, editor. Surgery of the thyroid and parathyroid glands. 3rd ed. Elsevier; 2021. p. 517–28.
28. Jinih M, O'Connell E, O'Leary DP, Liew A, Redmond HP. Focused versus bilateral parathyroid exploration for primary hyperparathyroidism: a systematic review and Meta-analysis. Ann Surg Oncol [Internet]. 2017;24(7):1924–34. https://doi.org/10.1245/s10434-016-5694-1.
29. Ishii H, Mihai R, Watkinson JC, Kim DS. Systematic review of cure and recurrence rates following minimally invasive parathyroidectomy. BJS Open [Internet]. 2018;2(6):364–70. https://doi.org/10.1002/bjs5.77.
30. Paspala A, Spartalis E, Nastos C, Tsourouflis G, Dimitroulis D, Pikoulis E, et al. Robotic-assisted parathyroidectomy and short-term outcomes: a systematic review of the literature. J Robot Surg [Internet]. 2020;14(6):821–7. https://doi.org/10.1007/s11701-020-01119-x.
31. Bagul A, Patel HP, Chadwick D, Harrison BJ, Balasubramanian SP. Primary hyperparathyroidism: an analysis of failure of parathyroidectomy. World J Surg [Internet]. 2014;38(3):1. https://doi.org/10.1007/s00268-013-2434-6.

32. Zaman M, Raveendran L, Senay A, Sayles H, Acharya R, Dhir M. Long-term recurrence rates after surgery in primary hyperparathyroidism. J Clin Endocrinol Metab [Internet]. 2023;108(11):3022–30. https://doi.org/10.1210/clinem/dgad316.
33. Harrison B. What steps should be considered in the patient who has had a negative cervical exploration for primary hyperparathyroidism? Clin Endocrinol (Oxf) [Internet]. 2009;71(5):624–7. https://doi.org/10.1111/j.1365-2265.2009.03597.x.
34. Busaidy NL, Jimenez C, Habra MA, Schultz PN, El-Naggar AK, Clayman GL, et al. Parathyroid carcinoma: a 22-year experience. Head Neck [Internet]. 2004;26(8):716–26. https://doi.org/10.1002/hed.20049.
35. Hundahl SA, Fleming ID, Fremgen AM, Menck HR. Two hundred eighty-six cases of parathyroid carcinoma treated in the U.S. between 1985-1995: a National Cancer Data Base report. Cancer. 1999;86(3):538–44.
36. Waldmann J, López CL, Langer P, Rothmund M, Bartsch DK. Surgery for multiple endocrine neoplasia type 1-associated primary hyperparathyroidism. Br J Surg [Internet]. 2010;97(10):1528–34. https://doi.org/10.1002/bjs.7154.
37. Nastos C, Papaconstantinou D, Kofopoulos-Lymperis E, Peppa M, Pikoulis A, Lykoudis P, et al. Optimal extent of initial parathyroid resection in patients with multiple endocrine neoplasia syndrome type 1: a meta-analysis. Surgery [Internet]. 2021;169(2):302–10. https://doi.org/10.1016/j.surg.2020.08.021.
38. Schreinemakers JMJ, Pieterman CRC, Scholten A, Vriens MR, Valk GD, Borel Rinkes IHM. The optimal surgical treatment for primary hyperparathyroidism in MEN1 patients: a systematic review. World J Surg [Internet]. 2011;35(9):1214. https://doi.org/10.1007/s00268-011-1068-9.
39. Bouriez D, Gronnier C, Haissaguerre M, Tabarin A, Najah H. Less than subtotal parathyroidectomy for multiple endocrine neoplasia type 1 primary hyperparathyroidism: a systematic review and meta-analysis. World J Surg [Internet]. 2022;46(11):1. https://doi.org/10.1007/s00268-022-06633-7.
40. Scholten A, Schreinemakers JMJ, Pieterman CRC, Valk GD, Vriens MR, Borel Rinkes IHM. Evolution of surgical treatment of primary hyperparathyroidism in patients with multiple endocrine neoplasia type 2A. Endocr Pract [Internet]. 2011;17(1):7–15. https://doi.org/10.4158/EP10050.OR.
41. Song Z, Wu C, Wang R, Gillis A, Fazendin J, Lindeman B, et al. The effects of parathyroidectomy vs medical treatments for secondary hyperparathyroidism in patients undergoing Dialysis: a Meta-analysis. Endocrine Practice [Internet]. 2024;30(6):569–76. Available from: https://www.sciencedirect.com/science/article/pii/S1530891X24004786.
42. Yuan Q, Liao Y, Zhou R, Liu J, Tang J, Wu G. Subtotal parathyroidectomy versus total parathyroidectomy with autotransplantation for secondary hyperparathyroidism: an updated systematic review and meta-analysis. Langenbecks Arch Surg [Internet]. 2019;404(6):669–79. https://doi.org/10.1007/s00423-019-01809-7.
43. Hou J, Shan H, Zhang Y, Deng X, Guo B, Kang J, et al. Network meta-analysis of surgical treatment for secondary hyperparathyroidism. Am J Otolaryngol [Internet]. 2020;41(2):102370. Available from: https://www.sciencedirect.com/science/article/pii/S0196070919310464
44. Liu ME, Qiu NC, Zha SL, Du ZP, Wang YF, Wang Q, et al. To assess the effects of parathyroidectomy (TPTX versus TPTX+AT) for secondary hyperparathyroidism in chronic renal failure: a systematic review and meta-analysis. Int J Surg Elsevier Ltd. 2017;44:353–62.
45. Tang JA, Friedman J, Hwang MS, Salapatas AM, Bonzelaar LB, Friedman M. Parathyroidectomy for tertiary hyperparathyroidism: a systematic review. Am J Otolaryngol [Internet]. 2017;38(5):630–5. Available from: https://www.sciencedirect.com/science/article/pii/S0196070917301758.
46. Dulfer RR, Franssen GJH, Hesselink DA, Hoorn EJ, van Eijck CHJ, van Ginhoven TM. Systematic review of surgical and medical treatment for tertiary hyperparathyroidism. Br J Surg [Internet]. 2017;104(7):804–13. https://doi.org/10.1002/bjs.10554.

Perioperative Imaging and Identification of Parathyroid Glands

27

Krishnakumar Thankappan, Lakshmi Ravunniarth Menon, and Sandhya Chirukandath Jayasankaran

Editorial

Dr. Thankappan and his colleagues have done an exhaustive review of parathyroid imaging and its identification, both preoperatively and intraoperatively. They have analyzed each and every imaging study, with its advantages and disadvantages. The ultrasound of the neck still remains the mainstay of evaluation. There is a considerable emphasis now on surgeon-performed ultrasound. It would be important for the operating surgeon to perform the ultrasound on the operating table and compare the findings with the intraoperative evaluation. This is the best way to learn and be an expert on parathyroid localization. The preoperative ultrasound will also define incidental findings of thyroid nodules, which should be worked up prior to surgical exploration.

There appears to be specific entity known as normocalcemic hyperparathyroidism. Institutional experience with this condition is generally quite limited, so patients should be referred to the centers of parathyroid excellence. Ultrasound evaluation and localization of the enlarged parathyroid gland just before surgery are good considerations. The weight of a normal parathyroid gland is 35–50 mg, and generally the parathyroid adenomas would be more than 500 mg. If the enlarged gland is 100–300 mg, one may consider this to be a part of multiglandular disease. The management of multiglandular disease is a complex subject, and most of the surgeons would consider subtotal parathyroidectomy.

There is a considerable interest now in four-dimensional CT scan, which provides highly detailed localization of the enlarged parathyroid gland and can even

K. Thankappan (✉) · L. R. Menon
Department of Head and Neck Surgery and Oncology, Amrita Institute of Medical Sciences and Research Centre, Amrita Vishwa Vidyapeetham, Kochi, India

S. C. Jayasankaran
Department of Radiology, Amrita Institute of Medical Sciences and Research Centre, Amrita Vishwa Vidyapeetham, Kochi, India

P. S. Pai et al. (eds.), *Controversies in Cancer of the Thyroid and Parathyroid Glands*, https://doi.org/10.1007/978-3-032-13130-0_27

describe the weight of enlarged parathyroid gland preoperatively. The authors have also discussed the newer advances in parathyroid identification, such as Niraf and PTEye, which are expensive tools. There appears to be considerable interest in Niraf and PTEye in Europe and the United States. From the preliminary results, it appears that these investigations are quite helpful in localizing the parathyroid gland during total thyroidectomy. The chapter is extremely well written, with considerable discussion about the advantages and disadvantages of each technique.

Ashok R. Shaha

Introduction

Perioperative imaging has revolutionized the management of parathyroid disorders, particularly in optimizing surgical outcomes for conditions such as primary hyperparathyroidism (PHPT). PHPT, caused by excessive secretion of parathyroid hormone, is most commonly due to a solitary adenoma, but multiglandular disease or ectopic adenomas can pose significant diagnostic and surgical challenges [1]. Successful parathyroidectomy, the definitive treatment for PHPT, depends on precise identification and localization of hyperfunctioning parathyroid tissue.

Historically, the surgical approach relied on bilateral neck exploration, requiring extensive dissection to identify all four glands. While effective, this approach carried higher morbidity and prolonged operative time. The advent of focused parathyroidectomy necessitated accurate preoperative localization and intraoperative validation, emphasizing the importance of robust perioperative imaging strategies [2]. Perioperative imaging not only guides surgical planning but also minimizes complications such as recurrent laryngeal nerve injury and persistent hyperparathyroidism.

In addition to anatomical localization, perioperative imaging addresses the unique challenges posed by re-operative parathyroid surgery, where scar tissue and altered anatomy increase the risk of surgical failure. The growing emphasis on minimally invasive techniques has further underscored the need for reliable imaging to achieve targeted and efficient interventions. Understanding the role of perioperative imaging is thus essential for improving the precision, safety, and success of parathyroid surgery.

Preoperative Identification of Parathyroid Glands

Objective of Preoperative Imaging

Preoperative imaging aims to identify abnormal parathyroid glands responsible for hyperparathyroidism, facilitating a focused surgical parathyroidectomy. This approach minimizes the need for bilateral neck exploration, thereby reducing the risk of complications such as bilateral recurrent laryngeal nerve injury. Figure 27.1 details the management of primary hyperparathyroidism.

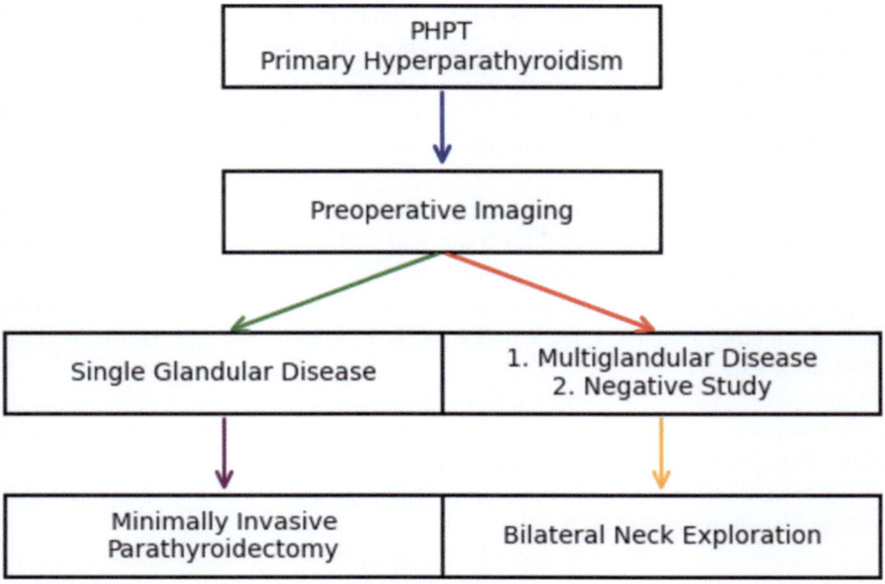

Fig. 27.1 Management algorithm in hyperparathyroidism

Imaging Modalities for Preoperative Localization
Preoperative imaging techniques for identifying parathyroid glands are categorized into first-line and cross-sectional imaging modalities [3, 4, 5].

First-line Imaging Modalities

First-line imaging modalities are typically employed as the initial step in localization and include the following:

1. *Ultrasound (USG)*: A non-invasive, readily available technique for neck assessment
2. *Sestamibi scintigraphy*: A nuclear medicine scan that detects hyperfunctioning parathyroid tissue with high sensitivity and specificity

Second-line Imaging Modalities

Second-line imaging modalities are utilized when first-line imaging is inconclusive, discordant, or negative. These include the following:

1. *Contrast-Enhanced Computed Tomography (CECT)*: Provides detailed anatomic visualization
2. *Contrast-Enhanced Magnetic Resonance Imaging (CEMRI)*: Useful for soft tissue differentiation and problem-solving in complex cases

3. *4D-Computed Tomography (4D-CT)*: Combines anatomical and functional imaging, offering superior localization of hyperfunctioning parathyroid glands
4. *Positron Emission Tomography-Computed Tomography (PET-CT)*: Often used with tracers like 18F-fluorocholine for cases where standard imaging fails

The European Association of Nuclear Medicine (EANM) practice guidelines for parathyroid imaging have shown that the first-line modality is the sestamibi scan with USG neck. The alternative to the first-line modality in case of negative, discordant, or inconclusive results is PET-CT with USG neck. The second line of imaging is 4D-CT neck or PET-CT. Problem-solving imaging will be MRI neck [6].

First-line Preoperative Imaging

Ultrasonography (USG) Neck

It is the most commonly performed initial imaging modality for preoperative localization of parathyroid glands. It employs a high-frequency linear transducer (10–12 MHz) and is conducted with the patient in a supine position with the neck hyperextended. Scanning typically covers the area from the carotid artery laterally to the midline and from the hyoid bone superiorly to the thoracic inlet inferiorly. Patients may be asked to swallow to visualize better the inferior parathyroid glands and their relationship to the clavicle [7]. Normal parathyroid glands are often not visible on ultrasound due to their small size relative to the thyroid gland. However, parathyroid adenomas typically appear as well-defined, ovoid, or bean-shaped hypoechoic lesions (Figs. 27.2 and 27.3). The hypoechoic appearance is attributed to the compact cellularity characteristic of parathyroid adenomas. Color Doppler imaging can identify a feeding vessel, often called the polar vessel, which most commonly originates from the inferior thyroid artery [8]. The feeder artery of a parathyroid adenoma frequently branches around the periphery of the gland before entering its center, creating a pattern known as rim vascularity. Color Doppler imaging (Fig. 27.4) can also reveal asymmetric hypervascularity, a helpful diagnostic feature for detecting adenomas. The method of graded compression is another valuable technique for differentiating adenomas from surrounding soft tissue. Parathyroid adenomas are typically less compressible than the surrounding tissue, which aids in their identification. A meta-analysis by Rudra et al. involving 54 studies demonstrated that ultrasound has a sensitivity of 79% in detecting parathyroid adenomas but only 35% in cases of hyperplasia [1]. Another prospective study with 98 patients showed that a polar feeding vessel significantly enhances the specificity for detecting parathyroid adenomas [10]. However, studies indicate poor sensitivity (20–40%) of ultrasound in identifying parathyroid lesions in cases of double adenomas [11].

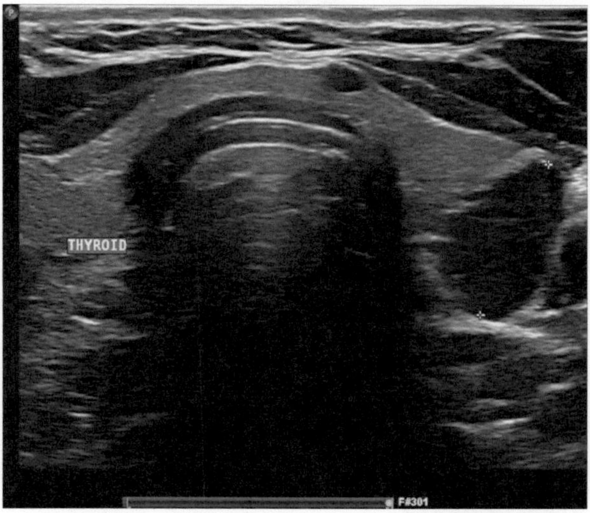

Fig. 27.2 Parathyroid adenoma on USG seen as hypoechoic area

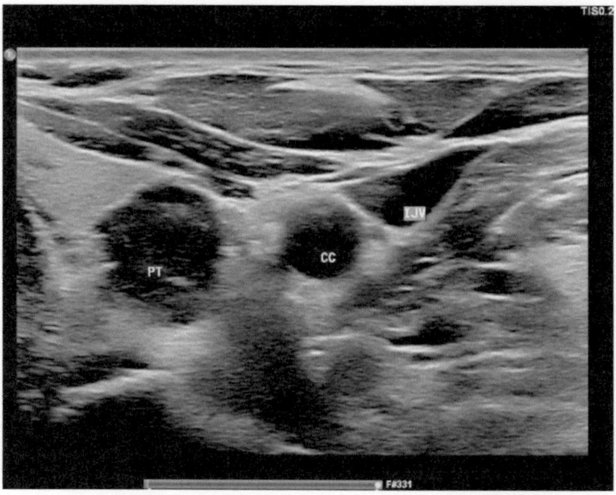

Fig. 27.3 Parathyroid adenoma and its relationship to surrounding structures. PT parathyroid; CC common carotid; IJV internal jugular vein

Advantages and Disadvantages of Ultrasound

Advantages

1. *No ionizing radiation:* This makes it safe for repeated use.
2. *Non-invasive:* Minimizes patient discomfort.
3. *Cost-effective and rapid:* Affordable and quick to perform.
4. *Short learning curve:* This can be mastered relatively quickly by clinicians.
5. *Widely available:* Accessible in most healthcare settings.
6. *Guidance for needle biopsy:* Facilitates fine-needle aspiration or core biopsy.
7. *Identification of concomitant thyroid nodules:* Useful for detecting additional thyroid abnormalities.

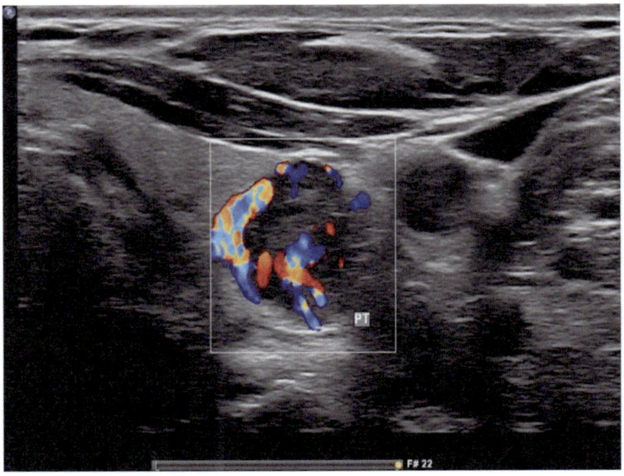

Fig. 27.4 Parathyroid adenoma, seen on color Doppler imaging showing asymmetric hypervascularity. PT parathyroid

Disadvantages

1. *Operator dependency:* Accuracy depends on the skill and experience of the clinician.
2. *Limited sensitivity in multiglandular disease:* Poor at detecting parathyroid hyperplasia in multiglandular disorders.
3. *Acoustic limitations:* Ineffective for imaging ectopic glands located behind air or bone, such as mediastinal ectopic parathyroid glands.
4. *Difficulty distinguishing from lymph nodes:* Challenges in differentiating parathyroid glands from nearby lymph nodes.
5. *Complications with nodular thyroid disease:* Difficulty in identifying parathyroid adenomas when thyroid nodules are present [9].

Additional Uses of Neck Ultrasound

1. *Combination with Fine-Needle Aspiration Cytology (FNAC):* Ultrasound can be combined with FNAC to confirm parathyroid lesions, particularly in challenging situations such as postoperative anatomical changes or a distorted neck. However, caution is advised as parathyromatosis—a rare condition caused by the seeding of abnormal parathyroid tissue along the FNAC track—can occur [12].
2. *Sonography-Guided Ethanol Ablation:* This technique is employed to treat tertiary hyperparathyroidism, particularly in patients with renal failure who are not suitable candidates for surgery. The procedure involves injecting ethanol into the parathyroid glands, with the volume of ethanol corresponding to 50% of the gland's volume. Injection continues until the absence of blood flow is confirmed using color Doppler imaging. Sonography-guided ethanol ablation is a viable alternative for patients who are not surgically fit for gland excision [13].

Sestamibi Scintigraphy

Nuclear imaging has been used for parathyroid localization since the 1980s and remains the most accurate and reliable diagnostic method. It is considered the first-line imaging tool in the era of focused parathyroidectomy. No radionuclide is specific to the parathyroid glands, as all available radionuclides accumulate in both parathyroid and thyroid tissues. The imaging process involves the oral or intravenous administration of a radiotracer, which is then captured by a gamma camera. Planar nuclear imaging produces two-dimensional images from a single perspective, while single-photon emission computed tomography (SPECT) captures multiple two-dimensional images from different angles to create a three-dimensional structural reference. Sestamibi (hexakis 2-methoxy-2-methylpropylisonitrile), also known as MIBI, was first introduced for parathyroid imaging in 1989. It is a lipophilic cation that localizes in hyperfunctioning parathyroid glands due to its affinity for the mitochondria-rich oxyphilic cells commonly found in parathyroid adenomas [14]. The washout rate of sestamibi from parathyroid adenomas varies depending on the mitochondrial content of the tissue. Although normal thyroid tissue also accumulates sestamibi, its lower mitochondrial content leads to a faster washout compared to parathyroid adenomas, aiding in their differentiation.

Variations of Sestamibi Scintigraphy

Dual-Phase MIBI Imaging:

Sestamibi is absorbed by both thyroid and parathyroid tissues, but adenomatous and hyperplastic parathyroid glands retain the tracer for a longer duration (Fig. 27.5). This technique involves early imaging (10 to 30 minutes post-injection) and delayed imaging (90 to 150 minutes post-injection). While the tracer washes out quickly from thyroid tissue, it is retained in hyperfunctioning parathyroid glands, enabling better identification. Double-phase imaging is the most commonly used variation of sestamibi scintigraphy.

MIBI with SPECT:

Planar imaging has largely been replaced by SPECT imaging, which involves capturing images from multiple angles to construct a three-dimensional representation. SPECT/CT enhances the anatomical localization (Fig. 27.6) of hyperfunctioning parathyroid glands, significantly improving the sensitivity of sestamibi scintigraphy [15].

Dual Isotope Subtraction Imaging:

This technique employs two radiotracers, such as I123 or Tc99 (thyroid-specific tracers), alongside sestamibi. The thyroid-specific tracer accumulates only in the thyroid gland. Images acquired from the two tracers are digitally subtracted to identify persistent focal uptake, indicating abnormal parathyroid tissue (Fig. 27.7). Although effective, this method exposes the patient to additional radiation. Studies

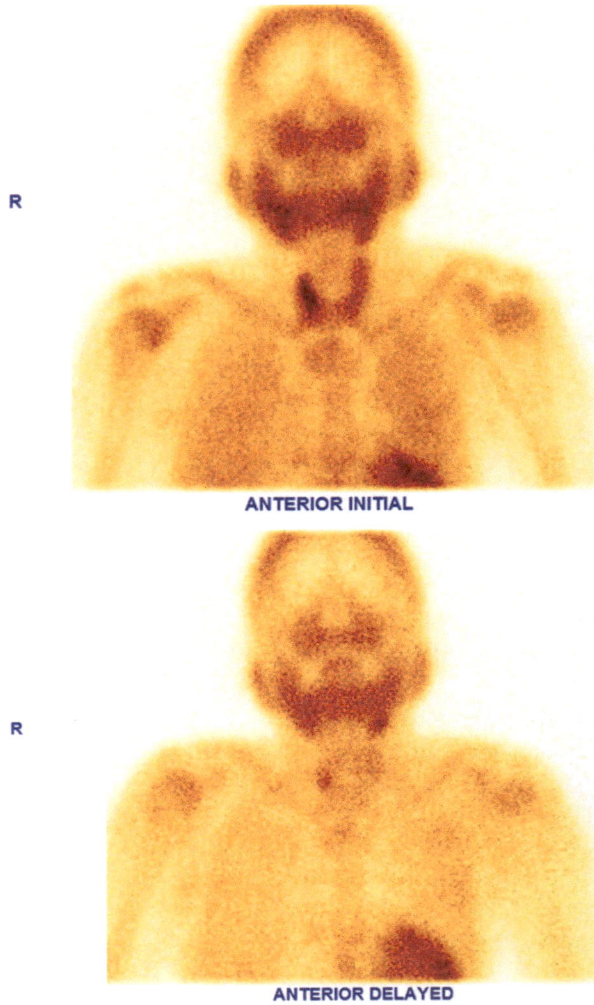

Fig. 27.5 Showing dual-phase MIBI with delayed image uptake in right inferior parathyroid. Initial image (upper) showing uptake both in thyroid and parathyroid, delayed image (lower) after 2 hours showing uptake only in the right parathyroid

report a sensitivity of 89% and specificity of 90–95% for detecting parathyroid adenomas [16]. A study by Civelek et al., involving 338 patients, demonstrated the sensitivity of Tc99 sestamibi scintigraphy to be 90% for adenomas, 73% for double adenomas, and 45% for hyperplasia [17].

Advantages and Disadvantages of Sestamibi Scintigraphy

Advantages

1. *Identification of ectopic glands:* Effective in detecting ectopic parathyroid glands, including deep or posterior glands that may be missed on ultrasound.

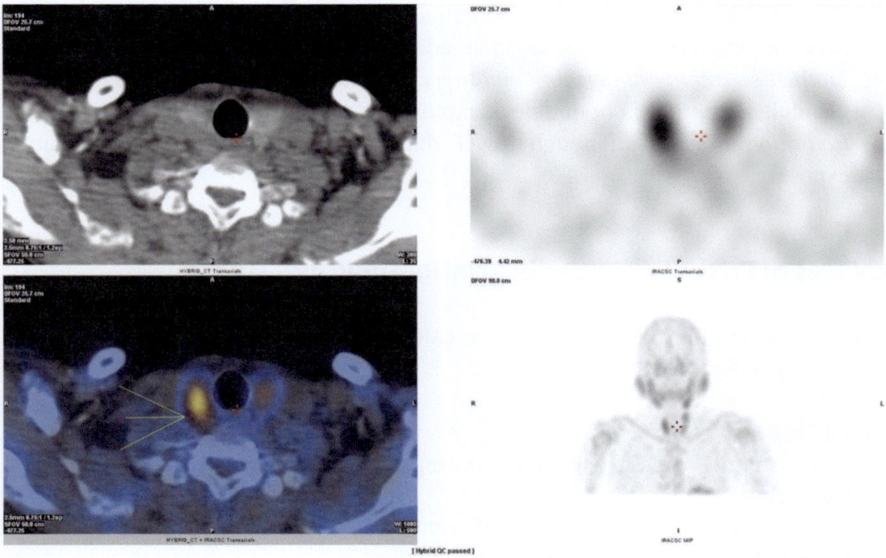

Fig. 27.6 Showing sestamibi scintigraphy with SPECT-CT showing right inferior PTH adenoma

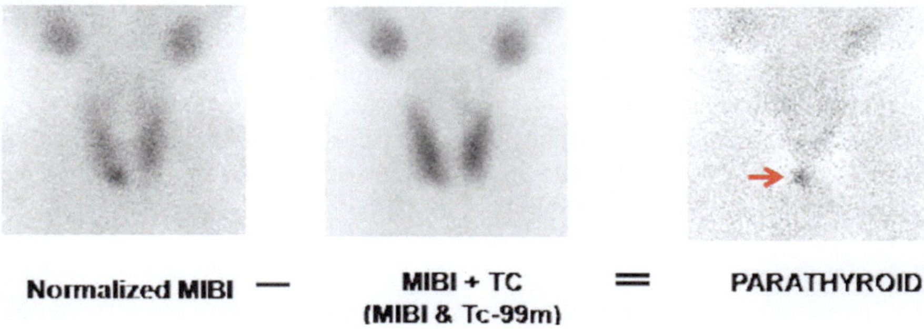

Fig. 27.7 Showing dual subtraction sestamibi scintigraphy showing right inferior PTH adenoma

2. *Alternative for contrast allergies:* Suitable for patients who cannot undergo iodinated CT contrast or 4D-CT due to allergies or renal failure.
3. *Lower radiation exposure:* Involves a lower radiation dose compared to 4D-CT.
4. *Better anatomical localization:* When combined with SPECT/CT, it provides enhanced anatomical detail.
5. *High sensitivity for adenomas:* Particularly useful for identifying solitary parathyroid adenomas.

Disadvantages

1. *Time-consuming:* Requires long image acquisition times, making it less convenient.
2. *Cost:* More expensive than ultrasound or 4D-CT.

3. *False-positive/negative results:* Potential for misdiagnosis due to factors such as concomitant thyroid disease or small adenomas.
4. *Limited sensitivity in certain conditions:* Reduced sensitivity in cases of multi-glandular hyperplasia or double adenomas.
5. *Radiation exposure:* Though lower than 4D-CT, it still involves radiation exposure.

Causes of Errors in Sestamibi Scintigraphy

Errors in sestamibi scintigraphy can be categorized into false negatives (17–25%) and false positives (5–10%):

False Negatives

1. *Patient-related issues:* Movement during imaging can cause misregistration of the images.
2. *Ectopic adenomas:* Misdiagnosis of adenomas located in atypical positions.
3. *Deep-seated lesions:* Lesions that are challenging to detect due to their location.
4. *Small adenoma volume (<500 mg):* Smaller adenomas may not retain enough tracer to be visualized.
5. *Mitochondrial characteristics:* Adenomas with low oxyphil cell content may exhibit rapid tracer washout.
6. *Hyperplasia:* Small size and reduced oxyphil cell content result in lower sensitivity (approximately 45%).
7. *Double adenomas:* The sensitivity drops to 30% in cases of multiple adenomas.
8. *Increased P-glycoprotein expression:* Elevated expression may lead to rapid tracer clearance, reducing visibility.

False Positives

1. *Thyroid-related conditions:* Conditions like oxyphil adenoma and Hashimoto's thyroiditis can mimic parathyroid uptake.
2. *Reactive lymph nodes:* Nodes with abnormal tracer uptake may lead to misinterpretation.
3. *Parathyroid carcinoma:* Can present tracer uptake resembling benign conditions.
4. *Lymphoma:* Certain lymphomas may also retain the tracer.
5. *Metastatic disease:* Metastatic lesions may exhibit radiotracer uptake, confounding results.
6. *Sarcoidosis:* Granulomatous diseases may mimic hyperparathyroid states.
7. *Thymoma:* Thymic tumors can cause false-positive uptake.
8. *Mediastinal veins:* Prominent veins may obscure the imaging.
9. *Ectopic thyroid tissue:* Thyroid tissue in ectopic locations may be mistaken for parathyroid glands.

These limitations underline the need to combine sestamibi scintigraphy with complementary imaging modalities, such as ultrasound or SPECT/CT, to improve diagnostic accuracy.

Combined Sonography with Scintigraphy for Preoperative Hyperparathyroidism

Combining sonography with scintigraphy significantly enhances the sensitivity for diagnosing preoperative parathyroid adenomas, making it the first-line investigative choice. While sonography is highly specific for identifying the side and site of the adenoma, scintigraphy proves invaluable for detecting ectopic glands. A study by Lumachi et al. demonstrated a combined sensitivity of 95% for this approach, compared to 80% for sonography alone and 87% for scintigraphy alone [18]. Concordant findings on sonography and scintigraphy facilitate planning for focused parathyroidectomy, achieving cure rates comparable to those of traditional bilateral neck exploration. However, both techniques exhibit reduced sensitivity for detecting multiglandular disease and double adenomas. Studies have reported a sensitivity of only 30% in cases involving multiglandular disease [19].

Cross-sectional Imaging for Parathyroid Glands

Indications for Cross-sectional Imaging

1. Suspicion of multiglandular disease (10–30%): Includes hyperplasia and double adenomas.
2. Detection of small lesions: The sensitivity of ultrasound and scintigraphy for small lesions ranges from 16 to 45%.
3. Recurrent or persistent cases of hyperparathyroidism.
4. Suspected parathyroid carcinoma.
5. Parathyromatosis.
6. Ectopic parathyroid lesions (20–25%).
7. Discordant, negative, or inconclusive results on ultrasound or scintigraphy.

Computed Tomography (CT) of the Neck

CT and MRI are often employed as second-line imaging modalities in cases of recurrent or persistent hyperparathyroidism or when initial parathyroidectomy fails. CT imaging extends from the skull base to the mediastinum, identifying parathyroid lesions as hypointense ovoid masses (Fig. 27.8a) that show contrast enhancement (Fig. 27.8b) relative to the thyroid gland. With the advent of 4D-CT, conventional CT neck imaging has become largely obsolete for parathyroid localization.

Advantages

1. Effective in detecting ectopic parathyroid glands
2. Rapid image acquisition time
3. Relatively cost-effective compared to other advanced modalities
4. Provides detailed anatomical visualization

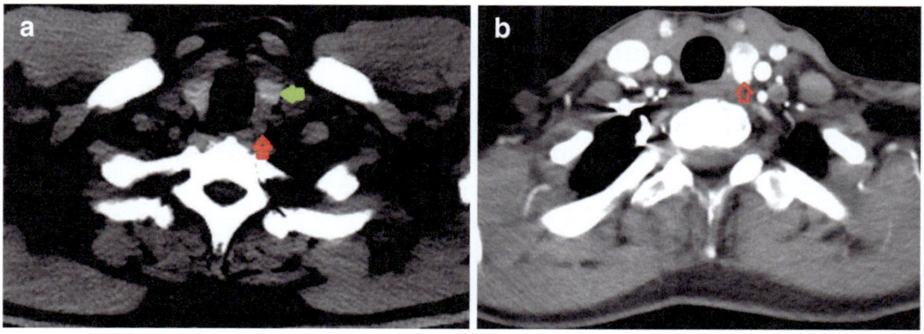

Fig. 27.8 (**a**) CT scan without contrast, normal thyroid tissue (green arrow) seen as hyperdense structure and parathyroid seen hypodense (**b**) CT scan with contrast, normal thyroid tissue (green arrow) seen as hyperdense structure and parathyroid seen hypodense

Disadvantages

1. Exposure to ionizing radiation
2. Limited sensitivity in identifying multiglandular disorders

Studies report that CT neck is sensitive to detecting parathyroid lesions, ranging between 46% and 87% [20]. Despite its limitations, CT remains valuable in selected cases where initial imaging is inconclusive or discordant.

Parathyroid 4D-CT

First introduced by Rogers et al. in 2006, 4D-CT was initially used as a complementary imaging modality alongside sestamibi scintigraphy and ultrasound. Over time, it has evolved into a primary imaging technique for the preoperative localization of parathyroid glands [21].

4D-CT involves a triple-phase neck and upper chest CT scan, capturing images during non-contrast, arterial, and delayed phases. The imaging extends from the angle of the mandible to the thoracic inlet, covering all potential ectopic locations of parathyroid glands. The scan is performed with the patient's neck hyperextended to optimize visualization of the thyroid and parathyroid glands.

The Concept of 4D-CT

The "four dimensions" in 4D-CT refer to the following:

1. Three anatomical planes: Axial, coronal, and sagittal views.
2. The fourth dimension is dynamic contrast enhancement over time during serial phases.

Parathyroid adenomas typically appear hypodense on non-contrast imaging (Fig. 27.9a) compared to the hyperdense thyroid gland, which has a high iodine content. Adenomas demonstrate intense enhancement on arterial-phase imaging

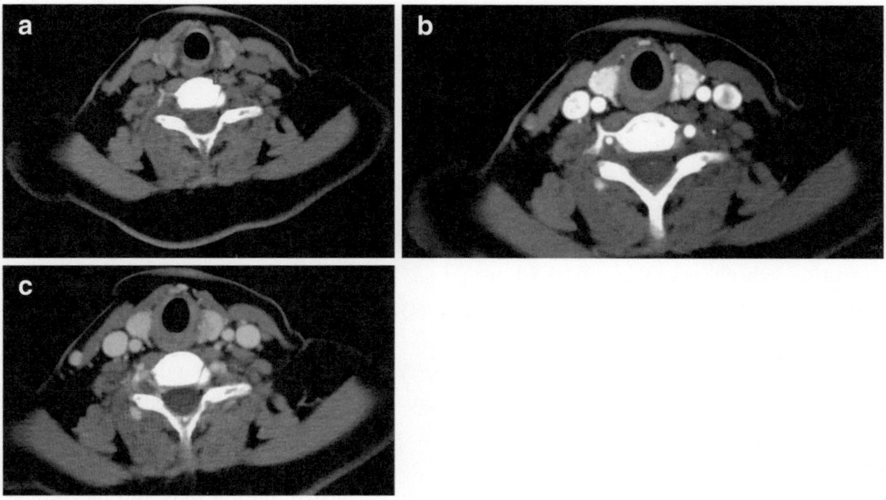

Fig. 27.9 (**a**) 4D-CT showing left inferior parathyroid adenoma (red arrow) in the non-contrast study. (**b**) 4D-CT showing left inferior parathyroid adenoma (red arrow) in the arterial phase of the study. (**c**) 4D-CT showing left inferior parathyroid adenoma (red arrow) in the delayed venous phase of the study

(Fig. 27.9b), followed by a rapid washout on delayed-phase imaging (Fig. 27.9c). In contrast, lymph nodes exhibit mild arterial-phase enhancement that increases in the delayed phase.

Imaging Protocol: A non-contrast scan is performed first, followed by intravenous administration of 75 mL iodinated contrast at 4.0 mL/second with a saline flush. Arterial-phase images are acquired 25–30 seconds after contrast injection, while delayed venous-phase images are captured 60–80 seconds post-injection. A late, delayed phase is optionally performed at 90–105 seconds. Axial images are reconstructed at 1 mm slice thickness for high-resolution detail. 4D-CT is widely accessible, as it can be performed at any imaging center equipped with a 16-slice or higher CT scanner and an intravenous contrast injector.

Key Imaging Features

- Parathyroid adenomas: Most conspicuous in the arterial phase across all three planes, with rapid contrast washout in delayed phases
- Polar vessel sign: Enlarged vessels at the superior or inferior poles of a parathyroid adenoma, aiding in differentiation from other structures
- Lymph nodes: Show progressively increasing enhancement across phases and typically exhibit a fatty hilum, distinguishing them from parathyroid adenomas4D-CT has become a cornerstone imaging modality, particularly in complex or challenging cases, offering high sensitivity and specificity for parathyroid localization.

Advantages and Disadvantages of 4D-CT

Advantages

1. *High spatial resolution:* Provides detailed imaging for precise localization of parathyroid glands.
2. *Superior anatomical detail:* Enables accurate differentiation between parathyroid adenomas, lymph nodes, and other structures.
3. *Fast imaging:* This can be completed within 2 minutes, unlike sestamibi scintigraphy, which may take up to 4 hours.
4. *Not operator-dependent:* Reduces variability associated with ultrasound interpretation.
5. *Detection of ectopic glands:* This modality offers excellent visualization of deep and ectopic parathyroid glands, which are often missed with other modalities.

Disadvantages

1. *Limited availability:* Requires radiological expertise, which may not be universally available.
2. *Atypical enhancement patterns:* Some parathyroid adenomas may not follow the classic enhancement and washout patterns.
3. *Lower accuracy in complex cases:* Sensitivity decreases in multiglandular disease and smaller adenomas.
4. *Higher radiation dose:* Involves greater radiation exposure than other imaging techniques like ultrasound and sestamibi scintigraphy.

A meta-analysis comparing 4D-CT with MIBI SPECT/CT reported a sensitivity and specificity of 85% and 93% for 4D-CT versus 68% and 98% for MIBI SPECT/CT, respectively [22]. This highlights the growing role of 4D-CT as a reliable and efficient imaging modality for parathyroid localization.

PET-CT for Parathyroid Gland Lesions

Positron emission tomography (PET), when combined with computed tomography (CT), provides both functional and anatomical imaging (Fig. 27.10). It involves the intravenous administration of a radioactive tracer, enabling the identification of metabolic and functional abnormalities alongside detailed anatomical visualization [23]. Common PET radiopharmaceuticals for parathyroid imaging are F-18 choline, C-11 choline, C-11 methionine, F-18 FDG (fluorodeoxyglucose), and Ga-68 dotatate. Abnormal parathyroid tissue, such as adenomas or hyperplastic glands, leads to increased secretion of parathyroid hormone, which in turn upregulates phospholipid-dependent choline kinase activity. This heightened activity results in increased uptake of radiotracers, particularly choline-based tracers, within abnormal parathyroid cells [24]. The *Standard Uptake Value (SUV max)* of parathyroid glands in PET-CT is typically more than four times that of adjacent thyroid tissue, providing a clear distinction between normal and abnormal tissues [25]. PET-CT is

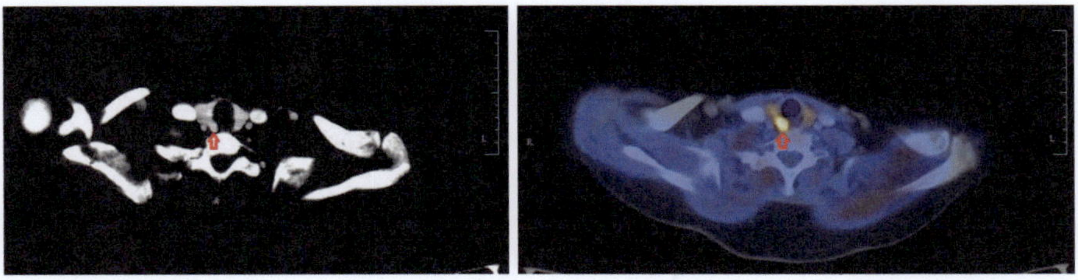

Fig. 27.10 Showing CT with contrast (left image), delayed venous phase showing right inferior parathyroid adenoma (red arrow). Also seen is the choline PET-CT (right image) with uptake (red arrow)

particularly valuable for complex cases, such as recurrent or persistent hyperparathyroidism, ectopic parathyroid glands, or cases where conventional imaging techniques are inconclusive.

Advantages and Disadvantages of Choline PET-CT

Advantages

1. *Effective in resolving discordant imaging results:* Particularly useful when sestamibi scintigraphy and neck ultrasound provide conflicting or inconclusive findings.
2. *Lower radiation dose:* Choline PET-CT involves less radiation exposure compared to MIBI-SPECT or 4D-CT.
3. *Shorter acquisition time:* Imaging is completed faster than many other modalities.
4. *Higher resolution:* Smaller lesions can be detected due to the superior spatial resolution of CT.

Disadvantages

1. *Lack of standardization:* There is no universally accepted protocol for choline PET-CT imaging, which can affect consistency.
2. *High cost:* The technique is expensive, making it less accessible in many settings.
3. *Limited availability:* Choline PET-CT is not widely available due to the need for specific equipment and expertise.
4. *Nonspecific uptake:* The radiotracer is not exclusive to parathyroid tissue, which can lead to challenges in interpretation.

A meta-analysis reported an overall sensitivity of 95% and a positive predictive value (PPV) of 97% for choline PET-CT in detecting parathyroid lesions [26]. Another meta-analysis by Sang-Woo et al. found that choline PET-CT had the highest odds ratio (5.22) for localizing primary hyperparathyroidism compared to other imaging modalities [27]. Choline PET-CT is a highly effective imaging modality for parathyroid localization, particularly in challenging cases, though its cost and limited availability may restrict its use to select cases.

Magnetic Resonance Imaging (MRI) for Parathyroid Localization

Magnetic resonance imaging (MRI) serves as a second-line imaging modality for preoperative localization of parathyroid glands. It operates by aligning protons in tissue when subjected to a magnetic field, producing a magnetic vector that forms the basis of image generation.

MRI is beneficial in cases where first-line imaging techniques, such as ultrasound or sestamibi scintigraphy, yield negative or discordant results. It is also indicated in situations involving persistent or recurrent primary hyperparathyroidism, previous neck surgery, or suspected ectopic parathyroid glands [28]. Studies report that MRI using a 3 T scanner achieves a sensitivity of over 80% for detecting parathyroid lesions [20]. Despite its limitations, MRI remains a valuable tool for complex cases, particularly in patients with recurrent disease or atypical gland locations.

Imaging Characteristics

- *Normal Parathyroid Glands:* Hypointense on T1-weighted images and hyperintense on T2-weighted images.
- *Contrast Enhancement:* Following intravenous gadolinium administration, rapid enhancement is observed during the arterial phase (Fig. 27.11).
- *Diffusion-Weighted Imaging (DWI):* Measures the random motion of water molecules within tissue. Parathyroid glands appear as bright signals due to their high cellularity.

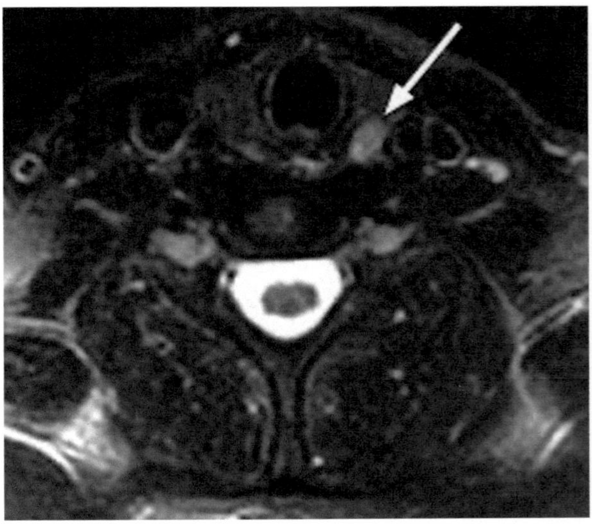

Fig. 27.11 Showing left superior parathyroid adenoma on contrast MRI head and neck

Table 27.1 Summary of diagnostic accuracy of the imaging in parathyroid disease

Imaging	Sensitivity (%)	Specificity (%)	PPV (%)	NPV (%)
USG [31]	70–76	90–93	85–90	80–85
Tc^{99m} sestamibi scintigraphy [31]	75–83	90–95	85–90	85–95
4D-CT [31]	85–89	90–95	90–95	90–96
F-18 [32] fluorocholine PET/CT	90–93	95–96	94	95

Table 27.2 Summary of showing radiation dose in imaging modality

Imaging modality	Radiation dose (mSv)	Cost in USD
Tc-99 m sestamibi SPECT/CT	8–14	1000–2500 dollars
4D-CT	15–25	1500–3500 dollars
F-18 fluorocholine PET/CT	11–15	3000–6000 dollars

Advantages

1. *No radiation exposure:* Ideal for patients who need repeated imaging or are radiation-sensitive.
2. *Superior soft tissue contrast:* Excellent for distinguishing soft tissue structures.
3. *Detection of ectopic glands:* Highly effective in identifying ectopic or deep-seated parathyroid glands [29].

Disadvantages

1. *Longer imaging time:* Requires significantly more time compared to CT or PET-CT
2. *Motion artifacts:* Susceptible to artifacts caused by breathing or patient movement, which can reduce image quality [30]

Table 27.1 summarizes the diagnostic accuracy of different imaging techniques, and Table 27.2 shows the radiation doses.

Intraoperative Parathyroid Imaging

Intraoperative imaging is crucial in accurately identifying parathyroid glands during surgery, especially in challenging cases of ectopic glands, reoperations, or multiglandular disease. These techniques are categorized into non-invasive and invasive methods.

Non-invasive Methods

1. Methylene Blue: A vital dye used to stain parathyroid tissue selectively.
2. Carbon Nanoparticles: Serve as tracers to assist in distinguishing parathyroid glands from surrounding tissues.

3. Raman Spectroscopy: Uses light scattering to identify biochemical signatures unique to parathyroid tissue.
4. Dynamic Optical Contrast Imaging: Provides high-resolution images of tissue vascularity and structure.
5. Laser Speckle Spectroscopy: Analyzes blood flow dynamics within parathyroid glands to distinguish them from other tissues.
6. Shear Wave Elastography: Measures tissue stiffness to differentiate parathyroid glands from adjacent structures.
7. Autofluorescence: Parathyroid glands emit intrinsic fluorescence when exposed to near-infrared light, enabling real-time identification without contrast agents.
8. Indocyanine Green (ICG) Imaging: A dye-based technique that highlights parathyroid glands under near-infrared fluorescence, aiding in their localization.

Invasive Methods

1. Parathyroid Venous Sampling: Involves sampling venous blood to measure parathyroid hormone levels, helping to localize hyperfunctioning glands
2. Parathyroid Arteriography: Uses contrast injection into arteries supplying the parathyroid glands to visualize their location
3. USG/CT-Guided Fine Needle Aspiration Cytology (FNAC): Involves sampling from suspected parathyroid tissue under imaging guidance to confirm its identity

Each method offers unique advantages and applications depending on the complexity of the case, the availability of technology, and the surgeon's expertise. Non-invasive techniques are preferred for safety and efficiency, while invasive methods are reserved for complex or recurrent cases where standard imaging fails.

Non-invasive Techniques of Intraoperative Parathyroid Imaging

Methylene Blue

Methylene blue, introduced by Heinrich Caro in 1876, is a dye with multiple medical applications [33]. Chemically known as *methylthioninium chloride*, it functions by converting ferric iron in hemoglobin to ferrous iron, making it effective for treating conditions such as methemoglobinemia, urinary tract infections, and cyanide poisoning. While methylene blue has established therapeutic uses, its common side effects include headache, confusion, vomiting, shortness of breath and hypertension, potential serotonin syndrome, hemolysis and allergic reactions, and discoloration of bodily fluids such as urine, sweat, and stool [34].

Intraoperative Use in Parathyroid Imaging

In 1971, Dudley proposed methylene blue as an exogenous contrast agent for parathyroid imaging. Parathyroid glands demonstrate the ability to absorb the dye, making them distinguishable during surgery (Fig. 27.10). However, the absorption and subsequent clearance rates differ between parathyroid and thyroid tissue. According to Sari et al., parathyroid glands regain their original color within 3 minutes, while the thyroid gland retains the stain for up to 15 minutes. Despite its availability and utility, methylene blue has limitations, mainly due to its *inconsistent identification rates* and potential *toxicity*, especially when administered intravenously. Reported complications include systemic side effects and rare instances of severe reactions, which have led to the declining use of methylene blue for routine intraoperative parathyroid imaging in favor of safer and more reliable methods. Given the risks and variability in effectiveness, methylene blue is no longer routinely recommended for parathyroid imaging during surgery. Its use is reserved for select cases where other imaging modalities are unavailable or inconclusive.

Carbon Nanoparticles

Carbon nanoparticles are effective tracers used for lymph node detection during surgical procedures. These particles, reduced to nanoscale dimensions of less than 100 nm, are confined to the lymphatic vessels and do not enter the bloodstream. Their strong affinity for the lymphatic system allows them to dye targeted tissues black, providing excellent contrast against the surgical field. A suspension containing 1 mL of 50 mg carbon nanoparticles is injected into the lower third of the thyroid gland. Careful injection technique is crucial to avoid extravasation, which could result in unintended staining of surrounding tissues. Once administered, the nanoparticles selectively stain the thyroid gland and lymph nodes black, leaving the parathyroid glands unstained. This clear contrast enables surgeons to differentiate between the thyroid and parathyroid glands during surgery. The advantages of using carbon nanoparticles include cost-effectiveness, a high detection rate, ease of administration, and a relatively low learning curve for surgeons. However, this method has limitations, such as its inability to differentiate between normal parathyroid glands and pathological conditions like adenomas or hyperplasia. Despite this drawback, carbon nanoparticles remain a valuable tool for enhancing surgical accuracy and are particularly useful as a supplemental technique in parathyroid surgeries.

A study by Shi et al. demonstrated a 100% detection rate of parathyroid glands using carbon nanoparticles. The rate of inadvertent parathyroid gland removal was significantly lower in the nanoparticle group (1.9%) compared to 15.6% in the non-nanoparticle group [35]. Similarly, Yan et al. reported that combining carbon nanoparticles with another modality, such as ultrasound-guided fine needle aspiration cytology (FNAC), allowed for identifying all parathyroid adenomas [36]. The injection of carbon nanoparticle suspension can also be combined with Technetium-99 m sestamibi scanning to enhance the localization of parathyroid glands. Studies have indicated that this combination significantly reduces operative time, improving surgical efficiency and outcomes [37].

Raman Spectroscopy

Raman spectroscopy is an optical diagnostic method that operates on the inelastic light scattering principle. The molecular vibrations or rotational frequencies within the tissue interact with light, producing unique spectral signatures specific to the tissue's molecular components. This technique is particularly advantageous for distinguishing between parathyroid adenomas and hyperplasia. In a study by Palermo et al., Raman spectroscopy demonstrated 100% accuracy in differentiating healthy parathyroid tissue from parathyroid adenomas [38].

Dynamic Optical Contrast Imaging

Dynamic optical contrast imaging uses light-emitting diodes (LEDs) at different wavelengths to illuminate tissues. The light generates pixel values and color diagrams unique to the tissue type. For instance, wavelengths between 465 and 594 nm effectively identify the thymus and parathyroid tissues. A study by Kim et al. showed that this technique provides a high detection rate for parathyroid glands [39].

Laser Speckle Contrast Imaging

Laser speckle contrast imaging is a real-time, contrast-free method to assess tissue vascularity. It works by detecting the movement of particles, such as red blood cells, beneath the tissue surface. The variation in particle velocity affects light scattering, creating a speckle pattern composed of bright and dark areas. Viable parathyroid glands exhibit lower speckle contrast compared to non-viable glands, making this technique useful in assessing parathyroid viability during surgery [40].

Shear Wave Elastography

Shear wave elastography identifies tissues based on their stiffness. Pathological parathyroid adenomas are stiffer due to reduced fat content and the presence of a hard capsule, distinguishing them from parathyroid hyperplasia and lymph nodes. A study reported significant differences in mean shear wave velocity, with parathyroid hyperplasia measuring 1.46 ± 0.23 m/s compared to 2.28 ± 0.5 m/s for parathyroid adenomas [41]. However, shear wave elastography has limitations, including an inability to determine lesion dimensions and difficulty distinguishing between thyroid nodules and parathyroid lesions.

Autofluorescence

Autofluorescence refers to the ability of certain substances or molecules to absorb light at a specific wavelength (excitation) and emit light at a longer wavelength (emission) with lower energy. This phenomenon allows tissues to be illuminated with a filtered light source at a defined wavelength, emitting a fluorescence band that can be captured by a camera [42, 43].

There are two approaches to highlight fluorescence in tissues:

1. Exogenous contrast agents: Administered externally and either localized in target cells/tissues or distributed via vascular supply
2. Intrinsic autofluorescence: A label-free optical technique that relies solely on the natural fluorescent properties of tissues

Parathyroid glands exhibit strong intrinsic autofluorescence in the near-infrared (NIR) spectrum, emitting a significantly stronger signal than the thyroid or surrounding tissues. This characteristic enables real-time, intraoperative identification of parathyroid glands with high accuracy, eliminating the need for exogenous contrast agents that may be non-specific or toxic. Figure 27.14 shows the identified parathyroid glands in the thyroid bed, and Fig. 27.14 b shows the same on parathyroid near-infrared imaging. Although the exact fluorophore responsible for parathyroid autofluorescence remains unknown, this technique provides a safe and effective method for detecting parathyroid glands during thyroidectomy and parathyroidectomy [44]. NIR fluorescence spectroscopy reliably identifies parathyroid tissue regardless of patient demographics or clinical characteristics [45]. The autofluorescence of parathyroid glands was first reported in 2011 by Paras et al., a team of biomedical engineers at Vanderbilt University, USA. Their studies demonstrated that parathyroid tissue in the NIR spectrum emits a fluorescence signal with greater intensity than the thyroid and other surrounding tissues, such as fat, muscle, and lymph. Fluorescence measurements were performed with room and surgical lights turned off, using a fiber optic probe placed in contact with the tissue to ensure consistency. Excess blood at the site was removed prior to analysis to avoid interference. The peak fluorescence intensity of parathyroid tissue was consistently higher than that of adjacent tissues. This heightened autofluorescence suggests either a greater concentration of fluorescent molecules in the parathyroid glands or a suppression of fluorescence in other tissues, such as the thyroid. Known fluorophores, such as porphyrins, typically emit light in the 600–700 nm range, whereas parathyroid autofluorescence peaks above 800 nm (Fig. 27.12). Melanin, another potential candidate, is absent in thyroid or parathyroid tissue. One hypothesis is that the calcium-sensing receptor, a protein found in parathyroid and thyroid tissues but not

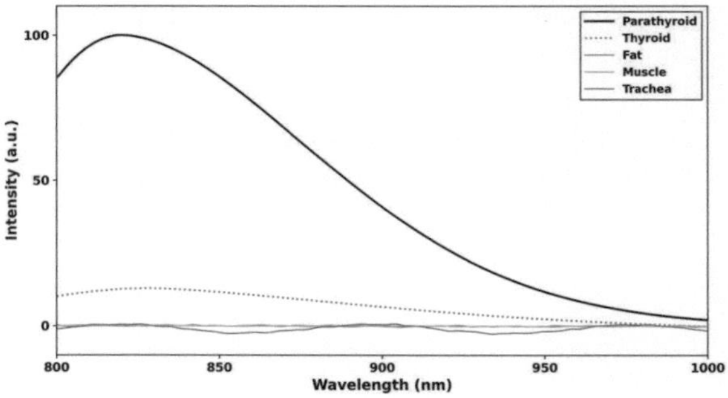

Fig. 27.12 Autofluorescence of parathyroid compared to surrounding structures. (Figure reproduced from Demarchi et al. [63], under the terms of the Creative Commons Attribution (CC BY 4.0) license)

elsewhere in the neck, may contribute to this unique autofluorescence property [46]. Further research is needed to identify the precise source of NIR autofluorescence in parathyroid glands.

Following the discovery by Paras et al. in 2011, McWade introduced the feasibility of near-infrared (NIR) imaging for intraoperative parathyroid identification in 2014, utilizing a modified Karl Storz camera. Subsequent studies have confirmed that NIR fluorescence is reliable for detecting parathyroid tissue during thyroid surgery [47].

Principle of Autofluorescence

Autofluorescence works on three key steps:

1. An external light beam at a specific wavelength excites the tissue.
2. The tissue absorbs the light.
3. The tissue emits light at a longer wavelength, which is captured by a camera.

Parathyroid tissue demonstrates a unique autofluorescence when excited at a wavelength of 785 nm, re-emitting light between 820 and 830 nm. This emission intensity is up to 11 times greater than surrounding tissues, such as the thyroid gland, enabling accurate detection and localization of the parathyroid glands.

Devices for Parathyroid Detection

1. *Fluobeam*: A non-contact optical system providing real-time grayscale imaging by enhancing autofluorescent tissues. The result is displayed as black-and-white images on a screen.
2. *PTeye*: A probe-based system that analyzes the optical properties of tissue at its tip, providing both video and audio signals upon contact with parathyroid tissue.
3. *Irillic NM*: A handheld near-infrared autofluorescence imaging system (Irillic Pvt. Ltd., Bangalore, India) designed to visualize and preserve parathyroid glands during surgery.
   Figure 27.13a shows the non-contact imaging system, and Fig. 27.13b shows the handheld imaging probe (Irillic Pvt. Ltd., Bangalore, India) that is used at the authors' institution.

Applications of NIR Autofluorescence (NIRAF)

NIRAF offers two main functionalities:

1. *Parathyroid Identification*: Detecting and localizing parathyroid glands during surgery(Fig. 27.14).
2. *Contrast-Enhanced NIR Fluorescence*: Combined with contrast agents to evaluate gland vascularity and perfusion, it assists in identifying and preserving parathyroid glands, maintaining vascular integrity, and assessing gland viability post-surgery.

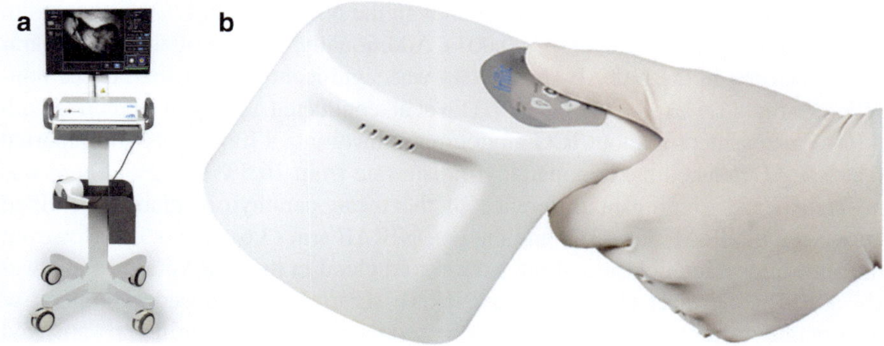

Fig. 27.13 (**a**) NIRAF imaging system. (**b**) Handheld probe for imaging

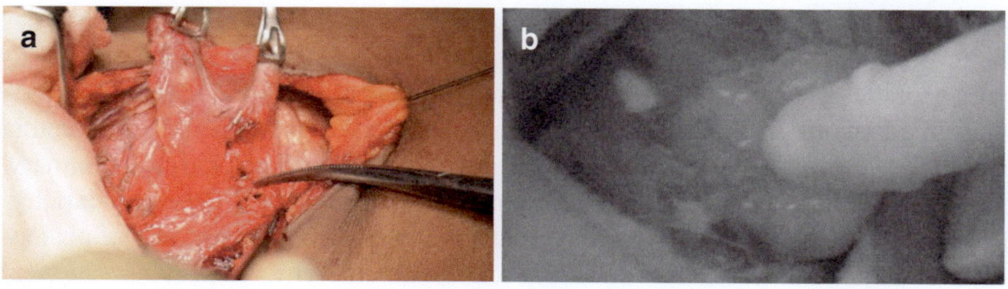

Fig. 27.14 (**a**) Shows the identified parathyroid glands in the thyroid bed. (**b**) Shows the same on parathyroid near-infrared imaging

Limitations of NIRAF

Although NIRAF's sensitivity ranges from 80% to 100%, false positives may occur due to [48] brown fat, metastatic lymph nodes, colloid nodules, Vicryl sutures, and muscle tissue.

Advances in Fluorescence Technology

Early studies required turning off operating room (OR) lights to reduce interference between ambient light and the light emitted by parathyroid autofluorophores. However, *fluorescence lifetime imaging (FLIm)*, a novel technique, utilizes a handheld laser-induced fluorescence probe to measure spectroscopic differences between tissues. Unlike NIR fluorescence imaging, FLIm operates in the visible spectrum following UV excitation and does not require contrast agents. Additionally, its pulsed operation is unaffected by OR lighting, enabling uninterrupted scanning of the surgical field [49].

Clinical Efficacy of NIRAF

Several studies have demonstrated the clinical utility of NIRAF: The ParaFluo Trial by Benmiloud et al. in France showed a statistically significant difference in the identification of all four parathyroid glands in the NIRAF arm (47%) compared to the non-NIRAF arm (19.2%) ($p < 0.001$). Additionally, the rate of accidental parathyroidectomy in the NIRAF arm (2.4%) was significantly lower than in the non-NIRAF arm (11.5%) ($p = 0.006$) [50]. Dip et al. conducted a study in Argentina with NIRAF assessment without ICG angiography involving 170 patients and reported that NIRAF reduced the hypoparathyroidism rate from 16.5% to 8.2%. There was no statistically significant difference in the mean parathyroid glands identified between the NIRAF arm (3.7) and the non-NIRAF arm (3.6) ($p = 0.32$). However, the auto-transplantation rate of the parathyroid gland in the NIRAF arm was lower (4.7%) [47]. Serra et al. found that NIRAF significantly reduced postoperative hypoparathyroidism ($P = 0.044$) and increased the number of identified parathyroid glands ($P < 0.001$). The technique demonstrated 100% sensitivity and 87.5% specificity in identifying inadvertently removed parathyroid glands [51]. Despite these findings, some studies have reported no significant reduction in postoperative hypocalcemia or inadvertent parathyroid resection using NIRAF [52]. A meta-analysis by Rao et al., which included nine randomized controlled trials, showed a statistically significant difference in the overall rate of hypocalcemia and temporary hypocalcemia favoring the NIRAF. The difference in the rate of permanent hypocalcemia was lower in the NIRAF arm but was not statistically significant [53]. In summary, many studies have validated the efficacy of NIRAF in accurately detecting parathyroid glands during surgery. Its application has been shown to reduce rates of postoperative hypoparathyroidism and hypocalcemia, thereby improving surgical outcomes. However, the technology has limitations, and further advancements may address its shortcomings.

Indocyanine Green (ICG)

ICG is the only clinically approved NIR fluorescent dye, with approval first received for clinical use in 1956. ICG was first used in the 1970s in ophthalmology for retinal angiography. In addition, ICG has most recently emerged as a technique for assessing the vascularization of the parathyroid glands, which is closely correlated with parathyroid function after thyroid resection. Indocyanine green is a tricarbocyanine dye having a molecular weight of 751.4 Da. Dry ICG is pharmacologically available and stable at room temperature. ICG is soluble in water (1 mg/mL) but is not readily soluble in saline, and hence, ICG should first be dissolved in distilled water. ICG is excreted via hepatic clearance and does not have any known metabolites. The principal advantages causing the rapid acceptance of ICG were the presence of the absorption maximum, around 800 nm, confined to the vascular compartment through binding with plasma proteins, resulting in low toxicity and rapid excretion, almost exclusively into the bile. ICG fluoresces at about 800 nm and longer wavelengths. ICG is approved for clinical use due to its safety; it is nontoxic and nonionizing. It binds efficiently to blood lipoproteins and does not leak from circulation—ideal for angiography.

There is a rapid washout, and hence, it can be given repeatedly. Autofluorescence by itself can only detect parathyroid glands. It cannot analyze the perfusion status of parathyroid glands. The viability of the parathyroid gland is paramount in thyroid surgery when aiming to reduce postoperative hypoparathyroidism, which remains the most common complication of thyroidectomy, occurring in as many as 30% of patients. Thus, ICG aids in identifying vascularity and perfusion of PTH glands. The disadvantages of ICG include [54] allergy, leakage of the dye, inability to localize de-vascularized parathyroid glands, and delayed response.

A study by Vidal et al. [55] gave the safe dosage for ICG. ICG (25 mg vial) was prepared by mixing ICG powder with 10 mL of sterile water. So, the concentration is 2.5 mg/mL. The dosage is 0.3 mg/kg, which is 4–6 mL. This injection could be repeated until a maximum dose of 5 mg per kg. The catheter is then rapidly purged after each infusion to acquire a rapid image gain. After approximately 30 s to 2 min, images are acquired with a NIRAF camera, showing the distribution of ICG in the explored tissue. There are many studies on ICG in thyroid surgery. A study by Rudin et al. with 210 patients found that at least two vascularized parathyroid glands may detect a good postoperative parathyroid function [56]. Another study by Razavi et al., comprising 111 patients, showed no significant changes in mean PTH levels or hypocalcaemia at the end of surgery. They commented that low-flow ICG did not necessitate auto transplantation [57]. A study by Jin et al. concluded that one parathyroid gland with an ICG score of 2 resulted in normal postoperative PTH [58]. These studies showed that ICG with reliable scoring was a good predictive marker for predicting postoperative hypoparathyroidism. The grading system of ICG used in the study was given by Benmiloud et al. [59]. There is grading for vascularity and perfusion. Vascularity grading is as follows:

iMAP 0, not informative; iMAP 1, general vascular pattern visible but no clear vascular pedicle flowing into the PG; and iMAP 2, clear vascular pedicle flowing into the PG. ICG-assisted perfusion scoring is given as Grade 0, no perfusion; Grade 1, moderate uptake; and Grade 2, intense uptake (Figs. 27.15, 27.16, and 27.17). The clinical utility of ICG angiography in thyroid surgery is debatable; unless there is a policy to auto-transplant the gland that has shown the worst grading in the assessment of perfusion and vascularity, the scorings may be irrelevant.

In a study by Silvia et al. [60], 39 consecutive patients undergoing total thyroidectomy for multinodular goiter were evaluated using the *4-ICG score* to assess parathyroid gland (PG) viability. The score was calculated by assigning a viability grade to each of the four PGs based on the following criteria: PG appears black, *1* PG appears gray and/or heterogeneous, and *2* PG appears white. The total score for all four glands ranged from 0 to 8. A *4-ICG score more excellent than 3* demonstrated a *negative predictive value of 95% for postoperative hypocalcemia*. The study concluded that the 4-ICG score effectively predicted postoperative hypocalcemia in patients undergoing total thyroidectomy.

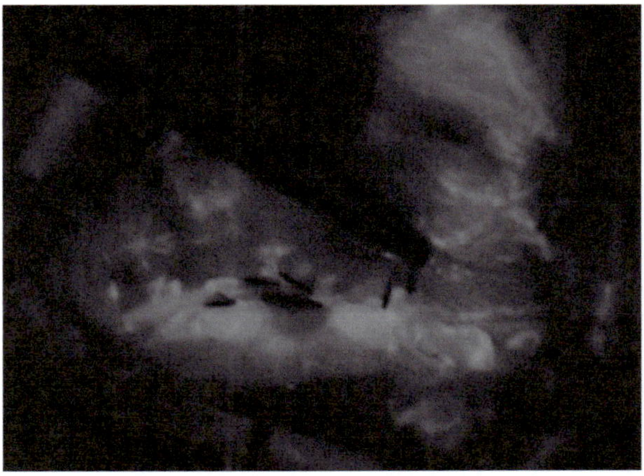

Fig. 27.15 Showing ICG with NIRAF showing good vascularity and perfusion of parathyroids

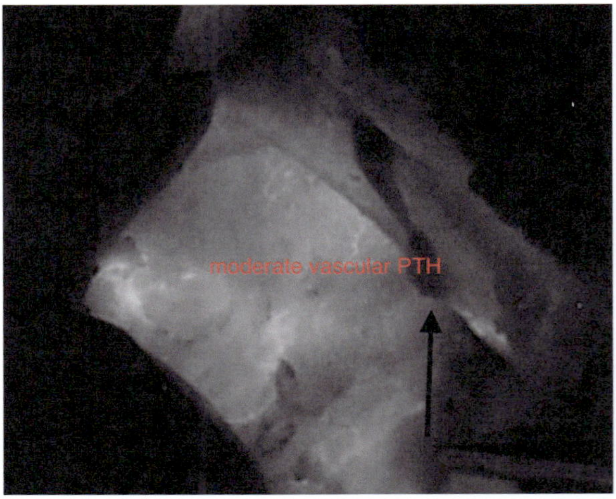

Fig. 27.16 Showing ICG with NIRAF showing moderate vascularity and perfusion of parathyroids

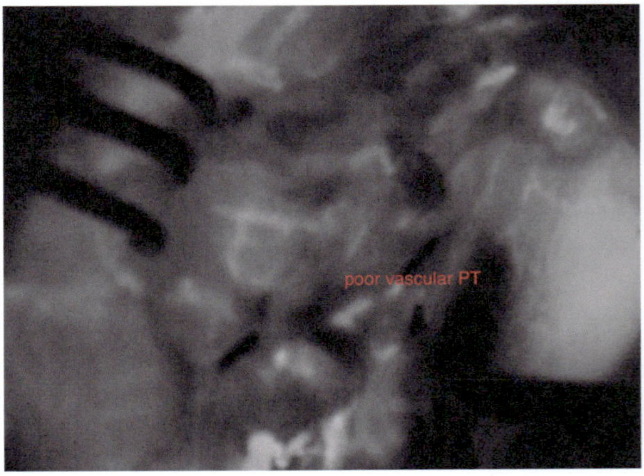

Fig. 27.17 Showing ICG with NIRAF showing poor vascularity and perfusion of parathyroids

At our institute, a prospective trial was conducted to compare near-infrared-aided fluorescence (NIRAF)-aided parathyroid detection with visual parathyroid detection in patients undergoing total thyroidectomy. A total of *151 patients* were included in the study, with 76 patients in the NIRAF group and 75 in the control group. Baseline clinicopathological characteristics were comparable between the two groups.

The results showed that postoperative hypoparathyroidism was significantly lower in the NIRAF group (14.5%) than in the control group (28%) ($p = 0.042$). NIRAF improved the visualization rate of parathyroid glands from *34.5% to 68%*. Univariate analysis revealed that NIRAF significantly reduced hypoparathyroidism in patients with larger thyroid nodules (>2 cm) ($p = 0.021$) and in those undergoing thyroidectomy combined with neck dissection ($p = 0.045$). This study highlighted the efficacy of NIRAF in enhancing parathyroid identification during thyroidectomy and its potential to reduce postoperative hypoparathyroidism, particularly in challenging cases such as larger nodules or combined neck dissections.

Parathyroid Venous Sampling

It is an invasive intraoperative localization technique used primarily in patients with persistent or recurrent hyperparathyroidism or those with negative or discordant imaging studies. This procedure is performed by an experienced interventional radiologist, who collects venous samples from veins surrounding the thyroid bed and those draining the anterior mediastinum. Commonly sampled veins include the internal jugular, brachiocephalic, internal mammary, vertebral, and thymic veins. The procedure is carried out via peripheral venous catheterization.

In some cases, selective sampling from the superior, middle, and inferior thyroid veins may be performed to achieve more precise localization of hyperfunctioning parathyroid glands. The parathyroid hormone (PTH) gradient is measured, and an abnormal gradient is defined as a twofold or greater increase in PTH levels compared to the inferior vena cava. The hypersecreting gland's location is then inferred based on the territory drained by the vein with the elevated PTH level.

Localization Based on Venous Territories

1. Superior thyroid vein: Drains into the internal jugular vein. An abnormal PTH gradient here suggests the presence of a superior parathyroid gland adenoma.
2. Middle thyroid vein: Drains into the internal jugular vein and can indicate a superior or inferior parathyroid lesion.
3. Inferior thyroid vein: Drains into the brachiocephalic vein. An abnormal gradient suggests an inferior parathyroid lesion.

4. Vertebral vein: An abnormal gradient may indicate an inferior or retroesophageal parathyroid gland.
5. Internal mammary vein: Elevated PTH levels in this vein are suggestive of a mediastinal or thymic parathyroid lesion.

Parathyroid venous sampling remains a valuable tool in complex cases where non-invasive imaging fails to provide sufficient information. While invasive, this method offers highly localized information that can guide surgical intervention and improve outcomes in challenging cases of parathyroid disease. An analysis of 12 pooled studies revealed that selective parathyroid venous sampling has a pooled sensitivity of *74%*, specificity of *41%*, and a positive likelihood ratio of *1.55* [61].

Advantages

- It serves as a valuable tool for guiding surgical intervention in patients with prior failed parathyroidectomy by localizing the hyperfunctioning parathyroid gland.
- This is particularly beneficial in cases where non-invasive imaging modalities yield negative or discordant results.

Disadvantages

- Limited availability due to the requirement for highly skilled radiologists experienced in performing this technique.
- Being an invasive procedure, it carries risks such as intravenous extravasation of contrast and catheter-related complications, including bleeding or thrombosis.

Despite its limitations, selective parathyroid venous sampling remains critical for challenging cases, especially when other diagnostic methods have been inconclusive.

Parathyroid Arteriography

Selective angiographic injection of the inferior thyroid artery can occasionally demonstrate a "parathyroid blush," with reported detection rates ranging from 25% to 70%. However, this procedure is rarely utilized due to the risk of severe complications, including quadriplegia and infarction [62]. These significant adverse events have largely replaced the procedure by safer, non-invasive, and less risky imaging modalities for parathyroid localization (Table 27.3).

Table 27.3 Advantages and disadvantages of intraoperative parathyroid detection methods

Method	Advantages	Disadvantages
Dynamic optical contrast imaging	1. Non-invasive 2. No admission of exogenous substances 3. Instant feedback	Not enough evidence
Laser speckle contrast imaging	1 No admission of exogenous substances 2. Instant feedback 3. Assess of viability of PGs	High susceptibility to Movement of the operation field
Spectroscopy	1. Non-invasive 2. no admission of exogenous substances 3. Instant feedback	1. No information about the viability of PGs 2. Requires the blackout of the operating room light 3. Limited ability to localize PGs covered deeply by other tissues
Autofluorescence imaging	Non-invasive No admission of exogenous substance Instant feedback Contactless Possibility to differentiate adenomas Possibility to display on the operation field	No information about the viability of PGs Requires the blackout of the operating room Limited ability to localize PGs covered deeply by other tissues
Raman spectroscopy	Non-invasive No admission of exogenous substance Possibility to differentiate adenomas	Requires additional time
Carbon nanoparticles	Do not penetrate to tissues Visible in the operation field Admission of exogenous substance	Requires precise injection Do not differentiate adenomas
Shear wave elastography	Non-invasive No admission of exogenous substance Possibility to differentiate adenomas	Dimensions of parathyroid adenomas cannot be estimated
Indocyanine green	Inexpensive Safe Possibility to differentiate adenomas Visible in the operation field	Admission of exogenous substance Contrast nonspecific for PGs Contains iodine

Special Considerations in Parathyroid Localization

Localization Studies During Pregnancy

Ultrasound (USG) is the imaging modality of choice for parathyroid localization during pregnancy due to its safety profile. It avoids ionizing radiation and provides adequate anatomical detail.

Localization in MEN1, Secondary, and Tertiary Hyperparathyroidism:

In cases of multiglandular disease, such as those associated with multiple endocrine neoplasia type 1 (MEN1) or secondary and tertiary hyperparathyroidism, USG and sestamibi (MIBI) scintigraphy often demonstrate low sensitivity. As discussed, multiglandular disease poses a diagnostic challenge due to the involvement of multiple glands. In such scenarios, cross-sectional imaging modalities like CT, 4D-CT, or MRI are recommended to enhance localization accuracy and guide surgical planning effectively.

Summary

Parathyroid localization techniques play a pivotal role in managing hyperparathyroidism, facilitating accurate diagnosis and guiding surgical treatment. Preoperative imaging typically begins with ultrasound (USG) and sestamibi scintigraphy, which are effective first-line modalities, particularly for solitary parathyroid adenomas. However, their sensitivity decreases in multiglandular disease, small adenomas, or ectopic glands. Advanced imaging techniques, such as 4D-CT, MRI, and PET-CT, offer improved localization accuracy in these challenging cases. For instance, 4D-CT provides high spatial resolution and rapid imaging, while PET-CT with choline tracers is particularly effective in discordant or inconclusive findings. With its excellent soft tissue contrast, MRI is reserved for second-line use in persistent or recurrent cases.

Intraoperative imaging enhances the identification and preservation of parathyroid glands during surgery. Near-infrared autofluorescence (NIRAF) has revolutionized intraoperative localization by providing real-time, label-free detection of parathyroid glands, significantly reducing postoperative hypocalcemia and inadvertent gland resection. Raman spectroscopy and laser speckle imaging also aid intraoperative detection by assessing tissue composition and vascularity. Invasive methods like selective parathyroid venous sampling and arteriography, while less common due to associated risks, are valuable in complex or recurrent cases. These preoperative and intraoperative imaging techniques improve surgical precision, minimize complications, and optimize outcomes, particularly in challenging cases like multiglandular disease, ectopic glands, or reoperations.

Conflict of Interests None

References

1. Ruda JM, Hollenbeak CS, Stack BC Jr. A systematic review of the diagnosis and treatment of primary hyperparathyroidism from 1995 to 2003. Otolaryngol Head Neck Surg. 2005;132(3):359–72. https://doi.org/10.1016/j.otohns.2004.10.005.

2. Patel N, Mihai R. Long-term cure of primary hyperparathyroidism after scan-directed parathyroidectomy: outcomes from a UK endocrine surgery unit. World J Surg. 2022;46(9):2189–94. https://doi.org/10.1007/s00268-022-06556-3.
3. Patel CN, Salahudeen HM, Lansdown M, Scarsbrook AF. Clinical utility of ultrasound and 99mTc sestamibi SPECT/CT for preoperative localization of parathyroid adenoma in patients with primary hyperparathyroidism. Clin Radiol. 2010;65(4):278–87. https://doi.org/10.1016/j.crad.2009.12.005.
4. Rodgers SE, Hunter GJ, Hamberg LM, Schellingerhout D, Doherty DB, Ayers GD, Shapiro SE, Edeiken BS, Truong MT, Evans DB, Lee JE, Perrier ND. Improved preoperative planning for directed parathyroidectomy with 4-dimensional computed tomography. Surgery. 2006;140(6):932–40; discussion 940–1. https://doi.org/10.1016/j.surg.2006.07.028.
5. Kunstman JW, Kirsch JD, Mahajan A, Udelsman R. Clinical review: parathyroid localization and implications for clinical management. J Clin Endocrinol Metab. 2013;98(3):902–12. https://doi.org/10.1210/jc.2012-3168.
6. Petranović Ovčariček P, Giovanella L, Carrió Gasset I, Hindié E, Huellner MW, Luster M, Piccardo A, Weber T, Talbot JN, Verburg FA. The EANM practice guidelines for parathyroid imaging. Eur J Nucl Med Mol Imaging. 2021;48(9):2801–22. https://doi.org/10.1007/s00259-021-05334.
7. American Institute of Ultrasound in Medicine AIUM practice guideline for the performance of a thyroid and parathyroid ultrasound examination. J Ultrasound Med. 2003;22:1126–30.
8. Wolf RJ, Cronan JJ, Monchik JM. Color Doppler sonography: an adjunctive technique in assessment of parathyroid adenomas. J Ultrasound Med. 1994;13(4):303–8. https://doi.org/10.7863/jum.1994.13.4.303. PMID: 7932996.
9. Berber E, Parikh RT, Ballem N, Garner CN, Milas M, Siperstein AE. Factors contributing to negative parathyroid localization: an analysis of 1000 patients. Surgery. 2008;144:74–9.
10. Rickes S, Sitzy J, Neye H, Ocran KW, Wermke W. High-resolution ultrasound in combination with colour-Doppler sonography for preoperative localization of parathyroid adenomas in patients with primary hyperparathyroidism. Ultraschallmed. 2003;24:85–9.
11. Haciyanli M, Lal G, Morita E, Duh QY, Kebebew E, Clark OH. Accuracy of preoperative localization studies and intraoperative parathyroid hormone assay in patients with primary hyperparathyroidism and double adenoma. J Am Coll Surg. 2003;197:739–46.
12. Gooding GA, Clark OH, Stark DD, Moss AA, Montgomery CK. Parathyroid aspiration biopsy un-der ultrasound guidance in the postoperative hyperparathyroid patient. Radiology. 1985;155:193–6.
13. Harman CR, Grant CS, Hay ID, et al. Indications, technique, and efficacy of alcohol injection of enlarged parathyroid glands in patients with primary hyperparathyroidism. Surgery. 1998;124:1011–9.
14. Eslamy HK, Ziessman HA. Parathyroid scintigraphy in patients with primary hyperparathyroidism: 99mTc sestamibi SPECT and SPECT/CT. Radiographics. 2008;28(5):1461–76.
15. Lorberboym M, Minski I, Macadziob S, Nikolov G, Schachter P. Incremental diagnostic value of preoperative 99mTc-MIBI SPECT in patients with parathyroid adenoma. J Nucl Med. 2003;44:904–8.
16. Nichols KJ, Tomas MB, Tronco GG, Palestro CJ. Sestamibi parathyroid scintigraphy in multigland disease. Nucl Med Commun. 2012 [cited 2019 Nov 29];33(1):43–50.
17. Civelek AC, Ozalp E, Donovan P, Udelsman R. Prospective evaluation of delayed technetium-99m sestamibi SPECT scintigraphy for preoperative localization of primary hyperparathyroidism. Surgery. 2002;131:149–57.
18. Lumachi F, Zucchetta P, Marzola MC, et al. Advantages of combined technetium-99m-sestamibi scintigraphy and high-resolution ultrasonography in parathyroid localization: comparative study in 91 patients with primary hyperparathyroidism. Eur J Endocrinol. 2000;143:755–60.
19. Sugg SL, Krzywda EA, Demeure MJ, Wilson SD. Detection of multiple gland primary hyperparathyroidism in the era of minimally invasive parathyroidectomy.
20. Gotway MB, Higgins CB. MR imaging of the thyroid and parathyroid glands. Magn Reson Imaging Clin N Am. 2000;8:163–82.

21. Rodgers SE, Hunter GJ, Hamberg LM, Schellingerhout D, Doherty DB, Ayers GD, Shapiro SE, Edeiken BS, Truong MT, Evans DB, Lee JE, Perrier ND. Improved preoperative planning for directed parathyroidectomy with 4-dimensional computed tomography. Surgery. 2006;140(6):932–40; discussion 940–1.
22. Messa C, Bettinardi V, Picchio M, Pelosi E, Landoni C, Gianolli L, Gilardi MC, Fazio F. PET/CT in diagnostic oncology. Q J Nucl Med Mol Imaging. 2004;48(2):66–75.
23. Hara T, Kosaka N, Kishi H. PET imaging of prostate cancer using carbon-11-choline. J Nucl Med. 1998;39(6):990–5. PMID: 9627331.
24. Parvinian A, Martin-Macintosh EL, Goenka AH, Durski JM, Mullan BP, Kemp BJ, Johnson GB. ^{11}C-Choline PET/CT for detection and localization of parathyroid adenomas. AJR Am J Roentgenol. 2018;210(2):418–22. https://doi.org/10.2214/AJR.17.18312. Epub 2017 Nov 15. PMID: 29140118.
25. Pretet V, Rotania M, Helali M, Ignat M, Vix M, Imperiale A. ^{18}F-fluorocholine PET and multiphase CT integrated in dual modality PET/4D-CT for preoperative evaluation of primary hyperparathyroidism. J Clin Med. 2020;9(6):2005.
26. Michaud L, Burgess A, Huchet V, Lefèvre M, Tassart M, Ohnona J, Kerrou K, Balogova S, Talbot JN, Périé S. Is 18F-fluorocholine-positron emission tomography/computerized tomography a new imaging tool for detecting hyperfunctioning parathyroid glands in primary or secondary hyperparathyroidism? J Clin Endocrinol Metab. 2014;99(12):4531–6.
27. Lee SW, Shim SR, Jeong SY, Kim SJ. Direct comparison of preoperative imaging modalities for localization of primary hyperparathyroidism: a systematic review and network meta-analysis. JAMA Otolaryngol Head Neck Surg. 2021;147(8):692–706.
28. Bley TA, Wieben O, François CJ, Brittain JH, Reeder SB. Fat and water magnetic resonance imaging. J Magn Reson Imaging. 2010;31(1):4–18. https://doi.org/10.1002/jmri.21895. PMID: 20027567.
29. Aschenbach R, Tuda S, Lamster E, Meyer A, Roediger H, Stier A, Conrad E, Basche S, Klisch J, Vogl TJ. Dynamic magnetic resonance angiography for localization of hyperfunctioning parathyroid glands in the reoperative neck. Eur J Radiol. 2012;81(11):3371–7.
30. Merchavy S, Luckman J, Guindy M, Segev Y, Khafif A. 4D MRI for the localization of parathyroid adenoma: a novel method in evolution. Otolaryngol Head Neck Surg. 2016;154(3):446–8.
31. Cheung K, Wang TS, Farrokhyar F, Roman SA, Sosa JA. A meta-analysis of preoperative localization techniques for patients with primary hyperparathyroidism. Ann Surg Oncol. 2012;19(2):577–83.
32. Reglia G, Piccardo A, Imperiale A, Strobel K, Kaufmann PA, Prior JO, Giovanella L. Diagnostic performance of choline PET for detection of hyperfunctioning parathyroid glands in hyperparathyroidism: a systematic review and meta-analysis. Eur J Nucl Med Mol Imaging. 2019;46(3):751–65.
33. Bewick J, Pfleiderer A. The value and role of low dose methylene blue in the surgical management of hyperparathyroidism. Ann R Coll Surg Engl. 2014;96:526–9. https://doi.org/10.1308/003588414X13946184903883.
34. Methylthioninium Chloride. 2020. https://bnf.nice.org.uk/drug/methylthioninium-chloride.html. Accessed 10 Sept 2020.
35. Shi C, Tian B, Li S, Shi T, Qin H, Liu S. Enhanced identification and functional protective role of carbon nanoparticles on parathyroid in thyroid cancer surgery: a retrospective Chinese population study. Medicine (Baltimore). 2016;95(46):e5148. https://doi.org/10.1097/MD.0000000000005148. PMID: 27861338; PMCID: PMC5120895.
36. Yan S, Zhao W, Wang B, Zhang L. A novel technology for localization of parathyroid adenoma: ultrasound-guided fine needle aspiration combined with rapid parathyroid hormone detection and nano-carbon technology. Surg Innov. 2018;25(4):357–63. https://doi.org/10.1177/1553350618779703. Epub 2018 Jun 12. PMID: 29890904.
37. Gencoglu EA, Aras M, Moray G, Aktas A. The effectiveness of low-dose versus high-dose 99mTc MIBI protocols for radioguided surgery in patients with primary hyperparathyroidism. Nucl Med Commun. 2014;35(4):398–404. https://doi.org/10.1097/MNM.0000000000000056. PMID: 24323310.

38. Chen J, Zhou Q, Feng J, Wang J. Combined use of a nanocarbon suspension and ^{99m}Tc-MIBI for the intra-operative localization of the parathyroid glands. Am J Otolaryngol. 2018;39(2):138–41. https://doi.org/10.1016/j.amjoto.2017.12.008. Epub 2017 Dec 13. PMID: 29336900.
39. Abbaci M, De Leeuw F, Breuskin I, Casiraghi O, Lakhdar AB, Ghanem W, Laplace-Builhé C, Hartl D. Parathyroid gland management using optical technologies during thyroidectomy or parathyroidectomy: a systematic review. Oral Oncol. 2018;87:186–96. https://doi.org/10.1016/j.oraloncology.2018.11.011. Epub 2018 Nov 16. PMID: 30527238.
40. Kazmi SM, Faraji E, Davis MA, Huang YY, Zhang XJ, Dunn AK. Flux or speed? Examining speckle contrast imaging of vascular flows. Biomed Opt Express 2015;6(7):2588–2608. https://doi.org/10.1364/BOE.6.002588. PMID: 26203384; PMCID: PMC4505712.
41. Hattapoğlu S, Göya C, Hamidi C, Taşdemir B, Alan B, Durmaz MS, Teke M, Ekici F. Evaluation of parathyroid lesions with point shear wave elastography. J Ultrasound Med. 2016;35(10):2179–82. https://doi.org/10.7863/ultra.15.10074. Epub 2016 Aug 29. PMID: 27573796.
42. Alander JT, Kaartinen I, Laakso A, Pätilä T, Spillmann T, Tuchin VV, Venermo M, Välisuo P. A review of indocyanine green fluorescent imaging in surgery. Int J Biomed Imaging. 2012;2012:940585. https://doi.org/10.1155/2012/940585. Epub 2012 Apr 22. PMID: 22577366; PMCID: PMC3346977.
43. De Boer E, Harlaar NJ, Taruttis A, Nagengast WB, Rosenthal EL, Ntziachristos V, Van Dam GM. Optical innovations in surgery. Br J Surg. 2015;102:56–72.
44. Perrier ND, Ituarte P, Kikuchi S, Siperstein AE, Duh QY, Clark OH, et al. Intraoperative parathyroid aspiration and parathyroid hormone assay as an alternative to frozen section for tissue identification. World J Surg. 2000;24(11):1319–22.
45. McWade MA, Sanders ME, Broome JT, Solórzano CC, Mahadevan-Jansen A. Establishing the clinical utility of autofluorescence spectroscopy for parathyroid detection. Surgery. 2016;159(1):193–202.
46. Lakowicz R. Fluorophores. In: Principles of fluorescence spectroscopy. New York: Springer; 2006. p. 63–95.
47. Falco J, Dip F, Quadri P, de la Fuente M, Prunello M, Rosenthal RJ. Increased identification of parathyroid glands using near infrared light during thyroid and parathyroid surgery. Surg Endosc. 2017;31(9):3737–42. https://doi.org/10.1007/s00464-017-5424-1. Epub 2017 Mar 31. PMID: 28364157.
48. Romero- Velez G, Elshamy M, Beber E. A review of parathyroid autofluorescence imaging in detection and preservation of parathyroid glands during thyroid surgery. Ann Thyroid. 2023.
49. Paras C, Keller M, White L, Phay J, Mahadevan-Jansen A. Near-infrared autofluorescence for the detection of parathyroid glands. J Biomed Opt. 2011;16(6):067012. https://doi.org/10.1117/1.3583571. PMID: 21721833.
50. Benmiloud F, Godiris-Petit G, Gras R, Gillot JC, Turrin N, Penaranda G, Noullet S, Chéreau N, Gaudart J, Chiche L, Rebaudet S. Association of autofluorescence-based detection of the parathyroid glands during total thyroidectomy with postoperative hypocalcemia risk: results of the PARAFLUO multicenter randomized clinical trial. JAMA Surg. 2020;155(2):106–12. https://doi.org/10.1001/jamasurg.2019.4613. PMID: 31693081; PMCID: PMC6865247.
51. Serra C, Silveira L, Canudo A, Lemos MC. Parathyroid identification by autofluorescence - preliminary report on five cases of surgery for primary hyperparathyroidism. BMC Surg. 2019;19(1):120. https://doi.org/10.1186/s12893-019-0590-9. PMID: 31455299; PMCID: PMC6712745.
52. DiMarco A, Chotalia R, Bloxham R, McIntyre C, Tolley N, Palazzo FF. Does fluoroscopy prevent inadvertent parathyroidectomy in thyroid surgery? Ann R Coll Surg Engl. 2019;101(7):508–13. https://doi.org/10.1308/rcsann.2019.0065. Epub 2019 Jul 15. PMID: 31305127; PMCID: PMC6667958.
53. Rao KN, Rajguru R, Dange P, Vetter D, Triponez F, Nixon IJ, Randolph GW, Mäkitie AA, Zafereo M, Ferlito A. Lower rates of hypocalcemia following near-infrared autofluorescence use in thyroidectomy: a meta-analysis of RCTs. Diagnostics (Basel). 2024;14(5):505.

54. Jitpratoom P, Anuwong A. The use of ICG enhanced fluorescence for the evaluation of parathyroid gland preservation. Gland Surg. 2017;6(5):579–86. https://doi.org/10.21037/gs.2017.09.01. PMID: 29142851; PMCID: PMC5676163.
55. Vidal Fortuny J, Belfontali V, Sadowski SM, Karenovics W, Guigard S, Triponez F. Parathyroid gland angiography with indocyanine green fluorescence to predict parathyroid function after thyroid surgery. Br J Surg. 2016;103:537–43.
56. Rudin AV, McKenzie TJ, Thompson GB, Farley DR, Lyden ML. Evaluation of parathyroid glands with indocyanine green fluorescence angiography after thyroidectomy. World J Surg. 2019;43:1538–43.
57. Razavi AC, Ibraheem K, Haddad A, Saparova L, Shalaby H, Abdelgawad M, Kandil E. Efficacy of indocyanine green fluorescence in predicting parathyroid vascularization during thyroid surgery. Head Neck. 2019;41(9):3276–81. https://doi.org/10.1002/hed.25837. Epub 2019 Jun 17. PMID: 31206817.
58. Jin H, Dong Q, He Z, Fan J, Liao K, Cui M. Research on indocyanine green angiography for predicting postoperative hypoparathyroidism. Clin Endocrinol. 2019;90(3):487–93. https://doi.org/10.1111/cen.13925. Epub 2019 Jan 7. PMID: 30585665.
59. Benmiloud F, Penaranda G, Chiche L, Rebaudet S. Intraoperative mapping angiograms of the parathyroid glands using Indocyanine green during thyroid surgery: results of the Fluogreen study. World J Surg. 2022;46(2):416–24. https://doi.org/10.1007/s00268-021-06353-4. Epub 2021 Nov 6. PMID: 34743241.
60. Gálvez-Pastor S, Torregrosa NM, Ríos A, Febrero B, González-Costea R, García-López MA, Balsalobre MD, Pastor-Pérez P, Moreno P, Vázquez-Rojas JL, Rodríguez JM. Prediction of hypocalcemia after total thyroidectomy using indocyanine green angiography of parathyroid glands: a simple quantitative scoring system. Am J Surg. 2019;218(5):993–9. https://doi.org/10.1016/j.amjsurg.2018.12.074. Epub 2019 Jan 4.
61. Ibraheem K, Toraih EA, Haddad AB, Farag M, Randolph GW, Kandil E. Selective parathyroid venous sampling in primary hyperparathyroidism: a systematic review and meta-analysis. Laryngoscope. 2018;128:2662–7.
62. Heller SJ. Parathyroid arteriography. Otolaryngol Clin N Am. 1980;13(1):161–7. PMID: 7367001.
63. Demarchi MS, Karenovics W, Bédat B, Triponez F. Intraoperative autofluorescence and indocyanine green angiography for the detection and preservation of parathyroid glands. J Clin Med. 2020;9(3):830. https://doi.org/10.3390/jcm9030830.

Surgical Management of Hyperparathyroidism

28

Shawn Thomas Sam and Deepak Thomas Abraham

Editorial

Drs. Sam and Abraham have described the surgical management of hyperparathyroidism including intraoperative and post-operative complications. The majority of the patients seen today are asymptomatic, diagnosed primarily by biochemical analysis. On detailed questioning, some of them may have mild symptoms, which are most likely to improve after surgical intervention. Several nuances have been described by the authors, including the role of appropriate imaging, ultrasound, sestamibi (MIBI) scan. There is an enormous interest in four-dimensional CT scan. This technological advancement is quite helpful to the operating surgeons to know the exact location of the enlarged parathyroid gland. The technology is so advanced now that the radiologist can practically tell us the approximate weight of the enlarged parathyroid gland. This is quite helpful to the operating surgeon for satisfactory and complete surgical procedures.

Even though several patients are asymptomatic, on detailed questioning, it is common to find vague symptoms related to mild hyperparathyroidism. However, these symptoms invariably improve after the surgical intervention. The intraoperative complications are related to the inability to find the enlarged parathyroid gland and post-operative persistent hypercalcemia. This can be quite a difficult problem as the families and the patients expect a complete cure. Management of persistent or recurrent thyroid cancer is quite complex, which involves complete diagnosis and localization studies. The risk of complications is much higher in pre-operative surgery, as to the risk of nerve injury and aberrant locations of the enlarged parathyroid gland.

S. T. Sam
Department of Endocrine Surgery, Christian Medical College, Vellore, Tamil Nadu, India

D. T. Abraham (✉)
Department of Endocrine Surgery, Christian Medical College, Vellore, Tamil Nadu, India

Department of Surgery, American Mission Hospital, Manama, Bahrain

P. S. Pai et al. (eds.), *Controversies in Cancer of the Thyroid and Parathyroid Glands*, https://doi.org/10.1007/978-3-032-13130-0_28

There has always been debate between focused parathyroidectomy with intraoperative PTH vs. bilateral exploration. There appears a paradigm shift toward bilateral exploration and removal of all enlarged parathyroid glands. Obviously, we will have to wait for long-term follow-up after surgical procedures, and some of these patients may come back with mild persistent hyperparathyroidism. However, this may not have major clinical implications. Parathyroid surgery has become a common surgical procedure due to incidental identification of primary hyperparathyroidism. The authors have done a splendid job on the evaluation and management of hyperparathyroidism.

Ashok R. Shaha

Medical management with cinacalcet, bisphosphonates, or denosumab is an option for non-surgical candidates with indications. Special considerations exist for PHPT in pregnancy, HPT-JT, multiple endocrine neoplasia, and familial hypocalciuric hypercalcemia. Effective communication and a multidisciplinary approach are vital for optimal patient outcomes.

Definition Primary hyperparathyroidism (PHPT) is defined as an elevated serum calcium adjusted for albumin in the presence of an elevated or inappropriately normal intact parathyroid hormone (iPTH) utilizing either a second- or third-generation assay on two occasions at least 2 weeks apart [1]. Parathyroid gland hyperactivity and the resultant overproduction of parathyroid hormone(PTH) are the hallmark of PHPT [2].

Etiology Incidence is significantly more in women than in men [2]. The most common etiology is a benign adenoma, seen in about 85%, followed by multi-gland disease (15%) and very rarely parathyroid carcinoma (1%) [2]. Mutations in the tumor suppressor genes such as MEN 1 and CDC73 and familial hypocalciuric hypercalcemia are rare variants and should be kept in mind when working on a diagnosis of PHPT [3].

Clinical Presentation The classical description of PHPT includes "stones, abdominal groans, bones and psychiatric overtones" indicating the presence of nephrolithiasis, peptic ulcer disease, bony pains or fractures, and severe neuropsychiatric symptoms [2]. Untreated PHPT causes significant cardiovascular morbidity such as hypertension, myocardial dysfunction, and hypertrophy of the cardiac muscles. It is associated with elevated circulating levels of angiotensin and renin and higher arterial pressure [4]. With more routine biochemical testing, the percentage of asymptomatic hyperparathyroidism has steadily been on the rise [2]. Untreated asymptomatic PHPT will progress to classical manifestations in about 30% of patients [2]. Hypercalcemic crisis is a potentially life-threatening emergency and presents with markedly elevated serum calcium >14 mg/dl and associated with signs of multi-organ dysfunction. Treatment initially is supportive and includes hydration and stopping of drugs such as thiazides that can contribute to hypercalcemia. Calcitonin, bisphosphonates, and cinacalcet can be used as a bridge to urgent parathyroidectomy [3].

Indications for parathyroidectomy even in asymptomatic HPT include the following:

- Age <50 years.
- Serum calcium >1 mg/dl (0.25 mmol/L) above the upper limit of normal.
- Skeletal involvement with fracture by vertebral fracture assessment (VFA) or vertebral X-ray or bone mineral density (BMD) ≤−2.5 at any site.
- Renal involvement with eGFR or creatinine clearance <60 mL/min or evidence of nephrocalcinosis or nephrolithiasis detected on abdominal imaging or hypercalciuria >250 mg/day in women and >300 mg/dl in men [1].

Localization studies Pre-operative localization—PHPT is always a biochemical diagnosis followed by imaging to localize and locate the most hyperfunctioning foci. Imaging is not recommended for diagnostic purposes [1, 2]. Current imaging modalities fail to detect multi-gland disease with certainty [2]. Localization procedures are also less sensitive in localizing posteriorly located, small glands and multiple adenomas as compared to a larger adenoma [5]. Non-localized parathyroids are more likely multi-gland disease and require more extensive surgery [6].

Ultrasound of the neck should be performed in all patients with PHPT to look for enlarged parathyroid and concurrent clinically relevant thyroid pathology which may require further evaluation. Ultrasound features of parathyroid adenomas include a well-defined, hypoechoic lesion close to the thyroid lobe and occasionally in the thyro-thymic tract at the tip of the thymus (Fig. 28.1) [2, 7]. Ultrasound maybe false negative in small or ectopic adenomas or when there is a large multinodular goiter or previous neck surgery [8].

99mTc-sestaMIBI is concentrated in hyperfunctioning parathyroid glands due to retention of the radio-tracer by mitochondria-rich oxyphil cells of parathyroid tissue, and this property is used to localize hyperfunctioning parathyroid glands [2]. SestaMIBI single-photon emission computed tomography (SPECT) gives a three-dimensional view by combining sestaMIBI SPECT and non-contrast neck CT and

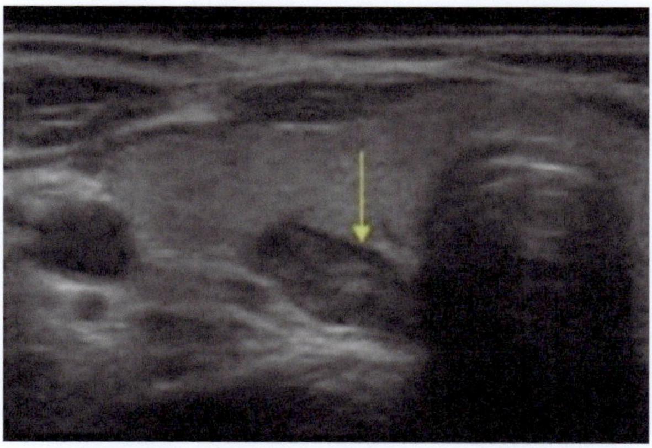

Fig. 28.1 Ultrasound of the neck showing typical appearance of parathyroid

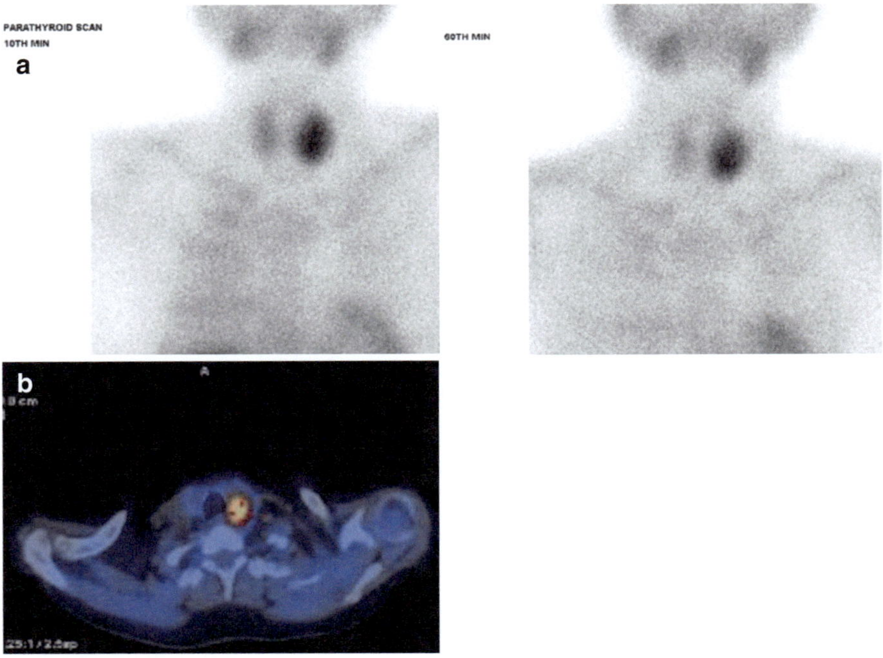

Fig. 28.2 (**a**) SestaMIBI scintigraphy, (**b**) SPECT CT

can improve the detection of hyperfunctioning parathyroids compared to SPECT alone [2]. Figure 28.2a (sestaMIBI scintigraphy) and 2b (SPECT CT) demonstrates typical appearance of parathyroid on these imaging modalities [7]. Ultrasound and sestaMIBI SPECT should be considered as first-line imaging in PHPT [9].

Newer imaging modalities include the use of four-dimensional computed tomography (4D-CT) and choline PET which are generally reserved for non-localized or discordant imaging [2]. Other rarely used imaging modalities include magnetic resonance imaging and selective venous sampling [9] (Fig. 28.3).

Anatomical considerations In-depth knowledge of anatomy and possible sites of ectopic parathyroids is paramount for a successful parathyroidectomy. The main supply for the parathyroid is from the inferior thyroid artery which is responsible for supply to the upper and lower glands in 80% of cases; however, 20% of superior and 5% of inferior parathyroids can also be supplied by the superior thyroid artery. Preserving blood supply to the normal parathyroid in a bilateral neck exploration is critical to avoid permanent hypoparathyroidism [9]. The superior parathyroid arises from the fourth branchial pouch, is usually found on the posterolateral aspect of the thyroid lobe or in the tracheoesophageal groove, and is located posterolateral to the RLN. The other ectopic locations include retropharyngeal or parapharyngeal spaces, intra-thyroidal, or in the middle mediastinum [10]. Inferior parathyroids arise from the third branchial pouch and have a more variable location due to a longer path of descent (Fig. 28.4) [11].

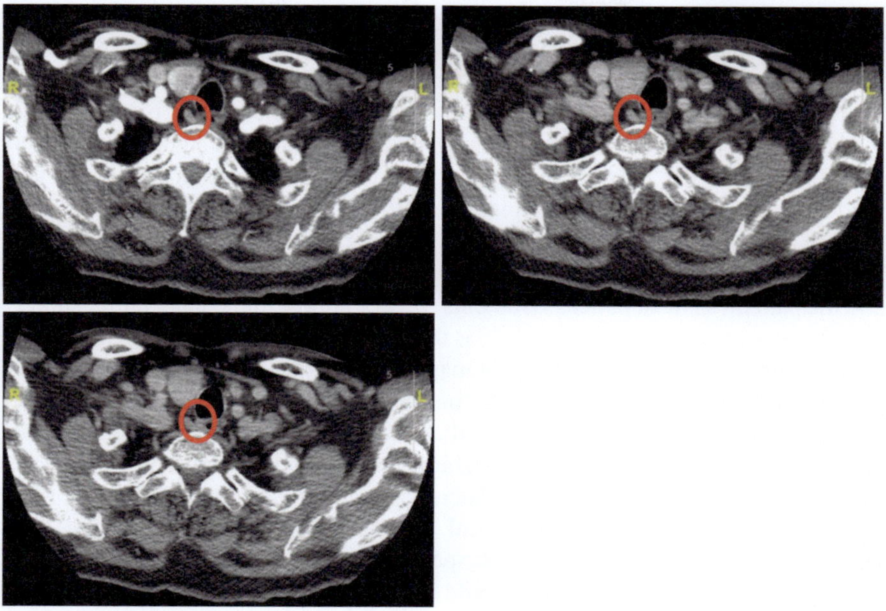

Fig. 28.3 4D CT—arterial, venous, and delayed venous phases, respectively, in a 4D CT showing an arterial enhancing lesion in the tracheoesophageal groove with rapid wash-out in the venous phase and complete wash-out in the delayed venous phase

Fig. 28.4 Path of descent of superior and inferior parathyroid glands [11]

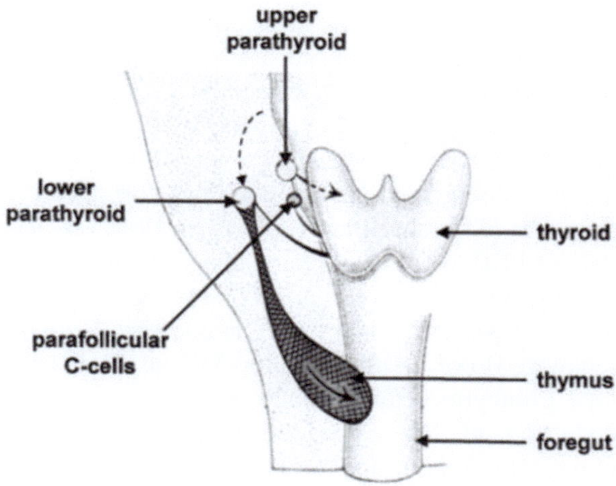

It is typically located in the thyro-thymic tract or near the inferior pole of the thyroid. The other locations include the cervical thymus, anterior mediastinum, or in the carotid sheath [10]. The weight of a normal parathyroid is about 40–60 mg. Parathyroid surgery requires a detailed understanding of the possible anatomical locations of the parathyroid, meticulous dissection, systematic deduction, and skill to estimate the weight of the parathyroid in vivo [10]. The expected surgical cure rate in PHPT is about 90–95%. This is achievable only if the surgical strategy is appropriate and attention is paid to genotype-phenotype correlation. Surgeons' familiarity with imaging tests is important to precisely predict the location intra-operatively in case of a descended superior parathyroid and ectopic parathyroids in the horn of the thymus [9]. Hence the surgeons' experience is a significant factor in predicting a cure [3]. Surgery of parathyroid should also be atraumatic and a clean field to avoid the risk of parathyromatosis [10].

Surgical Approaches Parathyroid surgery is highly satisfying to both, the surgeon and the patient, as most patient symptoms recover almost immediately after surgery [10]. Focused parathyroidectomy (FP) is the preferred surgical approach in primary hyperparathyroidism with concordant imaging [10]. The advantages of focused surgery are shorter operative time, smaller incision size, and less tissue scarring, lesser complication rates, and reduced hospital costs. Focused parathyroidectomy should be complemented ideally with intra-operative parathyroid hormone (IOPTH) monitoring assay to establish cure [1, 10]. Focused parathyroidectomy can be performed with a superficial cervical block, local anesthesia, and minimal sedation [12]. However, if multi-gland disease is suspected intra-operatively during a focused parathyroidectomy, the procedure should be converted to a bilateral neck exploration [10]. The success of focused parathyroidectomy without IOPTH has been shown to be inferior as compared to when it is combined with it [10].

Multi-gland disease is more common in non-localized PHPT; however, it should not deter from expert management [2]. Multi-gland involvement is more often seen in familial cases; however, it can also be seen in sporadic cases and requires a high index of suspicion to avoid persistent disease [10]. Bilateral neck exploration (BNE) involves visualization of all the parathyroids and comparing the gland size to remove the enlarged parathyroid(s), preserving adequate vascularized parathyroid tissue to prevent permanent hypoparathyroidism [10]. If the pre-operative localization studies show discordant imaging or are negative, then the preferred surgical approach should be bilateral cervical exploration. However, negative imaging in a confirmed case of PHPT with end-organ damage should proceed to surgery. If missing, the parathyroids should be searched first in their usual locations, then in ectopic sites, and lastly intra-thyroidal [9]. If an adenoma is found, the affected gland alone is removed. However, if there is multi-gland disease affecting all four glands, a subtotal parathyroidectomy should be performed leaving the most normal and least nodular gland [9]. Surgeons still rely occasionally on BNE because it is independent of pre-operative imaging and is not affected by IOPTH dynamics [13]. BNE is generally performed nowadays only on complex cases and hence is associated with longer operative times, a higher incidence of multi-gland disease, and has relatively higher incidence of surgical failure [13].

Unilateral neck exploration is the visualization of the ipsilateral parathyroid with the diseased gland in a localized parathyroid adenoma without the use of IOPTH. The rationale is visualization of a normal parathyroid to exclude multi-gland disease and avoid the need for bilateral neck exploration [13].

Remote access parathyroidectomy includes robotic or endoscopic parathyroidectomy. It has the advantage of better cosmetic outcomes, but requires more extensive dissection [13].

Sub-total parathyroidectomy involves identification of all parathyroids, thereafter preserving about 50–100 mg of the most normal appearing parathyroid and then removal of all the other parathyroids [10]. Some centers advocate routine cryopreservation of resected parathyroid tissue with variable results—viability at 24 months ~70% and failure of transplanted tissue of ~80% [10]. It involves storing minced parathyroid tissue in a buffered medium at 179–196 °C [10].

Total parathyroidectomy with immediate or delayed auto-transplantation is rarely performed due to the high risk of permanent hypoparathyroidism.

In parathyroid carcinoma, en bloc resection without rupture of the capsule is recommended to prevent recurrence. The role of external beam radiotherapy is debatable. These patients require regular follow-up and surveillance [3].

Re-operative parathyroidectomy may be required in persistent (if hypercalcemia persists after surgery) or recurrent disease (hypercalcemia recurs after documented cure and a 6-month period of normocalcemia). A thorough review of the previous surgical notes and histopathology should be done before proceeding to surgery. Re-operative surgery should ideally be focused. Localization studies should be performed again, and the surgical approach should be tailored to the findings. There is a higher risk of surgical complications such as recurrent laryngeal nerve injury and hypoparathyroidism in re-operative surgery in view of scar tissue and hence should be performed by a high volume experienced parathyroid surgeon. Use of IOPTH is strongly recommended in a re-operative setting [13].

Surgical Adjuncts

IOPTH is an important adjunct that helps confirm that all hypersecreting parathyroid tissue was excised, especially in a case of focused parathyroidectomy without looking at the other parathyroid glands [10]. It was first devised by George Irvin and team who came up with the Miami criteria to decide on unilateral versus bilateral exploration [14]. IOPTH utilizes the short half-life of PTH of 3–5 min to rapidly establish if surgery has been adequately completed [10]. There are several verified protocols which can help the surgeon decide if further exploration can be stopped [10]. Vienna criteria fairs slightly better than the Miami criteria in that the reoperation rates may be lower; however, more patients require BNE using the Vienna criteria [15]. A more than 50% fall in IOPTH and into the normal range confirms cure. However, there are several conflicting reports regarding its utility, especially in multi-gland disease. False-positive and false-negative reports can result in surgical failure in up to 16% of cases [16]. A recent systematic review has shown higher cure rates without the use of IOPTH (99.3%) as compared to the use of IOPTH (98.1%) [15]. PTH levels from bilateral jugular veins can also be compared to lateralize the side of the parathyroid [10]. The use of IOPTH is dictated by the philosophy—localization tells you where to start and IOPTH tells you when to stop [14].

Intra-operative frozen section helps to identify if the tissue is parathyroid or not and whether it is normal or hypercellular; however, it will not be able to differentiate if it is an adenoma or hyperplasia [5].

Intra-operative ultrasound helps the surgeon precisely make the incision for minimally invasive surgery and see relation of the parathyroid to adjacent structures [5].

Intra-operative gamma probe is based on the ability of the hyperfunctioning parathyroid glands to retain Tc99m-sestaMIBI during surgery and the use of hand-held probes to compare background activity to higher activity seen in the hypercellular parathyroid glands [5].

Near-infrared autofluorescence—NIRAF—diseased parathyroids are 30% less fluorescent than normal parathyroid glands. It may help visualize the diseased parathyroid and normal parathyroid and hence can help reduce the incidence of persistent hyperparathyroidism and more importantly permanent hypoparathyroidism [17].

The complications with parathyroidectomy include hematoma, injury to the recurrent laryngeal nerve, permanent hypoparathyroidism, hungry bone syndrome, and persistent hyperparathyroidism [10]. Post-operative hypocalcemia following FP is related to suppressed other normal parathyroids or bone hunger. However, in sub-total parathyroidectomy, hypocalcemia is generally due to ischemia of remanent parathyroids or inadequate volume. Other factors that can contribute to hypocalcemia is the degree of pre-operative hypercalcemia and vitamin D deficiency [10]. Hungry bone syndrome is defined as prolonged severe hypocalcemia, hypomagnesemia, and hypophosphatemia characteristically seen in patients with bad bone disease and is due to post-operative influx of calcium into the bone after parathyroid surgery. Treatment of hungry bone disease involves supplementation of calcium, activated vitamin D, and magnesium [5].

Medical management of PHPT can be offered to those who do not choose surgery, but have indications for surgery as listed above. The available options include the use of cinacalcet, alendronate, or denosumab. Calcium intake should be restricted to 1000 mg/ day for women >50 and men >70 years old and 800 mg/day for women <50 and men <70 years old [1]. Bi-annual measurement of calcium and bone mineral density is recommended in patients who do not undergo surgery [3].

Special Considerations

Pregnancy: Pre-operative imaging should be limited to ultrasound, and surgery should be considered in the second trimester if serum calcium >11.0 mg/dl [1]. There is a higher risk of obstetric and neonatal complications such as pregnancy loss, preterm delivery, and pre-eclampsia, transient post-partum hypocalcemia, tetany, and convulsions, in patients who are conservatively managed without surgery as compared to those who undergo successful parathyroidectomy [18].

HPT-JT: Bilateral neck exploration is recommended due to a higher risk of parathyroid carcinoma [1].

Multiple endocrine neoplasia: Bilateral neck exploration is the surgery of choice because of multi-gland disease [1].

Familial hypocalciuric hypercalcemia: Surgery is contraindicated in most cases [1].

Effective and timely communication between the healthcare provider and patient positively impacts trust, adherence to treatment plans, and satisfaction [19]. Treatment for PHPT requires a multi-disciplinary approach and early referral to surgery in confirmed cases of PHPT to optimize patient quality of life and outcomes and reduce morbidity [4].

References

1. Bilezikian JP, Khan AA, Silverberg SJ, Fuleihan GEH, Marcocci C, Minisola S, et al. Evaluation and management of primary hyperparathyroidism: summary statement and guidelines from the fifth international workshop. J Bone Miner Res. 2020;37(11):2293–314.
2. Kurtom S, Carty SE. Primary hyperparathyroidism. Surg Clin North Am. 2024;104(4):791–8.
3. Nilsson I-L. Primary hyperparathyroidism: should surgery be performed on all patients? Current evidence and residual uncertainties. J Intern Med. 2019;285(2):149–64.
4. Ramonell KM, Liou R, Zheng X, Song Z, Lee JA, Sedrakyan A, et al. Effect of delayed parathyroidectomy on risk of future cardiovascular and nephrolithiasis interventions in adults with primary hyperparathyroidism [Original Study]. Ann Surg [Internet]. 2024 [cited 2024 Nov 21]. Available from: https://journals.lww.com/10.1097/SLA.0000000000006508
5. Perrier N, Lang BH, Farias LCB, Poch LL, Sywak M, Almquist M, et al. Surgical aspects of primary hyperparathyroidism. J Bone Miner Res. 2020;37(11):2373–90.
6. Miller AB, Frank E, Simental AA, Feng M. Surgery for nonlocalizing hyperparathyroidism in high volume center. Head Neck. 2024;46(7):1788–94.
7. Maceri DR, Tai T. Parathyroid disease: a paradigm for disease management.
8. Kochman M. Primary hyperparathyroidism: clinical manifestations, diagnosis and evaluation according to the Fifth International Workshop guidelines. Rheumatology. 2023;61(4):256–63.
9. Gómez-Ramírez J, Arranz Jiménez R. Surgical tactics of parathyroidectomy: should we abandon the use of ioPTH? Am J Surg. 2024;235:115709.
10. Kurtom S, Carty SE. Primary hyperparathyroidism. Surg Clin North Am. 2024;104(4):799–809.
11. Mariani G, Gulec SA, Rubello D, Boni G, Puccini M, Pelizzo MR, et al. Preoperative localization and radioguided parathyroid surgery.
12. Insogna KL. Primary hyperparathyroidism. Solomon CG, editor. N Engl J Med. 2018;379(11):1050–9.
13. Neves MCD, Santos RO, Ohe MN. Surgery for primary hyperparathyroidism. Arch Endocrinol Metab. 2022;66(5):678–88.
14. Scott-Coombes D, Stechman M, Patel N, Egan R. Intraoperative parathyroid hormone assay benefits surgery for primary hyperparathyroidism when preoperative localisation is negative or not performed. Ann R Coll Surg Engl. 2024:rcsann.2024.0051.
15. Bátora D, Iskandar R, Gertsch J, Kaderli RM. Impact of perioperative diagnostic tools on clinical outcomes and cost-effectiveness in parathyroid surgery: a decision model-based analysis. BMJ Open. 2024;14(9):e082901.
16. Dahiya D, Abuji K, Kumari P, Gautam A, Bhadada S, Sood A, et al. Surgical outcome after focused parathyroidectomy: experience from a tertiary care centre in North India. Pol J Surg. 2021;93(5):39–43.
17. Demarchi MS, Triponez F. Advancing parathyroid surgery: a critical examination of probe-based near-infrared autofluorescence technology. Gland Surg. 2024;13(6):1137–40.
18. Eli S, Gal SG, Adnan Z. Comparison between surgical and non-surgical management of primary hyperparathyroidism during pregnancy: a systematic review. Endocrine. 2024;86(1):101–8.
19. Phillips W, Stallworth J, Gillis A, Lindeman B, Chen H, Fazendin J, et al. Patient perspectives on barriers to obtaining surgery for primary hyperparathyroidism: a qualitative review. Am J Surg. 2024;228:122–5.

Decision in Management of Primary Hyperparathyroidism

29

Brendan C. Stack

Editorial

Primary hyperparathyroidism (pHPT) is the most common disorder of the parathyroid glands. Yet this condition is improperly managed, leading to inappropriate diagnosis, surgical failures, multiple surgeries, and morbidity. We need to simplify the diagnosis and incorporate standard practices that will improve the outcomes and quality of life of our patients. The author has laid out a systematic approach starting with basic understanding of calcium physiology along with appropriate utilization of imaging to ensure successful diagnosis and treatment of pHPT.

Diagnosing and localizing the affected gland are fraught with issues. Taking a standardized approach may help, especially using functional and axial imaging notwithstanding their lack of universal availability. The best form of diagnosis and localization is still elusive, and clinical correlation and surgical judgment are critical. Focused surgery is possible due to concordant localization but is still not foolproof. Misses and recurrences are a reality, and stress is on reducing the morbidity. Finally, a team effort is required to improve diagnose, minimize surgical morbidity, and improve the quality of life of the patient.

Prathamesh S. Pai

Introduction

The leading cause of hypercalcemia in an ambulatory population is primary hyperparathyroidism (pHPT) [1]. The basic physiologic concept is that when calcium levels decrease, parathyroid hormone (PTH) levels increase to restore the desired

B. C. Stack (✉)
Department of Otolaryngology-Head and Neck Surgery, Southern Illinois University School of Medicine, Springfield, IL, USA

P. S. Pai et al. (eds.), *Controversies in Cancer of the Thyroid and Parathyroid Glands*, https://doi.org/10.1007/978-3-032-13130-0_29

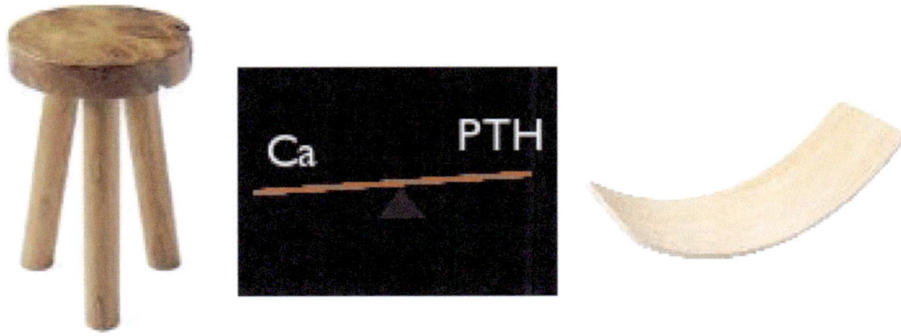

Fig. 29.1 The "three-legged stool" to diagnose primary hyperparathyroidism (pHPT) (left); the physiologic balance of calcium and PTH (center); the straight cantilever of calcium/PTH physiology is "functionally curved" in pHPT (right)

Table 29.1 Incidence of types of surgical parathyroid pathology from successfully operated cases

Parathyroid histopathologies	"Prevalence (%)"	95% CI
Solitary adenomas	88.90	88.89–88.92
Multiple gland disease	9.84	9.84
Multiple gland hyperplastic disease	5.74	5.33–6.15
Double adenomas	4.14	3.74–4.53
Carcinomas	0.74	0.53–0.95

From Ruda et al. [2]

calcium homeostasis (Fig. 29.1). When PTH production from parathyroid gland(s) is chronically increased, concordant with elevated calcium levels, a pathophysiologic state is achieved known as pHPT. The majority of pHPT results from a single parathyroid adenoma [2] (Table 29.1). Likewise, the majority of hypercalcemia noted in electronic medical records (EMR) go unaddressed, thereby creating a pool of untreated patients likely to have undiagnosed pHPT [3].

The underpinnings of the diagnosis of pHPT have been described as a "three-legged stool," referring to the historically three required synchronous elements to diagnose classical pHPT. These elements include elevations of serum calcium, intact parathyroid hormone, and urinary calcium occurring at the same time (Fig. 29.1, left panel). The physiologic balance of calcium and PTH is represented as a cantilever (center). The straight cantilever of the calcium/PTH relationship is functionally "curved" in cases of pHPT (right).

Understanding the Physiology of Calcium and PTH

The diagnosis of pHPT starts with a sound understanding of parathyroid physiology and diseases (Fig. 29.2). In addition, one must be aware of, and always consider, the broad list of differential diagnoses that can affect the key elements of pHPT, namely calcium and PTH (Fig. 29.3).

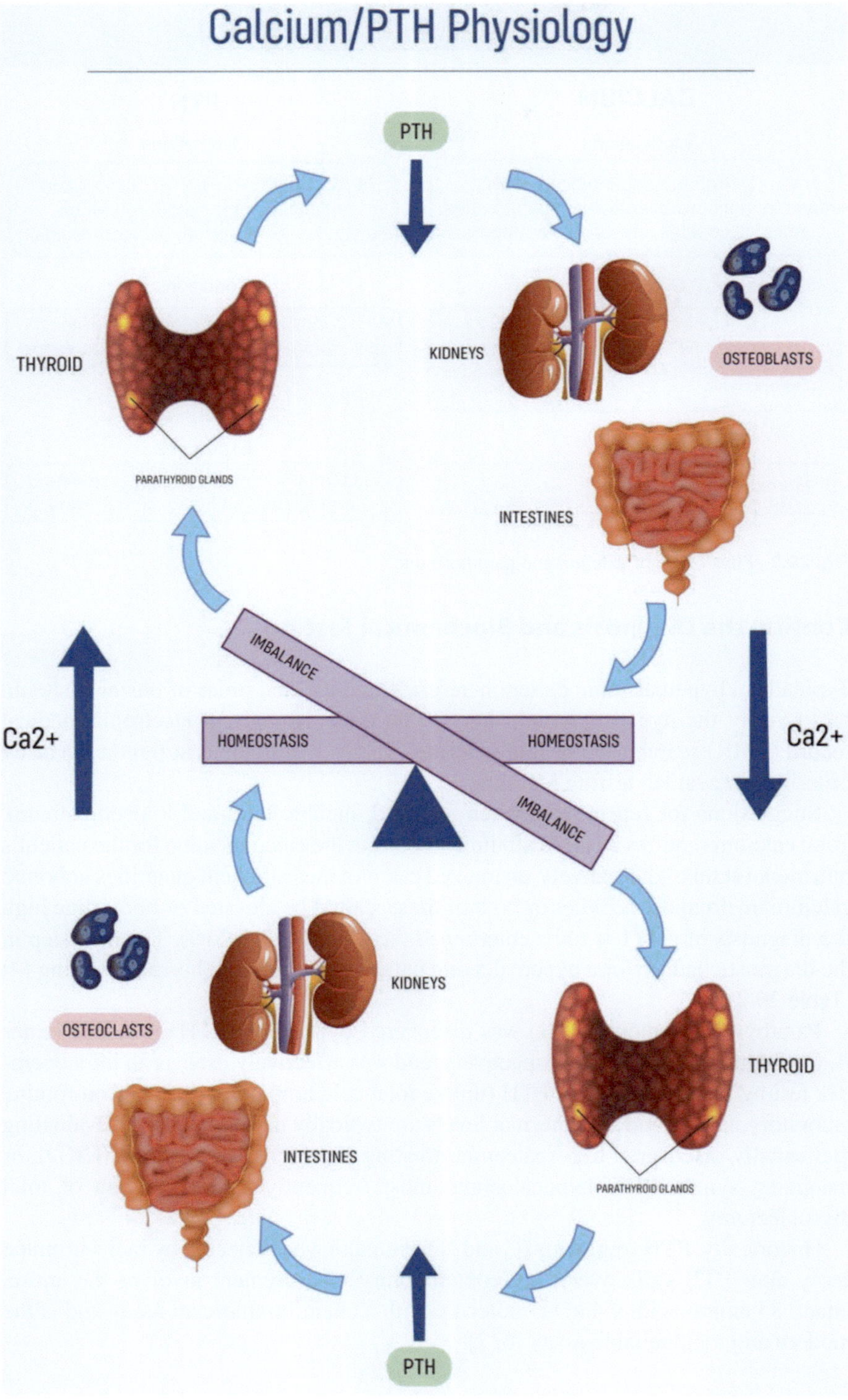

Fig. 29.2 Figure designed for author (BCS) previously published in Stack [9]

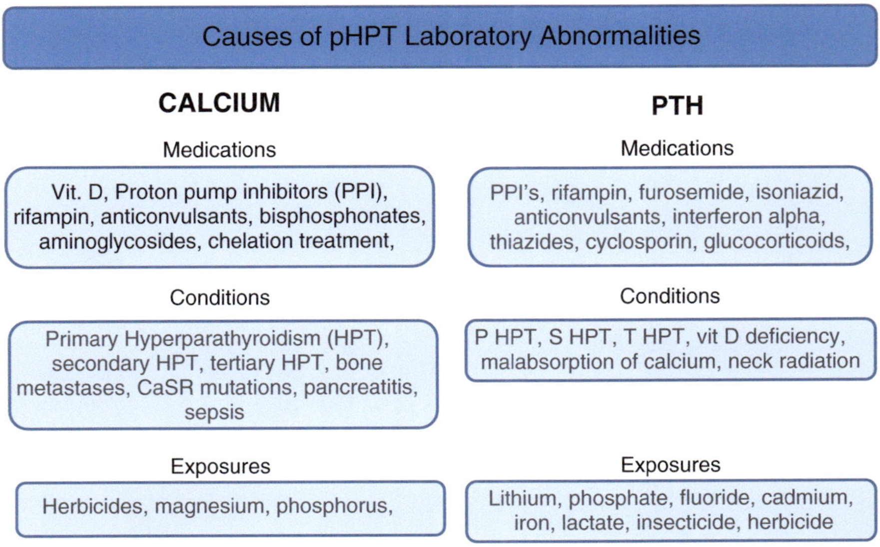

Fig. 29.3 Physiology of calcium and parathormone

Confirm the Diagnosis and Biochemical Testing

Typically, a hypercalcemic patient is referred and the first order of business should be to verify the hypercalcemia. This can be done through an electronic medical record (EMR) search (two or more elevated values within the past 6 months) or by ordering a repeat lab testing real time.

Suggestions for repeat labs, when required, include total and ionized calcium. Total calcium requires a paired albumin to correct the calcium value for the patient's nutritional status. Alternatively, an ionized calcium measurement quantifies unbound calcium in circulation. Either or both of these should be elevated or borderline high if a diagnosis of pHPT is to be entertained (see "variants" below). The next step in the diagnostic ladder for a hypercalcemic patient is parathyroid hormone testing [4] (Table 29.2).

Parathyroid hormone (PTH) was discovered by Adolph M. Hanson and James B. Collip in 1923 and 1925, respectively, and was effectively used as an intra operative test by Irvin in 1988 [5]. PTH (unlike total calcium) is not screened on routine laboratory panels, and its abnormal levels are typically discovered when evaluating incidentally discovered hypercalcemia, treating chronic kidney disease (CKD), or managing symptomatic hypocalcemia, most frequently a complication of total thyroidectomy.

Historically, PTH fragments (C and N terminals) were detected by radio-immune assay after PTH's discovery, but contemporary measurement involves the entire, intact, 84 amino acid, 9.4 kDa, molecule with a chemiluminescent assay and is the modern and most reliable assay [6, 7].

Table 29.2 Costs (2016, in USD) of comprehensive calcium testing for pHPT diagnosis, postoperative surveillance, or hypocalcemia management

Test	Costs (US Dollars)[a]
Intraoperative PTH	4.10[b]
Intact PTH	4.10[c]
lonized calcium	2.41
Serum calcium	0.51
Magnesium	4.10
Chloride	4.10
Phosphate	2.41
Creatinine	0.51
25-Hydroxyvitamin D	4.10

Nelson et al. [4]
[a]Cost reflects charge for patients at the University of Arkansas for Medical Sciences, 2016
[b]Run in 15 min
[c]Run in 30 min

Classical primary hyperparathyroidism is defined by hypercalcemia (10.4 mg/dL or greater), hyperparathyrohormonemia (greater than 65 or 88 ug/mL, depending on the assay), and hypercalcuria (in excess of 350 mg/24hs, depending on local laboratory standards). Historically, clinical indications for pHPT included "bones, stones, moans, and psychic overtones." This cliche acknowledges pHPT's impact on the skeleton (osteopenia/osteoporosis), kidney stones, musculoskeletal and joint pain, and depression and neurocognitive decline.

The classical pHPT phenotype has increasingly given way to "borderline" cases, partially due to widespread calcium testing prompting pre- or early symptomatic investigation and diagnosis, which has been observed in many industrialized societies. In these cases, suspicion for multigland disease must be increased and concern for masquerading conditions of the kidney, which are unaddressed by parathyroid surgery. These include familial hypercalcemic hypocalcuria (FHH) and renal causes of hypocalcemia. The former can result in hypercalcemia but is identified by hypocalcuria in a 24 h urine collection that can subsequently be confirmed by genetic testing. The latter results from a calcium resorption kidney defect, which can also be genetically tested, and can normalize serum calcium levels through calcium hyperexcretion while PTH is elevated. This is a nephrology entity and will not be further explored in this chapter.

Sporadic pHPT

The majority of pHPT are not inherited (MEN (multiple endocrine neoplasia) or familial) but are sporadic. The majority of pHPT are also the result of single-gland parathyroid adenomas [2]. Statistics on the types of parathyroid pathology causing pHPT have varied in reports over time, largely due to the deployment and evolution of novel imaging technologies. This has led, in part, to a focused parathyroidectomy approach for a majority of patients (Table 29.1).

Vitamin D

The leading cause of secondary HPT (sHPT) is vitamin D deficiency. This often coexists with pHPT. Vitamin D deficiency is widespread in developed nations due to limited sun exposure from prevalent lifestyles. Reduced vitamin D results in less dietary calcium being absorbed or less renal filtered calcium being retained, which promotes an elevation in PTH levels. Vitamin D insufficiency or deficiency should be treated when diagnosed as part of hyperparathyroidism management [8]. Chronic elevation of PTH is the stimulus for parathyroid gland hyperplasia, which can result in multiple gland enlargement (Fig. 29.4).

Renal

The spectrum of kidney failure [chronic kidney disease (CKD)] demonstrated by elevations of creatinine, blood urea nitrogen (BUN), and decreasing glomerular filtration rate (GFR) reduces vitamin D activation (1 hydroxylation) and provides an increased demand on parathyroid glands for PTH production, leading toward hyperplasia [9] (Fig. 29.2 and Table 29.3). Further discussion of CKD exceeds the scope of this chapter.

Lithium

Chronic lithium use for bipolar depression is a known cause for hyperparathyroidism. Lithium use has decreased as of late due to the proliferation of many novel psychotropic medicines. Lithium-induced hyperparathyroidism is most frequently

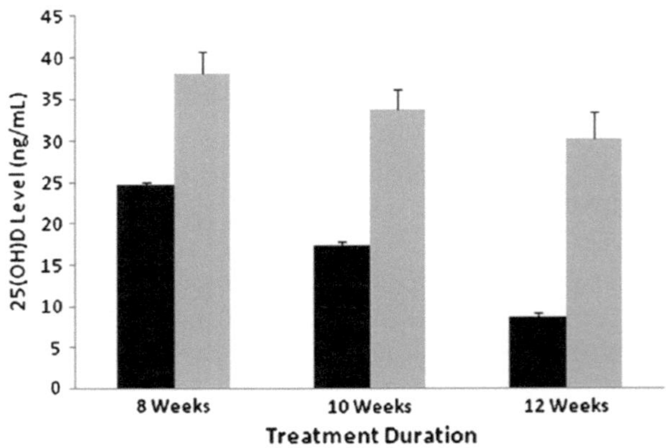

Fig. 29.4 Effect of vitamin D repletion regimen on 25 OH levels. 25-Hydroxyvitamin D levels before and after treatment with 50,000 IU on vitamin D2. Average initial level (black box) and final level (gray box), for three treatment periods of 8, 10, and 12 weeks. (From Middleton et al. [8])

Table 29.3 Differential diagnosis of hypercalcemia with normal parathyroid hormone level

Entity	Test(s)
Familial hypocalciuric hypercalcemia	24 h urine calcium Functional excretion calcium
Malignancy Humoral Multiple myeloma Lymphoma	PTHrp Serum or urine protein electrophoresis 25-OH vit D and 1,25-OH vit D
Granulomatous disease	25-OH vit D and 1,25-OH vit D
Medications (HCTZ, Ca, vit D, vit A, lithium)	Discontinue medication(s) and recheck calcium and PTH
Hyperalbuminemia	Calculate corrected serum calcium Ionized calcium
Hyperthyroidism	Thyroid function tests
Normohormonal hypercalcemia Primary hyperparathyroidism	Trial cinacalcet Repeat calcium and PTH

From Gillis et al. [44]

from parathyroid hyperplasia but adenomas can be found. Some patients have been on lithium for decades, have achieved symptom control and stability, and are reluctant to change their medication. This may prove to be a challenge for both patients and surgeons for managing these concurrent diseases [10].

Variants

"Variants" or "borderline" designations refer to cases that may represent early or developing pHPT and have biochemical data that deviates from classic pHPT (hypercalcemia concurrent with hyperparathormonemia). These variant/borderline patients still bear the risks of classic pHPT (Fig. 29.5). When these cases present, there are strategies to examine biochemical data to diagnose pHPT (Fig. 29.6). This should be done diligently, and patients SHOULD NOT be reflexively sent for imaging prior to a solid diagnosis. Imaging in these cases may return as nonlocalized for parathyroid(s) [11, 12].

Testing

Ideally a simultaneous measurement of all analytes of calcium physiology is obtained to most effectively diagnose and manage pHPT over the short and medium term. Elements that should be tested include calcium (total and ionized), intact PTH, 25-OH vitamin D, magnesium, phosphate, creatinine [which usually comes with estimated glomerular filtration rate (EGFR)], and bone-specific alkaline phosphatase. The rationale for each of these follows [4]:

Variable	Normocalcemic (NC)[a]			Normohormonal (NH)[a]			Classic (C)[a]			P value[b]	
	N_{study}	N_{subj}	% (n)	N_{study}	N_{subj}	% (n)	N_{study}	N_{subj}	% (n)	NC vs C	NH vs C
Nephrolithiasis	23	1285	21.7 (279)	6	276	25.4 (70)	16	5767	15.9 (915)	0.313[c]	0.605[d]
Neuropsychiatric symptoms	4	359	23.4 (84)	4	456	29.6 (135)	5	2697	21.9 (591)	—	—
DM/impaired fasting glucose	7	340	24.1 (82)	0	—	—	5	480	26.5 (127)	0.174[e]	—
Hypertension	9	406	48.5 (197)	3	376	22.0 (112)	7	1181	41.7 (492)	0.009[f]	—
Chondrocalcinosis	3	107	3.7 (4)	0	—	—	2	43	16.3 (7)	—	—
Fracture	13	376	18.1 (68)	1	232	45.3 (105)	5	404	4.2 (17)	0.962[g]	—
↓ BMD (total)	23	1255	49.7 (624)	5	273	40.3 (110)	17	5562	39.7 (2210)	0.264[h]	0.271[i]
Osteopenia	?	650	10.3 (670	?	111	4.5 (5)	?	2213	35.2 (779)	—	—
Osteoporosis	?	624	49.2 (307)	?	110	18.2 (20)	?	2213	22.1 (489)	—	—
↓ BMD (unspecified)	?	623	40.1 (250)	?	110	77.3 (85)	?	2211	42.6 (942)	—	—

Abbreviations: BMD, bone mineral density; DM, diabetes mellitus; —, no data was available or could be calculated.
[a]Summaries for these groups includes data from all studies reporting the variable of interest.
[b]*P* values are from meta-analysis that only includes studies reporting information for both groups being compared; thus, the number of studies upon which the meta-analysis *P* value is based will always be less than or equal to the number of studies reported for the group summaries. For instance, the *P* value resulting from the NC vs C comparison of nephrolithiasis is based on 13 studies.
[c]n = 13 studies.
[d]n = 6 studies.
[e]n = 5 studies.
[f]n = 5 studies.
[g]n = 5 studies.
[h]n = 13 studies.
[i]n = 5 studies.

Variable	Normocalcemic (NC)[a]			Normohormonal (NH)[a]			Classic (C)[a]			P value[b]	
	N_{study}	N_{subj}	Mean (SD)	N_{study}	N_{subj}	Mean (SD)	N_{study}	N_{subj}	Mean (SD)	NC vs C	NH vs C
Total calcium, mg/dL	25	927	9.71 (0.43)	9	638	10.59 (0.43)	28	5700	11.11 (0.77)	<.001[c]	0.035[d]
Corrected calcium, mg/dL	19	579	9.58 (—)	2	23	10.11 (—)	7	491	10.95 (—)	—	—
Ionized calcium, mmol/L	4	233	1.29 (0.08)	1	46	1.40 (—)	4	682	1.44 (0.12)	<.001[e]	—
Phosphorus, mg/dL	14	538	2.97 (0.61)	4	292	3.09 (0.44)	13	1523	2.66 (0.94)	<.001[f]	0.336[g]
PTH, pg/mL	28	1575	112.6 (72.2)	9	638	51.8 (9.9)	31	7862	166.5 (303.6)	<.001[h]	0.018[i]
25-OHD, ng/mL	23	1227	31.6 (14.8)	8	537	30.0 (10.4)	24	4930	28.0 (18.2)	0.003[j]	0.008[k]
Urine calcium, mg/24 h	8	217	243.7 (113.6)	4	212	322.4 (137.7)	10	2075	324.0 (175.5)	0.036[l]	0.405[m]
Creatinine, mg/dL	14	435	0.84 (—)	2	127	0.93 (—)	7	2098	0.85 (—)	—	—

Abbreviations: PTH, parathyroid hormone; 25-OHD, 25-hydroxvitamin D; —, no data was available or could be calculated.
[a]Summaries for these groups include data from all studies reporting the variable of interest.
[b]*P* values are from a meta-analysis that only includes studies reporting information for both groups being compared; thus, the number of studies upon which the meta-analysis *P* value is based will always be less than or equal to the number of studies reported for the group summaries. For instance, the *P* value resulting from the NH vs C comparison of total calcium is based on 9 studies.
[c]n = 25 studies.
[d]n = 4 studies.
[e]n = 4 studies.
[f]n = 13 studies.
[g]n = 3 studies.
[h]n = 28 studies.
[i]n = 9 studies.
[j]n = 22 studies.
[k]n = 7 studies.
[l]n = 8 studies.
[m]n = 4 studies.

Fig. 29.5 pHPT variants. Normocalcemic (NC), Normohormonal (NH), and classical pHPT demonstrating comorbidities (above) and lab values (below). (From Hollowoa et al. [11])

Calcium should always be ordered to confirm the first report of hypercalcemia. This can be done as total, which requires albumin for adjustment, or ionized, which is a direct measurement of all unbound calcium.

PTH is ordered as intact (sometimes referred to as third generation) to avoid the confusion of PTH fragment assays, which each have varying half-lives in circulation and potentially confound the study of the Ca:PTH relationship, which is the keystone of the classic pHPT diagnosis [4].

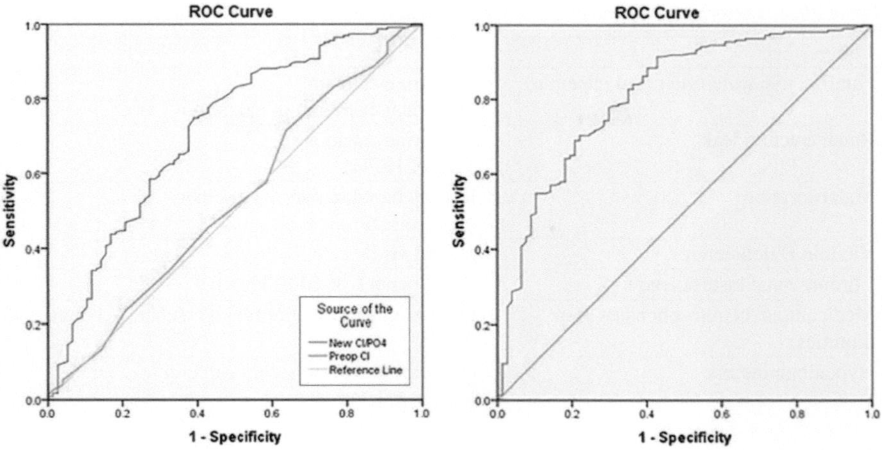

Fig. 29.6 Proxies used to diagnose "borderline" pHPT: Cl and Cl/PO4 (left) and Ca/PO4 (right). (From Wright et al. [12])

Divalent (double charged) ions are often abnormal when calcium levels are altered. *Magnesium* (+2) can be elevated in cases of hypercalcemia, and its supplementation should be avoided. Its replenishment can be useful in cases of hypoparathyroidism. *Phosphate* (−2) can be low in cases of hypercalcemia but is often corrected with successful treatment of pHPT. Elevated phosphate can herald renal compromise as is the case in renal sHPT or can place the patient at risk of calciphylaxis (Ca X P > 55) [13]. Hyperphosphatemia can be treated with intestinal phosphate binders.

Creatinine, and calculated EGFR by extension, is a marker of renal dysfunction as is the case in renal sHPT. *Bone-specific alkaline phosphatase* (AP) can be elevated in conditions of heightened osteoclastic activity, which may result from pHPT. Chronically, pHPT can lead to osteopenia or osteoporosis, which may require a bone(DXA) scan for complete evaluation (Table 29.2).

Laboratory proxies that have been studied to diagnose pHPT in "borderline" cases have included Cl, Cl:P, and Ca:P. Ca:P appears the most robust. Proxies are useful to help resolve laboratory ambiguity in "borderline" cases and should be pursued prior to ordering imaging [12] (Fig. 29.6 and Table 29.4).

Table 29.4 Differential diagnosis of hyperparathyroidism with normal calcium

Entity	Test(s)
Familial hypocalciuric hypercalcemia	24 h urine calcium Fractional excretion of calcium
Renal calcium leak	24 h urine calcium Trial of HCTZ
Malabsorption	History bariatric surgery or other (e.g., celiac)
Vitamin D deficiency	25-OH vit D
Chronic renal insufficiency	Renal panel (Cr, GFR, Phos)
Medications (bisphosphonates loop diuretics)	Discontinue medication(s) and recheck calcium and PTH
Hypoalbuminemia	Calculate corrected serum calcium Ionized calcium
Normocalcemic primary hyperparathyroidism	Trial Ca BID/TID + HCTZ Repeat Ca and PTH

From Gillis et al. [44]

Imaging

One of the greatest advances in the treatment of pHPT has been the application of new imaging modalities with high degrees of resolution, which have been further refined with advanced hardware, processing/computational power, and the addition of machine learning most lately. Not all imaging are available in all health systems and locales, so their selection by surgeons is based on experience and availability. For this reason, which is compounded by evolving technology, many guidelines on pHPT have deferred from exclusively singling out one technology. We will review salient history and features to aid clinicians in their selection of the POST-diagnostic, PRE-procedural imaging (Fig. 29.7) [14, 15].

Additional imaging modalities have been added to the parathyroid imaging armamentarium over time, largely driven by a desire for accuracy and precision of parathyroid localization, with an overarching desire to focus and minimize central neck surgery, thereby decreasing complications (Fig. 29.7). These innovations have leveraged, in parallel, features of parathyroid gland anatomy and hyperfunctionality. Eventually, this resulted in a fusion of anatomic and functional images into a single image set with a goal of increased precision and accuracy.

Ultrasound

Ultrasound (US) is commonly the first line of parathyroid imaging due to its low cost, ambulatory accessibility, universal availability, absence of ionizing radiation, or the need for infusion of radio isotopes, also a source of ionizing radiation. Training for US has proliferated from the radiology department to many patient-facing clinics across specialties over the last few decades. Multiple certification programs have been created for the same.

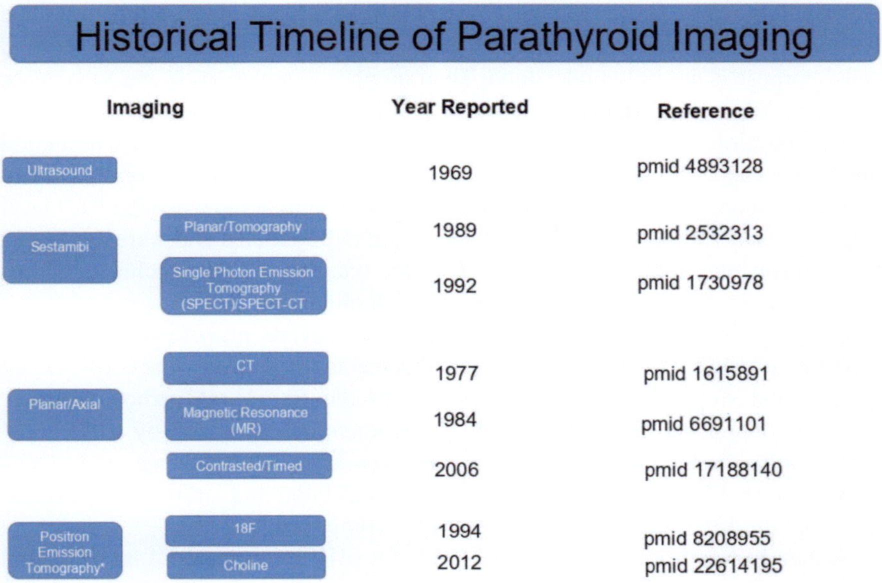

Fig. 29.7 History of parathyroid imaging

First reported in the 1970s [16], US was incidentally noted to image pathologically enlarged parathyroid glands. With increased experience and hardware and software innovations, the accuracy of the technique has steadily improved. Many centers that value multimodality parathyroid images to seek concordant parathyroid imaging result in their clinical pathways. Those centers initiate the imaging process with an US, often at the time of first surgical consultation.

An underappreciated advantage of US is surgeon-driven neck examination. Unique to the surgeon is the "muscle memory" that can develop over time between the activities of surgeon-performed ultrasound preoperatively and open surgical exploration and successful resection of parathyroid lesions. A mental (memory) connection of the preoperative image and the gross anatomic encounter with the gland during surgery creates a positive, reinforcing, learning loop. The benefits of this memory develop over a surgical career [17].

Functional Imaging

This form of imaging derives its origins from leveraging a specific isotope that exploits physiologic properties of a hyperfunctional parathyroid gland(s) in order to locate it (them). Parathyroid glands are heterogeneous in their cell constituents, chief cells, oxyphil cells, and adipocytes. Chief cells (C cells) are responsible for producing and secreting parathyroid hormone (PTH) and calcitonin (80% of parathyroid mass). They are smaller than oxyphil cells (20% of parathyroid of mass) but are more abundant. Chief cells have a well-developed endoplasmic reticulum and prominent Golgi apparatus to help with the synthesis and secretion of PTH. Oxyphil cells' purpose is not fully understood. Their number (population) seems to increase with age. Adipocytes are lipid-ladened cells without a known function [18].

This physiologic attribute of chief cells is leveraged by radio-labeled sestamibi images (planar, SPECT, etc.). Sestamibi attaches to the inner mitochondrial membrane. It is more likely to be positive and detectable on imaging when the PTH level is greater than 150 pg/dL [19]. Other tracers are radio-labeled and were developed for positron emission tomography (PET) for oncology. These included fluoro-deoxy-glucose (FDG) and isotopic variants of choline.

Oxyphil cells are rich in mitochondria, which coverts glucose into adenosine triphosphate (ATP). Deoxy glucose enters this metabolic pathway like conventional glucose and stops prior to the completion of the Embden–Myerhoff reaction. 2-Deoxy-glucose labeled with 18F (FDG) is, therefore, taken up by these cells' mitochondria preferentially because of their increased metabolic rate, and FDG's conversion to ATP is arrested. FDG remains intracellular and emits positron radiation from the 18F until its radioactive decay is completed [20, 21].

Sestamibi was first reported in the 1980s for pHPT as a result of an incidental finding of a parathyroid adenoma during a nuclear cardiac scan. Sestamibi [22–24] interacts with parathyroid mitochondria through binding to its inner membrane. The sestamibi half-life is 6 h. It is taken up by the thyroid and parathyroid tissues. It washes out of the thyroid in 15–30 min and is retained in the parathyroid 60–180 min following injection. This differential washout allows the ability to distinguish thyroid vs. parathyroid uptake [22].

Tc 99 Sestamibi Imaging

A two-dimensional image of a patient is taken from a conventional gamma camera (Fig. 29.8). This type of image can be helpful in determining the side of neck for location and eventual resection. This scan also indicates superior vs. inferior vs. ectopic and can be improved by the addition of oblique images [25].

SPECT is a single-photon emission tomography [14]. This is taken with a panoramic camera gantry that provides a three-dimensional localization of the parathyroid adenoma(s) in the neck. This is particularly helpful in distinguishing superior vs. inferior parathyroid glands. This imaging technique is useful in cases of low-lying superior (posterior or deep) glands.

SPECT CT is a single-photon emission tomography digitally fused with a co-registered CT scan. This is superior to SPECT by providing greater anatomic detail around the area of sestamibi uptake by an adenoma(s) [26, 27].

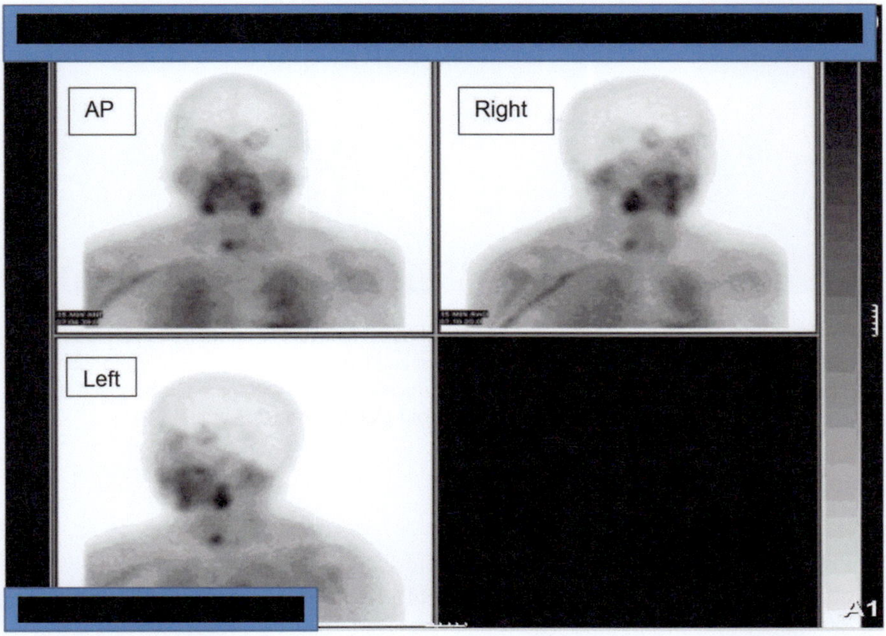

Fig. 29.8 A two-dimensional image of a patient is taken from a conventional gamma camera, Anterior-posterior (AP), right oblique, and left oblique. Solo parathyroid adenoma appears to change sides, which reflects parallax classically seen with a low-lying superior parathyroid

PET

PET imaging for malignancies started in the 1990s but was not reported and applied to pHPT until the 2000s and then continued to develop with the addition of CT to PET and focus upon isotopes with specificity for parathyroids. Focus has been upon FDG (18F being the principal isotope used for malignancies) and choline. Choline has been used with 11C and 18F isotopes. The availability of these radio tracers, short half-life, and cost have been a rate-limiting step in the clinical adoption of this imaging [28–30]. The scarcity of choline isotopes and their short half-lives have limited their use to centers that have their own cyclotron for isotope synthesis.

Radioguided Surgery

Immediate pre-op Sestamibi and PET isotope administration have been used to guide surgeons to locate parathyroid adenoma(s) intraoperatively. This can be done with a isotope specific hand-held gamma detecting probe [31] or using an intraoperative gamma camera apparatus [32] (Fig. 29.9).

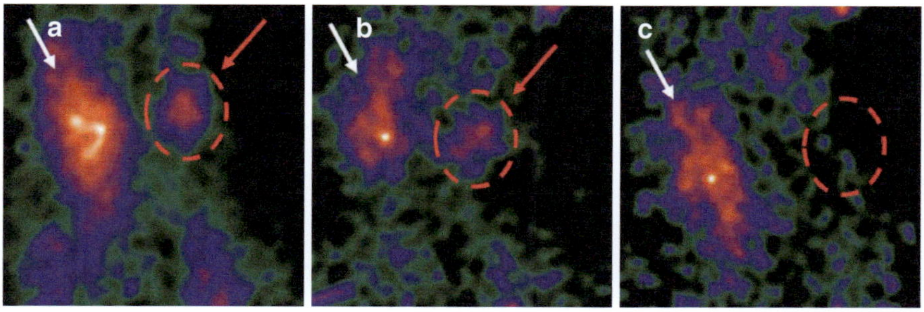

Fig. 29.9 An intraoperative gamma scintigraphy image. Patient with primary hyperparathyroidism with uptake in the thyroid gland (white arrow) and hyperfunctioning parathyroid gland (red arrow and circle). (**a**) Pre-incision image; (**b**) post-incision image with parathyroid gland in vivo; and (**c**) post-excision of hyperfunctioning parathyroid gland. (Creighton et al. [32])

Axial Imaging

Preoperative axial imaging for parathyroid surgery has surged in popularity as nuclear imaging techniques have disappointed expectations for the discovery of smaller and multigland lesions. Parathyroid-focused protocols have been created for both axial imaging modalities and are primarily based on multiple, sequenced images based on contrast enhancement. These tests are rarely first-line exams but serve to confirm findings from more cost-effective scans such as ultrasound in centers that seek concordant scan localization prior to surgery. They are also deployed to find nonvisualized parathyroid in biochemically confirmed cases [33] of pHPT or reoperative settings [15].

4D CT

All axial parathyroid imaging that is "4D" leverages the differential enhancement with intravenous contrast over a short interval of time [34]. With 4D CT, the patient is scanned 3–4 times per contrast infusion. Disadvantages include contrast costs and complications, as well as ionizing radiation exposure from multiple passes through the CT gantry [35].

4D MR

The principles outlined under 4D CT apply to 4D MR. This modality has the advantage of no ionizing radiation exposure [36]. The disadvantages include the scarcity of scanners, scan-related expenses, and possible complications.

Cases with Images

A 69-year-old with hypercalcemia and elevated parathormone levels. Nuclear medicine Tc-99 m sestamibi scan with planar (Fig. 29.10a) and SPECT/CT (Fig. 29.10b) images were interpreted as positive for focal retention at the region of the right inferior thyroid lobe (arrows), not well seen on SPECT/CT; query thyroid adenoma or parathyroid adenoma. 4D-CT performed 2 months later confirmed probable parathyroid adenoma posterior to the right thyroid lobe (Fig. 29.10c, arrows); a second lesion within the thyroid gland on 4DCT was considered likely a thyroid nodule (arrowhead).

Preoperatively, intact was PTH 128 pg/mL (normal 15–65) with total calcium of 10.3 mg/dL (normal 8.6–10.0). The patient underwent removal of an 891-gram right lower parathyroid adenoma. The IOPTH went from 105 (pre-), to 46 (post- #1), to 31 (#2), to 28 (#3), and the outpatient postoperative intact PTH was 16 pg/mL with calcium of 8.5 mg/dL.

Courtesy of Tracy L. Yarbrough, MD, PhD, MAEd, California Northstate University

A 27-year-old with sporadic hypercalcemia in the setting of multiple endocrine neoplasia (MEN) type 2a status post adrenalectomy. Labs revealed total serum calcium of 10.5 mg/dL (normal 8.6–10.0 mg/dL), 24-h urine calcium of 315.0 mg/24 h (normal 100–300/24 h), and intact PTH of 54 pg/mL (normal 15–65 pg/mL) in the setting of normal/mildly low vitamin D and no abnormal PTHrp. There was no calcitonin elevation or other evidence of medullary thyroid carcinoma.

Tc-99 m sestamibi scan was nonlocalizing on planar images (Fig. 29.11a), but demonstrated asymmetry along the posterior aspect of the mid-to-upper left thyroid bed on SPECT/CT (Fig. 29.11b, arrows). Focal uptake was seen in this same region of a hypodense soft tissue lesion along the posterior left thyroid gland on DOTATATE PET/CT (Fig. 29.11c, arrows), suggestive of left-sided parathyroid adenoma. Clinically diagnosed with concurrent mild primary and secondary hyperparathyroidism, on active surveillance; declined thyroidectomy (no RET mutation).

Courtesy of Tracy L. Yarbrough, MD, PhD, MAEd, California Northstate University

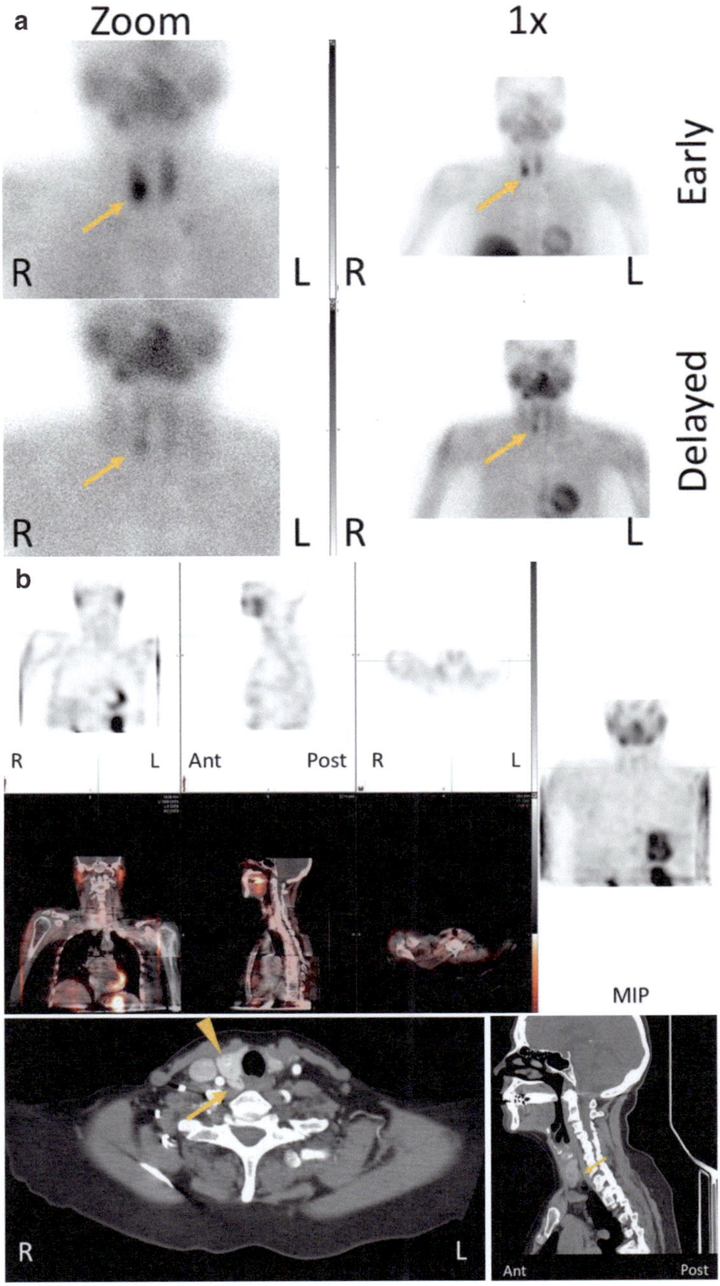

Fig. 29.10 Tc-99 m sestamibi scan with planar (**a**) and SPECT/CT (**b**) focal retention at the region of the right inferior thyroid lobe (arrows). 4D-CT performed 2 months later confirmed probable parathyroid adenoma posterior to the right thyroid lobe (**c**, arrows); a second lesion within the thyroid gland on 4DCT was considered likely a thyroid nodule (arrowhead). (Courtesy of Tracy L. Yarbrough, MD, PhD, MAEd, California Northstate University)

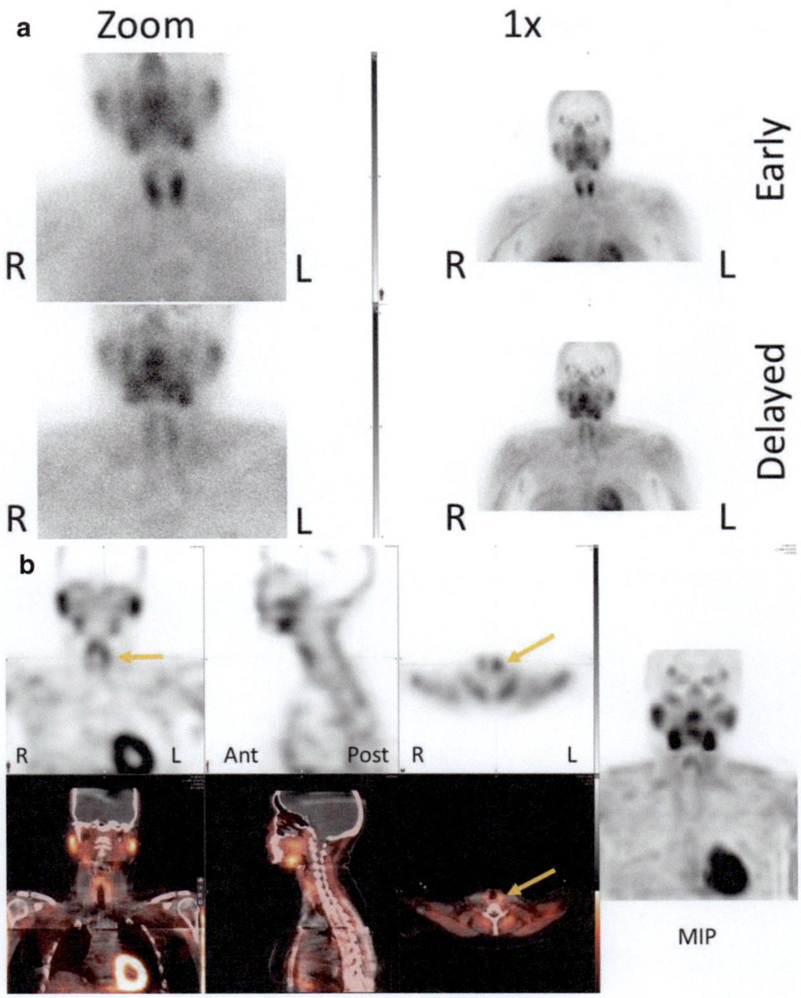

Fig. 29.11 Tc-99 m sestamibi scan was nonlocalizing on planar images (**a**) but demonstrated asymmetry along the posterior aspect of the mid-to-upper left thyroid bed on SPECT/CT (**b**) arrows. Focal uptake was seen in this same region as a hypodense soft tissue lesion along the posterior left thyroid gland on DOTATATE PET/CT (**c**) arrows suggestive of left-sided parathyroid adenoma. (Courtesy of Tracy L. Yarbrough, MD, PhD, MAEd, California Northstate University)

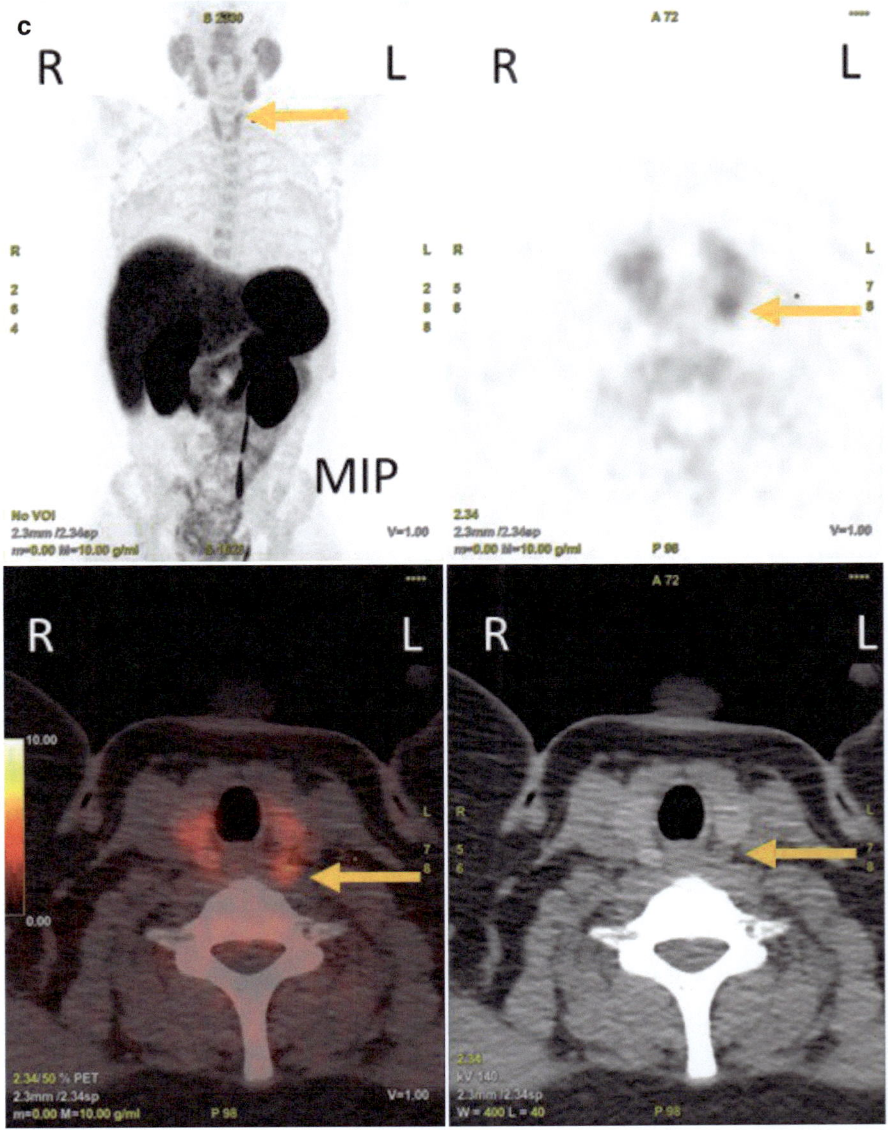

Fig. 29.11 (continued)

Therapeutic Approach

Open surgery in its various forms has been the gold standard for central neck surgery (Fig. 29.12). This has also been the case for the definitive treatment of pHPT. There has been an evolution in recent years from the historical standard for central neck surgery, with the 6 cm Kocher incision toward lesser invasive approaches

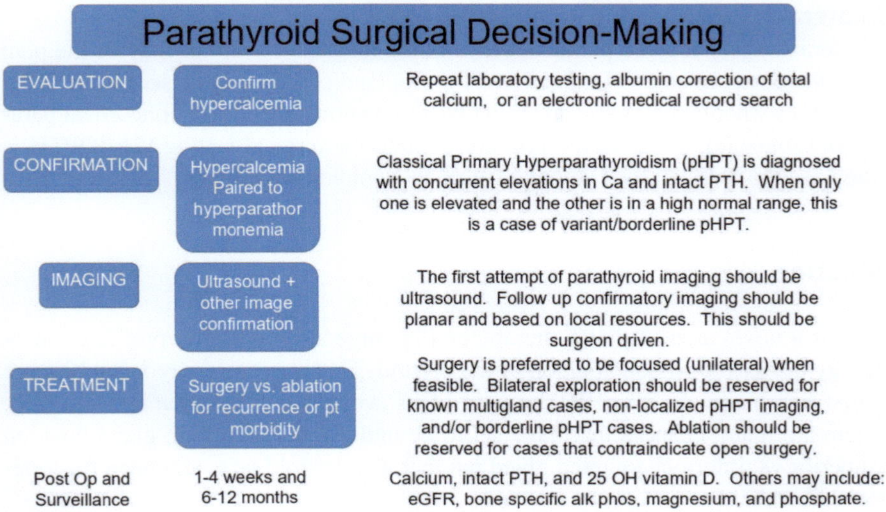

Fig. 29.12 Surgical decision-making flowchart

[37]. These have included smaller incisions such as minimally invasive (MIVAP, MIRP) [31, 38], which have leveraged endoscopes or gamma radiation with probe detection. Further efforts to hide evidence of external neck surgery have included remote access incisions such as the trans-axillary, breast incisions, and trans-oral approaches. Finally, we have arrived at an age where ultrasound-guided delivery of per cutaneous needle-directed energy that ablates tissue lesions. Each of the approaches will be briefly described below.

Surgery

Open surgeries have been classified based on their extent and their goal regarding parathyroid examination. This classification is not arbitrary but has the goal of reducing operative time and complications.

Focused

Focused surgery is only possible and practicable in a setting of precision preoperative parathyroid imaging, which indicates single-gland pHPT. Optimally this is via two concordant image modalities (US + another). Focused surgery attempts to strike a balance between an open surgical approach with limited recurrent laryngeal nerve (RLN) dissection (unilateral vs. bilateral) and limited manipulation of all four parathyroid glands. It also has the advantage of a smaller neck incision (2–3 cm) [31]. The goal of this approach is cure of the pHPT while reducing the risk for bilateral vocal cord dysfunction and hypoparathyroidism. This approach does not preclude an intraoperative decision to perform bilateral exploration. These approaches often utilize intraoperative PTH measurement (IOPTH).

Bilateral

Bilateral surgery may be pursued after a failed focused attempt or may be the plan from the outset in cases of contralateral multigland pHPT disease, secondary HPT, or in cases where preoperative imaging fails to demonstrate any or concordant parathyroid image(s), either in the primary or revision surgical setting [2]. IOPTH is often used to reassure the surgeon of surgical completeness.

Ablation

This is a novel area of pHPT therapy and is burgeoning with the proliferation of energy devices for tissue ablation of the thyroid. This approach may 1 day become a first-line treatment for pHPT because of its avoidance of an open incision [39]. There are many nuances that have yet to be understood, including gland position (superior vs. inferior), targeted gland number, parathyroid size, and need for long-term surveillance.

Parathyroid Carcinoma

Although this entity is a departure from the most common reason for ambulatory hypercalcemia (99% vs. >1%), it deserves mention in this chapter, which addresses decision-making in what needs to be entertained in the differential diagnosis of primary hyperparathyroidism. The historical clinical vignette that was considered unique to parathyroid carcinoma was hypercalcemia in the presence of a palpable neck mass. This assertion has become less emphatic as hypercalcemia currently presents earlier in the course of parathyroid diseases as a result of calcium screening and because of an increased attention to and/or prevalence of nodular thyroid disease [2, 40, 41].

If parathyroid carcinoma is considered preoperatively, axial imaging is important for operative planning of the extent of surgery to be performed and the decision to include a neck dissection. If this diagnosis is discovered during surgery, most often by the discovery of a firm, enlarged, and pale parathyroid mass, then the surgeon must decide on performing an ipsilateral hemi-thyroidectomy plus/minus level VI nodal excision. On occasion, the diagnosis of parathyroid carcinoma is not contemplated/acted upon until the return of the surgical pathology report (Fig. 29.13), at which time considerations should be made as to the need for revision surgery, adjuvant treatment, and/or close surveillance.

Surgery

Surgery for parathyroid carcinoma suspected preoperatively or appreciated intraoperatively has traditionally been managed with mass excision en bloc with ipsilateral hemi-thyroidectomy. Level VI is typically added if there is visual/palpable evidence

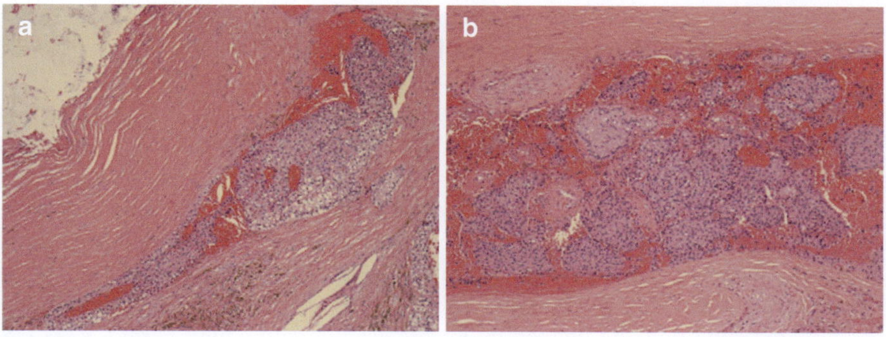

Fig. 29.13 (**a**) Parathyroid carcinoma exhibiting lymphovascular invasion (H and E), original magnification. (**b**) Parathyroid carcinoma exhibiting lymphovascular invasion (H and E), original magnification. (Dudney et al. [40]. Figure 7, p. 447)

of adenopathy in the tracheoesophageal groove. Adjuncts such as intraoperative nerve monitoring and IOPTH may be helpful if available. IOPTH changes may be less useful than when deployed for standard pHPT (i.e., modified Miami criteria) yet, but witnessing a significant intraoperative PTH decrease, can be reassuring.

Surveillance

PTH is the primary biomarker of parathyroid carcinoma. Elevations of PTH can result in hypercalcemia from renal retention or osteolysis. Therefore, paired PTH and calcium should be monitored quarterly the first year and then less frequently thereafter if levels are stable. If there is concern for de-differentiation and/or PTH levels do not match the clinical picture, chorioembryonic antigen (CEA) can be added to the surveillance panel.

Follow-Up

Follow-up can vary widely based on the setting in which treatment is delivered. It may involve the primary caregiver, referring endocrinologist, or surgeon. No one type of following provider is superior but, more importantly, follow-up is very important. Follow-up should focus on the resolution of hypercalcemia in classic pHPT cases. Resolution of parathyroid hormone levels should be achieved in both cases of classic and borderline pHPT as well as sHPT [42].

Avoidance of Reoperative Procedures

Meticulous evaluation of patient data in a systematic fashion is the most significant hedge against treatment failure. When presented with a case of postoperative persistent hypercalcemia/pHPT, it is important to assiduously follow reoperative parathyroid best practices and be aware of presentation of complications and possibility of revision-related complications [43].

Summary

Decision management in primary hyperparathyroidism starts with making the correct diagnosis. The correct diagnosis is based on calcium and PTH levels. This is optimally determined when both tests are drawn simultaneously. Classic pHPT has simultaneously elevated calcium and PTH. Variants of pHPT are an increasingly encountered condition and defined by hypercalcemia with a high normal PTH *OR* elevated PTH concurrent with a high normal calcium.

Decision management in pHPT continues with methodical preoperative imaging and then continues with a treatment plan, which may include surgery or ablation. Finally, a disciplined and consistent follow-up is required to ensure the treatment of pHPT was successful and will achieve desired health-related benefits regarding arthralgias, osteopenia/porosis, renal impairment, and/or cardiovascular diseases.

References

1. Walker MD, Silverberg SJ. Primary hyperparathyroidism. Nat Rev Endocrinol. 2018;14(2):115–25. https://doi.org/10.1038/nrendo.2017.104. Epub 2017 Sep 8
2. Ruda JM, Hollenbeak CS, Stack BC Jr. A systematic review of the diagnosis and treatment of primary hyperparathyroidism from 1995 to 2003. Otolaryngol Head Neck Surg. 2005;132(3):359–72. https://doi.org/10.1016/j.otohns.2004.10.005.
3. Quilao RJ, Greer M, Stack BC Jr. Investigating the potential underdiagnosis of primary hyperparathyroidism at the University of Arkansas for Medical Sciences. Laryngoscope Investig Otolaryngol. 2020;5(4):773–7. https://doi.org/10.1002/lio2.415.
4. Nelson KL, Hinson AM, Lawson BR, Middleton D, Bodenner DL, Stack BC Jr. Postoperative calcium management in same-day discharge thyroid and parathyroid surgery. Otolaryngol Head Neck Surg. 2016;154(5):854–60. https://doi.org/10.1177/0194599816631732. Epub 2016
5. Irvin GL 3rd, Dembrow VD, Prudhomme DL. Operative monitoring of parathyroid gland hyperfunction. Am J Surg. 1991;162(4):299–302. https://doi.org/10.1016/0002-9610(91)90135-z.
6. Hawker CD. Parathyroid hormone: radioimmunoassay and clinical interpretation. Ann Clin Lab Sci. 1975;5(5):383–98.
7. Hawker CD, Di Bella FP. Radioimmunoassay for intact and carboxyl-terminal parathyroid hormone: clinical interpretation and diagnostic significance. Ann Clin Lab Sci. 1980;10(1):76–88.
8. Middleton L, Stack BC Jr, Riggs AT, Bodenner DL. Vitamin D deficiency: a simple algorithm employing weekly administration of 50,000 IU of vitamin D. Am J Otolaryngol. 2014;35(2):85–8. https://doi.org/10.1016/j.amjoto.2013.12.002. Epub 2013 Dec 12
9. Stack BC Jr. Secondary hyperparathyroidism. Otolaryngol Clin N Am. 2024;57(1):99–110. https://doi.org/10.1016/j.otc.2023.07.010. Epub 2023 Aug 25
10. Nilsson IL, Thorsteinsson D, Nylén C, Koman A, Granath F, Bränström R. Surgical strategy in lithium-associated hyperparathyroidism: a population-based study. World J Surg. 2024;48(2):408–15. https://doi.org/10.1002/wjs.12071. Epub 2024 Jan 12
11. Hollowoa BR, Spencer HJ 3rd, Stack BC Jr. Normocalcemic and normohormonal primary hyperparathyroidism: laboratory values and end-organ effects. Otolaryngol Head Neck Surg. 2021;165(3):387–97. https://doi.org/10.1177/0194599820983728. Epub 2021 Jan 19

12. Wright C, King D, Small M, Gibson C, Gardner R, Stack BC Jr. The utility of the cl:PO4 ratio in patients with variant versions of primary hyperparathyroidism. Otolaryngol Head Neck Surg. 2021;164(2):308–14. https://doi.org/10.1177/0194599820947009. Epub 2020 Aug 4
13. Beus KS, Stack BC Jr. Calciphylaxis. Otolaryngol Clin N Am. 2004;37(4):941–8, xii. https://doi.org/10.1016/j.otc.2004.03.001.
14. Morris MA, Saboury B, Ahlman M, Malayeri AA, Jones EC, Chen CC, Millo C. Parathyroid imaging: past, present, and future. Front Endocrinol (Lausanne). 2022;12:760419. https://doi.org/10.3389/fendo.2021.760419.
15. Zafereo M, Yu J, Angelos P, Brumund K, Chuang HH, Goldenberg D, Lango M, Perrier N, Randolph G, Shindo ML, Singer M, Smith R, Stack BC Jr, Steward D, Terris DJ, Vu T, Yao M, Tufano RP. American Head and Neck Society Endocrine Surgery Section update on parathyroid imaging for surgical candidates with primary hyperparathyroidism. Head Neck. 2019;41(7):2398–409. https://doi.org/10.1002/hed.25781. Epub 2019 Apr 19
16. Solorzano CC, Carneiro-Pla DM, Irvin GL 3rd. Surgeon-performed ultrasonography as the initial and only localizing study in sporadic primary hyperparathyroidism. J Am Coll Surg. 2006;202:18–24. https://doi.org/10.1016/j.jamcollsurg.2005.08.014.
17. Wilson M. Head and neck ultrasonography: essential and extended applications, Second Edition. Lisa A. Orloff. ISBN13: 978-1-59756-858-6. J Laryngol Otol. 2017;131(08):749.
18. https://www.ncbi.nlm.nih.gov/books/NBK537203/#:~:text=Structure%20and%20Function,increase%20in%20number%20with%20age
19. Norman JG, Jaffray CE, Chheda H. The false-positive parathyroid sestamibi: a real or perceived problem and a case for radioguided parathyroidectomy. Ann Surg. 2000;231(1):31–7. https://doi.org/10.1097/00000658-200001000-00005.
20. Andrew M. Hinson, Brendan C. Stack J. Applied embryology, molecular genetics, and surgical anatomy of the parathyroid glands. In: Stack Jr BC, Bodenner DL, editors. Medical and surgical treatment of parathyroid diseases - an evidence-based approach. Cham: Springer; 2017. p. 17–26. ISBN 978-3-319-26794-4.
21. Andrew M. Hinson, Brendan C. Stack J. Parathyroid physiology and molecular biology. In: Stack Jr BC, Bodenner DL, editors. Medical and surgical treatment of parathyroid diseases - an evidence-based approach. Cham: Springer; 2017. p. 27–40. ISBN 978-3-319-26794-4.
22. Taillefer R, Boucher Y, Potvin C, Lambert R. Detection and localization of parathyroid adenomas in patients with hyperparathyroidism using a single radionuclide imaging procedure with technetium-99m-Sestamibi (double-phase study). J Nucl Med. 1992;33:1801–7.
23. Hiromatsu Y, Ishibashi M, Nishida H, Okuda S, Miyake I. Technetium-99ma new agent for parathyroid imaging. Nucl Med Commun. 1989;10:791–4. https://doi.org/10.1097/00006231-198911000-00003.
24. Coakley AJ, Kettle AG, Wells CP, O'Doherty MJ, Collins RE. 99Tcm sestamibi--a new agent for parathyroid imaging. Nucl Med Commun. 1989;10(11):791–4. https://doi.org/10.1097/00006231-198911000-00003.
25. Arveschoug AK, Bertelsen H, Vammen B, Brøchner-Mortensen J. Preoperative dual-phase parathyroid imaging with tc-99m-sestamibi: accuracy and reproducibility of the pinhole collimator with and without oblique images. Clin Nucl Med. 2007;32(1):9–12. https://doi.org/10.1097/01.rlu.0000249401.48030.9c.
26. Wong KK, Fig LM, Gross MD, Dwamena BA. Parathyroid adenoma localization with 99mtc-Sestamibi SPECT/CT: a meta-analysis. Nucl Med Commun. 2015;36:363–75. https://doi.org/10.1097/MNM.0000000000000262.
27. Yarbrough TL, Bartel TB, Stack Jr. BC. Single-photon scintigraphic imaging of the parathyroid glands: planar, tomography (SPECT), and SPECT-CT. Chapter 12. In Medical and surgical treatment of parathyroid diseases - an evidence-based approach 1st ed, Brendan C. Stack Jr, Donald L. Bodenner, editors. Cham: Springer, 2017. ISBN 978-3-319-26794-4.
28. Quak E, Lasne-Cardon A, Cavarec M, et al. F18-choline PET/CT or MIBI SPECT/CT in the surgical management of primary hyperparathyroidism: a diagnostic randomized clinical trial. JAMA Otolaryngol Head Neck Surg. 2024;150(8):658–65. https://doi.org/10.1001/jamaoto.2024.1421.

29. Tay D, Das JP, Yeh R. Preoperative localization for primary hyperparathyroidism: a clinical review. Biomedicine. 2021;9(4):390. https://doi.org/10.3390/biomedicines9040390.
30. Bartel TB, Stack BC Jr, Yarbrough TL. Advanced imaging of the parathyroids. Chapter 15. In: Stack Jr BC, Bodenner DL, editors. Medical and surgical treatment of parathyroid diseases - an evidence-based approach. 1st ed. Cham: Springer; 2017. ISBN 978-3-319-26794-4.
31. Cox MD, Stack JBC. Minimally invasive radioguided parathyroidectomy. Chapter 17. In: Stack Jr BC, Bodenner DL, editors. Medical and surgical treatment of parathyroid diseases - an evidence-based approach. 1st ed. Cham: Springer; 2017. ISBN 978-3-319-26794-4.
32. Creighton EW, Dunlap Q, Peckham MM, Elms C, King D, Stack BC Jr. Utility of intraoperative digital scintigraphy in radioguided parathyroidectomy. Head Neck. 2021;43(10):2967–72. https://doi.org/10.1002/hed.26780. Epub 2021 Jun 19
33. Hinson AM, Lee DR, Hobbs BA, Fitzgerald RT, Bodenner DL, Stack BC Jr. Preoperative 4D CT localization of nonlocalizing parathyroid adenomas by ultrasound and SPECT-CT. Otolaryngol Head Neck Surg. 2015;153(5):775–8. https://doi.org/10.1177/0194599815599372. Epub 2015 Aug 6
34. Lawson BR, Fitzgerald RT, Hinson AM, Bodenner DL, Stack JBC. How to perform 4D CT for parathyroid localization. VideoEndocrinol. 2(4) https://doi.org/10.1089/ve.2015.0048.
35. Hairston H, Gardner JR, Gibson AC, Wright C, Small M, King D, Fitzgerald R, Spencer HJ, Bodenner DL, Stack BC Jr. Four-dimensional computed tomography and ultrasonography for prediction of pathological parathyroid location: a retrospective review of a single surgeon's patients at a single institution. Gland Surg. 2024;13(8):1459–68. https://doi.org/10.21037/gs-24-141. Epub 2024 Aug 28
36. Scheepers MHMC, Al-Difaie Z, Brandts L, Peeters A, Winkens B, Al-Taher M, Engelen SME, Lubbers T, Havekes B, Bouvy ND, Postma AA. Diagnostic performance of magnetic resonance imaging for parathyroid localization of primary hyperparathyroidism: a systematic review. Diagnostics (Basel). 2023;14(1):25. https://doi.org/10.3390/diagnostics14010025.
37. Berber E, Bernet V, Fahey TJ 3rd, Kebebew E, Shaha A, Stack BC Jr, Stang M, Steward DL, Terris DJ, American Thyroid Association Surgical Affairs Committee. American thyroid association statement on remote-access thyroid surgery. Thyroid. 2016;26(3):331–7. https://doi.org/10.1089/thy.2015.0407.
38. Miccoli P, Berti P, Materazzi G, Donatini G. Minimally invasive video assisted parathyroidectomy (MIVAP). Eur J Surg Oncol. 2003;29(2):188–90. https://doi.org/10.1053/ejso.2002.1313.
39. Yue W, Jiang T, Ai Z, Deng E, Chai H, Li X, He H, Zhang Z, Weng N, Qin X, Fan J, Tang X, Heng W, Li Y, Sun L, Peng C, Xu H. US-guided percutaneous radiofrequency ablation for secondary hyperparathyroidism: long-term outcomes and prognostic factors. Radiology. 2024;311(1):e231852. https://doi.org/10.1148/radiol.231852.
40. Dudney WC, Bodenner D, Stack BC Jr. Parathyroid carcinoma. Otolaryngol Clin N Am. 2010;43(2):441–53, xi. https://doi.org/10.1016/j.otc.2010.01.011.
41. Beus KS, Stack BC Jr. Parathyroid carcinoma. Otolaryngol Clin N Am. 2004;37(4):845–54, x. https://doi.org/10.1016/j.otc.2004.02.014.
42. Redman C, Bodenner D, Stack B Jr. Role of vitamin D deficiency in continued hyperparathyroidism following parathyroidectomy. Head Neck. 2009;31(9):1164–7. https://doi.org/10.1002/hed.21082.
43. Stack BC Jr, Tolley NS, Bartel TB, Bilezikian JP, Bodenner D, Camacho P, Cox JPDT, Dralle H, Jackson JE, Morris JC 3rd, Orloff LA, Palazzo F, Ridge JA, Scott-Coombes D, Steward DL, Terris DJ, Thompson G, Randolph GW. AHNS Series: do you know your guidelines? Optimizing outcomes in reoperative parathyroid surgery: definitive multidisciplinary joint consensus guidelines of the American Head and Neck Society and the British Association of Endocrine and Thyroid Surgeons. Head Neck. 2018;40(8):1617–29. https://doi.org/10.1002/hed.25023. Epub 2018 Aug 2
44. Gillis A, Lindeman B, Russell MD, Jawad BA, Steward DL, Stack BC Jr. The difficult parathyroid: advice to find elusive gland(s) and avoid or navigate reoperation. Curr Probl Surg. 2023;60(3):101262. https://doi.org/10.1016/j.cpsurg.2022.101262. Epub 2022 Dec 15

Parathyroid Carcinoma

30

Supriya Sen, Anish Jacob Cherian, and Deepak Thomas Abraham

Editorial

Abraham et al. have summarised the complex subject of parathyroid carcinoma. It is a rare endocrine neoplasm with limited experience in any major institution. The clinical hallmarks of presentation are very high calcium and parathyroid hormone levels. Occasionally, the patients might be quite symptomatic due to hypercalcaemia. A clinically palpable lump in the thyroid lesion with hypercalcaemia needs further investigation to rule out parathyroid carcinoma. A fine-needle biopsy is quite helpful, along with complete imaging studies such as ultrasound and CAT scan. It is important to distinguish between thyroid and parathyroid masses, and fine-needle aspiration biopsy will be of great help.

During surgery, it is very important to make sure the lesion is not adherent to the thyroid. The majority of parathyroid carcinomas are generally attached to or infiltrating the thyroid, which will necessitate resection of the thyroid, along with enlarged parathyroid gland. Most of the time, it is uniglandular pathology, and intraoperative parathyroid hormone (PTH) will be of great help. Occasionally, the lesion may be invading the recurrent laryngeal nerve and may necessitate resection. The sine qua non of parathyroid carcinoma is local recurrence, nodal metastasis or distant metastasis. The pathological diagnosis rests on mitosis, local invasion or invasion into the thyroid gland. Microscopic features include necrosis, invasion into surrounding tissue and lymphovascular invasion.

The staging has been described in the recent American Joint Committee on Cancer (AJCC) system. The postoperative follow-up includes calcium and

S. Sen · A. J. Cherian
Christian Medical College, Vellore, Tamil Nadu, India
e-mail: anish@cmcvellore.ac.in

D. T. Abraham (✉)
American Mission Hospital, Manama, Bahrain
e-mail: deepak.abraham@amh.org.bh

P. S. Pai et al. (eds.), *Controversies in Cancer of the Thyroid and Parathyroid Glands*, https://doi.org/10.1007/978-3-032-13130-0_30

parathyroid hormone assays and ultrasound evaluation. The decision to use postoperative radiation therapy is a complex subject and should be determined after discussion in a multidisciplinary tumour board. There are several review articles on this subject, which may help the surgeon to make these critical decisions.

Ashok R. Shaha

Introduction

Parathyroid carcinoma is an uncommon cause of PTH-dependent hypercalcaemia. In view of the rarity of this entity, there have been limited reports and experience with regard to its presentation, diagnosis and management. However, patients with parathyroid carcinoma possess a distinctive clinical profile that can distinguish them from other benign causes of primary hyperparathyroidism (PHPT). In this chapter, we aim to review the etiopathogenesis, clinical profile, diagnostic modalities and prognosis in patients with parathyroid carcinoma. In addition, the surgical approaches to parathyroid carcinoma as well as medical strategies for the management of hypercalcaemia have been outlined.

Incidence

Parathyroid carcinoma is a rare endocrine malignancy, with an incidence of 0.005% of all cancers. The reported incidence among patients with PHPT is 0.5–1%, with a few reports claiming a higher incidence of up to 5% [1–5]. The majority are sporadic, while a minority are part of a genetic syndrome. Somatic mutations of CDC73 account for 80% of apparently sporadic parathyroid carcinoma, while germline mutations of CDC73 are seen in about 30% [6, 7].

Etiopathogenesis

The central role in the molecular pathogenesis of parathyroid carcinoma has been attributed to pathogenic variants of HRPT2 tumour suppressor gene (also known as CDC73). CDC73 is located on chromosome 1 and encodes a protein called parafibromin. Parafibromin is involved in the regulation of gene expression and inhibition of cell proliferation.

Sporadic parathyroid carcinoma: The majority are attributed to somatic and clonal mutations in HRPT2/CDC73 variants [8–10].

Hereditary syndromes: Germline mutations in the HRPT2/CDC73 gene lead to an autosomal-dominant disorder called hyperparathyroidism jaw– tumour syndrome (HPT-JT syndrome). The clinical features of this syndrome include ossifying fibromas of the jaw, cystic and neoplastic renal lesions, uterine tumours and parathyroid neoplasms. Parathyroid neoplasms in this condition are at an increased risk of parathyroid carcinomas. The reported incidence of parathyroid carcinoma in HPT-JT syndrome is 15–20%. Other reported hereditary associations, though not very common, are MEN-1 and MEN-2 syndromes [2, 6, 7, 11, 12].

Other genetic implications: Germline missense mutations of parathyroid transcription factor gene GCM2 have been reported in patients with sporadic parathyroid carcinoma [13]. Other genes that have been implicated in the pathogenesis of sporadic parathyroid carcinoma include mutations in retinoblastoma (Rb), p53, BRCA-2 and cyclin D1/PRAD1 genes. Epigenetic modifications as well like DNA methylation, histone modifications, microRNA misregulations and circular RNA have also been reported. Few parathyroid carcinomas also showed genetic alterations in core components of P13K/AKT/ mTOR pathway [14, 15].

Clinical Presentation

Patients with parathyroid carcinomas present in the fourth or fifth decades with no gender predilection. The majority are functional. The symptom complex is similar to that seen in PHPT due to a parathyroid adenoma; however, the symptoms may be more severe at presentation and may involve multiple organ systems due to the severity of hypercalcaemia [4, 6, 7, 16, 17].

Among the symptomatic patients, the most common organ systems involved are the musculoskeletal (up to 90%) and renal (up to 80%). Both the musculoskeletal and the renal system involvement may be seen in up to 50% of patients. The common clinical manifestations of musculoskeletal involvement include muscle and bone pain, osteopenia, osteoporosis, osteofibrosis, osteitis fibrosa cystica and pathological fractures. While the clinical features of the involvement of the renal system include loin pain or recurrent urinary tract infections secondary to ureteric calculi, nephrocalcinosis, nephrolithiasis and renal insufficiency. Less commonly, patients may present with bloating, constipation, peptic ulcers and pancreatitis from the involvement of gastrointestinal system and anxiety, fatigue and neurocognitive deficits [3, 5, 6, 17, 18].

A palpable neck mass is present in about 40–70% of patients with functional parathyroid carcinoma [2, 3, 5, 19]. These patients may in addition present with symptoms of local invasion such as hoarseness of voice or dysphagia. Associated cervical lymphadenopathy has been reported in up to 15%. Rarely (3–4%), parathyroid carcinoma may be metastatic at presentation, the sites of metastasis being the lungs, bone, liver and brain [3, 5–7, 11, 20, 21].

Less than 10% of patients with parathyroid carcinoma are non-functional and present with a palpable neck mass with or without the involvement of adjacent structures. In addition, this subset of patients may present at a more advanced stage with metastasis to the cervical nodes, bone, lung or liver [6, 17, 21].

Apart from symptoms secondary to organ damage, patients with parathyroid carcinoma may present with symptoms due to hypercalcaemia. These include nausea, vomiting, dehydration, constipation, myopathy, fatigue, disorientation and neurocognitive deficits. A rare presentation is in the form of parathyrotoxicosis or hypercalcaemic crisis (7–12%) [3, 4, 7, 15, 20, 21].

Diagnosis

Laboratory Investigations

Patients with parathyroid carcinoma present with symptoms suggestive of PHPT. The diagnosis of primary hyperparathyroidism is based on biochemical evaluation. PHPT is diagnosed by finding an elevated serum calcium, inappropriately elevated PTH, low or low normal serum phosphorous, with increased 24 hour urinary calcium excretion. Parathyroid carcinoma is suspected when serum calcium levels are greater than 14 mg/dl and the serum PTH values are 3–10 times the reference range [2, 4, 6, 15, 22].

Imaging

Once a diagnosis of primary hyperparathyroidism is made, the next step in management is to localise the lesion. Most commonly, two imaging modalities are performed to determine.

concordance. These include a structural imaging modality, commonly a neck ultrasound and a functional imaging modality ^{99m}Tc sestamibi scan. The features on a neck ultrasound that might raise the suspicion of parathyroid carcinoma include size more than 3 cm, heterogeneous nature, hypo echogenicity, lobulated lesion, irregular borders, calcifications, thick capsule, doubtful vascularity, invasion of adjacent structures and presence of adjacent lymph nodes [5, 7, 11, 15, 21, 23].

Contrast-enhanced computed tomography and/or magnetic resonance imaging are indicated in situations where local infiltration is clinically suspected. In addition, patients in whom parathyroid carcinoma has been suspected preoperatively, these modalities may help in the detection of metastasis. FDG-PET scan may be indicated in the postoperative follow-up algorithm for the detection of local recurrence and distant metastatic disease. The role of FDG PET in the preoperative work is not well established [5, 6, 11, 24].

The following table shows features which will raise a clinical suspicion of parathyroid carcinoma:

- Severe symptoms with the involvement of multiple organ systems
- Palpable neck mass
- Presence of significant cervical lymph nodes
- RLN palsy
- Serum calcium higher than 14 mg/dl (hypercalcaemic crisis)
- Serum PTH more than 3–10 times the laboratory reference range
- Imaging showing features of possible local invasion

Pathology

Role of Fine Needle Aspiration Cytology (FNAC)

The differentiation between parathyroid adenoma and carcinoma is not possible on FNAC, and in addition, FNAC carries the risk of seeding of tumour which preclude the chance of cure. Therefore, FNAC is not recommended for the evaluation of parathyroid carcinoma.

Gross Pathology

Parathyroid carcinomas are large tumours of 3 cm or more in size. They most often involve a single gland. They may appear grey or white as opposed to tan brown in parathyroid adenoma (Fig. 30.1). They exhibit a loss of plane or infiltration of adjacent structures such as strap muscles, adjacent thyroid lobe, RLN, oesophagus and pre-vertebral fascia. These features may be suggestive though not diagnostic as atypical parathyroid adenomas may have similar findings [6, 11, 25].

Histology

The histological diagnosis of parathyroid carcinoma is challenging. The absolute criteria include the presence of metastatic cervical lymph node or distant metastasis. The core elements for the diagnosis of parathyroid carcinoma as established by the WHO classification (2022) include

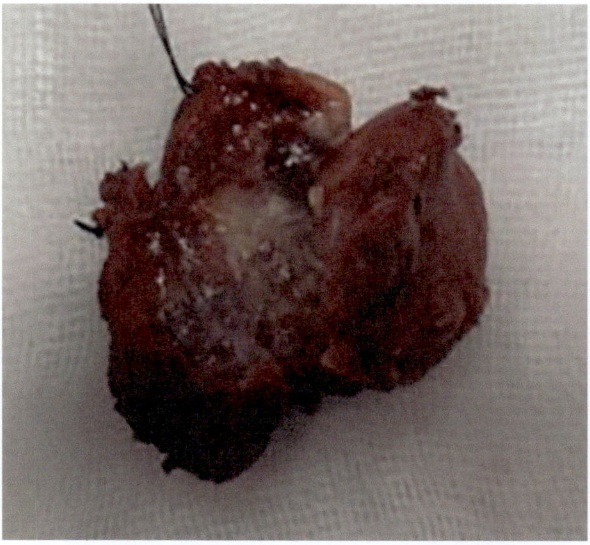

Fig. 30.1 A parathyroid carcinoma

- Lymphovascular invasion
- Neoplastic infiltration of adjacent tissues
- Perineural invasion
- Histological confirmation of metastasis

Certain features suggest a carcinoma, however, are insufficient for a diagnosis. They are currently labelled as atypical parathyroid tumour. These patients have been recommended to be kept on a close surveillance.

Atypical features include

- Trabecular growth
- Band-like fibrosis
- Cell nests in thickened connective tissue
- Tumour cells in capsule
- Increased mitotic activity (>5/10 mm^2)
- Atypical mitotic figures
- Coagulative necrosis
- Adherence to adjacent structures without frank invasion
- Parafibromin loss
- Ki67 > 5%.

The use of immunohistochemical (IHC) panel, including parafibromin, galactin-3, PGP 9.5 and Ki67, has been suggested to aid in the diagnosis of parathyroid carcinoma, reporting sensitivity of 80% and specificity of 100% [25, 26]. WHO recommends parafibromin IHC staining in patients with parathyroid carcinoma and also suggests CDC73 gene sequencing in patients with a high risk of recurrence [27]. Recently, there has been emerging evidence regarding the diagnostic role of epigenetic markers like 5hmc and microRNA 342-3p in the diagnosis of parathyroid carcinoma. However, these need further research to be established as tools for confirmation of diagnosis [25, 26].

Staging

The AJCC, eighth edition of parathyroid staging, has staged parathyroid carcinoma based on the extent of local invasion and presence of the distant metastasis. The TNM staging is as follows:

T1: localised to parathyroid gland with limited extension to soft tissue
T2: direct invasion into thyroid gland
T3: direct invasion into RLN, tracheal wall, oesophagus, thymus, skeletal muscles and adjacent lymph nodes
T4: direct invasion into a major blood vessel or spine
N0: no regional lymph node metastasis
N1: metastasis to regional lymph nodes

M0: no distant metastasis
M1: evidence of distant metastasis
Stage I: T1 or T2N0M0
Stage II: T3N0M0
Stage III: any T N1M0 or T4
Stage IV: any T any N M1

However, there is not much data available on prognosis depending on TNM staging. Hence, its use has been limited [28–30].

Treatment

Surgical Management

Management of Primary

Surgery is the mainstay of treatment for parathyroid carcinoma. Effective surgical management is dependent on preoperative and intraoperative suspicion of malignancy (large size, grey/white hard mass, local invasion and presence of significant cervical lymph nodes). The goal of surgery is en bloc resection of all adjacent tissue without capsular breech to achieve microscopically negative margins. This may encompass removal of ipsilateral thyroid lobe, adjacent fibrofatty or muscular soft tissue and recurrent laryngeal nerve. Regional lymph node dissection should be performed when there is suspected nodal involvement.

The following are the principles of the surgery:

- Minimal manipulation of the tumour preventing rupture of capsule or spillage of tumour.
- Careful inspection to detect strap muscle adherence, involvement of adjacent fibrofatty tissue, prevertebral fascia, thyroid lobe RLN, oesophagus and trachea.
- En block resection of the tumour with any involved structure. Though en block dissection does not improve survival, it has been shown to decrease the rates of local recurrence.
- Preservation of a preoperative functioning RLN if not infiltrated by the tumour (Fig. 30.2).
- Therapeutic central/lateral compartment neck dissection.

Role of Frozen Section

In patients where there is an intraoperative doubt regarding the nature of the tumour, frozen section may be used to confirm parathyroid origin. However, it is difficult to differentiate parathyroid carcinoma from adenoma on frozen section. In addition, frozen section may be used to confirm the presence of metastasis in a cervical lymph node and, therefore, necessity for a neck dissection.

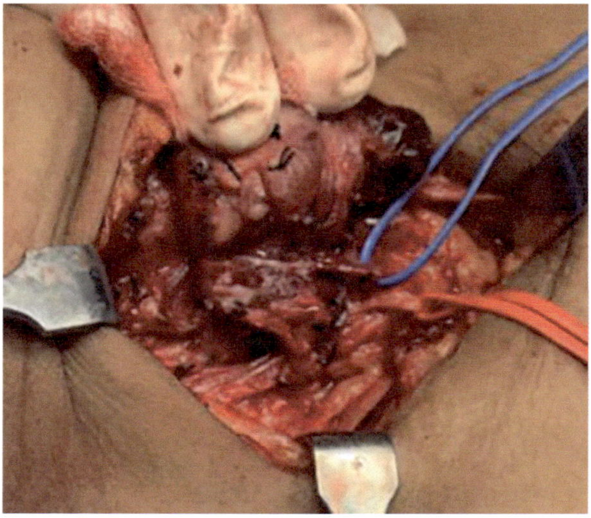

Fig. 30.2 Parathyroid carcinoma with preservation of recurrent laryngeal nerve (blue vessiloop)

Postoperative Management

These patients are prone to hungry bone syndrome and therefore require close monitoring of symptoms and signs of hypocalcaemia in addition to serum levels of calcium. They may require supplementation with oral and intravenous calcium along with active vitamin D. Hospitalisation may be prolonged till their calcium stores are adequately replete [1, 6, 7, 11, 16, 18].

Management of Recurrence

The reported local recurrence rates in patients with parathyroid carcinoma who have not undergone an oncological resection is 50–65%. Most recurrences are detected within the first 2–5 years of surgery; however, delayed recurrences have also been reported [3, 5, 6, 15, 21]. Optimal primary surgery in the form of en bloc resections has been shown to result in lower local recurrence rates. Patients who develop local recurrence present with symptoms suggestive of hypercalcaemia or gradually increasing levels of serum calcium and PTH. CECT or MRI is recommended for the assessment of operability. PET scan is an alternative imaging modality that may be performed in this situation to confirm a recurrent lesion, and in addition, detect metastatic disease. Following medical control of hypercalcaemia, if resectable, an en bloc resection is recommended [3, 4, 7, 15].

Management of Metastasis

The most common site of metastasis are lungs and bone. Surgery is recommended for lesions that are amenable for the same as this will palliate symptoms of hypercalcaemia [3, 4, 6, 7, 11, 20]. Inoperable lesions may be considered for ablative therapy in the form of ethanol or radiofrequency [5, 17].

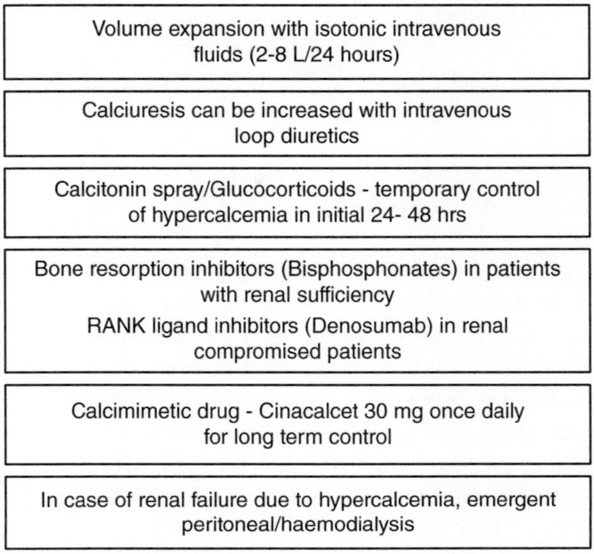

Fig. 30.3 Algorithm for the management of hypercalcaemia

Medical Treatment

Medical management is directed toward the treatment of hypercalcaemia. This may be either for preoperative optimisation or for palliation in patients with unresectable primary/metastatic disease with hypercalcaemic crisis. The agents used for medical management include (Fig. 30.3).

- Volume expansion: Isotonic saline infusion to cause rapid and complete volume re-expansion to help in maintaining a urine output of 100–150 ml/hour. This mechanism enhances renal calcium excretion. Depending on the clinical setting, 2–8 litres of fluid over 24 hours may be used.
- Loop diuretics (furosemide): Aid in renal calcium excretion (calciuresis). These drugs should be used judiciously in patients with cardiac and renal failure. It should be used in combination with high fluid volume replacement, or else, it may promote sodium excretion rather than calciuresis.
- Bone resorption inhibitors: Bisphosphonates (pamidronate and zolendronic acid) and denosumab (RANK- ligand inhibitor) inhibit calcium release. Bisphosphonates, which inhibit osteoclast action, have a slower onset of action but their effect lasts for a longer duration. Denosumab, also an osteoclast inhibitor, is indicated in patients who have hypercalcaemia refractory to cinacalcet and bisphosphonates.
- Calcitonin sprays, which are also bone resorption inhibitors, can be used in the initial stage of management as the effect is transient due to tachyphylaxsis.
- Other bone resorption inhibitors like glucocorticoids and gallium nitrate may be used.

- Calcimimetic drugs: These are allosteric modulator of calcium sensing receptor and inhibit PTH secretion (Cinacalcet).
- Peritoneal dialysis or haemodialysis may be considered in patients with renal insufficiency [6, 7, 11, 25, 31].

Adjuvant Treatment

External Beam Radiotherapy (EBRT)

There have been contrasting reports with regard to EBRT and disease-free/overall survival; however, the majority of reports have shown no significant benefits. Similarly, there have been contrasting reports regarding the effect of EBRT on local recurrence. When used in patients with a high risk of local recurrence such as those with infiltrative local disease, intraoperative tumour spillage, suspected R1 resection or cervical lymph node involvement, EBRT has been shown to reduce the rates of local recurrence. Therefore, EBRT may be considered in selected patients who are at a high risk of local recurrence [6, 11, 15, 32, 33]. In the adjuvant setting, EBRT is administered at a dose of 50–70 Gy over 6 weeks.

Chemotherapy is not effective in the treatment of parathyroid carcinoma, especially when it is metastatic or locally aggressive. The commonly used chemotherapy agents reported in the past include dacarbazine, 5-FU and cyclophosphamide.

Targeted Therapy

The overexpression of MAPK, PI3K and VEGF in parathyroid carcinoma has led to the trial of multitarget tyrosine kinase inhibitors (cabozantinib, sorafenib, lenvatinib, everolimus and reorafenib) in the treatment of parathyroid carcinoma. The oral alkylating agent, temozolomide, has been reported to be useful in the management of metastatic disease [19]. Newer biological agents based on parafibromin and telomerase inhibitors such as azidothymidine are being tested to see their effectivity in treatment of parathyroid carcinoma [4, 6, 7, 15].

Prognosis

Parathyroid carcinoma, though an indolent disease which is slowly progressive, may present with local recurrence or distant metastasis. The heterogeneity among this patient cohort results in its variable prognosis. Moreover, the lack of a standard, universally accepted staging system makes prognostication of the disease difficult. Poor prognostic factors include increased age at presentation, R2 resection, tumour spillage at the time of surgery, close or positive margins, shorter time to first recurrence, multiple recurrences and lymph node metastasis [3, 6, 7, 15]. The reported overall 5- and 10-year survival is 76–85% and 49–77%, respectively. The cause of mortality among patients with functional parathyroid carcinoma is secondary to complications of hypercalcaemia, whereas in non-functional parathyroid carcinoma it is due to the burden of metastatic disease [2, 5, 6].

Follow-Up

A 3-monthly follow-up for the first year following surgery has been recommended, followed biannually for the next 5 years and annually thereafter. Apart from history and clinical examination, serum calcium, PTH and a neck ultrasound should be performed. In view of reported delayed recurrences, surveillance has been recommended to continue lifelong [6, 16].

References

1. Kebebew E. Parathyroid carcinoma. Curr Treat Options in Oncol. 2001;2(4):347–54.
2. Zheng Y, Wen J, Lin W, Lin L, Chen G. Approach to parathyroid carcinoma (PC): seven cases and a review of the literature. Transl Cancer Res. 2020;9(8):4982–7.
3. Givi B, Shah JP. Parathyroid carcinoma. Clin Oncol (R Coll Radiol). 2010;22(6):498–507.
4. Alberti A, Smussi D, Zamparini M, Turla A, Laini L, Marchiselli C, et al. Treatment and outcome of metastatic parathyroid carcinoma: a systematic review and pooled analysis of published cases. Front Oncol. 2022;12:997009.
5. Ferraro V, Sgaramella LI, Di Meo G, Prete FP, Logoluso F, Minerva F, et al. Current concepts in parathyroid carcinoma: a single Centre experience. BMC Endocr Disord. 2019;19(Suppl 1):46.
6. Cetani F, Pardi E, Torregrossa L, Borsari S, Pierotti L, Dinoi E, et al. Approach to the patient with parathyroid carcinoma. J Clin Endocrinol Metab. 2024;109(1):256–68.
7. Ullah A, Khan J, Waheed A, Sharma N, Pryor EK, Stumpe TR, et al. Parathyroid carcinoma: incidence, survival analysis, and management: a study from the SEER database and insights into future therapeutic perspectives. Cancers (Basel). 2022;14(6):1426.
8. Digonnet A, Carlier A, Willemse E, Quiriny M, Dekeyser C, De Saint Aubain N, et al. Parathyroid carcinoma: a review with three illustrative cases. J Cancer. 2011;2:532–7.
9. Howell V, Haven C, Kahnoski K, Khoo S, Petillo D, Chen J, et al. HRPT2 mutations are associated with malignancy in sporadic parathyroid tumours. J Med Genet. 2003;40(9):657–63.
10. Betea D, Bradwell AR, Harvey TC, Mead GP, Schmidt-Gayk H, Ghaye B, et al. Hormonal and biochemical normalization and tumor shrinkage induced by anti-parathyroid hormone immunotherapy in a patient with metastatic parathyroid carcinoma. J Clin Endocrinol Metab. 2004;89(7):3413–20.
11. Selvan B, Paul MJ, Seshadri MS, Thomas N, Paul T, Abraham D, et al. High index of clinical suspicion with optimal surgical techniques and adjuvant radiotherapy is critical to reduce Locoregional disease progression in parathyroid carcinoma. Am J Clin Oncol. 2013;36(1):64.
12. Torresan F, Iacobone M. Clinical features, treatment, and surveillance of hyperparathyroidism-jaw tumor syndrome: an up-to-date and review of the literature. Int J Endocrinol. 2019;(2019):1761030.
13. Guan B, Welch JM, Sapp JC, Ling H, Li Y, Johnston JJ, et al. GCM2-activating mutations in familial isolated hyperparathyroidism. Am J Hum Genet. 2016;99(5):1034–44.
14. Kang H, Pettinga D, Schubert AD, Ladenson PW, Ball DW, Chung JH, et al. Genomic profiling of parathyroid carcinoma reveals genomic alterations suggesting benefit from therapy. Oncologist. 2019 Jun;24(6):791–7.
15. Machado NN, Wilhelm SM. Parathyroid cancer: A review. Cancers (Basel). 2019;11(11):1676.
16. Pelizzo MR, Piotto A, Bergamasco A, Rubello D, Casara D. Parathyroid carcinoma. Therapeutic strategies derived from 20 years of experience. Minerva Endocrinol. 2001;26(1):23–9.
17. Contemporary evaluation and management of parathyroid carcinoma. JCO Oncol Pract [Internet]. [cited 2024 Dec 28]. Available from: https://ascopubs.org/doi/10.1200/JOP.19.00540

18. Parathyroid Carcinoma: analysis of patient characteristics and outcomes in a retrospective review of eight cases seen in a single center. PMC [Internet]. [cited 2024 Oct 14]. Available from: https://www.ncbi.nlm.nih.gov/pmc/articles/PMC7784160/
19. Viswanath A, Drakou EE, Lajeunesse-Trempe F, Grossman AB, Dimitriadis GK. Parathyroid carcinoma: new insights. Best Pract Res Clin Endocrinol Metab. 2024:101966.
20. Hundahl SA, Fleming ID, Fremgen AM, Menck HR. Two hundred eighty-six cases of parathyroid carcinoma treated in the U.S. between 1985–1995. Cancer. 1999;86(3):538–44.
21. Healy SJ, Soe KK. Parathyroid cancer cases: a single center's experience. AACE Clin Case Reports. 2016;2(3):e221–7.
22. Mukherjee S, Arya AK, Bhadada SK, Saikia UN, Sood A, Dahiya D, et al. Parathyroid carcinoma: an experience from the Indian primary hyperparathyroidism registry. Endocr Pract. 2021;27(9):881–5.
23. de Almeida Vital JM, de Farias TP, Vaisman F, Fernandes J, Moraes ARL, José de Cavalcanti Siebra P, et al. Two case reports of parathyroid carcinoma and review of the literature. J Oncol Sci. 2017;3(1):22–8.
24. Evangelista L, Sorgato N, Torresan F, Boschin IM, Pennelli G, Saladini G, et al. FDG PET/CT and parathyroid carcinoma: review of literature and illustrative case series. World J Clin Oncol. 2011;2(10):348–54.
25. Diagnosis and management of parathyroid carcinoma: a state-of-the-art review. Endocr-Relat Cancer. 2023;30(4). [Internet]. [cited 2024 Oct 14]. Available from: https://erc.bioscientifica.com/view/journals/erc/30/4/ERC-22-0287.xml
26. Bergero N, De Pompa R, Sacerdote C, Gasparri G, Volante M, Bussolati G, et al. Galectin-3 expression in parathyroid carcinoma: immunohistochemical study of 26 cases. Hum Pathol. 2005;36(8):908–14.
27. Erickson LA, Mete O, Juhlin CC, Perren A, Gill AJ. Overview of the 2022 WHO classification of parathyroid tumors. Endocr Pathol. 2022;33(1):64–89.
28. Amin MB, Greene FL, Edge SB, Compton CC, Gershenwald JE, Brookland RK, et al. The Eighth Edition AJCC Cancer Staging Manual: Continuing to build a bridge from a population-based to a more "personalized" approach to cancer staging. CA Cancer J Clin. 2017;67(2):93–9.
29. Akirov A, Asa SL, Larouche V, Mete O, Sawka AM, Jang R, et al. The clinicopathological spectrum of parathyroid carcinoma. Front Endocrinol (Lausanne). 2019;10:731.
30. Parathyroid carcinoma: Current management and outcomes—A systematic review - ScienceDirect [Internet]. [cited 2024 Oct 14]. Available from: https://www.sciencedirect.com/science/article/pii/S0196070923000571?via%3Dihub
31. Johnson JT, George A, John JR, David N, Singh A, Abraham D, et al. Metastatic parathyroid carcinoma: a tale of refractory hypercalcemia. J Clin Transl Endocrinol Case Rep. 2023;(29):100151.
32. Limberg J, Stefanova D, Ullmann TM, Thiesmeyer JW, Bains S, Beninato T, et al. The use and benefit of adjuvant radiotherapy in parathyroid carcinoma: a National Cancer Database Analysis. Ann Surg Oncol. 2021;28(1):502–11.
33. Christakis I, Silva AM, Williams MD, Garden A, Grubbs EG, Busaidy NL, et al. Postoperative local-regional radiation therapy in the treatment of parathyroid carcinoma: the MD Anderson experience of 35 years. Pract Radiat Oncol. 2017;7(6):e463–70.

Index

P. S. Pai et al. (eds.), *Controversies in Cancer of the Thyroid and Parathyroid Glands*, https://doi.org/10.1007/978-3-032-13130-0

B

C

MIX
Papier aus verantwortungsvollen Quellen
Paper from responsible sources
FSC® C105338

If you have any concerns about our products,
you can contact us on
ProductSafety@springernature.com

In case Publisher is established outside the EU,
the EU authorized representative is:
Springer Nature Customer Service Center GmbH
Europaplatz 3, 69115 Heidelberg, Germany

Printed by Libri Plureos GmbH
in Hamburg, Germany